HADIDI · AZMY   Hypospadias Surgery

Springer
Berlin
Heidelberg
New York
Hong Kong
London
Milan
Paris
Tokyo

Ahmed T. Hadidi · Amir F. Azmy (Eds.)

Hypospadias Surgery

An Illustrated Guide

With 173 Figures in 482 Separate Illustrations,
Mostly in Color

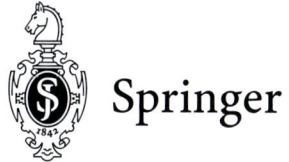

Professor Dr. Ahmed T. Hadidi
Cairo University Hospital
32 Haroon Street 32, El Messaha Dokki
Cairo 12311, Egypt

Mr. Amir F. Azmy
Royal Hospital for Sick Children
Yorkhill, Glasgow G3 8SJ, United Kingdom

ISBN 3-540-43041-5 Springer-Verlag Berlin Heidelberg New York

Library of Congress Cataloging-in-Publication
Hypospadias surgery: an illustrated guide/[edited by] Ahmed T. Hadidi, Amir F. Azmy. p.; cm.
Includes bibliographical references and index.
ISBN 3-540-43041-5 (alk. paper)
1. Hypospadias-Surgery. 2. Genitourinary organs-Surgery. 3. Pediatric urology. 4. Children-Surgery. I. Hadidi, Ahmed T. (Ahmed Taher),1958- II. Azmy, A.A.F.   [DNLM: 1. Hypospadias-surgery. 2. Hypospadias-complications. 3. Surgical Procedures, Operative-methods.   WJ 600 H998 2004]   RD137.H976 2004   617.4'63-dc21   2003045746

This work is subject to copyright. All rights are reserved, whether the whole or part of the material is concerned, specifically the rights of translation, reprinting, reuse of illustrations, recitation, broadcasting, reproduction on microfilm or in any other ways, and storage in data banks. Duplication of this publication or parts thereof is permitted only under the provision of the German Copyright Law of September 9, 1965, in its current version, and permission for use must always be obtained from Springer-Verlag. Violations are liable for prosecution under the German Copyright Law.

Springer-Verlag Berlin Heidelberg New York
a member of BertelsmannSpringer Science+Business Media GmbH
http://www.springer.de

© Springer-Verlag Berlin Heidelberg 2004
Printed in Germany

The use of descriptive names, registered names, trademarks, etc. in this publication does not imply, even in the absence of a specific statement, that such names are exempt from the relevant protective laws and regulations and therefore free for general use.

Product liability: The publisher can not guarantee the accuracy of any information about dosage and application contained in this book. In every individual case the user must check such information by consulting the relevant literature.

Cover-Design: Erich Kirchner, Springer-Verlag, Heidelberg, Germany
Drawings: Reinhold Henkel, Heidelberg, Germany
Typesetting: Fotosatz-Service Köhler GmbH, Würzburg, Germany
Printing and binding: H. Stürtz AG, Würzburg, Germany

Printed on acid-free paper.   24/3150 ih - 5 4 3 2 1 0

To
my father, *Taher*,
  for leading his children into intellectual pursuits;
my mother, *Mawaheb*,
  for devoting her life to her children;
my uncle, *Helmy*,
  for setting an outstanding example to follow;
my professors, *A. Loutfi* and *N. Kaddah*,
  for showing me the excitement and joy of paediatric surgery;
my mentors, *Dan Young* and *John Duckett*,
   for paving the way to international recognition.
A. T. H.

To
my wife, *Fatma*,
  for her love, encouragement and continuing support;
my daughter, *Iman*, and my son, *Ayman*,
  for their understanding;
my mentor, *Herbert Eckstein*,
  for introducing me to paediatric urology.
A. F .A.

Foreword

The challenge of hypospadias correction has always tested the ingenuity of surgeons and, although many of the older methods have been discredited and discarded, the diversity of procedures in current practice suggests that the perfect operation has yet to be devised. Evidently there have been important advances during the past 30 years, and the results now obtained would be the envy of older surgeons. It is instructive to note that particular attention is now given to securing a meatus at the tip of the glans (even in those minor degrees of hypospadias which would formerly have been left untreated), reflecting the pursuit of physical perfection which now fuels the popularity of cosmetic surgery.

There was undoubtedly a need for a comprehensive text dealing with all aspects of the abnormal development and its consequences as well as giving guidance on methods of surgical correction. The editorial duo of Hadidi and Azmy are to be congratulated on assembling a distinguished and expert team to fulfil this requirement. This volume will be indispensable reading for all those called upon to treat hypospadias, but it is gratifying to see that although the techniques of plastic surgery have contributed to the newer methods, it is the paediatric urologists who are now principally concerned. Hopefully they will ensure that hypospadias is fully corrected early in life and that adult urologists will no longer be asked to rescue sadly mismanaged young men with serious sexual and psychological handicaps.

Sir David Innes Williams

Foreword

An illness or abnormality that attracts a continuing bibliography of many hundreds of journal articles implies that there are unresolved problems. Such is the situation in hypospadias. And yet, at first glance, this is very surprising. Here is a deformity in an organ so overtly recognisable for clinical and epidemiological study, so easily accessible for tissue histology and histochemistry, and so amenable, one could assume, to the simplest of plastic surgical repair, given that there is total surgical access and exposure, surrounded by ample available tissues, and with a rich blood supply for healing; it should be a "gift" for even moderate surgical prowess! Yet nothing could be further from the truth.

In almost every facet we lack complete understanding. We have gaps in genetic information; the embryology is unsettled as to the nature of the tissue organizers, the relative contributions of the ectodermal folds and mesothelium, or whether the deformity is not "developmental" at all, but rather, as Douglas Stephens asserts, the result of distortion and displacement of early foetal cells by external pressure; why the great variation in clinical types, e.g. variations in orifice size and site and degree of chordee, or a large penile shaft orifice but no chordee, or a coronal orifice with complete prepuce, or a normally sited terminal orifice but marked chordee? We have incomplete understanding of the pathology of chordee, from the simplistic and probably mythical "white band" of Denis Browne to the varying contributions of skin, fascial layers and corpora, and what determines their contributions. The confusion is even more marked in the surgical management. With a lesion in which over 200 different repairs have been described, a cynic may be excused in claiming that none can be very satisfactory! We have proceeded through Browne repairs and scrotal flaps, to Duplay tubes, to free skin grafts, to island flaps and onlays, to bladder and buccal mucosal repairs, to a host of single-stage innovations, to different concepts of chordee correction and with all manner of bladder drainage systems. Although the penile repairs can be grouped into five or six major principles, depending on the tissues used, each has been subject to countless variations as one surgeon after another adds yet another modification to an already thrice-modified variation of a procedure adapted from a principle derived from the original! Further, some repairs are successful only in the hands of the original proponent, and the subtleties escape the novice, who, in frustration, flips to yet another technique. Hypospadias is bedevilled by surgeons who swap to the latest gimmick and never acquire the expertise of a practiced technique, which is essential for good results. We still debate the place of one- or two-stage repairs. Some repairs frankly offend major surgical principles in their complexity, in the fashioning of flaps, in disrespect for blood supply, and in inadequate layers and tension. What are the indications to use a specific repair in a given clinical situation? Do we need ten different procedures for ten different situations, with the attendant risk of insufficient volume of experience to acquire the necessary expertise in any of them, or can we reduce these to a manageable and well-practiced two or three adequate techniques with appropriate adaptations? In what circumstances is urinary diversion required and by means of which technique?

The problems do not stop with the completion of apparently successful surgery. I know of no surgery that can quite humble a surgeon as much as hypospadias–it carries a vicious bite with its list of complications, most galling when they can occur years later, such as a very late fistula or the manifestation of recurrent chordee. Add to this list problems of ejaculation or sexual function and the psychological effects before and after surgery or in later life, and we have a lesion to test the ingenuity, inventiveness and resilience of surgeons as much as any in surgery.

These are just some of the unresolved problems in the surgery of hypospadias. Given this maelstrom there could be no better time for the compilation of a volume bringing together the very best authorities in a critical analysis of all aspects of the malformation. Under the stimulating editorship of Ahmed Hadidi and Amir Azmy, themselves leaders in this field, the contributions of an international faculty of world leaders have been assembled. As a perusal of the table of contents will show, the book covers all the major operative repairs, described in many cases by their originators, but the book is much more than a collection of techniques. It rightly also covers the general aspects of history, epidemiology, genetics, embryology and pathology; surgical principles, ancillary aids and anaesthesia; the long-term evaluation of results, including early and late complications; and, importantly, an overview of management to bring perspective to this complex lesion.

In a subject with reports spread so widely throughout a vast list of publications, the book is a major contribution to the effort to reduce to manageable proportions the current accumulated knowledge of hypospadias, with each area being assessed and analysed by experts. We surely need such a volume. I have every expectation that the breadth of cover and the quality of the contributors are such that our puzzling unknowns will be addressed, and surgeons will have at hand an authoritative guide to practical management.

E. Durham Smith, AO, MD, MS, FRACS, FACS,
Hon.FRCS (Eng., Edin., Glas., Ire.)
Emeritus Consultant Surgeon
Royal Children's Hospital, Melbourne, Australia

Preface

Hypospadias Surgery: An Illustrated Guide

> Hypospadias is a grievous deformity which must ever move us to the highest surgical endeavour. The refashioning of the urethra offers a problem as formidable as any in the wide field of our art. The fruits of success are beyond rubies - the gratitude of a boy has to be experienced to be believed.
>
> T. Twistington Higgins, London, 1941
>
> Hypospadiology, defined as the in-depth study of the art and science of the surgical correction of hypospadias, is currently flourishing. Recently, heated debates have ensured, challenging the age-old truth ingrained in the historic teachings on this fascinating anomaly.
>
> These new concepts have prompted this treatise as a contribution to this anthology on the subject. Appropriate to the moment are two of our favourite quotations: "Scepticism blossoms on the compost of experience" and "Opinions abound where truths are hard to prove".
>
> John Duckett, Philadelphia, 1995

The purpose of this comprehensive, well-illustrated textbook is to help interested surgeons to develop vision, philosophy and talent, rather than just enumerate techniques. In this way we aim to provide an up-to-date global view of the management of the child with hypospadias, focusing primarily on the care of the condition and its associated problems. The book will be of specific interest to paediatric and adult urologists, paediatric and general surgeons and plastic surgeons.

The book is an example of international cooperation. Forty-six experts from 12 countries on five continents have contributed to it.

Each of the chapters in the book is written by an authority in the field of hypospadiology. A team of world class contributors present their expert opinions. The authors are members of major urological and paediatric surgical associations in the USA, UK, Australia, Japan and Europe.

Some of the chapters are written by non-surgeons and present new and important knowledge concerning epidemiology, genetics, and child psychology.

The book is well illustrated with ample colour diagrams and photographs of various operations together with many technical tips. There is a wide diversity of opinion and a large number of operations are described. Information is occasionally intentionally repeated when the circumstances demand.

The book consists of three sections.

Section 1 contains chapters dealing with the historical perspective: the evolution of hypospadias surgery, the basic principles of repair, the detailed embryology and anatomical studies, the epidemiology and genetics of hypospadias. Further contributions deal with general principles, including examination, imaging, intersexuality, preoperative preparation and hormonal stimulation, assessment of the results of hypospadias surgery, principles of plastic surgery and general principles of hypospadias surgery. Sutures, stenting materials and dressings are described, and a comprehensive chapter covers pain control.

Section 2 includes chapters describing the operative techniques for correction of the proximal and distal types of hypospadias. There is emphasis on the use of single-stage repair in severe types of hypospadias. However, the need for two-stage repair is discussed in detail. Current controversial issues such as the relative merits of single- versus two-stage repair, flaps versus grafts, dressings and urinary diversion are debated in depth.

Section 3 deals with the complications of hypospadias surgery and their management, complex redo repairs, long-term results in adolescence, and psychological adjustments.

Lastly, the editors present their personal overview of the current surgical techniques and potential developments in hypospadias surgery.

In addition, the text features a glossary for any readers who may not be familiar with the meanings of certain terms, as well as an appendix clarifying commonly used abbreviations.

The editors wish to thank all the contributing authors for the time and the hard work expended in producing their chapters and participating in the development of this textbook.

We are especially grateful to Pamela Clayton (lecturer, Glasgow University) for reviewing the manuscript and to our secretarial staff (Eleanor Watson, Caroline Hepburn and Mahmoud Saad), for their enormous help and support. Particular thanks are due to the Department of Medical Illustrations (Alistair Irwin and Jean Hyslop). Our deep appreciation and special thanks go to Reinhold Henkel, art designer working with Springer-Verlag, for his major contribution in designing all the illustrations within the book. We are also indebted to Gabriele Schroeder, Executive Medical Editor, Stephanie Benko, David Roseveare and Ingrid Haas of Springer-Verlag for their constructive criticism, help and advice.

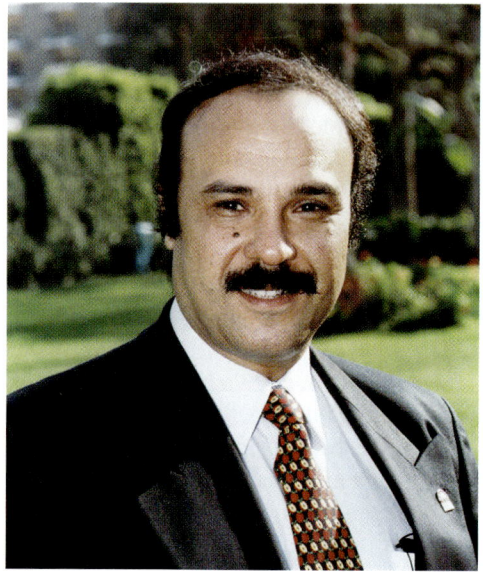

Ahmed T. Hadidi

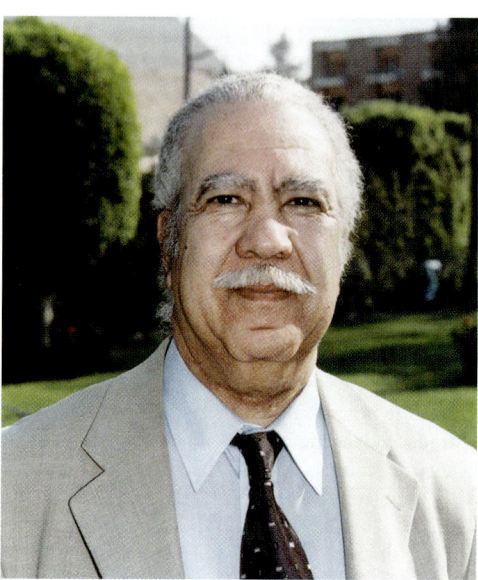

Amir F. Azmy

Contents

I General 1

1 Evolution of Hypospadias Surgery: Historical Perspective
Cenk Büyükünal 3

Egyptian Civilisation and Religious Documents 3
Greek, Ionian and Alexandrian Civilisations ... 3
The Byzantine Period 4
Islamic Medicine 4
The Renaissance Period 4
The Seventeenth to Eighteenth Centuries 5
The Nineteenth Century 5
    Creation of a Neourethra 5
        Efforts to Create an Urethra
        by Using Local Flaps 5
        Techniques for Reconstructing
        the Urethra by Using
        Vascularised Island Flaps 9
        Urethral Construction with Free Grafts 9
        Urethral Elongation 9
    The Concept of Chordee Correction 9
The Twentieth Century 10
    Creation of Neourethra 10
        Efforts to Create Urethra by Local Flaps 10
        Techniques for Reconstruction
        of the Urethra by Using
        Vascularised Island Flaps 11
        Urethral Construction with Free Grafts 13
        Urethral Elongation 13
    The Concept of Chordee Correction 14
Milestones in Modern Hypospadiology 14
References 15

2 Men Behind Principles and Principles Behind Techniques
Ahmed T. Hadidi 19

Abnormal Ventral Curvature of the Penis
and Orthoplasty 19
Abnormal Proximal Meatal Insertion
and Urethroplasty 23
    Urethral Mobilisation 23
    Use of Ventral Skin Distal to the Meatus .. 25
    Use of Ventral Skin Proximal to the Meatus
    (Meatal-Based Flaps) 29
    Use of Preputial Skin 33
    Combined Use of Prepuce and Skin
    Proximal to the Meatus 37
    Use of Scrotum 37
    Use of Dorsal Penile Skin 37
    Use of Grafts 43
    Use of a Protective Intermediate Layer ... 43
Abnormal Looking Glans Penis
and Glanuloplasty and Meatoplasty 43
References 48

3 Epidemiology of Hypospadias
Helen Dolk 51

The Prevalence of Hypospadias 51
Endocrine-Disrupting Chemicals
and Hormonal Aetiological Factors 54
Conclusion 56
References 56

4 Genetic Aspects of Hypospadias
Margo Whiteford 59

Hypertelorism with Oesophageal Abnormality
and Hypospadias 60
McKusick–Kaufman Syndrome 60
Pallister–Hall Syndrome 60
Smith–Lemli–Opitz Syndrome 60
Other Associations 61
References 61

5.1 Embryology and Anatomy of Hypospadias
John M. Hutson, E.C Penington 63

Normal Embryology of External Genitalia 63
    The Cloacal Cavity and the Cloacal Plate . 63
    The Fate of the Cloacal Plate 64
    The Urethral Plate and Formation
    of the Urethra 67
Phallus and Prepuce 68
Abnormal Development in Hypospadias 68
    Ectopic Orifice 68
    Dorsal Hood and Raphe 68
    Chordee 71
References 71

5.2 Blood Supply of the Penile Skin
Zacharias Zachariou 73

Introduction 73
Embryology 73
Preputial Arterial Supply and Venous Drainage . 73
Surgical Considerations 76
Conclusions 76
References 77

5.3 Classification of Hypospadias
Ahmed T. Hadidi 79

6.1 Timing of Elective Hypospadias Repair
Athanasios Zavitsanakis,
Ewagelia Gougoudi 83

Emotional Development 83
Sexual Development 83
Psychological Effects of Surgery
and Anaesthesia 84
Improvement in Technical Aspects of Surgery
and Advances in Paediatric Anaesthesia 84
Editorial Comment 84
References 85

6.2 General Principles
Amir F. Azmy 87

History 87
Examination 87
The Role of Imaging 87
Associated Anomalies 88
Hypoplasia of the Penis 88
Preoperative Evaluation 88

Preoperative Preparation 88
Preoperative Hormonal Stimulation 88
Consent 89
Penoscrotal Transposition 90
Ambiguous Genitalia 90
Incidence of Intersexuality in Children
with Cryptorchidism and Hypospadias 90
Assessment of Results of Hypospadias Surgery . 91
Meatal and Urethral Calibration 91
Assessment Using Uroflowmetry 91
Objective Scoring System for Results
of Hypospadias Surgery 92
Analysis of Cosmetic Outcome
Using Photography 92
References 92

7 Plastic Surgery Principles
Ahmed T. Hadidi 93

Skin Grafts 93
    Split Skin Grafts 93
    Full-Thickness Skin Grafts 94
Skin Graft Survival 95
Flaps 96
    Random Flaps 97
    Axial Flaps 98
    Fasciocutaneous Flaps 98
References and Suggested Reading 98

8 Principles of Hypospadias Surgery
Ahmed T. Hadidi 99

Positioning 99
Magnification 99
Traction, Retraction and Tension 99
Tissue Handling and Viability 100
Instruments 100
Suture Material and Knots 100
Suturing Techniques 101
Haemostasis 101
Urinary Diversion 102
    Perineal Urethrostomy 102
    Suprapubic Cystotomy 103
    Urethral Catheterisation 103
    Transurethral Drainage (Dripping Stent) . 103
Dressings 104
References 104

9 Analgesia and Pain Control
John Currie 107

Preparation 107
The Preanaesthetic and Preoperative Visits 107
Premedication 108
The Parent in the Anaesthetic Room 108
Pre-emptive Analgesia 109
Local Anaesthetic Techniques 109
    Caudal Analgesia 110
    Epidural Analgesia 110
    Penile Block 110
    Local Application 111
    Summary of Agents Used 111
Preparation for Subsequent Surgery 111
References 112

II Operative 113

10 Chordee (Penile Curvature)
Amir F. Azmy 115

Chordee With Hypospadias 115
Chordee Without Hypospadias 115
Artificial Erection Test 115
Operative Correction of Chordee
Without Hypospadias 115
    Correction of Short Urethra 115
    Correction of Glanular Tilt 116
    Correction of the Paper-Thin Urethra 116
Correction of Chordee With Hypospadias 116
    Correction of Penile Curvature
    with the Essed–Schroder Technique 117
Chordee Without Hypospadias in Men 117
Late-Onset Recurrent Penile Chordee
After Successful Correction
of Hypospadias Repair 118
References 118

11 Meatal Advancement and Glanuloplasty (MAGPI) Procedure
Yegappan Lakshmanan, John P. Gearhart . 119

Introduction 119
Selection of Patients 119
Operative Technique 119
    Meatoplasty 119
    Glanuloplasty 121
Modifications 121
Results 121
Complications 122
Conclusions 122
References 122

12 Urethral Advancement, Glanuloplasty and Preputioplasty in Distal Hypospadias
Dimitris Keramidas, Michael Soutis 123

Operative Technique 123
Complications 125
Comments 125
References 125

13.1 Thiersch–Duplay Principle
Moneer Hanna, Adam C. Weiser 127

Introduction 127
Preoperative Evaluation 128
Patient Selection 128
Operative Management 128
Results 130
Conclusions 132
References 133

13.2 Megameatus Intact Prepuce Variant
Amir F. Azmy 135

14.1 The Meatal-based Flap "Mathieu" Technique
Cenk Büyükünal 139

Introduction 139
The Mustardé Procedure 139
The Horton–Devine Flip-Flap Procedure 139
The Mathieu Procedure 142
    Preoperative Evaluation
    and Patient Selection 142
    Contraindications
    of the Mathieu Procedure 142
    Operative Technique 142
    The Steps of Mathieu's Procedure 142
The Mathieu Technique
and Relevant Modifications and Controversies . 144
    Stenting 144
    Reinforcement of the Neourethra
    Using Local Tissues 145
    How To Improve the Appearance
    of the Meatus in Mathieu Cases 145
    Chordee 145
    Hinging of Urethral Plate 145
    Mathieu as a Rescue Operation 145
Results and Complications 145
Our Experience 146
References 146

14.2 The Y-V Glanuloplasty Modified "Mathieu" Technique
Ahmed T. Hadidi 149

Introduction 149
Patient Selection 149
Operative Technique 149
    Steps 4, 5, 6: Y-V Glanuloplasty 149
    Parameatal Flap Design 151
    Neourethra Reconstruction 152
    Meatoplasty and Glanuloplasty 152
    Urinary Diversion 153
    Dressing 153
Results and Conclusion 153
References 154

15 Tubularized Incised Plate Urethroplasty
Warren Snodgrass 155

Introduction 155
Preoperative Evaluation 155
Operative Technique 157
    Distal Hypospadias Repair 157
        Degloving the Penis 157
        Urethroplasty 157
        Glanuloplasty 158
        Skin Closure 158
    Proximal Hypospadias Repair 158
        Degloving the Penis 158
        Urethroplasty 159
    Reoperations 159
        Urethroplasty 159
Results 159
Complications 160
Conclusions 161
References 161

16.1 The Island Onlay Hypospadias Repair
Howard Snyder 163

Introduction 163
Operative Technique 163
    Timing 163
    Design of Glanuloplasty 163
    Incisions 165
    Penile Skin Dropped Back 166
    Elevation of Glans Wings 166
    Artificial Erection 166
    Design of Island Onlay Flap 166
    Glanuloplasty 166
    Skin Closure 167

    Urethral Stenting 167
    Dressing 167
    Aftercare 167
Outcome 168
Conclusion 168
Referencess 168

16.2 Tubularised Preputial Island Flap
Ahmed T. Hadidi, Amir F. Azmy 169

Operative Steps 169
References 172

17 Single-Stage Procedure for Severe Hypospadias: Onlay-Tube-Onlay Modification of the Transverse Island Preputial Flap
Jyoti Upadhyay, Anthony Khoury 173

Introduction 173
Surgical Treatment 174
    Choice of Repair 175
    General Principles 175
Spongioplasty/Glanuloplasty 177
Repair of Chordee 177
Urethroplasty 179
    Preputial Transverse Island
    Combined Onlay-Tube-Onlay Flap 179
Skin Coverage 181
Stents/Dressings 181
Follow-up 182
Results 182
References 184

18 The Modified Asopa (Hodgson XX) Procedure to Repair Hypospadias with Chordee
Jeffrey Wacksman 187

Introduction 187
Operative Technique 187
Conclusion 189
References 190

19 Koyanagi–Nonomura One-Stage Repair for Severe Perineal Hypospadias
Tomohiko Koyanagi, Katsuya Nonomura, Hidehiro Kakizaki, Masashi Murakumo, Takashi Shibata 191

Introduction 191
Operative Technique 191
   Step 1: Outlining the Skin Incision and Dartos Mobilization 191
   Step 2: Chordectomy and Creation of Parameatal Foreskin Flap 194
   Step 3: Bisecting the Glans and Creation of Glanular Wings 194
   Step 4: One-Stage Urethroplasty with Parameatal Foreskin Flaps (Koyanagi et al. 1987, 1994) 195
   Step 5: Glanulomeatoplasty 197
   Step 6: Byarsization of the Dorsal Foreskin and Its Subcutaneous Tissue for Skin Closure 197
   Step 7: Skin Closure 198
   Postoperative Care 199
Results 199
Comments 200
Editorial Comment 200
References 201
Recommended Reading 202

20 The Yoke Hypospadias Repair
Brent W. Snow 203

Technique 203
References 207

21 Lateral-based Flap With Dual Blood Supply: A Single-Stage Repair for Proximal Hypospadias
Ahmed T. Hadidi 209

Introduction 209
Surgical Technique 209
   Step 1: Stay Suture, Erection Test and Meatal Dilatation or Incision 209
   Step 2: Y-shaped Deep Incision of the Glans 209
   Step 3: Chordectomy 209
   Step 4: Outlining Skin Incision and Flap Mobilisation 209
   Step 5: Formation of the Neourethra 212
   Step 6: Glanulomeatoplasty 212
   Step 7: Protective Intermediate Layer 212
   Step 8: Skin Closure 212
   Step 9: Formation of Penoscrotal Angle . . . 212
   Step 10: Insertion of a Percutaneous Suprapubic Cystostomy Catheter 212
Results 212
Comments 213
Discussion 213
References 216

22 Grafts for One-Stage Repair
Seif Asheiry, Ahmed T. Hadidi 217

Preputial Skin Graft 217
Buccal Mucosa Graft 219
   Surgical Technique 220
   Onlay Patch 221
   Tube Urethroplasty 221
   Compound Tube 221
   Clinical Experience and Results 221
Bladder Mucosal Grafts 222
   Surgical Technique 222
   Results 223
Editorial Comments 223
References 223

23 Two-Stage Urethroplasty
Madan Samuel, Patrick G. Duffy 225

Free Full-Thickness Wolfe Graft 225
   Introduction 225
   Graft Material and Biology 225
      Full-Thickness Skin Free Graft (Wolfe) . 225
      Buccal Mucosa Free Graft 225
      Bladder Mucosa 226
   Operative Technique 226
      First Stage 226
      Second Stage 233
   Complications 233
      First stage 233
      Second Stage 234
Vascularised Preputial Skin Onlay Graft 234
   Introduction 234
   Operative Technique (Dundee Modification of the Bretteville Procedure) 234
      First Stage 234
      Second Stage 235
      Dundee Modification 235
      Complications 235
   Comments 235
References 235

24 Protective Intermediate Layer
Ahmed T. Hadidi 237

Skin De-epithelialisation 237
The Tunica Vaginalis Flap 237
The Dorsal Subcutaneous Flap 240
The Dartos Flap 240
External Spermatic Fascia Flap 240
Fibrin Sealants 241
References 241

25 Procedures to Improve the Appearance of the Meatus and Glans
Ahmed T. Hadidi, Mahmoud Zaher 243

Y-V Glanuloplasty 245
    Surgical Technique 245
        Step 1: Y-shaped Incision of the Glans . 245
        Step 2: V Excision of the Tip
        of the Neourethra 249
        Step 3: Glanuloplasty and Meatoplasty . 249
    Results and Complications 249
References 249

26 Penoscrotal Transposition Associated With Hypospadias
Amir F. Azmy 251

Mori–Ikoma Technique 252
Shanberg–Rosenberg Technique 252
Bifid Scrotum 254
Penile Torsion 255
References 255

27.1 Flaps Versus Grafts
Ahmed T. Hadidi 257

Flaps 257
Grafts 257
References 258

27.2 Single-Stage Versus Two-Stage Repair
Ahmed T. Hadidi 261

Thiersch–Duplay Technique as Modified
by Byars and Durham Smith 262
    First Stage 262
    Second Stage 262
    Results 266

Denis Browne Technique 266
    Results 267
References 267

27.3 Stenting Versus No Stenting
Ahmed T. Hadidi 269

27.4 Dressing Versus No Dressing
Ahmed T. Hadidi 271

III Complications and Late Sequelae ... 273

28.1 Early Complications
Ahmed T. Hadidi, Wael El-Saied 275

Infection 275
Meatal Stenosis 275
Loss of Skin Flaps 275
Oedema 275
Haemorrhage 275
Erection 275
Retrusive Meatus 276
Bladder Spasm 276
Catheter Blockage 276
References 276

28.2 Fistula Repair
Ahmed T. Hadidi 277

Incidence of Fistula Formation 277
Causes of Fistula Formation 277
Fistula Prevention 277
Types and Sites of Fistula 278
Treatment of Fistula 278
References 282

28.3 Cecil–Culp Operation
Amir F. Azmy 283

Modifications 283
References 283

28.4 Modified Cecil–Culp Technique for Repair of Urethrocutaneous Fistula
Christopher S. Cooper, Charles E. Hawtrey 289

Introduction and Patient Selection 289
Preoperative Evaluation 289
Operative Technique 290
Modifications of Original Technique 290
Results 292
Complications 292
References 293

29 Meatal Stenosis and Urethral Strictures After Hypospadias Surgery
Pat Malone 295

Introduction 295
Aetiology and Prevention 295
    Meatal Stenosis 295
    Urethral Stricture 296
Presentation and Assessment 296
Treatment 298
Conclusions 299
References 300

30 Urethral Diverticula and Acquired Megalourethra
Paolo Caione, Simona Nappo 301

31 Management of Failed Hypospadias Repairs
Pierre Mouriquand, Pierre-Yves Mure, Smart Zeidan, Thomas Gelas 305

Introduction 305
The Principles of Hypospadias "Re-do" Surgery 306
    Ascertainment and Correction of Chordee 306
    Repeated Urethroplasty 306
    Reconstruction of the Ventral Radius of the Penis 307
    Preoperative Care 307
    Postoperative Care and Follow-up 307
The Various Techniques of Re-do Urethroplasty 307
    The Salvage Mathieu Procedure 307
    Koff Urethral Mobilisation 308
    Thiersch–Duplay/Snodgrass Urethroplasty 308
    Onlay Island Flap Urethroplasty 308
    The Asopa–Duckett Tube 308
    Bladder Mucosa Graft Urethroplasty 308
    Buccal Mucosa Graft Urethroplasty 309
    Two-Stage Procedures 310
    Other Urethroplasties and Composite Urethroplasties 311
References 311

32 The Long-Term Consequences of Hypospadias
Christopher Woodhouse 313

Introduction 313
Surgical Results 313
    Appearance 313
    Voiding 315
    Chordee 316
Sexual Function 317
    Sexual Activity 317
    Ejaculation 318
    Psychological Aspects of Intercourse 318
Endocrine Function in Hypospadias 319
Fertility 319
Psychological Consequences 319
Hypospadias in Adults 320
    Late Complications 320
    New Adult Patients 321
References 322

33 Psychological Problems and Adjustment
Christina Del Priore, Kathleen McHugh, Sita Picton, Elizabeth Haldane 325

Introduction 325
Specific Findings 325
    Psychological Adjustment to Hypospadias 325
    Childhood and Hypospadias 326
    Selfhood and Genital and Gender Awareness 326
    Gender and Society 327
    Gender and Behaviour 327
    Gender and Parenting 328
    Parental Perceptions of Maleness 328
    The Phallus 328
    Decision Taking, the Rights of the Child, Law on Capacity for Consent 328
    Empowerment and Partnership 329
    Coping Styles 329
    Pain 329
    Adherence 329
    Talking to Children About Elimination Function, About Future Fertility and Sexual Function 330
    Cosmetic Challenge 330
    Solution Focus and Positive Psychology .. 330
Goals for Public Policy and Research 330
References 331

34 Uncommon Conditions and Complications
Amir F. Azmy 333

Uncommon Conditions 333
    Iatrogenic Hypospadias 333
    Genitourinary Injuries in the Newborn . . . 333
    Congenital Urethrocutaneous Fistula
    Without Hypospadias 333
    Urethral Duplication With Hypospadias . . 334
    Concealed Penis 334
    Congenital Buried Penis 334
    Accessory Scrotum 335
    Hair Coil 335
    Female Hypospadias 335
    Congenital Megalourethra 336
Uncommon Complications 337
    Partial Dissection of the Epithelium
    of the Urethral Wall 337
    Lymphoedema of the Penis
    After Hypospadias Surgery 337
    Adenoma After Hypospadias Repair 338
    Squamous Cell Carcinoma
    After Hypospadias Repair 338
    Hairy Urethra 338
References 338

35 Editorial Overview of the Current Management of Hypospadias
Ahmed T. Hadidi, Amir F. Azmy 339

Preservation of the Urethral Plate 339
Technical Surgical Details 339
Protective Intermediate Layer 339
New Methods for Glanuloplasty
and Meatoplasty 340
Single-Stage Repair 340
Flaps Rather Than Grafts 340
The Role of Stenting 340
The Role of Dressing 340
Preoperative Hormonal Treatment 340
References 341

36 Potential Techniques and Future Research
Arup Ray, Amir F. Azmy 343

Microsurgical Free Tissue Transfers 343
Tissue Expansion 344
Tissue Expansion for Urethral
and Penile Reconstruction 344
    Penile Enhancement 344
    Liposculpturing Procedures 345
Laser Tissue Soldering for Hypospadias Repair . 345
Reconstruction of Neourethra
from Cultivated Keratinocytes 345
    Harvesting Human Urothelial Cells
    for Urethral Reconstruction 346
Inert Collagen Matrix for Hypospadias Repair . 346
References 346

References 349

Subject Index 371

Contributors

Amir F. Azmy
Consultant Paediatric Urologist
Royal Hospital for Sick Children
Honorary Clinical Senior Lecturer
University of Glasgow
Glasgow, UK

Seif Asheiry
Senior Registrar, Department of Paediatric Surgery
University Hospitals
Cairo, Egypt

Cenk Büyükünal
Professor of Paediatric Urology
Cerrahpasa Medical Faculity
34301, P.O. Box 37, Cerrahpasa, Istanbul, Turkey

Paolo Caione
Professor of Paediatric Urology
Bambino Gesu Children's Hospital
Piazza S. Onofrio, 4, 00165 Rome, Italy

Christopher S. Cooper
Assistant Professor, Division of Pediatric Urology
Children's Hospital of Iowa
200 Hawkins Drive, 3 RCP
Iowa City, IA 52242-1089, USA

John Currie
Consultant Paediatric Anaesthetist
Director of Pain Relief
Royal Hospital for Sick Children
Glasgow, UK

Christina Del Priore
Consultant Paediatric Psychologist
Head of Department of Psychology
Royal Hospital for Sick Children
Glasgow, UK

Helen Dolk
Professor of Epidemiology
and Health Services Research, Room 1F08
Faculty of Life and Health Services,
University of Ulster at Jordanstown
Shore Road, Newtown Abbey, Co. Antrim, BT3 0QB, UK

Patrick G. Duffy
Consultant Paediatric Urologist
Hospital for Children, NHS Trust
Great Ormond Street, London, WC1N 3JH, UK

Wael El-Saied
Lecturer of Urology, Cairo University
Cairo, Egypt

John P. Gearhart
Professor of Pediatric Urology
Director of Pediatric Urology, Johns Hopkins Hospital
Baltimore, MD 21205, USA

Thomas Gelas
Department of Paediatric Urology, Hospital Debrousse
Claude-Bernard University
29 Rue Soeur Bouvier, 69322 Lyon Cedex 05, France

Ewagelia Gougoudi
Resident, Department of Paediatric Surgery
Hospital for Sick Children "St. Sofia"
Athens, Greece

Ahmed T. Hadidi
Professor of Paediatric & Plastic Surgery
Cairo University and Benha Children's Hospital
Cairo, Egypt
(mailing address: 32 Haroon Street, El Messaha,
Dokki, Cairo 12311, Egypt)

Elizabeth Haldane
Clinical Psychologist, Yorkhill NHS Trust
Glasgow, G3 8SJ, UK

Moneer Hanna
Professor of Urology
935 Northern Boulevard, Suite 303
Great Neck, NY 10021, USA

Charles E. Hawtrey
Department of Urology, Division of Paediatric Urology
Children's Hospital of Iowa
200 Hawkins Drive, 3 RCP
Iowa City, IA 52242-1089, USA

John M. Hutson
Professor of General Surgery
Royal Children's Hospital, Parkville
Victoria 3052, Australia

Hidehiro Kakizaki
Hokkaido University
Sapporo, Japan

Dimitris Keramidas
Professor of Paediatric Surgery,
Director of Paediatric Surgery
Aghia Sophia Children's Hospital
Athens, Greece

Anthony Khoury
Professor of Paediatric Urology
Hospital for Sick Children
Toronto, Canada

Tomohiko Koyanagi
Professor of Paediatric Urology, Hokkaido University
Sapporo, Japan

Yegappan Lakshmanan
Brady Urological Institute, Marburg 1
Johns Hopkins Hospital
600 North Wolfe Street, Baltimore, MD 21287, USA

Pat Malone
Consultant Paediatric Urologist
Southampton General Hospital
Tremona Road, Southampton, SO16 6YD, UK

Kathleen McHugh
Consultant Clinical Psychologist
Royal Hospital for Sick Children
Yorkhill, Glasgow, G3 8SJ, UK

Pierre Mouriquand
Professor of Paediatric Urology
Claude-Bernard University, Hospital Debrousse
29 Rue Soeur Bouvier, 69322 Lyon Cedex 05, France

Masashi Murakumo
Kokkaido University
Sapporo, Japan

Pierre-Yves Mure
Department Of Paediatric Urology
Claude-Bernard University, Hospital Debrousse
29 Rue Soeur Bouvier, 69322 Lyon Cedex 05, France

Simona Nappo
Paediatric Urologist Assistant,
Division of Paediatric Urology
Bambino Gesu Children's Hospital
Piazza S. Onofrio, 4, 00165 Rome, Italy

Katsuya Nonomura
Kokkaido University
Sapporo, Japan

E.C. Penington
F. Douglas Stephens Surgical Research Laboratory
Murdoch Children's Research Institute
and Department of Paediatrics
University of Melbourne, Royal Children's Hospital
Melbourne, Australia

Sita Picton
Consultant Clinical Psychologist, Yorkhill NHS Trust
Glasgow, G3 8SJ, UK

Arup Ray
Consultant Plastic Surgeon, Canniesburn Hospital
Glasgow, UK

Madan Samuel
Consultant Paediatric Surgeon
Children's Hospital Birmingham
29 Brookhill Way
Rushmere, St. Andrews
Ipswich, IP4 SUL, UK

Takashi Shibata
Hokkaido University
Sapporo, Japan

Warren Snodgrass
Professor of Pediatric Urology
The University of Texas South Western Medical Centre
at Dallas and Children's Medical Center of Dallas 6300
Harry Hines Boulevard, Suite 1401
Dallas, TX 75235, USA

Brent W. Snow
Professor of Pediatric Urology
Primary Children's Medical Centre
100 North Medical Drive, #2200
Salt Lake City, UT 84113, USA

Howard Snyder
Professor of Pediatric Urology
Children's Hospital of Philadelphia
Philadelphia, PA, USA

Michael Soutis
Paediatric Surgeon, Aghia Sophia Children's Hospital
Athens, Greece

Jyoti Upadhyay
Paediatric Urology, The Hospital for Sick Children
M299-555 University Avenue,
Toronto, M5G1X8, Canada

Jeffrey Wacksman
Professor of Pediatric Urology
University of Cincinnati College of Medicine
Associate Director of Pediatric Urology
Children's Hospital Medical Center
Cincinnati, OH, USA

Adam C. Weiser
Paediatric Fellow, Schneider Children's Hospital
Long Island Medical Centre
New Hyde Park, New York, NY, USA

Margo Whiteford
Consultant Clinical Geneticist
Department of Medical Genetics,
Duncan Guthrie Institute of Medical Genetics
Royal Hospital for Sick Children, NHS Trust
Glasgow, UK

Christopher Woodhouse
Reader in Adolescent Urology
The Institute of Urology & Nephrology
University College,
48 Riding House Street, London, W1N 8AA, UK

Zacharias Zachariou
Professor of Paediatric Surgery
University of Heidelberg
Im Neuenheimer Feld 110
69120 Heidelberg, Germany

Mahmoud Zaher
Senior Registrar,
Department of Paediatric and Plastic Surgery
Ahmed Maher Teaching Hospital, Cairo, Egypt

Athanasios Zavitsanakis
Associate Professor of Paediatric Surgery
University of Thessaloniki School of Medicine
Thessaloniki, Greece

Smart Zeidan
Department Of Paediatric Urology
Claude-Bernard University, Hospital Debrousse
29 Rue Soeur Bouvier, 69322 Lyon Cedex 05, France

General

Hypospadias Surgery

Evolution of Hypospadias Surgery: Historical Perspective

Cenk Büyükünal

The term hypospadias is derived from the Greek. "*Hypo*" means under and "*spadon*" means a rent or fissure (Duckett and Baskin 1996; Zaontz and Packer 1997). Durham Smith (1997) mentioned the dictum "There is nothing new in surgery not previously described", and this exactly summarises the efforts which were made in the past for the description, classification, pathology and treatment of hypospadias. Many modern surgeons mention the originality of their ideas, but an investigation of historical papers, documents and books indicates that all current techniques, theoretical and practical knowledge were described centuries ago by various surgeons.

Egyptian Civilisation and Religious Documents

Man's interest in learning the treatment of genital abnormalities began with a simple procedure: circumcision. The first documentation on this subject was found in Egypt. The circumcision procedure as a ritual is shown in the famous relief in the tomb of Ankhmahor at Saqqara, dating from the sixth dynasty, c. 2345 BC. This relief shows two young men or adolescents being circumcised. This is probably one of the best preserved documents that we have. There is a similar relief, severely damaged, in the temple of Muten Asheru at Karnak (Filler 1995; Nunn 1996; Reeves 2001). In the Eber papyrus, discovered in 1872 near Luxor, there is a recipe for the treatment of bleeding resulting from circumcision (Rogers 1973). Bettmann and Hinch (1956) mention the application of fresh meat to stop the haemorrhage. In these documents, the anaesthetic action of carbon dioxide resulting from the acetic effect of vinegar put on Memphis limestone was used to relieve the pain of children during circumcision procedures. Analysis of these documents, however, reveals neither description nor treatment of hypospadias, with the single exception of a finding in the temple of Kom Ombo. On one of the outer walls of this temple there is a relief of surgical instruments, including metal shears, surgical knives, spatulas, small hooks and forceps (Nunn 1996; Portman 2001; Reeves 2001). Although there are no scientifically acceptable data specifying the use of these tools for penile surgery, these tiny and fine surgical instruments would seem to be efficacious for circumcision and similar surgical procedures. The ancient Jews may have learned the surgical technique of circumcision from Egyptian civilisation; and circumcision is the only surgical procedure mentioned in the Old Testament (Ellis 2001). According to Zeis, in ancient Jewish practice a deficient prepuce due to extensive circumcision or tumour may have been treated by reconstructive surgical procedures (Zeis 1963). In the texts of the Bible, the Apochrypha Pseudoepigrapha and the Talmud, any male whose penis was cut off or any man suffering an abnormal opening could not marry (Sussman 1967). Penile amputation was an operation practised in the past. Amputation of the male organ was a fairly common form of punishment or sign of degradation into slavery, especially after wars. In 1300 BC the Egyptian pharaoh Merneptah had inscribed on the walls of the Temple of Karnak the story of the amputation of more than 13,000 phalluses of his enemies (Bitschai and Brodny 1956).

Greek, Ionian and Alexandrian Civilisations

Infibulation was another interesting procedure. Infibulation means a "narrowing procedure in the preputium" by using a ring, pin, clamp, or a leather thong passed through two artificial holes created surgically to prevent coition or masturbation (Schwarz 1970). In ancient Greece, this surgical technique was especially performed among the professional athletes to cover the glans during the Olympic games as well as to immobilise and protect the naked organ (Barcat 1973; Dingwall 1925). In ancient Greek civilisation, the goddess Hermaphrodite was described as half man and half woman. In many antique Greek statues, genitalia resembling hypospadias may represent a kind of admiration of the goddess Hermaphrodite. Therefore nobody tried to treat this condition until the advent of two Alexandrian surgeons named Helidorus and Antyllus, who lived in the first and second centuries AD. According to the recorded data, they were the pioneers who described, classified and defined pathophysiology and the treatment of hypospadias. They mentioned the problem of proper, straightforward ejaculation in hypospadias and described the problem of "acquired hypospadias" due to severe inflammatory and ulcerative disease of the penis. Helidorus and Antyllus made a rough classification of hypospadias according to the location of the ectopic meatus, and declared the proximal form of the disease as incurable. They were the first to describe the partial resection of glans penis to locate the orifice more centrally. Bandaging, cauterisation and the local application of vinegar were recommended to stop the haemorrhage (Antyl 1984; Bitschai and Brodny 1956; Bussmaker and Daremberg 1851–1876). Amputation beyond the orifice was also recommended by Paul of Aegina (625–690 AD) (Aeginata 1844; Smith 1997). Galen (130–199 AD), born in Pergamon, Western Anatolia, was the first physician to use the term "hypospadias". He mentioned the problems of chordee and difficulty in ejaculation towards the uterus during sexual intercourse (Galen; Rogers 1973; Smith 1997).

The Byzantine Period

Oribasius (325–403 AD) showed the same concerns, reiterated the problems mentioned by Helidorus and Antyllus and gave the details of the operation called "cutting the glans a little above the coronary sulcus" for those patients with the distal type of hypospadias. By means of this operation he was able to bring the neo-meatus to the tip and centre of the remnant of the glans (Lascaratos et al. 1999).

Islamic Medicine

Albucasis from Cordoba (963–1013) was a well-known Arab surgeon who made enormous contributions to the field of paediatric surgery. He used a scalpel for the treatment of an imperforate urethra during the new-born period. He used a solid non-tubularised lead sound in order to prevent stricture formation after treatment of imperforated urinary meatus. He removed this sound intermittently to allow the child to urinate easily (Herrlinger 1970; Montagnani 1986; Spinks and Lewis 1973).

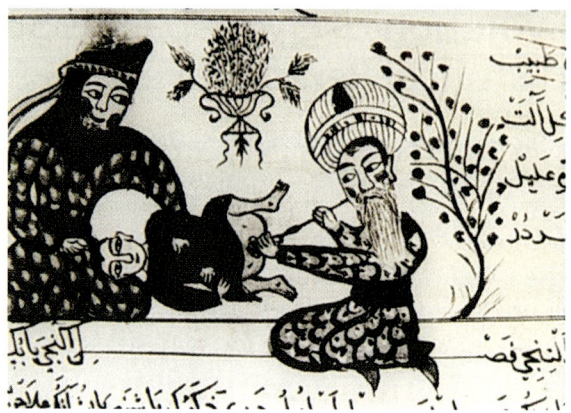

Fig. 1.1. Serafeddin using an instrument to dilate meatal stenosis

Sabuncuoglu şerafeddin (fifteenth century) was a surgeon from Central Anatolia, one of the master surgeons of the Ottoman Period in all aspects of surgery. The miniature in Fig. 1.1 shows him and one of his trainees (a female physician, not a midwife!). In his book *Cerrahiye-i Ilhaniye*, chapter 55, he describes the fine scalpel "*mibza*" used for the treatment of meatal stenosis in hypospadias (or imperforate urinary meatus). This scalpel was more straight than the scalpel used by Albucasis. şerafeddin's most important contribution was to use a sound with a patent canal. This was very practical for children, enabling them to urinate through it instead of removing it for every urination. In his famous manuscript, he describes the importance of the location of the urinary meatus and gives a detailed classification of hypospadias. He also mentions different repair methods for the correction of erroneous circumcision performed by unqualified people (chapter 57). This book also contains many miniature drawings concerning the operative procedures, surgical instruments and technical details. The paediatric surgical part of this book can be accepted as the first paediatric surgical atlas, with its various colourful, informative pictures (Büyükünal and Sary 1991; Numanoğlu 1973; Sabuncuoğlu 1465; Uzel 1992; Unver 1939).

The Renaissance Period

Since the Renaissance period, several historical anecdotes and scientific data related with the social problems created by "hypospadias" have been recorded. In 1556, Amatus Lusitanus from Portugal (Rogers 1973) treated a 2-year-old boy with penoscrotal hypospadias. He created a canal by using a silver cannula that he directed from the proximal ectopic urinary meatus up to the penile shaft as far as a surgically created meatus in the imperforate glans. This was the first real scientific development since the primitive techniques of Antyllus, Helidorus, Oribasius and Paul of Aegina. In the mid-sixteenth century, Henry II became king of France. Despite his active sexual life and his robust and athletic appearance, he had severe chordee. This was the reason why he had no children during the first 10 years of his marriage. Jean Fernel, the private surgeon of the king, corrected his problem and the king went on to father ten children by his queen, Catherine de Medici (Duckett and Baskin 1996; Smith 1997).

According to the records of the University of Rome (Cassar 1974; Duckett and Baskin 1996), the case of Maltese woman called Mathia seems very interesting. She applied for the annulment of her marriage due to her husband's problem: severe hypospadias with chordee. This case was discussed in the Bishop's Court; two medical witnesses examined her husband and his penis was reported as "inept", "incapable" and "useless for perforation". As a result, the Court annulled the marriage. This was the normal procedure in sixteenth-century Europe, and the Common Law established by religious authorities conferred the right for a patient to be examined in the presence of Court officials and medical authorities without any respect to individual privacy. Ambrois Paré, the famous French surgeon of the sixteenth century, was one of the first in medical history to describe the details of chordee malformation and its surgical treatment. He advised cutting off all fibrotic tissue to make the penis more straight (Johnson 1968; Paré 1575). This was a very scientific and reliable contribution.

The Seventeenth to Eighteenth Centuries

Fabricius of Aquapendente (1533–1619) mentioned the importance of "carving glans tissue" until the normal meatus appears (Fabricii ab Aquapendente 1619, 1641). This technique was recommended for the distal forms and is not considered relevant to modern surgery. Pierre Dionis, the author of the famous book *Cours d'opérations*, published in 1707, advised the technique of Albucasis for the treatment of an imperforated glans in the neonate, but he refused to use a lead sound. He thought that frequent urination in a neonate would suffice to prevent the reunion of the edges of the wound or adhesions. He used a lead catheter only for older patients, in the postoperative period after urethroplasty. His technique for the excision of chordee was similar to Paré's technique. He simply incised the fibrous bands to make the shaft more straight (Dionis 1710, 1718). Lorenz Heister (1683–1758), a German surgeon, developed a technique for the treatment of the chordee problem which, albeit logical, was practically inapplicable. To make the penile shaft more straight, he advised the application of emollients to the contracted side and astringents to the opposite side of the penis. He also advised small skin incisions in the ventral side of the shaft. In addition, he recommended a special bandage technique after chordee correction. He found a positive correlation between paternity rates and the location of the ectopic hypospadiac meatus (Heister 1743).

The Nineteenth Century

Significant improvements in the understanding of the precise pathology of hypospadias were achieved and the fundamental characteristics of modern surgical techniques were created in the nineteenth century.

Creation of a Neourethra

Efforts to Create an Urethra by Using Local Flaps

In 1838, Dieffenbach perforated the glans down to the urethral meatus and inserted a cannula in between, until the neourethra was covered by normal urothelium (Dieffenbach 1837, 1847) (Fig. 1.2). Although it was a clever idea, the operation was not successful. In 1861, Bouisson suggested a ventral transverse incision to straighten the penile shaft and thus alleviate the chordee problem (Bouisson 1869, 1861). This was not a radical way to treat chordee. In addition, Bouisson was the first surgeon to use a rotated local pedicled scrotal flap in order to cover the ventral defect. The inner surface of this scrotal flap was used to create the anterior part of the neourethra with a technique resembling the Mathieu operation (Fig. 1.3).

In 1869, Karl Thiersch started for the first time to use local tubularised skin flaps to repair epispadias (Horton et al. 1973; Thiersch 1869). Théophile Anger adopted this technique to repair hypospadias. He used longitudinal flaps on either side of the urethral groove and permitted them to overlap without "denuding". Although the result was unsuccessful (Anger 1874a, b, 1875), Anger was the real initiator of the modern urethroplasty technique in hypospadias surgery. He performed two parallel but asymmetrical incisions in the skin of the ventral shaft. This manoeuvre theoretically prevented the overlapping between the urethral and skin closures and thus reduced the rate of fistula formation (Fig. 1.4).

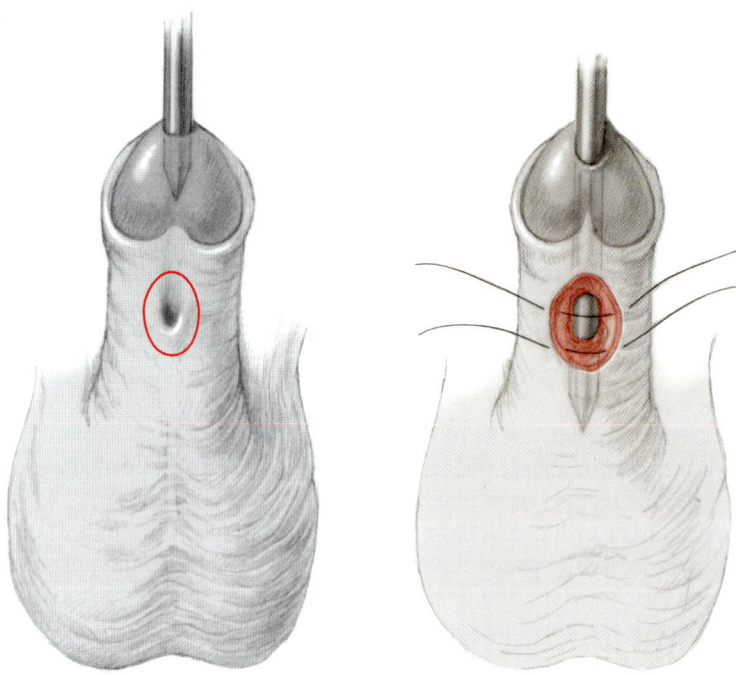

Fig. 1.2. Dieffenbach pierced the glans and left a catheter in place until the channel became epithelialised. The operation was not successful

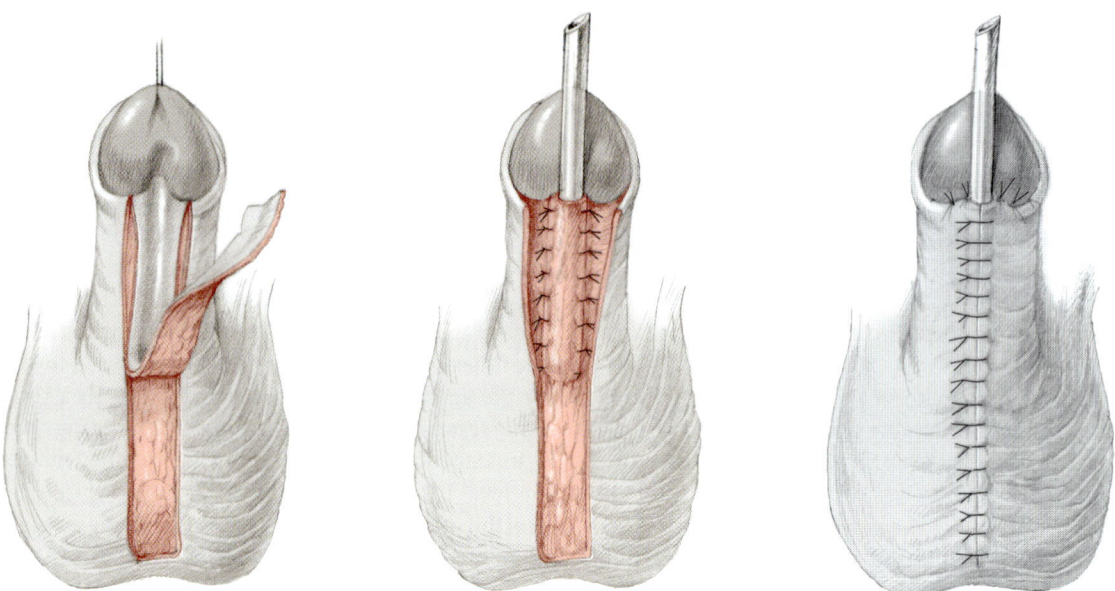

Fig. 1.3. Bouisson (1861) used scrotal tissue to reconstruct the urethra

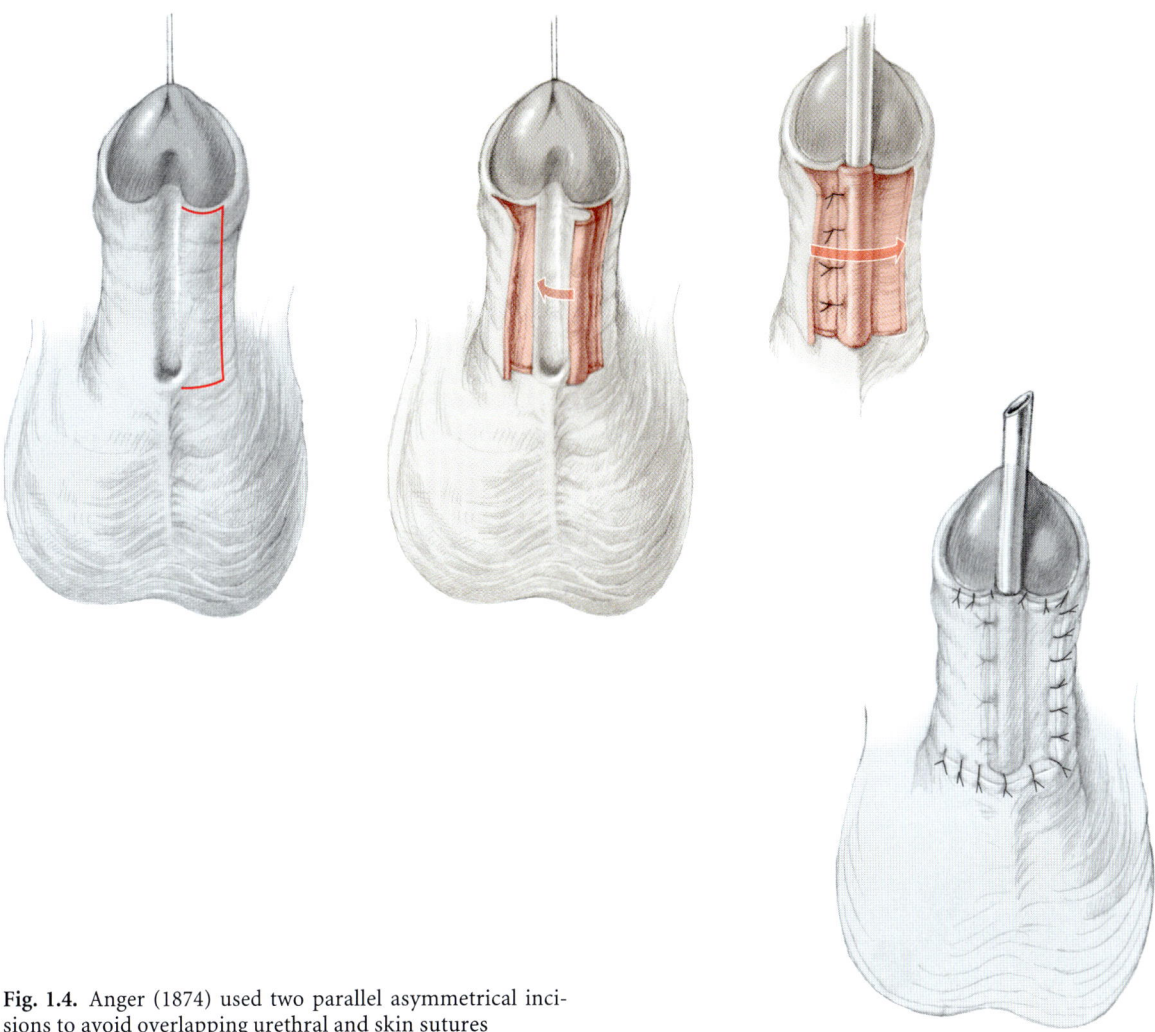

Fig. 1.4. Anger (1874) used two parallel asymmetrical incisions to avoid overlapping urethral and skin sutures

In 1870 Moutet used scrotal tissue to reconstruct the urethra (Moutet 1870). The ventral penile skin defect over the raw surface of the neourethra was covered by bipedicled suprapubic abdominal skin flaps.

In 1874 Duplay used the Bouisson technique to release the chordee (Duplay 1874; Smith 1981) (👁 Fig. 1.5a–c). In the second stage he incised the ventral skin on either side of the urethral groove. This flap, namely the "urethral groove", was tubularised. The edges of the outer skin were sutured over the tube (👁 Fig. 1.5d, e). In 1880 Duplay described a second procedure (Duplay 1880) where a narrower strip was used. This was a real buried strip which would be popularised by Browne 69 years later. Duplay did not consider suturing the outer skin edge-to-edge to the sides of the urethral strip.

Wood, in 1875 (quoted by Mayo 1901), presented a "meatal-based flap" technique to create a neourethra (👁 Fig. 1.6). Basically, his proposal was similar to the technique of Mathieu. He also introduced the idea of the buttonhole flap to cover the ventral surface of the penis and the raw surface of the newly created urethra. The buttonhole technique had originally been mentioned by Thiersch for the coverage of a dorsal shaft defect in epispadias surgery (Thiersch 1869).

Rosenberg (1891), Landerer (1891) and Bidder (1892) used basically similar principles of treatment for proximal types of hypospadias. Their modification was to bury the ventral part of the penis into the scrotum by using penoscrotal sutures to create a neourethra from the inner part of the scrotal tissue. In the second stage they divided this surgically created penoscrotal fusion and covered the raw surface in the ventral part of the neourethra using lateral skin flaps from the penile shaft.

Rochet (1899) used a distally created meatal-based scrotal flap to create a complete scrotal-urethral channel. This tube was buried in a subcutaneous tunnel which was created in the ventral part of the penile shaft.

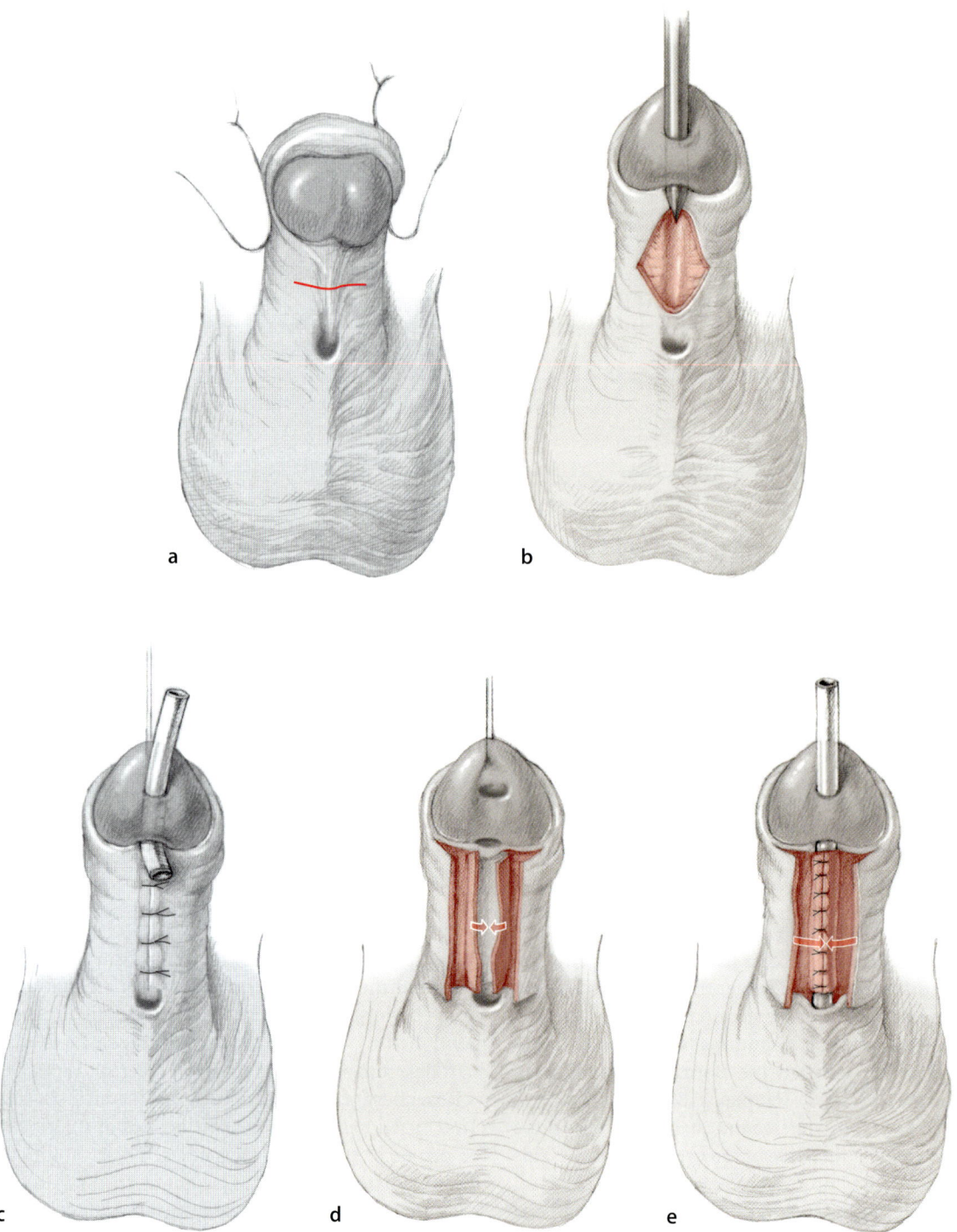

Fig. 1.5. a–c Duplay (1874) used a transverse incision closed longitudinally to correct chordee. **d, e** A U-shaped incision to tubularise the skin distal to the meatus

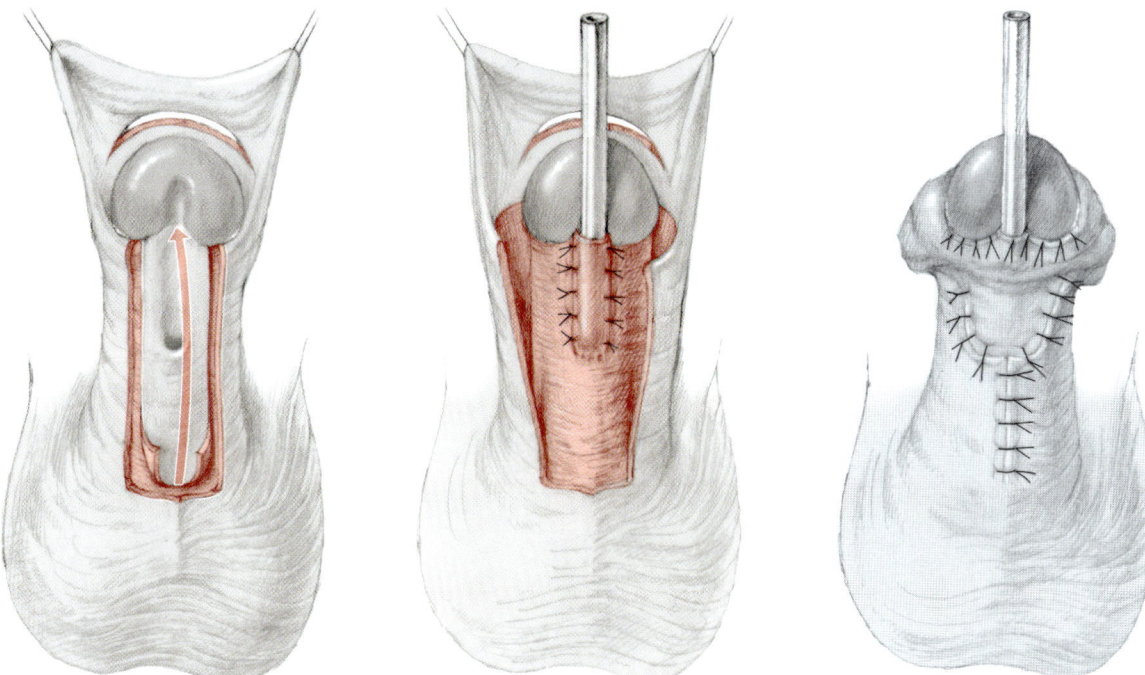

Fig. 1.6. Wood (1875) described the "meatal-based flap". He also buttonholed the prepuce to cover the neourethra

Techniques for Reconstructing the Urethra by Using Vascularised Island Flaps

In 1896 Van Hook described for the first time the creation of vascularised dorsal preputial flaps to reconstruct the urethra. In addition, he suggested using lateral oblique vascularised flaps from the lateral part of the preputium and penile skin. This was a proximally based pedicled tube derived from the preputium. These techniques were performed in two stages. To our knowledge, he is the first surgeon to describe and use vascularised island flaps in hypospadias surgery.

Urethral Construction with Free Grafts

In 1897 Nové-Josserand described the application of split-thickness free skin grafts for the reconstruction of the urethra (Fig. 1.7). This was a two-stage procedure. He reported his results again in 1914 (Nové-Josserand 1914). He was the first to successfully use a free graft to create urethra.

Urethral Elongation

Beck (1898) and Hacker (1898) presented a special technique for the distal type of hypospadias without chordee. They undermined and mobilised the urethra and advanced it into the glans. Tunnelisation of the glans was performed with the help of a trochar-like instrument (Fig. 1.8). For deeper grooves they advised cutting the glans medially and reapproximating it over the advanced urethra.

The Concept of Chordee Correction

In 1842, Mettauer advocated making many subcutaneous incisions to treat skin tethering. Although this was a very modern and scientific concept for the mid-nineteenth century it was ignored and instead a misconception pointed out by Bouisson in 1860 continued for more than a century. Duplay (1874a,b; 1880) mentioned the importance of chordee release even before urethroplasty. Lauenstein in 1892 used pubic skin flaps to treat skin deficiency in the ventral surface of the hypospadiac penile shaft. In 1844 Pancoast resected a small part from the dorsal corpora to correct a bending problem, almost a century before the so-called Nesbit's procedure (Pancoast 1844, 1972).

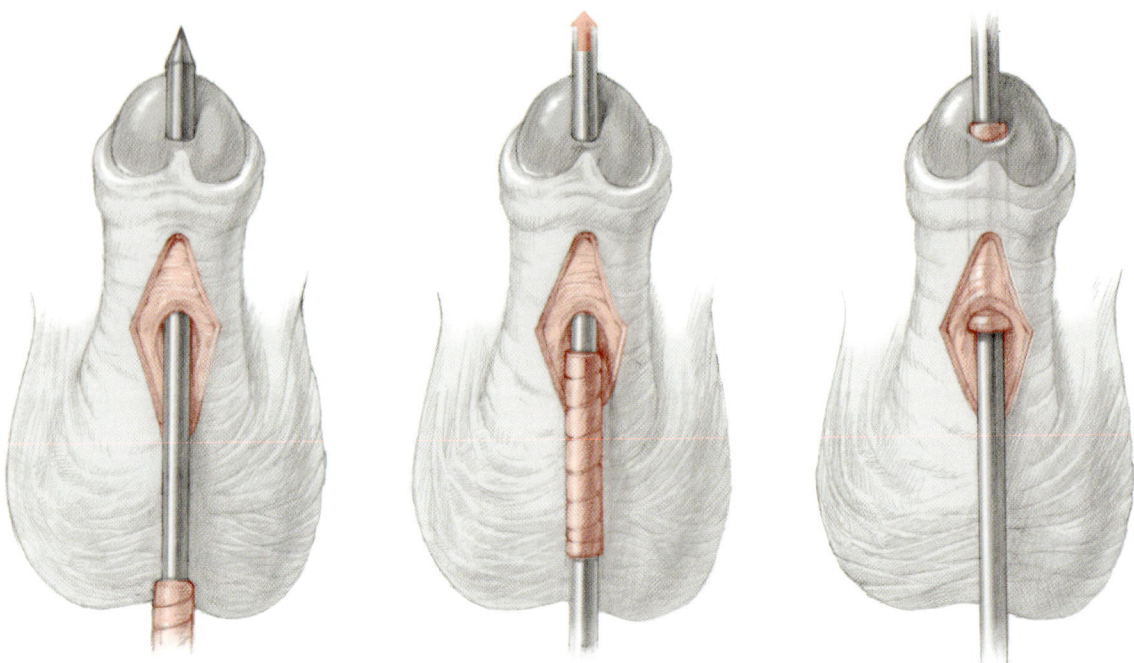

Fig. 1.7. Nové-Josserand (1897) used split-thickness skin graft to reconstruct the neourethra

The Twentieth Century

Creation of Neourethra

Efforts to Create Urethra by Local Flaps

Ombrédanne, a real scientific pioneer, reached one of the milestones of hypospadiology. In his reports and his famous book (Ombrédanne 1911, 1925, 1932) he advised performing a large round flap to create an urethra (👁 Fig. 1.9a, b, p. 12). After the creation of the urethra, the defect in the ventral penile shaft was covered by a dorsal preputial flap which was brought down by the philosophy of the buttonhole technique (👁 Figs. 1.9c, d, 1.10, p. 13). This was a single-stage repair with a reasonable rate of complication. In 1913 credit was given to Edmunds (DeSy and Oesterlinck 1980) as the first surgeon to transfer the dorsal preputial flap to cover the ventral penile skin after an extensive chordee release. This extensive chordee release was performed in the first stage, followed by the second stage where healthy and abundant skin was easily manipulated into a Duplay-type urethroplasty.

Bevan in 1917 created a rectangular-shaped meatal based flap and carried it through the surgically created glanular channel aiming to treat distal types of hypospadias. According to the author, this technique is considered the initial version of flip-flap techniques. In 1917 Beck presented his two-stage technique for proximal hypospadias plus severe chordee. In the first stage he released the chordee and brought a bipediculated preputial flap to cover the ventral skin defect. In the second stage, a Duplay-type urethroplasty was performed and was covered by a pediculated lateral penoscrotal rotation flap.

In 1932, Mathieu used a meatal-based penile skin flap technique for the treatment of distal hypospadias. The flap was rotated superiorly and sutured to the internal lips of the two paramedian glanular and shaft incisions. The ventral skin defect was closed by suturing external edges of the glans and skin.

In 1950, Denis Browne popularised his "buried strip of skin" method (Browne 1936, 1949, 1953). Until recent times this technique was favoured by most paediatric surgeons and paediatric urologists.

Davis (1940, 1950) developed a tube from the dorsal penile skin. The pedicle of the tube was situated in the proximal part of the dorsal penile shaft. The penis was bent in the dorsal direction to bring the tip of the glans to the base of the pedicle of the tubularised flap, whose tip was anastomosed to the edges of the hypospadiac meatus. The base of the flap was divided as a second-stage operation.

For treatment of distal hypospadias, Horton and Devine (1959) created a flip flap from the ventral surface of the shaft adjacent to the urethral meatus, and a triangular midline glanular flap to form the distal urethra (Devine 1961; Dieffenbach 1837). The ventral

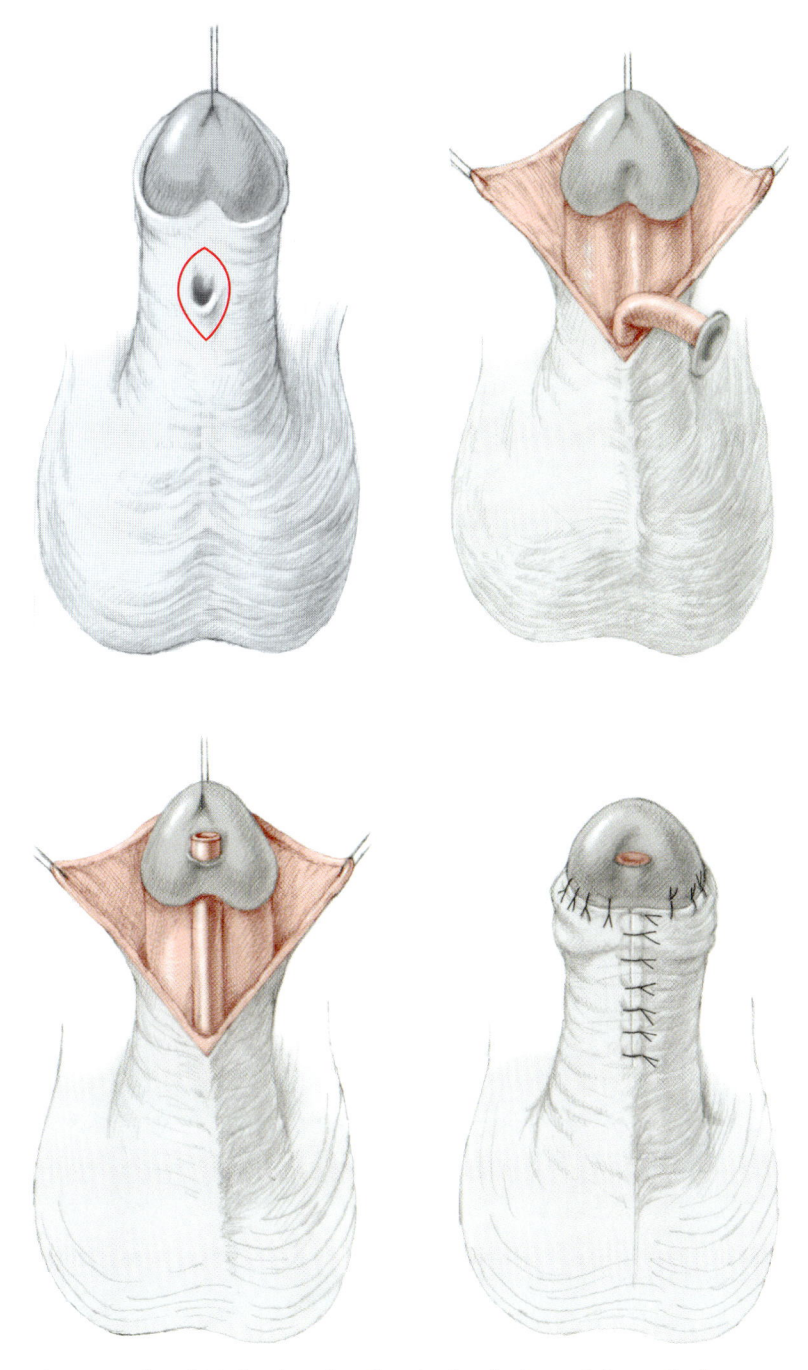

Fig. 1.8. Beck and Hacker (1897) undermined and advanced the urethral meatus into the glans

surface could easily be covered by lateral glanular flaps. In 1965, Mustardé combined the Bevan rectangular flap technique and midline glanular triangular flap techniques. Instead of incising the glans, he passed the tube through a surgically created glanular tunnel. He also benefited from the preputial buttonhole technique to cover the ventral skin defect.

Techniques for Reconstruction of the Urethra by Using Vascularised Island Flaps

In 1961, Des Prez et al. and Broadbent et al. presented a single-stage technique for severe proximal forms (Broadbent et al. 1961; Des Prez et al. 1961). They used a lateral vascularised preputial island flap for urethral reconstruction. The new urethral meatus was anasto-

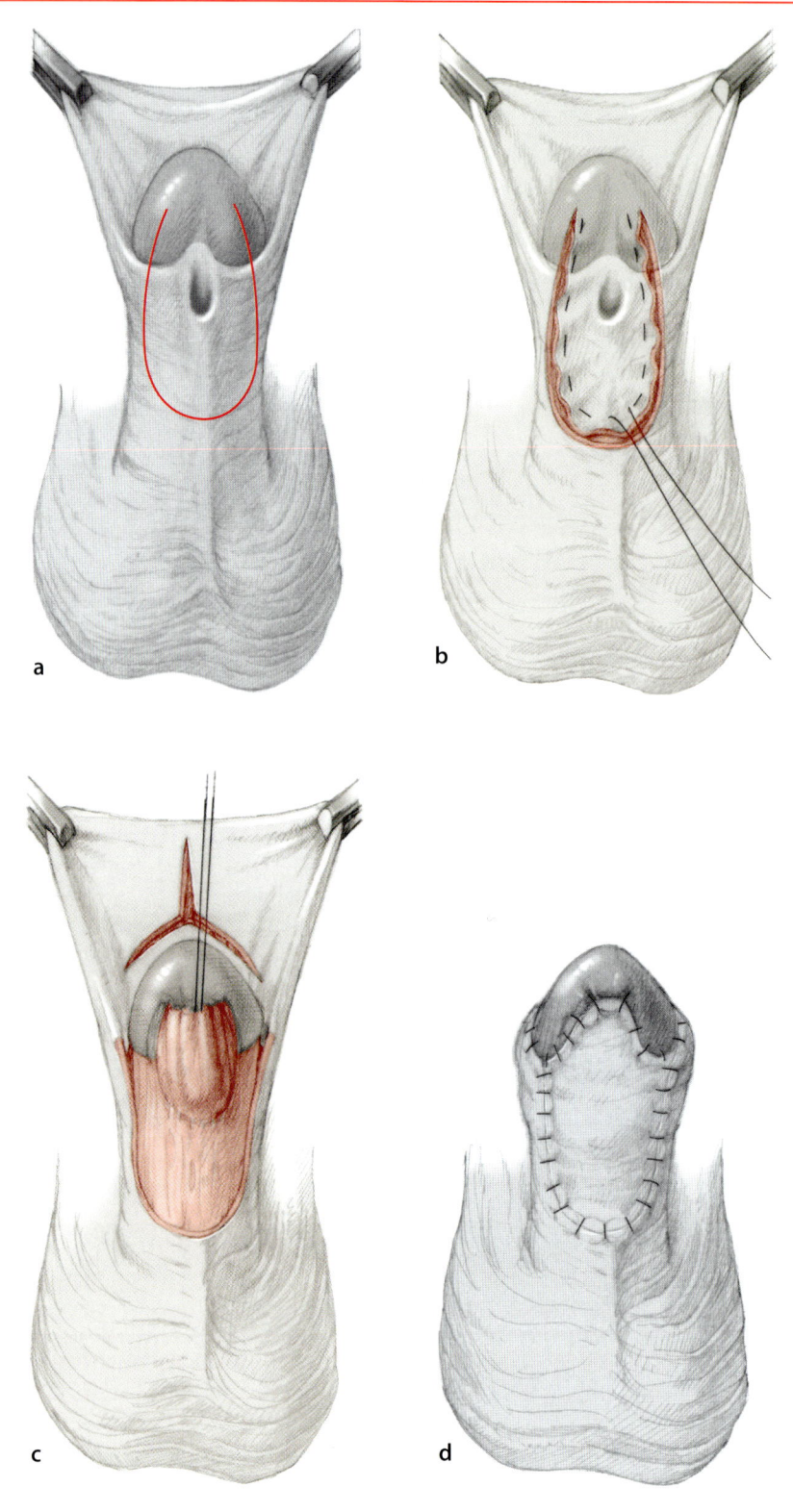

Fig. 1.9a–d. Ombredanne (1911) designed a large round flap and used a purse-string suture to reconstruct the neourethra

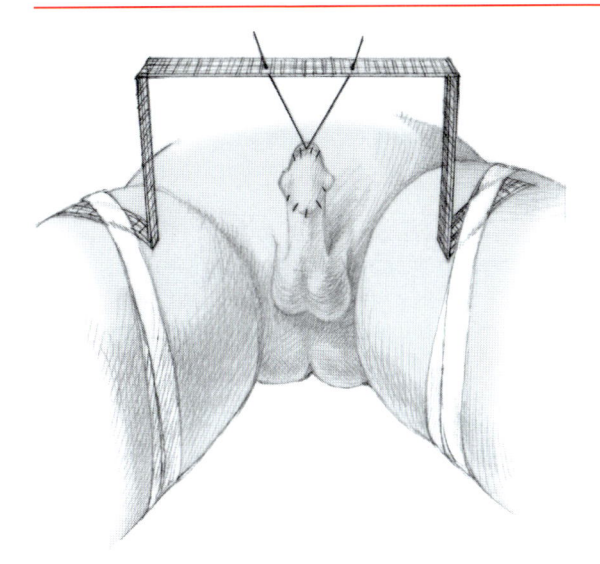

Fig. 1.10. The Ombredanne method of fixation of the penis after hypospadias repair

mosed to the tip of the glans by either splitting or tunnelling the glans tissue.

Toksu (1970) and Hodgson (1970) created a technique based on a vertical preputial vascularised flap from the inner preputial surface in 1970. This single-stage procedure was indicated only for distal cases.

In 1971, Asopa presented a similar technique which is applicable to severe proximal hypospadias (Asopa et al. 1971). In this technique, a horizontal preputial flap is prepared from the inner surface and tubularised to form a neourethra. This urethra was brought down to the ventral surface by means of a Byars flap.

In 1968 Hinderer presented a technique which is applicable for all types of hypospadias (Hinderer 1971, 1975). A vascularised flap beginning from the hypospadiac meatus extending beyond the midline to the inner surface of the preputium was prepared to form the urethral canal. Instead of splitting, the glans is tunnelled by a special type of trochar in order to bring the pediculated flap through it.

Standoli (1979, 1982) created a neourethra by using a vascularised island flap which is horizontally prepared from the outer surface of the preputium. This was a real island flap with its intact vascular pedicle and this pedicle was rotated around the penis to bring the neourethra to the ventral side of the shaft.

In 1980 Duckett popularised his preputial island flap which is created from the inner surface of the preputium in horizontal direction (Duckett 1980, 1981a). A ventral skin defect was covered by the outer preputial skin using the Byars technique.

Asopa popularised his double-face prepuce flap in order to create a neourethra and to cover the ventral skin defect (Asopa and Asopa 1984). This approach, presented in 1984, is still used by many hypospadiologists.

Urethral Construction with Free Grafts

Free Skin Grafts ▸ McIndoe (1937) used Nové-Josserand's split-thickness graft method by using a special type of trochar to introduce the graft under the penile skin and through the glans. This was a two-stage technique.

In 1961 Horton and Devine created a single-stage procedure which can be used for all types of proximal cases (Devine and Horton 1961; Horton and Devine 1959). They used a full-thickness inner preputial free skin graft to create an urethra. A triangular glanular flap was used for the anastomosis between the graft and glanular meatus. A notable initiator of this technique was Humby (1941), who used a full-thickness preputial flap years before Horton and Devine in 1941.

Other Free Grafts ▸ Free grafts prepared from tissues such as the appendix, the urethra and other vessels were used by various authors yet without significant clinical success (Smith 1997). On the other hand, bladder mucosa and buccal mucosa are associated with higher consistency and are still used by various surgeons with reasonable complication rates. Bladder mucosa was used by Memmelaar in 1947 and by Marshall and Spellman in 1955. This method was popularised by Hendren and Reda (1986) and Ransley et al. (1987). Buccal mucosa for the creation of a neourethra was used by Humby in 1941 and Mirabet in 1964, but popularised by Duckett (1986), Dessanti et al. (1992) and Ransley from the UK.

Urethral Elongation

In 1981, Duckett presented a meatal advancement and glanuloplasty (MAGPI) technique for subcoronal and glanular cases without chordee (Duckett 1981b). In 1982, Baran used a modification of the Beck and Hacker technique by elongating the distal urethra to the tip of the penis through a surgically created tunnel (Baran and Çenetoğlu 1993). A glanular triangular flap was used in the meatal anastomosis in order to prevent stricture formation. This was an operation especially advised for circumcised hypospadiac patients.

The Concept of Chordee Correction

In 1913, Edmunds transferred preputial skin to the ventrum of the penis in order to stabilise the deficient skin. In 1917 Beck had used the buttonhole technique by passing the glans through the preputium in order to transfer the dorsal skin easily to the ventral part. This was popularised by Nesbit (1941, 1965, 1966). Blair and Byars in 1938 and Byars in 1955 used the relevant model of dorsal preputial flaps to treat the "deficient skin problem" in the ventral surface of the shaft. Byars in 1955 drew attention to the extensive removal of the fibrous tissues from the entire ventral half of the penile circumference down to the corpus cavernosum.

The modern concept of chordee correction, mentioned in 1842 by Mettauer, was rediscovered by Smith of the USA in 1967. Smith's work contributed in a major way to the realisation of the "importance of tethering and shortening of the skin and subcutaneous tissues".

In 1968 Allen and Spence and in 1970 King used the same concept in the operative treatment of chordee problems. In 1965 Nesbit reported the successful results of his dorsal plication technique in three consecutive cases of chordee without hypospadias (Nesbit 1965, 1966). During the past 15 years J.W. Duckett's philosophy of "corporal disproportion" has enlarged the horizons of our knowledge and surgical philosophy of chordee problems (Baskin et al. 1994; Duckett 1987; Duckett and Baskin 1996).

During the last quarter of the 20th century, there were a couple of innovative techniques and important discoveries regarding the pathologic anatomy and treatment modalities in hypospadiology. According to the anatomical studies of Baskin et al. (1998), since there are no neural elements in the dorsal midline (12 o'clock position) of the penile shaft, a mid-dorsal single plication suture could be recommended for the treatment of corporal disproportion. In 1973 Barcat made a modification in the Mathieu procedure by mobilising the glans flap in addition to the parameatal flap and splitting the glans dorsally to bury the urethral tube. In 1984 Koyanagi et al. created an ingenious technique (Koyanagi et al. 1984, 1995). This is a meatal-based flap which can be easily and circumferentially extended to the glans to form a foreskin flap to be converted to an urethral plate. In their experience, this technique could be used universally for the treatment of all types of hypospadias.

In 1994 Snodgrass from the USA presented his "tubularised incised plate technique" for the treatment of distal hypospadias. Recently it has been shown that this technique could be applicable to proximal hypospadias (Snodgrass et al. 1998, 2002). In 1998 Perovic from Yugoslavia presented his penile disassembly technique for the treatment of severe penile curvatures and especially for glans tilt and curvatures that are located distally (Perovic et al. 1998).

Milestones in Modern Hypospadiology

Browne (1936), Smith (1938), and Schaffer and Erbes (1950) made an anatomical classification of hypospadias according to the localisation of the ectopic meatus. Barcat in 1973 presented a new concept related to the new localisation of the meatus after the chordee release procedure.

In 1974, Gittes and McLaughlin popularised the "artificial erection test" by injecting saline solution after placing a tourniquet at the base of the penis. This was a real advance in the diagnosis and treatment of chordee.

In 1980 DeSy and Oosterlinck introduced silicone foam dressing, which was considered a significant improvement for paediatric patients and solved the issue of various postoperative care problems. Jensen, in 1981, presented the idea of "supplemental local block for postoperative pain relief" by using 0.5% bupivacaine solution. This was a revolution in the anaesthesia of hypospadias and postoperative pain problems.

Surgical correction became more effective and less complicated after improved optic magnification techniques and new suture materials (Manley and Epstein 1981).

After the declaration of the Section of Urology of the AAP in 1975 and the paper of Schultz et al., the operation age for hypospadias decreased to between 6 and 18 months (Schultz et al. 1983; Shokeir and Hussein 1999).

Monfort and Lucas (1982) recommended testosterone stimulation in the preoperative period to increase the size and the vascularity of the penile shaft and skin. This was found to be extremely useful for the patient as well as the surgeon.

Among modern diversion techniques, a simple method, "Silastic tubing placed through the repair into the bladder allowing a constant dripping from the catheter into the diaper", which was popularised by Duckett and Snyder (1985; Duckett 1992), was another revolution. Oral intake of oxybutinin made this application even more tolerable by the young patients (Duckett 1987; Duckett and Baskin 1996).

In 1994, Snow used tunica vaginalis as an additional protective tissue to cover the urethra to prevent fistula formation. Since the 1990s, subcutaneous tissues prepared from the dorsal preputial skin or dartos has been used for the same purpose.

From the historical perspective, it can be concluded that, in the twenty-first century, no paediatric surgeon or paediatric urologist can claim originality for any of the techniques and principles for the treatment of hypospadias. Most of the modern techniques of reconstructive procedures were developed through the work of innovative and pioneer surgeons of previous centuries. Recent improvements are due not only to developments in paediatric anaesthesia, antibiotics, suture materials and catheters, but to the incredible efforts of the old masters.

References

Aeginata P: Seven books of Paulus Aeginata. Sydenham Society, London, 1844.
Allen TD, Spence HM: The surgical treatment of coronal hypospadias and related problems. J Urol. 1968; 100:504–508.
Anger MT: Hypospadias. Bull Soc Chir Paris. 1874a; p 32.
Anger MT: In: Murphy LJT (ed): (1972) The history of urology. Thomas, Springfield, Illinois. 1874b; p 454.
Anger MT: Hypospadias péno-scrotal, compliqué de coudure de la verge: redressment du pénis et uréthro-plastie par inclusion cutanée:guérison. Bull Soc Chir Paris. 1875; p 179.
Antyl (1st century AD) In: Hauben DJ (ed): The history of hypospadias. Acta Chir Plast. 1984; 26:196–199.
Asopa R, Asopa HS: One stage repair of hypospadias using double island preputial skin tube. Int J Urol. 1984; 1:41–43.
Asopa HS, Elhence EP, Atria SP, et al: One stage correction of penile hypospadias using a foreskin tube: a preliminary report. Int Surg. 1971; 55:435–448.
Baran NK, Çenetoğlu S: Pictorial history of hypospadias repair techniques. Gazi Medical Faculty, Plast Reconstr Surg. 1993; pp 1–50.
Barcat J: Current concepts of treatment of hypospadias. In: Horton CE (ed): Plastic and reconstructive surgery of the genital area. Little Brown, Boston, 1973; pp 249–263.
Baskin LS, Duckett JW, Ueoka K, et al: Changing concepts of hypospadias curvature lead to more onlay island flap procedures. J Urol. 1994; 151:191–196.
Baskin LS, Erol A, Li YW, et al: Anatomic studies of hypospadias. J Urol. 1998; 160:1108–1115.
Beck C: A new operation for balanic hypospadias. NY Med J. 1898; 67:147.
Beck C: Hypospadias and its treatment. Surg Gynecol Obstet. 1917; 24:511.
Bettmann OL, Hinch PS: A pictorial history of medicine, 2nd edn. Thomas, Springfield, Illinois. 1956; pp 4–5.
Bevan AD: A new operation for hypospadias. JAMA. 1917; 68:1032.
Bidder A: Eine Operation der Hypospadie mit Lappenbildung aus dem Scrotum. Dtsch Med Wochenschr. 1892; 10:208.
Bitschai J, Brodny ML: A history of urology in Egypt. Riverside, New York, 1956.
Blair VP, Byars LT: Hypospadias and epispadias. J Urol. 1938; 40:814.
Bouisson MF: Remarques sur quelques variétés de l'hypospadias et sur le traitement qui leur convient. Bull Ther. 1860; 59:349–362.
Bouisson MF: De l'hypospadias et de son traitment chirurgical. Trib Chir. 1861; 2:484.
Broadbent TR, Woolf RM, Toksu E: Hypospadias – one stage repair. Plast Reconstr Surg. 1961; 27:154–159.
Browne D: A comparison of the Duplay and Denis Browne techniques for hypospadias operation. Surgery. 1953; 34:787.
Browne D: An operation for hypospadias. Lancet. 1936; 1:141.
Browne D: An operation for hypospadias. Proc R Soc Med. 1949; 41:466–468.
Bussemaker UC, Daremberg CV: Ouvres d'Oribase, texte Grec en Grande Partie Inédit. Imprimerie Nationale, Paris, 1851– 1876 (6 vols).
Büyükünal SNC, Sary N: Şarafeddin Sabuncuoğlu,the author of the earliest pediatric surgical atlas: Cerrahiye-i Ilhaniye, J Pediatr Surg. 1991; 26:1148–1151.
Byars LT: A technique for consistently satisfactory repair of hypospadias. Surg Gynecol Obstet. 1955; 100:184–190.
Cassar P: A medico-legal report of the 16th century from Malta. Med Hist. 1974; 18:354–359.
Davis DM: The pedicle tube graft in the surgical treatment of hypospadias in the male. Surg Gynecol Obstet. 1940; 71:790.
Davis DM: The surgical treatment of hypospadias,especially scrotal and perineal. Plast Reconstr Surg. 1950; 5:373.
Des Prez JD, Persky L, Kiehn CL: One stage repair of hypospadias by island flap technique. Plast Reconstr Surg. 1961; 28:405–411.
Dessanti A, Rigamonti W, Merulla V et al: Autologous buccal mucosa graft for hypospadias repair: an initial report. J Urol. 1992; 147:1081–1084.
De Sy WA, Oosterlinck W: Silicone foam elastomer: A significant improvement in postoperative penile dressing. J Urol. 1982; 128:39–41.
Devine CJ, Horton CE: A one stage hypospadias repair. J Urol. 1961; 85:166–172.
Dieffenbach JF: Die operative Chirurgie. Brockhaus, Leipzig, 1845.
Dieffenbach JF: Guérison des fentes congénitales de la verge, de l'hypospadias. Gaz Hebd Med. 1837; 5:156.
Dingwall EJ: Male infibulation. Bale and Danielson, London, 1925.
Dionis P: In: Haeger K (ed) The illustrated history of surgery. Harold Strake, London, 1718; pp 132–134.
Dionis PA: Course of chirurgical operations demonstrated in Royal Garden at Paris, 2nd edn. J Tonson, London. 1710; pp 137–155.
Duckett JW: Transverse preputial island flap technique for repair of severe hypospadias. Urol Clin North Am. 1980; 7:423–431.
Duckett JW: The island flap technique for hypospadias repair. Urol Clin North Am. 1981a; 8:503–511.
Duckett JW: MAGPI (meatal advancement and glanuloplasty): a procedure for subcoronal hypospadias. Urol Clin North Am. 1981b; 8:513–520.
Duckett JW: Use of buccal mucosa urethroplasty in epispadias. Meeting of Society of Pediatric Urology, Southampton, England. 1986.
Duckett JW: Hypospadias. In: Gillenwater JY, Grayhack JT, Howards SS, Duckett JW (eds): Adult and pediatric urology, vol II, 2nd edn. Year Book Medical Publishers, Chicago. 1987; pp 1880–1915.
Duckett JW: Successful hypospadias repair. Contemp Urol. 1992; 4:42–55.
Duckett JW, Snyder HM: Hypospadias "pearls". Soc Pediatr Urol Newslett. 1985; 7:4.

Duckett JW, Baskin LS: Hypospadias. In: Gillenwater JY, Grayhack JT, Howards SS, Duckett JW (eds) Adult and pediatric urology, vol 3, 3rd edn. Mosby, St Louis. 1996; pp 2549–2589.

Duplay S: De l'hypospadias périneo-scrotal et de son traitement chirurgical. Arch Gen Med. 1874a; 1:613, 657.

Duplay S: De l'hypospadias périnéo-scrotal et de son traitment chirurgical. Asselin, Paris, 1874b.

Duplay S: Sur le traitement chiurgical de l'hypospadias et de l'epispadias. Arch Gen Med. 1880; 5:257.

Edmunds A: An operation for hypospadias. Lancet. 1913; 1:447.

Elder JS, Duckett JW, Snyder HM: Onlay island flap in the repair of mid and distal hypospadias without chordee. J Urol. 1987; 138:376.

Ellis H: A history of surgery. Greenwich Medical Media, London. 2001; pp 4–5.

Fabricii ab Aquapendente H: Opera Chirurgica Patavii: Franciscum Bolzettam, 1641.

Fabricii ab Aquapendente H: Opera Chirurgica Venetiis: Apud Robertum Megliettum, 1619.

Filler J: Disease. British Museum Press, London. 1995; p:90.

Galen (c. 130–201 AD). In: Opera Omnia vol 10. Kühn, Leipzig, Cnobloch, p 1001

Gittes RF, McLaughlin AP III: Injection technique to induce penile erection. Urology. 1974; 4:473–474.

Hacker V: Zur operativen Behandlung der Hypospadia Glandis. Beitr Z Klin Chir. 1898; 22:271–276.

Heister L: General system of surgery in three parts. Winnys, London. 1743; pp 129–138; 243–250.

Hendren WH, Reda EF: Bladder mucosa graft for reconstruction of male urethra. J Pediatr Surg. 1986; 21:189.

Herrlinger R: History of medical illustration: from antiquity to 1600. Medicina Rara, New York, 1970.

Hinderer U: Behandlung der Hypospadie und der inkompletten Hypospadieformen nach eigenen Methoden von 1966 bis 1975. In: Schmied E, Widmaier W, Reichert H (eds) Wiederstellung von Form und Funktion organischer Einheiten der verschiedenen Körperregionen: Jahrestagung der Deutschen Gesellschaft für Plastische und Wiederherstellungschirurgie. Thieme, Stuttgart. 1975; pp 263–290.

Hinderer U: New one-stage repair of hypospadias (technique of penis tunnelization). In: Hueston JT (ed) Transactions of the 5th International Congress of Plastic and Reconstructive Surgery. Butterworth, Stoneham. 1971; pp 283–305.

Hodgson NB: A one-stage hypospadias repair. J Urol. 1970; 104:281–284.

Horton CE, Devine CJ, Baran NK: Pictorial history of hypospadias repair techniques.In: Horton CE (ed) Plastic and reconstructive surgery of the genital area. Little Brown, Boston. 1973; pp 237–248.

Horton CE, Devine CJ: Film: a one-stage hypospadias repair. Eaton Laboratories, 1959.

Humby G: A one stage operation for hypospadias. Br J Surg. 1941; 29:84–92.

Jensen BH: Caudal block for postoperative pain relief after genital operations. A comparison between morphine and bupivacaine. Acta Anesthesiol Scand. 1981; 25:373–375.

Johnson T: The works of that famous chirurgion Ambrose Paré, translated out of Latine and compared with the French by T Johnson. Cotes TH, Young R, London, 1634. Reprinted by Milord, Boston, 1968.

King LR: Hypospadias – a one-stage repair without skin graft based on a new principle: chordee is sometimes produced by skin alone. J Urol. 1970; 103:660–662.

Koyanagi T, Nonomura H, Kakizaki H, et al: Hypospadias repair. In: Thüroff JW, Hohenfellner M (eds): Reconstructive surgery of the lower urinary tract in children. Isis Medical Media, Oxford. 1995; pp 1–21.

Koyanagi T, Nonomura K, Gotoh T et al: One stage repair of perineal hypospadias and scrotal transposition. Eur J Urol. 1984; 10:364–367.

Landerer: Dtsch Z Chir. 1891; p 32.

Lascaratos J, Kostakopoulos A, Louras G: Penile surgical techniques described by Oribasius (4th century CE). BJU Int. 1999; 84:16–19.

Lauenstein C: Zur Plastik der Hypospadie. Arch Klin Chir. 1892; 43:203.

Manley CB, Epstein ES: Improved optical magnification have made surgical correction at an earlier age more successful. J Urol. 1981; 125:698–700.

Marshall VF, Spellman RM: Construction of urethra in hypospadias using vesical musocal grafts. J Urol. 1955; 73: 335–342.

Mathieu P: Traitement en un temps de l'hypospadias balanique et juxta-balanique. J Chir. 1932; 39:481.

Mayo CH: JAMA. 1901; 36:1157.

McIndoe AH: An operation for cure of adult hypospadias. Br Med J. 1937; 1:385.

Memmelaar J: Use of bladder mucosa in a one stage repair of hypospadias. J Urol. 1947; 58:68–73.

Mettauer JP: Practical observations on those malformations of the male urethra and penis,termed hypospadias and epispadias, with an anomalous case. Am J Med Sci. 1842; 4:43.

Mirabet Ippolito V: Modification de la técnica de McIndoe para el tratamiento de los hipospadias. Doctoral thesis, Valencia, 1964.

Monfort G, Lucas C: Dihydrotestosterone penile stimulation in hypospadias surgery. Eur Urol. 1982; 8:201–203.

Montagnani CA: Pediatric surgery in Islamic medicine from the middle ages to renaissance. In: Rickam PP (ed) Historical aspects of pediatric surgery. Prog Pediatr Surg, vol 20. Springer, Berlin Heidelberg New York. 1986; pp 39–51.

Moutet: De l'uréthroplastie dans hypospadias scrotal. Montpellier Méd, May, 1870.

Mustardé JC: One stage correction of distal hypospadias and other people's fistulae. Br J Plast Surg. 1965; 18:413–420.

Nesbit RM: Congenital curvature of the phallus: report of three cases with description of correction operation. J Urol. 1965; 93:230–232.

Nesbit RM: Operation for correction of distal penile ventral curvature with and without hypospadias. Trans Am Assoc Genitourin Surg. 1966; 58:12–14.

Nesbit RM: Plastic procedure for reconstruction of hypospadias. 1941; 45:699–707.

Nové-Josserand G: Traitment de l'hypospadias; nouvelle méthode. Lyon Méd. 1897; 85:198.

Nové-Josserand G: Résultates éloignés de l'uréthroplastie par la tunnelisation et la greffe dermo-épidermique dans les formes graves de l'hypospadias et de l'épispadias. J Urol Med Chir. 1914; 5:393.

Numanoğlu Y: Cerrahiye-i Ilhaniye: The earliest known book containing pediatric surgical procedures. J Pediatr Surg. 1973; 8:547–548.

Nunn JF: Ancient Egyptian medicine. Chapter 8: Surgery, trauma and dangerous animals. British Museum Press, London. 1996; pp 163–190.

Ombrédanne L: Hypospadias pénien chez l'enfant. Bull Mem Soc Chir Paris. 1911; 37:1076.

Ombrédanne L: Précis clinique et opératoire de chirurgie infantile. Masson, Paris. 1925; pp 654–689.

Ombrédanne L: Précis clinique et opératoire de chirurgie infantile. Masson, Paris. 1932; p 851.

Pancoast J: Hypospadias. In: Treatise on operative surgery. Carey and Hart, Philadelphia. 1844; p 317.

Pancoast J: In: Murphy LJT (ed): The history of urology. Thomas, Springfield, Illinois. 1972; p 456.

Paré A: Les oeuvres de M. Ambroise Paré. Chez Gabriel Buon, Paris, 1575.

Perovic SV, Vukadinovic V, Djordjevic MLJ, et al: The penile disassembly technique in hypospadias repair. Br J Urol. 1998; 81:479–487.

Portman I: A guide to the Temple of Kom Ombo. Palm Press, Cairo. 2001; p 19.

Ransley PG, Duffy PG, Oesh IL et al: The use of bladder mucosa and combined bladder mucosa/preputial skin grafts for urethral reconstruction. J Urol. 1987; 138:1096.

Reeves C: Egyptian medicine. Shire Publications, Buckinghamshire, UK. 2001; pp 26–27, 29–31.

Rochet V: Nouveau procédé pour réfaire le canal pénien dans l'hypospadias. Gaz Hebd Med Chir. 1899; 4:673.

Rogers BO: History of external genital surgery. In: Horton CE (ed): Plastic and reconstructive surgery of the genital area. Little Brown, Boston. 1973; pp 3–47.

Rosenberger: Dtsch Med Wochenschr. 1891; 9:1250.

Sabuncuoğlu Ş: Cerrahiye-i Ilhaniye, Istanbul Fatih National library, 1465; no 79 (1st manuscript).

Schaeffer DD, Erbes J: Hypospadias. Am J Surg. 1950; 80:183.

Schultz JR, Klykylo WM, Wacksman J: Timing of elective hypospadias repair in children. Pediatrics. 1983; 71:342–351.

Schwartz GS: Infibulation, population control and the medical profession. Bull NY Acad Med. 1970; 46:964.

Section of Urology, American Academy of Pediatrics: The timing of elective surgery on genitalia of male children with particular reference to undescended testis and hypospadias. Pediatrics. 1975; 56:479.

Shokeir AA, Hussein MI: The urology of Pharaonic Egypt. BJU Int. 1999; 84:755–761.

Smith CK: Surgical procedures for correction of hypospadias. J Urol. 1938; 40:239.

Smith DR: Repair of hypospadias in pre-school child. A report of 150 cases. J Urol. 1967; 97:723–730.

Smith ED: Durham Smith repair of hypospadias. Urol Clin North Am. 1981; 8:451–455.

Smith ED: The history of hypospadias. Pediatr Surg Int. 1997; 12:81–85.

Snodgrass W: Tubularized incised plate urethroplasty for distal hypospadias. J Urol. 1994; 151:464–465.

Snodgrass W, Baskin LS, Mitchell ME: Hypospadias. In: Gillenwater JY, Grayhack JT, Howards SS, Mitchell ME (eds): Adult and pediatric urology, vol III, 4th edn. Lippincott, Williams and Wilkins, Philadelphia. 2002; pp 2509–2532.

Snodgrass W, Koyle M, Manzoni G, et al: Tubularized incised plate hypospadias repair for proximal hypospadias. J Urol. 1998; 159:2129–2131.

Snow BW: Use of tunica vaginalis to prevent fistula in hypospadias surgery. J Urol. 1986; 136:861.

Spinks MS, Lewis GL: Albucasis: On surgery and instruments. A definitive edition of the Arabic text with English translation and commentary. The Wellcome Institute of the History of Medicine, London. 1973; pp:170:827.

Standoli L: Correzione dell'ipospadia in tempo unico: technica dell'uretroplastica con lembo ad isola prepuziale. Rass IT Chir Ped. 1979; 21:82–91.

Standoli L: One-stage repair of hypospadias: Preputial island flap technique. Ann Plast Surg. 1982; 9:81–88.

Sussman M: Diseases in the bible and the Talmud. In: Brothwell D, Sandison AT (eds): Diseases in antiquity: a survey of the diseases. Injuries and surgery of early population. Thomas, Springfield, Illinois. 1967; p 209.

Thiersch C: Über die Entstehungsweise und operative Behandlung der Epispadie. Arch Heilkunde. 1869; 10:20.

Toksu E: Hypospadias: one-stage repair. Plast Reconstr Surg. 1970; 45:365.

Ünver AS: Şerafeddin Sabuncuoğlu: Kitabül Cerrahiye-i Ilhaniye (Cerrahname), Istanbul, Y.Ü Typ Tarihi Enstitüsü, Adet. 1939; 12:870–1465.

Uzel I: Şerafeddin Sabuncuoğlu: Cerrâhiyyetü'l-hâniyye, vol-I, Atatürk Kültür Dil ve Tarih Yüksek Kurumu Yayynlary, III. Dizi. 1992; pp 280–281.

Van Hook W: A new operation for hypospadias. Ann Surg. 1896; 23:378.

Wood J: cited by Mayo CH: JAMA. 1901; 36:1157

Zaontz MR, Packer MG: Abnormalities of the external genitalia. Pediatr Clin North Am. 1997; 44:1267–1297.

Zeis E: Die Literatur und Geschichte der plastischen Chirurgie. Wilhelm Englemann, Leipzig. 1963; pp 145–173.

Men Behind Principles and Principles Behind Techniques

Ahmed T. Hadidi

The philosopher Santayana (1863–1952) said: "Those who cannot remember the past are condemned to repeat it". In an address to the Royal College of Surgeons, Winston Churchill remarked: "The longer you look back, the further you can look forward" (McCarthy 1990).

As Durham Smith mentioned in his forward to this book, "Although the penile repairs can be grouped into five or six major principles, depending on the tissues used, each has been subject to countless variations as one surgeon after another adds yet another modification to an already thrice-modified variation of a procedure adapted from a principle derived from the original!"

From Alexandria, Egypt came the first hypospadias pioneers, Helidorus and Antyllus. Living in the first century, they were the first to describe and define the pathophysiology and treatment of hypospadias (Bussemaker and Daremberg 1851).

The aim of this chapter is to reduce the enormous variety of techniques in hypospadias to a few basic principles and to give credit to the great pioneers who first described these concepts (Table 2.1). The following account is by no means exhaustive, nor does it include all the techniques described for hypospadias repair.

In dealing with a boy with hypospadias, the surgeon has to correct the following major abnormalities:
1. Abnormal ventral curvature or chordee, by orthoplasty
2. Abnormal proximal meatal insertion, by urethroplasty
3. abnormal looking glans penis, by glanuloplasty and meatoplasty
4. abnormal looking prepuce, either by circumcision or prepuce reconstruction

Abnormal Ventral Curvature of the Penis and Orthoplasty

Gittes and McLaughlin, writing in 1974, described intraoperative saline inflation of the corpora cavernosa. This guided and ensured successful orthoplasty. This artificial erection test has been refined with Normosol and transglanular needle placement (Fig. 2.1).

There are two types of chordee associated with hypospadias. The first is the chordee that is occasionally present in patients with distal hypospadias (skin chordee). This superficial chordee is subcutaneous, proximal to the meatus and can be corrected by mobilisation of the skin proximal to the meatus (King 1970, 1981) (Fig. 2.2).

The other type of chordee is commonly associated with proximal hypospadias. It is usually deep, fibrous and located distal to the meatus. There are three basic techniques to correct this type of deep, fibrous chordee (Fig. 2.3): (a) the abnormal ventral curvature can be corrected by *dorsal plication*, first described by Physick (Pancoast 1844) and popularised as the Nesbit procedure (1965), but this has the disadvantage of shortening the penis. (b) More commonly, the chordee can be corrected by *excision of the ventral subcutaneous fibrous bands*, usually proximal to the meatus in distal hypospadias (skin chordee). In proximal forms, the contractions are usually distal to the meatus and a transverse incision and excision of the fibrous bands can be carried out as first described by Pancoast (1844) and commonly called the Heineke–Mikulicz technique. (c) Another way of correcting chordee is by *corporal rotation*, first described by Koff and Eakins (1984). Decter (1999) added midline ventral splitting and called it the "split and roll" technique. Various skin and fascial grafts and flaps have been used to cover the resultant defect in multistage repair.

Table 2.1. Short list of men behind principles

Contributor	Date	Contribution
Helidorus and Antyllus	First century AD	First description of pathophysiology and repair of hypospadias
Galen	130–199 AD	First to use the term "hypospadias" and to emphasise significance of penile curvature
Paré	1510–1590	Extensive discussion of hypospadias and penile curvature and treatment
Dieffenbach	1837	Attempted urethroplasty by piercing the glans to the normal urethra
Mettauer	1842	"Arrest of development" theory for hypospadias aetiology; "skin tethering" theory for curvature aetiology
Physick	1844	First described chordee correction by dorsal plication
Pancoast	1844	First described chordee correction by transverse incision and longitudinal closure
Bouisson	1861	First to use scrotal skin for urethral reconstruction
Thiersch	1869	U-shaped urethroplasty for epispadias; buttonholing of the prepuce
Wood	1875	Described meatal-based flap with buttonhole of prepuce
Duplay	1880	Acknowledged Thiersch; described incomplete urethroplasty
Van Hook	1896	First description of "preputial vascular island flap" and lateral oblique flap
Beck	1898, 1917	First to describe urethral mobilisation; used rotation flap from scrotum for coverage; used a bipedicled preputial flap to resurface ventral penile skin
Nové-Josserand	1897	First description of tubularised free skin graft urethroplasty
Edmunds	1913	Three-stage ventral repositioned prepuce via buttonholed pedicle followed by tubularised urethroplasty
Ombredanne	1932	Described meatal-based flap and a purse-string suture for urethroplasty and button hole of prepuce for skin coverage
Mathieu	1932	U-shaped flap from proximal skin and two suture lines
Davis	1940	Utilised a tube of skin from the dorsal penile skin for urethral reconstruction
Humby	1941	Tubularised free skin graft urethroplasty; donor sites: inner upper arm, thigh, "mucous membrane from lower lip"
Cecil	1946	Popularised staged scrotal skin incorporation into urethroplasty
Memmelaar	1947	First description of bladder mucosa use for one-stage urethroplasty
Browne	1949	"Buried incomplete urethral plate" urethroplasty
Byars	1955	Popularised midline incision and transposition of the prepuce with second-stage tubularised urethroplasty
DesPrez et al.	1961	Described "island pedicle flap" that circumscribes the meatus and extends along the inner aspect of the prepuce
Devine and Horton	1961	Popularised one-stage free skin graft urethroplasty and V incision of the glans
Broadbent et al.	1961	One-stage urethroplasty with dorsolateral penile skin
Mustarde	1965	Recommended V incision of the glans and large proximal meatal-based flap
Barcat	1969	Described balanic groove technique
Smith	1973	Described de-epithelialisation of skin as a second protective layer
Gittes and Maclaughlin	1974	First described artificial erection test
DeSy and Oosterlinck	1980	Introduced silicon foam dressing
Duckett	1981b	Described MAGPI procedure, transverse preputial island flap
Monfort and Lucas	1982	Recommended testosterone stimulation preoperatively
Koyanagi et al.	1983	Described parameatal foreskin flap
Koff and Eakins	1984	Described chordee correction by corporal rotation
Snow	1986, 1994	Described use of tunica vaginalis wrap, yoke repair
Elder et al.	1987	Described onlay island flap
Retik et al.	1988	Preputial vascular fascia as a second protective layer
Rich et al.	1989	Described hinging of the urethral plate combined with Mathieu repair
Snodgrass	1994	Described tubularised incised plate urethroplasty
Bracka	1995a, b	Popularised two-stage repair with free skin graft
Hadidi	1996, 2003	Described Y-V glanuloplasty for distal hypospadias, lateral-based flap for proximal hypospadias and questioned the role of dressing and stenting
Decter	1999	Described chordee correction by split and roll technique
Boddy and Samuel	2000	Described excision of a triangle from apex of Mathieu flap for distal types

Men Behind Principles and Principles Behind Techniques 21

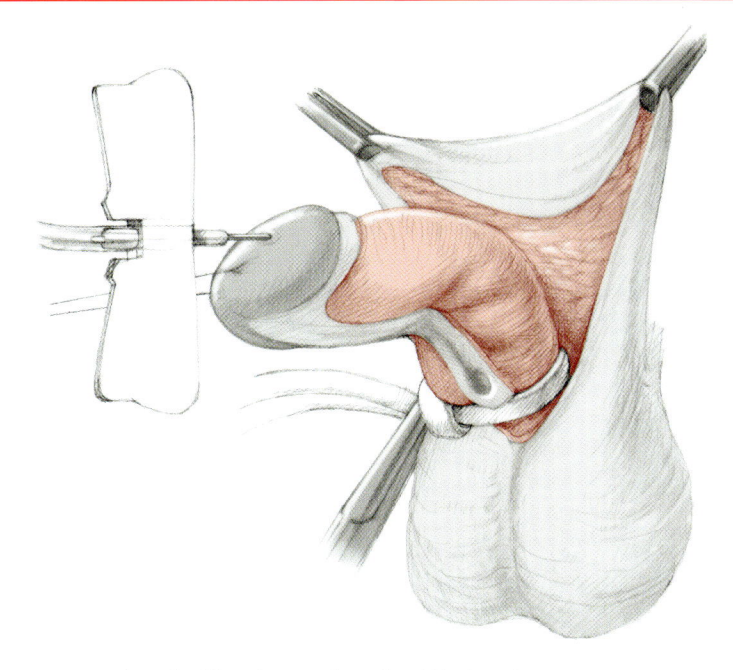

Fig. 2.1. Artificial erection test described by Gittes and Maclaughlin (1974)

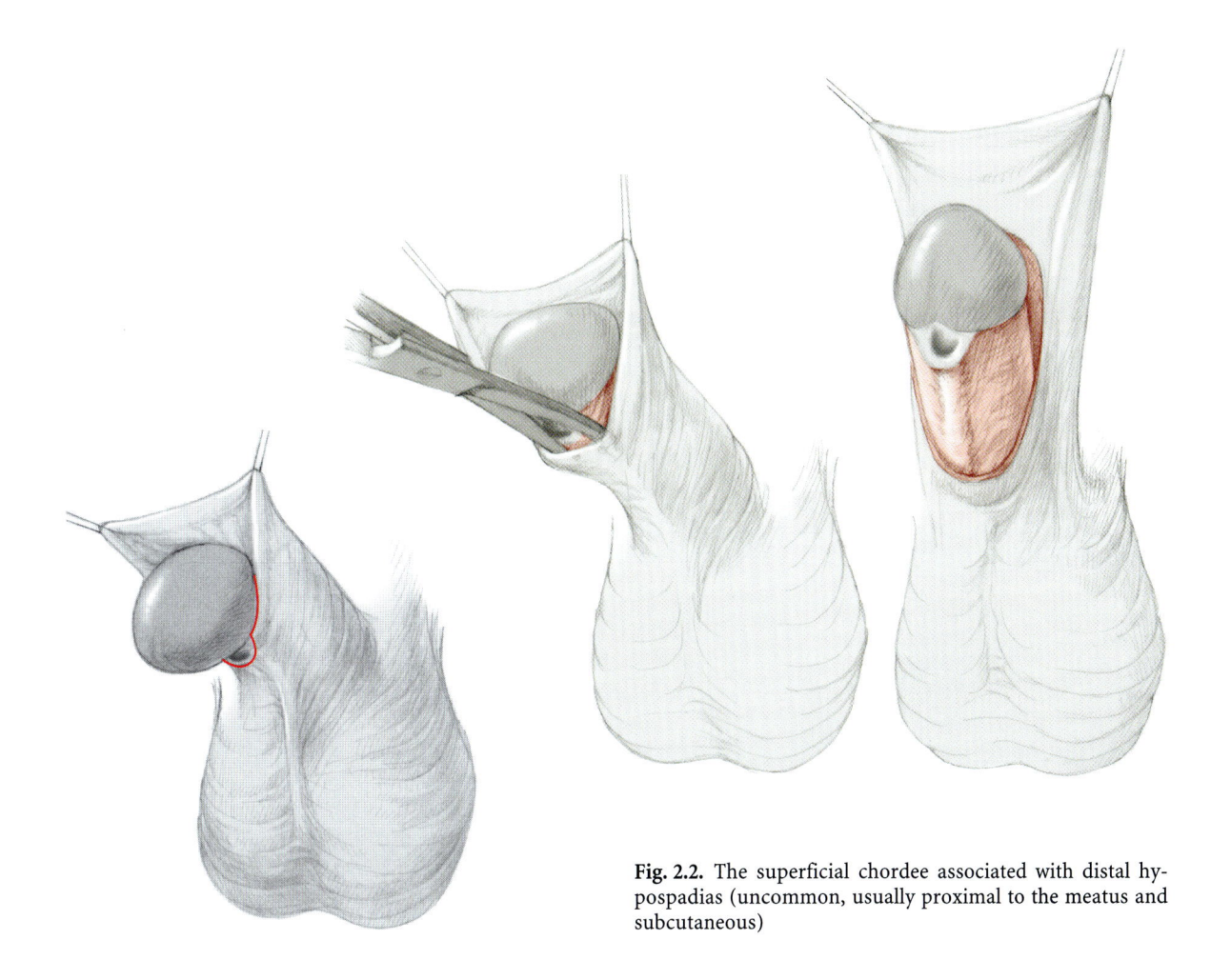

Fig. 2.2. The superficial chordee associated with distal hypospadias (uncommon, usually proximal to the meatus and subcutaneous)

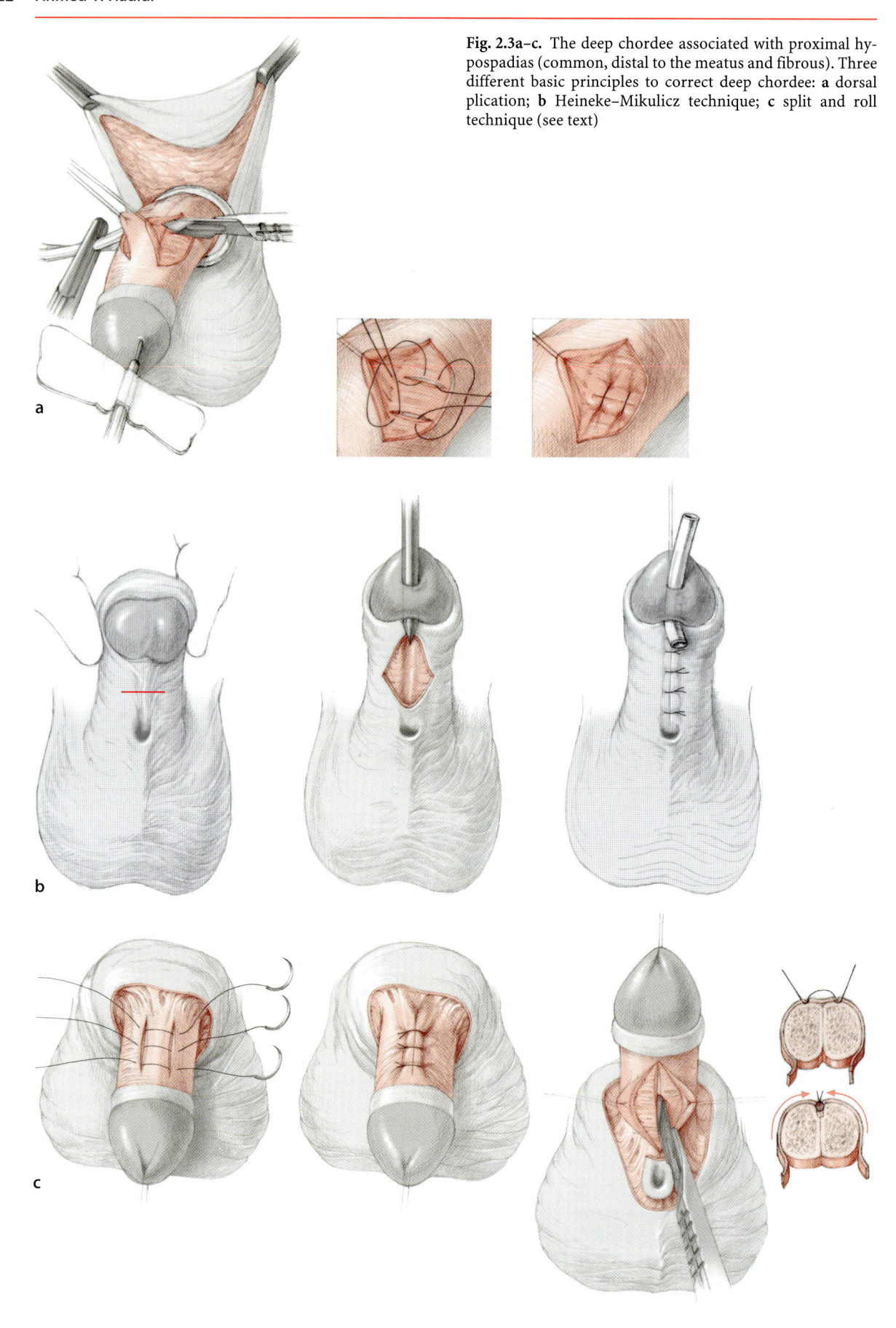

Fig. 2.3a–c. The deep chordee associated with proximal hypospadias (common, distal to the meatus and fibrous). Three different basic principles to correct deep chordee: **a** dorsal plication; **b** Heineke–Mikulicz technique; **c** split and roll technique (see text)

Abnormal Proximal Meatal Insertion and Urethroplasty

The first attempt to make the meatus terminal was by Helidorus and Antyllus in Alexandria, Egypt in the first century AD. They simply amputated the penile tissue distal to the existing meatus in distal forms of hypospadias.

To correct hypospadias and achieve a terminal meatus, one may use one of the following basic principles or tissues: (1) mobilisation of the urethra; (2) skin distal to the meatus; (3) skin proximal to the meatus;(4) preputial skin; (5) combined prepuce and skin proximal to the meatus; (6) scrotal skin; (7) dorsal penile skin; (8) different grafts; a protective intermediate layer (Fig. 2.4).

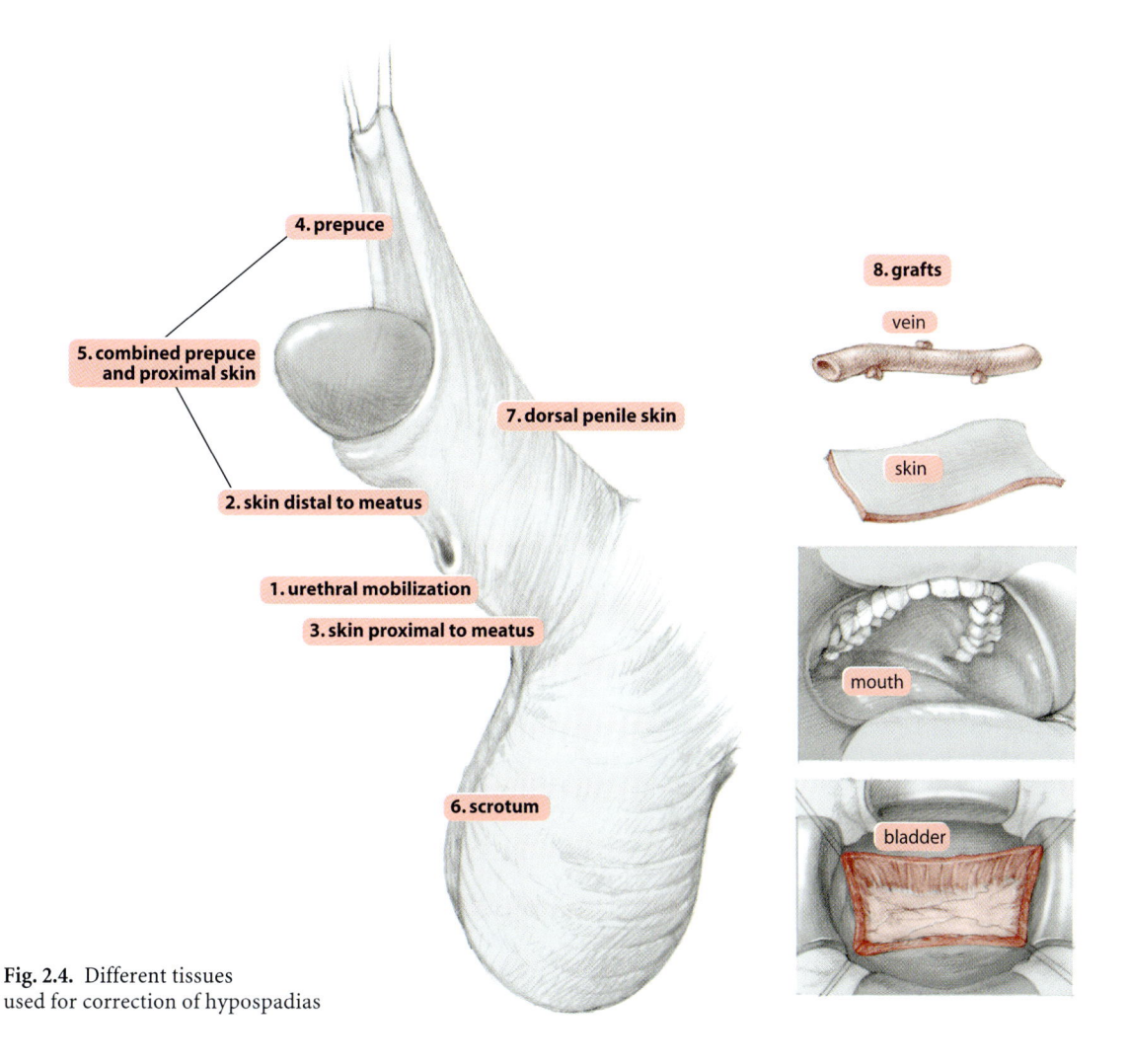

Urethral Mobilisation

Urethral mobilisation and meatal advancement was first described by Beck and Hacker in 1898 (quoted in Horton 1973) for balanic hypospadias (Fig. 2.5). The idea is to make use of the elasticity of the urethra. The procedure has the advantage that it is theoretically "risk-free" as the urethra remains completely intact. It has the drawbacks that it can only be applied to very distal forms of hypospadias. There is always the argument that you may be bringing the glans to the urethra rather than the urethra to the tip of the glans, as the penis is not a rigid structure. Some surgeons reported good results with urethral mobilisation (McGowan and Waterhouse 1964; Waterhouse and Glassberg 1981; Belman 1977; Koff 1981). This technique is still popular in some parts of Europe (Keramidas and Soutis 1995; Haberlik et al. 1997).

Fig. 2.4. Different tissues used for correction of hypospadias

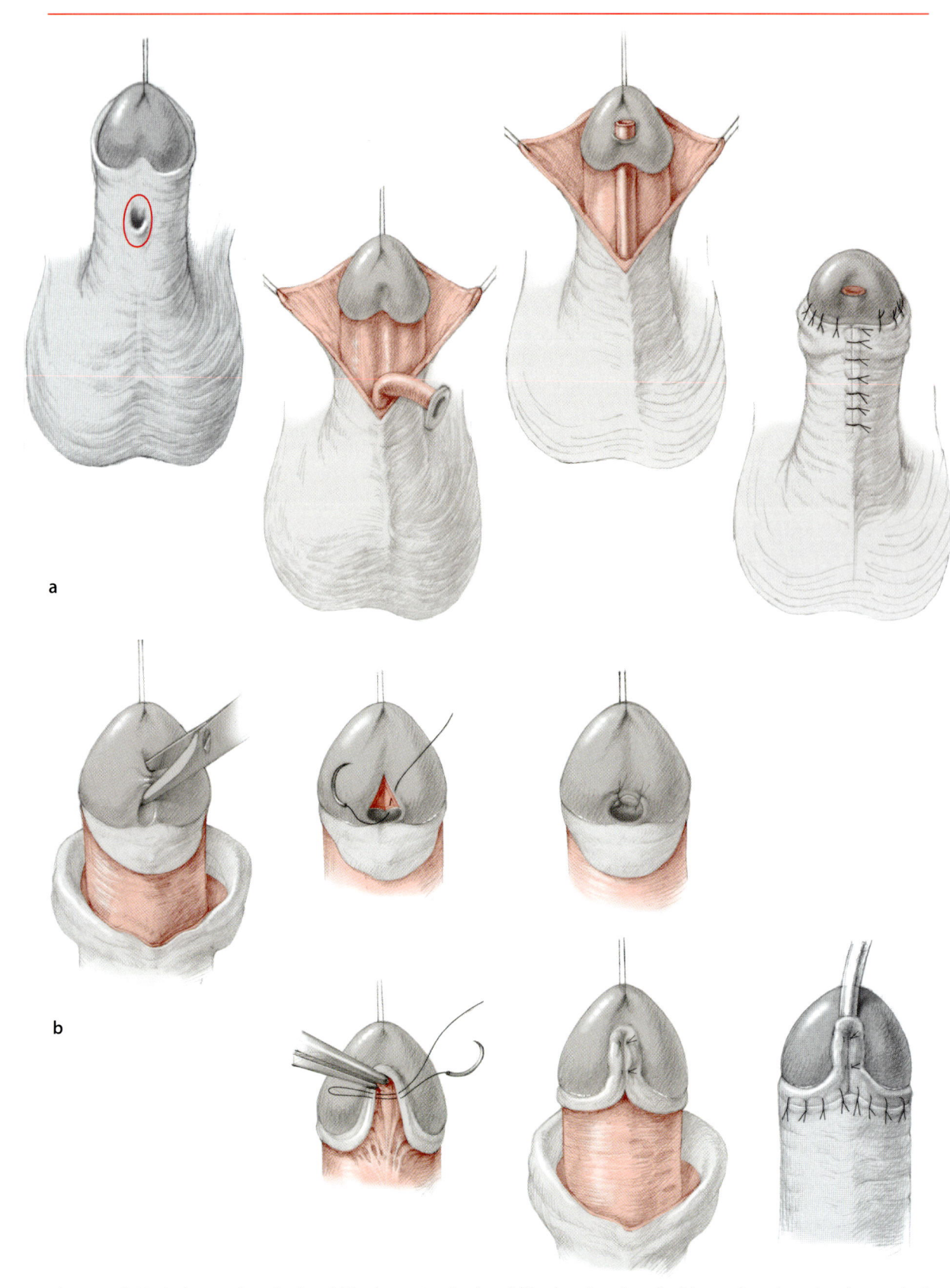

Fig. 2.5a–d. Techniques of urethral mobilisation. **a** Urethral mobilisation first described by Beck and Hacker (1897; cited in Horton 1973). **b** MAGPI described by Duckett (1981) (midline vertical incision closed transversely and mobilisation). **c, d** see p. 25

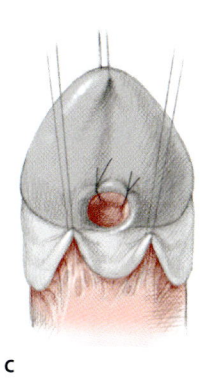

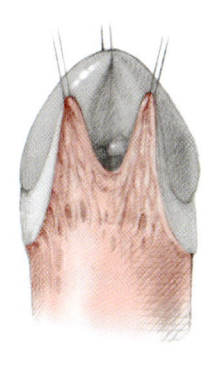

Fig. 2.5 (*continued*). **c** The M configuration by Arap et al. (1984), a modification of MAGPI by placing two sutures on the ventral edge. **d** UGPI modification of MAGPI by Harrison and Grobbelaar (1997), with a V-shaped incision around the original meatus and with deep glanular wings before urethral advancement and upward rotation of the glanular wings

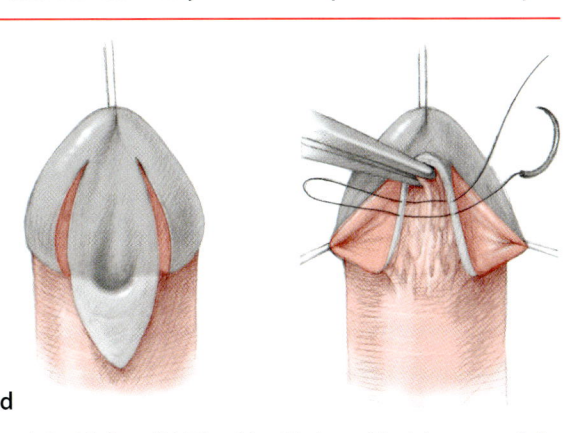

Duckett (1981b) described the "meatal advancement and glanuloplasty incorporated" (MAGPI) procedure, which combines the use of the Heineke–Mikulicz technique with urethral mobilisation in glanular hypospadias characterised by mobile urethra. Arap and his colleagues, in 1984, modified the MAGPI procedure by placing two sutures on the ventral skin edge and forming an "M" configuration. Harrison and Grobbelaar (1997) described the urethral advancement and glanuloplasty procedure (UGPI), which modifies MAGPI by having a V-shaped incision around the original meatus before mobilisation and having deep glanular wings. The meatus is advanced to the tip of the glans and two deep glanular wings are rotated upwards and wrapped around the urethra.

Use of Ventral Skin Distal to the Meatus

Reconstruction of a completely epithelialised neourethra may make use of the ventral skin distal to the meatus as in the Thiersch technique (1869), pyramid repair as described by Duckett and Keating (1989) for "megameatus intact prepuce", the glans approximation procedure (GAP) by Zaontz (1989) and distal urethroplasty and glanuloplasty (DUG) by Stock and Hanna (1997) (👁 Fig. 2.6).

Thiersch used two parallel vertical incisions to wrap the ventral skin distal to the meatus around a catheter. This was originally described for repair of epispadias (Thiersch 1869). Then Theophile Anger (1874, 1875) applied Thiersch's concepts for epispadias to hypospadias. In the same edition of the *Bulletin of the Surgical Society of Paris* (1874) Duplay of Paris described the three-stage procedure for release of chordee and creation of the ventral tube, which was later joined to the functional meatus. The same principle was adopted by Zaontz (1989) for patients with cleft glans and glanular hypospadias. Also, Duckett and Keating used the same principle to correct the defect known as megameatus intact prepuce (MIP), present in about 6% of cases of distal hypospadias, and called it pyramid repair. Stock and Hanna in 1997 combined the Thiersch–Duplay principle with the longitudinal midline incision of MAGPI, closed transversely (Heineke–Mikulicz).

Another principle recommended the use of the ventral skin distal to the meatus to form an incompletely epithelialised neourethra. Techniques adopting this principle include those of Duplay (1874), Denis Browne (1949), Rich et al. (1989) and Snodgrass (1994).

Duplay (1880) was the first to state that it did not matter whether the central tube was incompletely formed. He believed that epithelialisation would occur to form a channel if the incomplete tube was buried under the lateral flaps. The same principle was adopted by Denis Browne in his technique described in 1949. In both techniques, the defect was ventral. In 1989, Rich et al. described an incision in the glanular urethral plate to obtain a cosmetically acceptable vertical slit meatus for Mathieu repair. This dorsal midline incision was subsequently adopted for the entire length of the urethral plate as a complement to the Thiersch–Duplay urethroplasty for distal hypospadias by Snodgrass in 1994. The Snodgrass technique, also called the tubularised incised plate (TIP) urethroplasty, differs in that the defect is dorsal and the suture line is protected by a preputial subcutaneous fascial flap (👁 Fig. 2.7).

26　Ahmed T. Hadidi

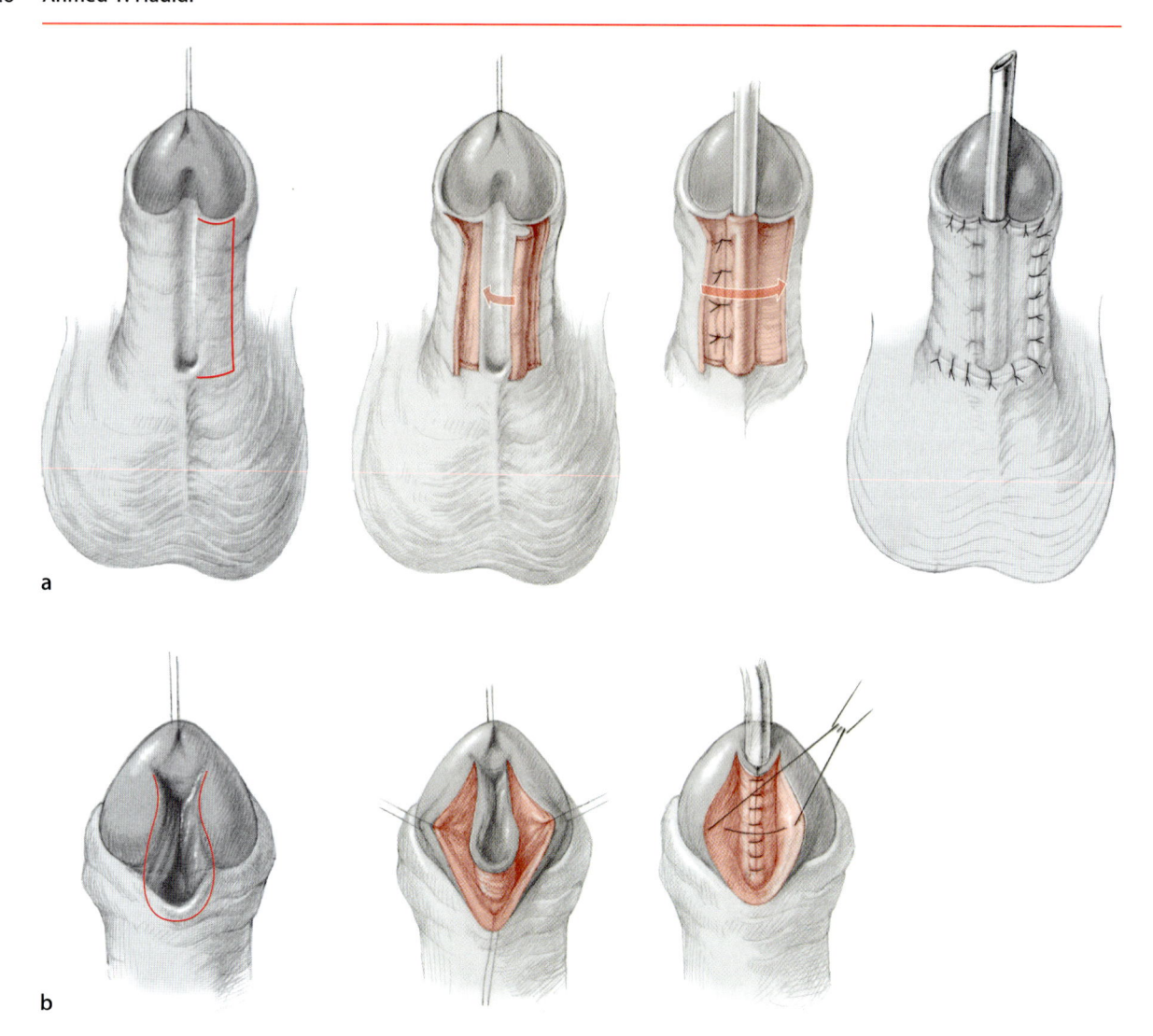

Fig. 2.6a–d. Use of ventral skin distal to the meatus to reconstruct a completely epithelialised neourethra. **a** U-shaped incision as first described by Thiersch (1869). Notice the U incision is not central in order to avoid suture lines on top of each other. **b** Pyramid repair by Duckett and Keating (1989) for megameatus intact prepuce (MIP). **c, d** see p. 27

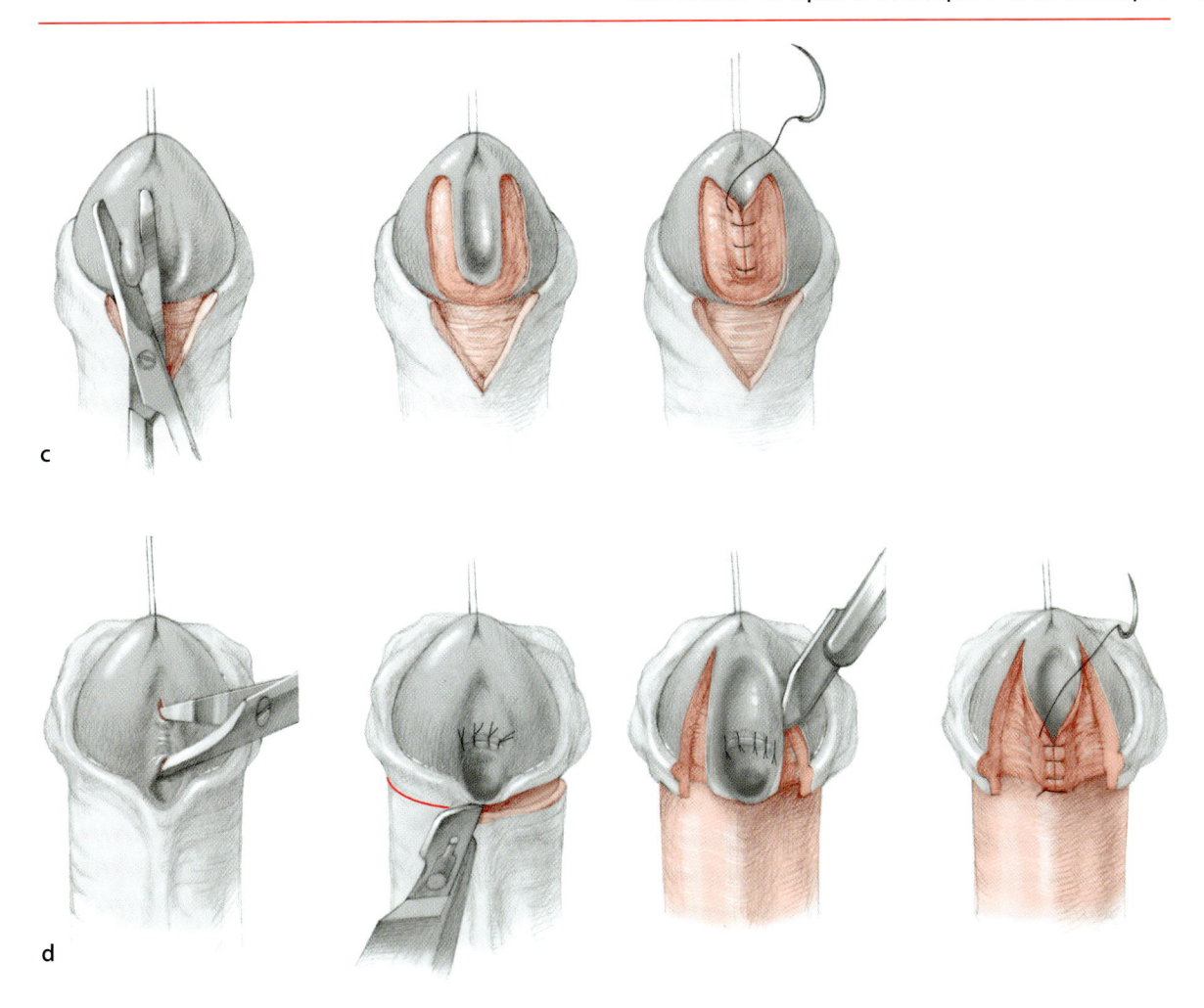

Fig. 2.6 (*continued*). **c** GAP repair by Zaontz (1989) for glanular hypospadias with cleft glans. **d** DUG repair by Stock and Hanna (1997) combining a U-shaped incision with a vertical midline incision closed transversely

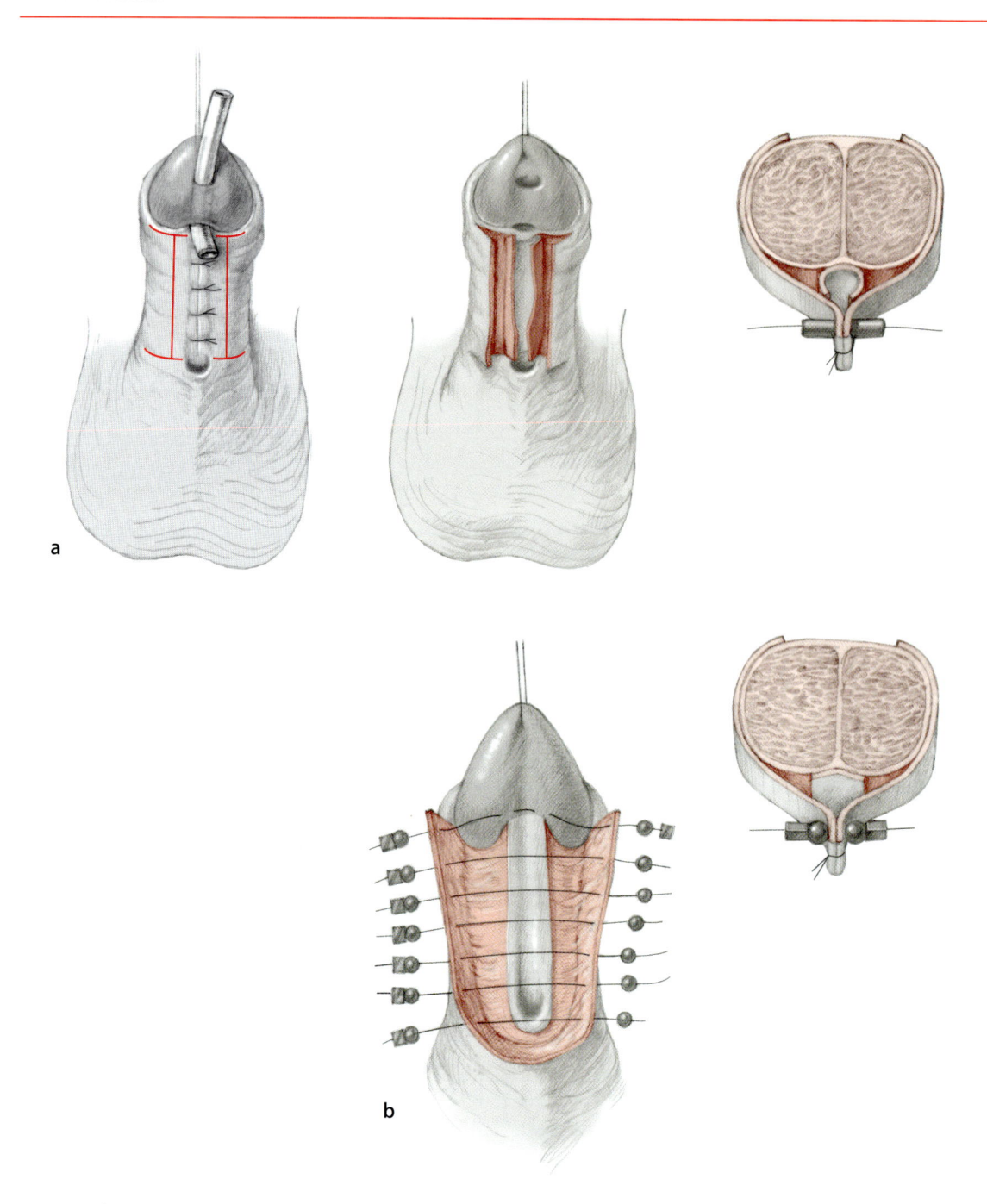

Fig. 2.7a–d. Use of ventral skin distal to the meatus to reconstruct a partially epithelialised neourethra: **a** Duplay incomplete urethroplasty (1880); **b** Denis Browne technique (1949); **c** hinging of the urethral plate (Rich et al. 1989); **d** Snodgrass TIP urethroplasty (1994). **c, d** see p. 29

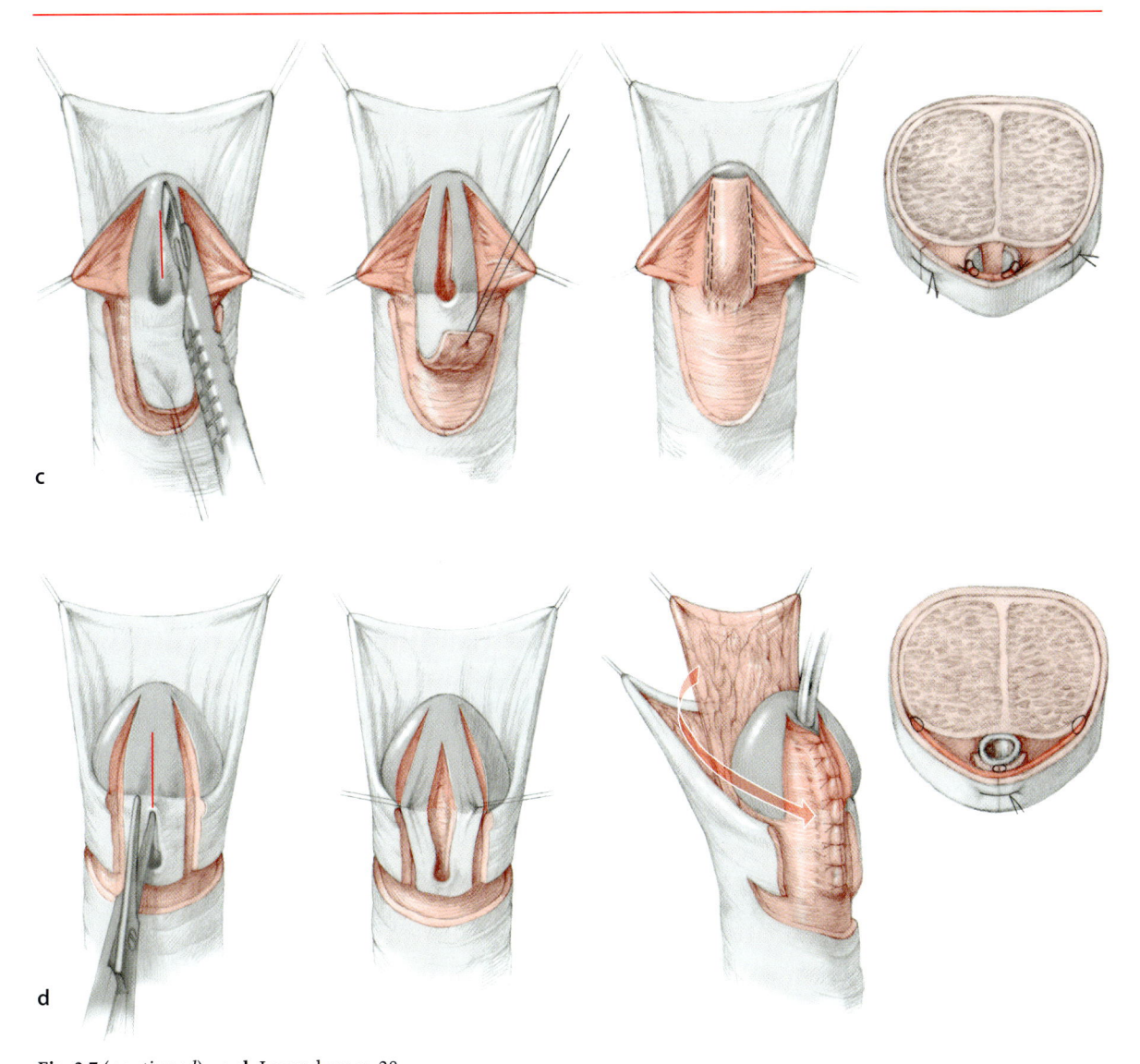

Fig. 2.7 (*continued*). **c, d** Legend see p. 28

Use of Ventral Skin Proximal to the Meatus (Meatal-Based Flaps)

A well-established group of techniques used the ventral skin *proximal* to the meatus as a meatal-based flap. This flap was used to form the ventral part of the neourethra as in the technique first described by Wood (1875), Ombrédanne (1911, 1932) and Bevan (1917) and popularised by Mathieu in 1932. Fevre (1961), Mustarde (1965), Barcat (1969, 1973) and Hadidi (1996) described techniques using the same principle.

Wood (1875) described a flap based distally on the meatus to be turned over to form the ventral surface of the neourethra. Omberdanne (1911) used a perimeatal flap but fashioned the neourethra using a purse-string suture. The repair was too baggy. Mathieu (1932) used a perimeatal flap and constructed the neourethra using two lateral suture lines. Mustarde used the same flap but differed in that he used the perimeatal flap to form the whole neourethra, not just the ventral surface. This bore the advantage of having a single suture line deep to the urethra. Barcat modified the Mathieu technique by mobilising the urethral plate and making a midline incision to push the neourethra deeper between the corpora. The goal was always advancement of the neourethra to the glans tip. Stenosis and fistula were frequently the price. Fevre (1961) used a longer meatal-based flap and folded it between the glanular wings. Mustarde (1965) included a V incision at the glans to achieve a wider meatus. Hadidi (1996) included a Y incision at the tip of the glans closed as a V. He also excised a V from the distal end of the flap to yield a terminal wide slit-like meatus (Fig. 2.8).

30   Ahmed T. Hadidi

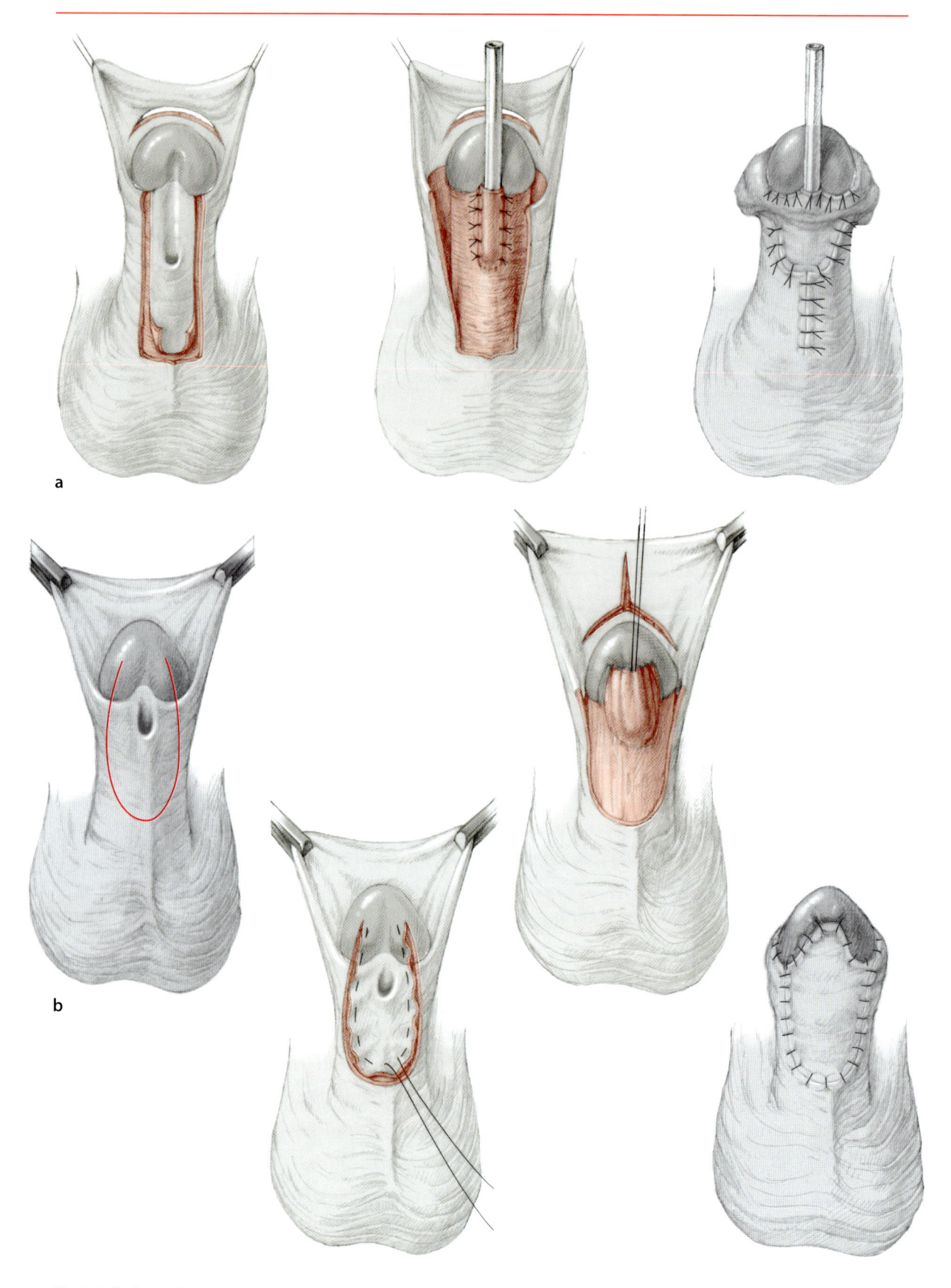

Fig. 2.8a, b. Legend see p. 31

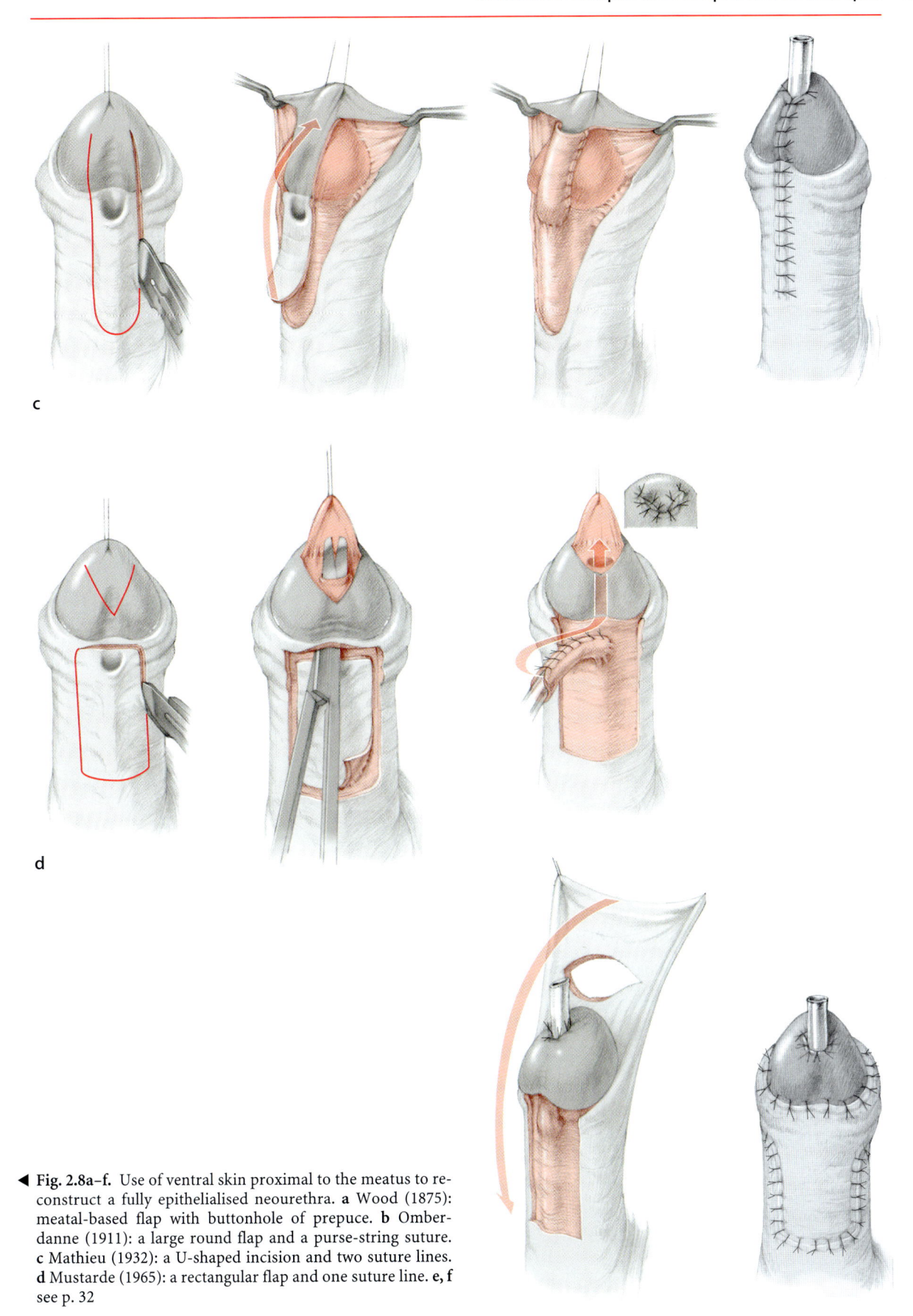

Fig. 2.8a–f. Use of ventral skin proximal to the meatus to reconstruct a fully epithelialised neourethra. **a** Wood (1875): meatal-based flap with buttonhole of prepuce. **b** Omberdanne (1911): a large round flap and a purse-string suture. **c** Mathieu (1932): a U-shaped incision and two suture lines. **d** Mustarde (1965): a rectangular flap and one suture line. **e, f** see p. 32

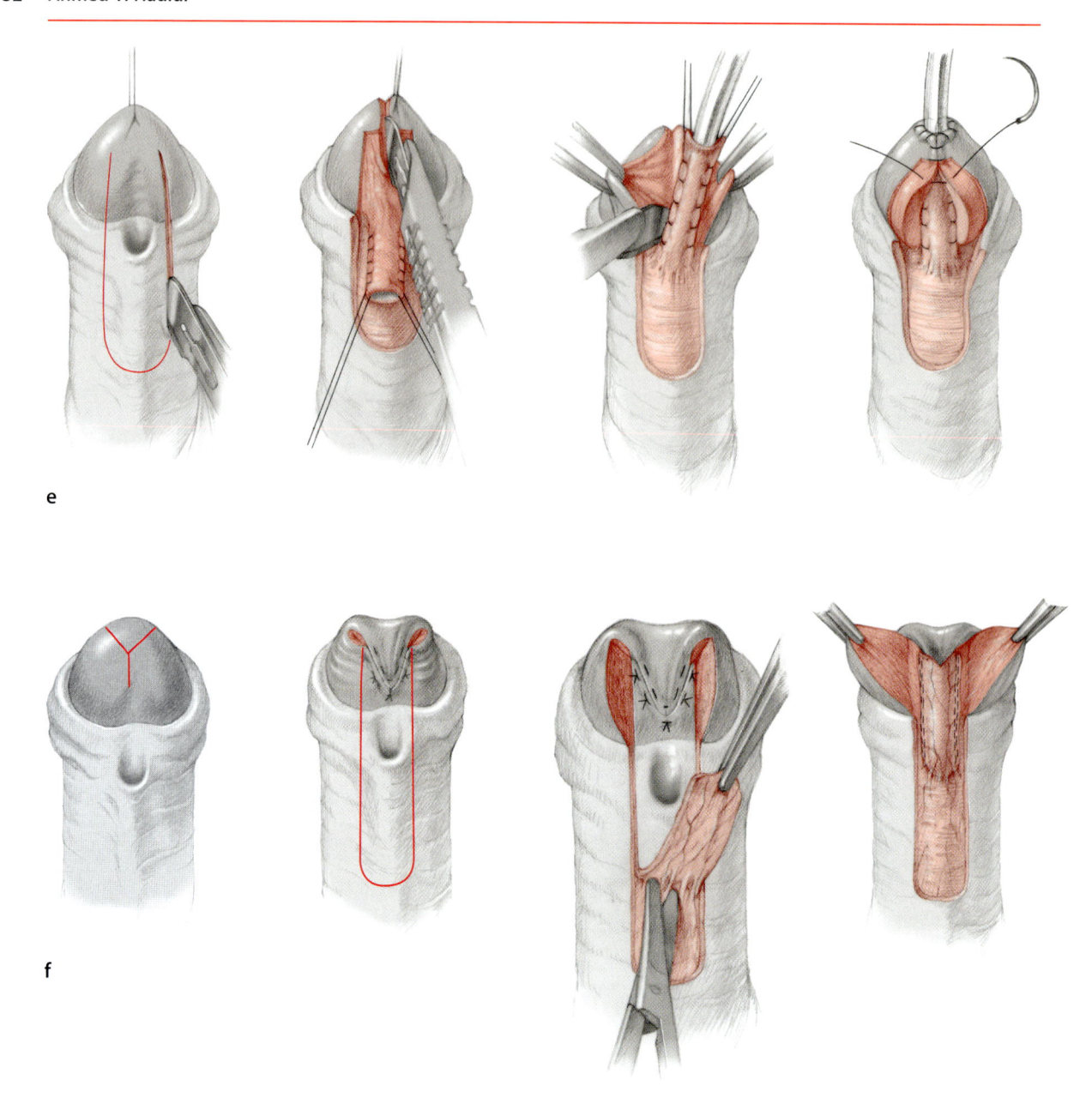

Fig. 2.8 (*continued*). **e** Barcat (1969): balanic groove technique and a deep midline incision. **f** Hadidi (1996): Y-V glanuloplasty, modified Mathieu – a Y incision in the glans, the centre at the tip of glans, closed as a V and dog-ears opened. A small V is excised from the distal end of the flap

Use of Preputial Skin

The preputial skin plays a very important role in the management of hypospadias (Fig. 2.9). It may be used in eight different ways;

1. The preputial skin may be mobilised ventrally to cover skin and fascial defects following excision of chordee in two-stage repair. Thiersch (1869) did the first buttonhole flap in the prepuce to allow resurfacing of the penis with the prepuce.
2. The preputial skin may be divided in the midline to form two flaps to cover the skin deficiency of the penis after chordee resection and after urethroplasty. This was described by Edmonds (1913) and popularised by Byars (1955).
3. The preputial skin may be used as a free skin graft to cover ventral defect after excision of ventral chordee as the first stage of two-stage repair. This was first described by Nové-Josserand in 1897 and popularised by Bracka (1995a, b).
4. The preputial skin may be used as a free skin graft to form the neourethra in single-stage urethroplasty as first described by Devine and Horton in 1961.
5. The preputial skin may be used as a pedicled flap for reconstruction of the neourethral tube. This may be vertical as described by Van Hook (1896), Toksu (1970) and Hodgson (1970) or horizontal and double-faced as described by Asopa et al. (1971). Duckett (1980a) adopted this technique using the inner face of the prepuce in a horizontal manner now known as the tubularised preputial island flap technique (TPIF). Standoli (1982) described the same technique but used the outer face of the prepuce.
6. The preputial skin may be used as a pedicled flap to form the ventral wall of the neourethra (not the whole neourethra), as described by Elder et al. in the technique known as onlay island flap (OIF) in 1987.
7. The preputial vascular fascia without skin may be used as a protective second layer to protect urethroplasty in the same way as after Mathieu and Snodgrass procedures, as first described by Retik et al. in 1988.
8. The preputial skin may be used in continuation with a parameatal skin flap as in Koyanagi et al. (1983), yoke repair (Snow 1994) and along with its fascia in the lateral-based flap technique (Hadidi 2003).

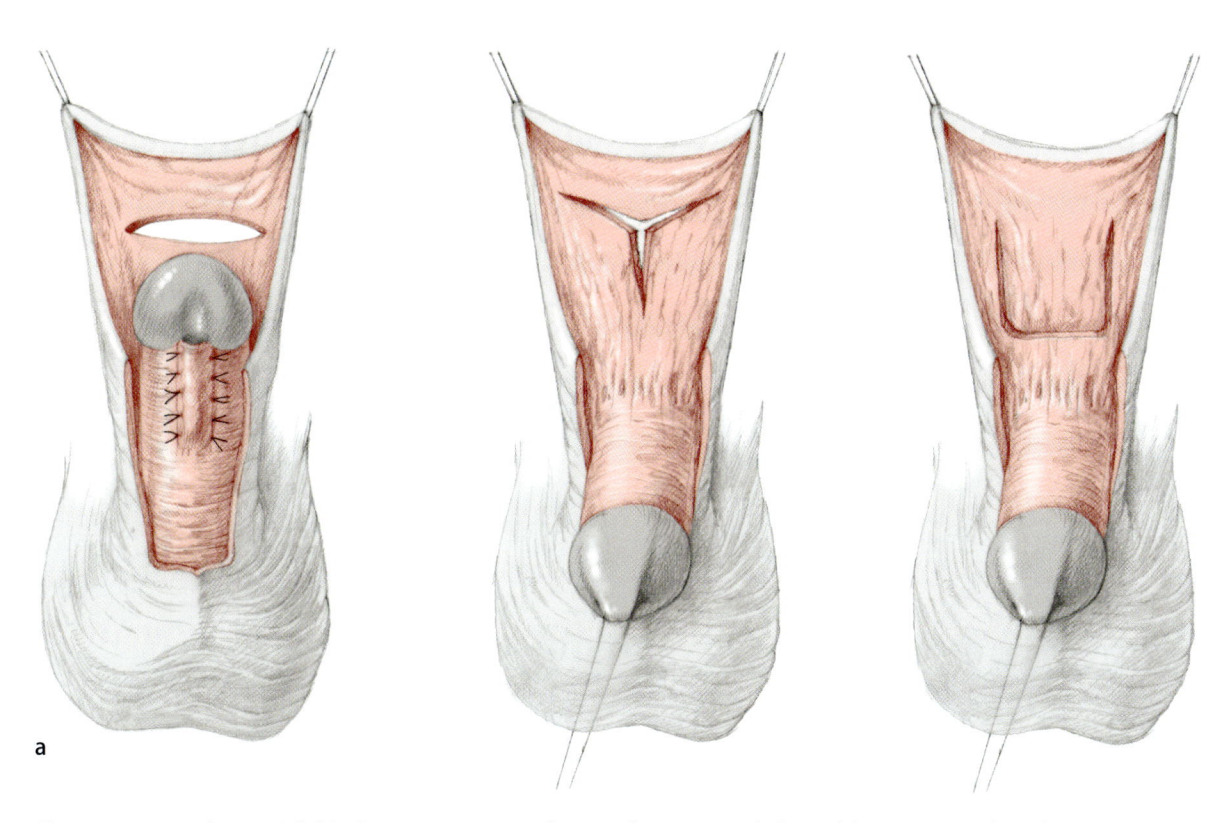

Fig. 2.9a–g. Use of preputial skin for reconstruction of neourethra. **a** Buttonholing of the prepuce as described by Thiersch (1869). **b-g** see pp. 34-36

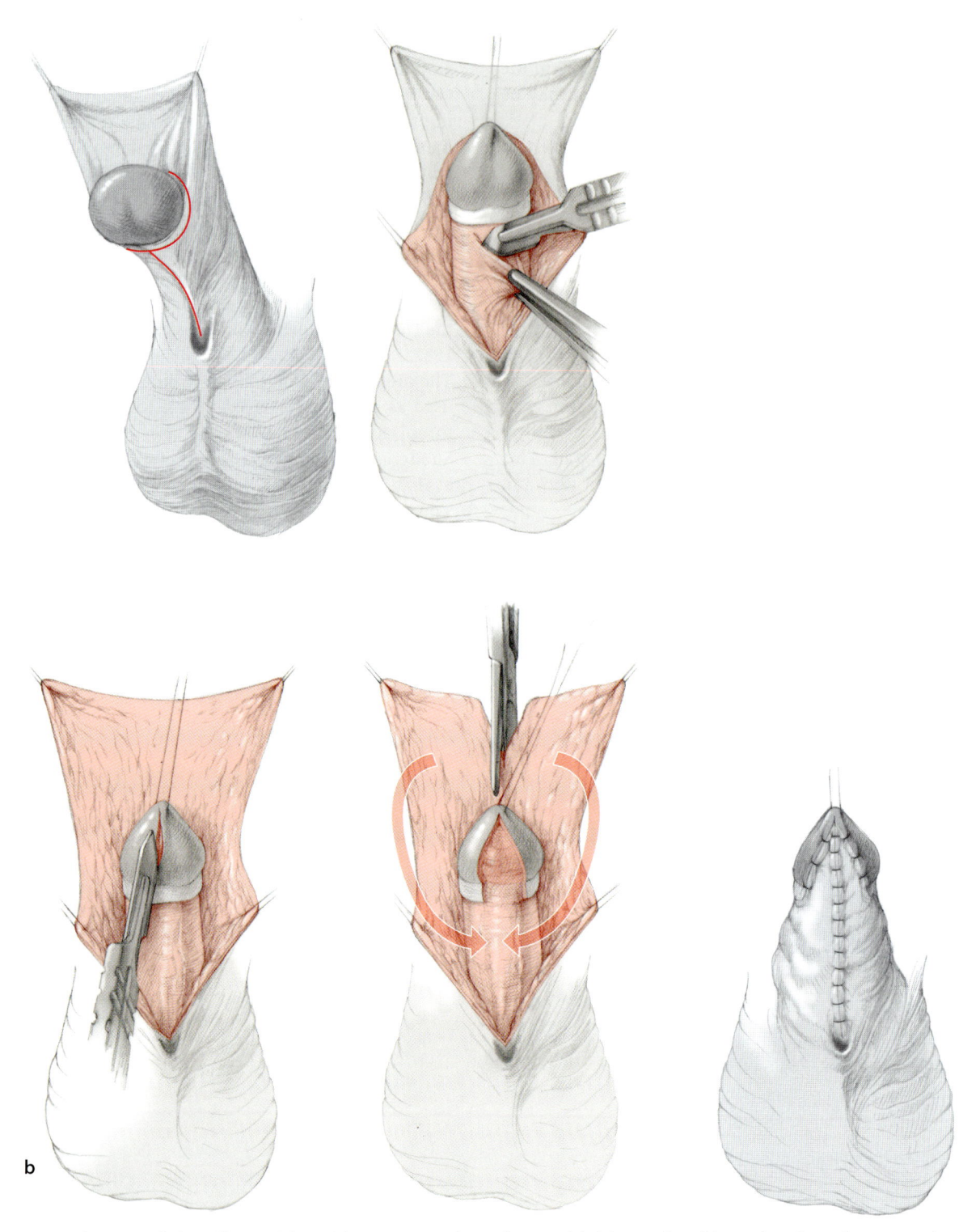

Fig. 2.9 (*continued*). **b** Midline incision of the prepuce as described by Edmunds (1913) and Byars (1955). **c** Preputial skin as a skin graft to cover the ventral defect of the penis as described by Nové-Josserand (1897) and Bracka (1995). **d** Preputial skin as a free skin graft to form the neo-urethra as described by Devine and Horton (1961). **e** Preputial island flap as described by Hook (1896), Toksu (1970), Hodgson (1970), Asopa and Duckett et al. (1980). **f, g** see p. 36

Fig. 2.9c–e. Legend see p.34

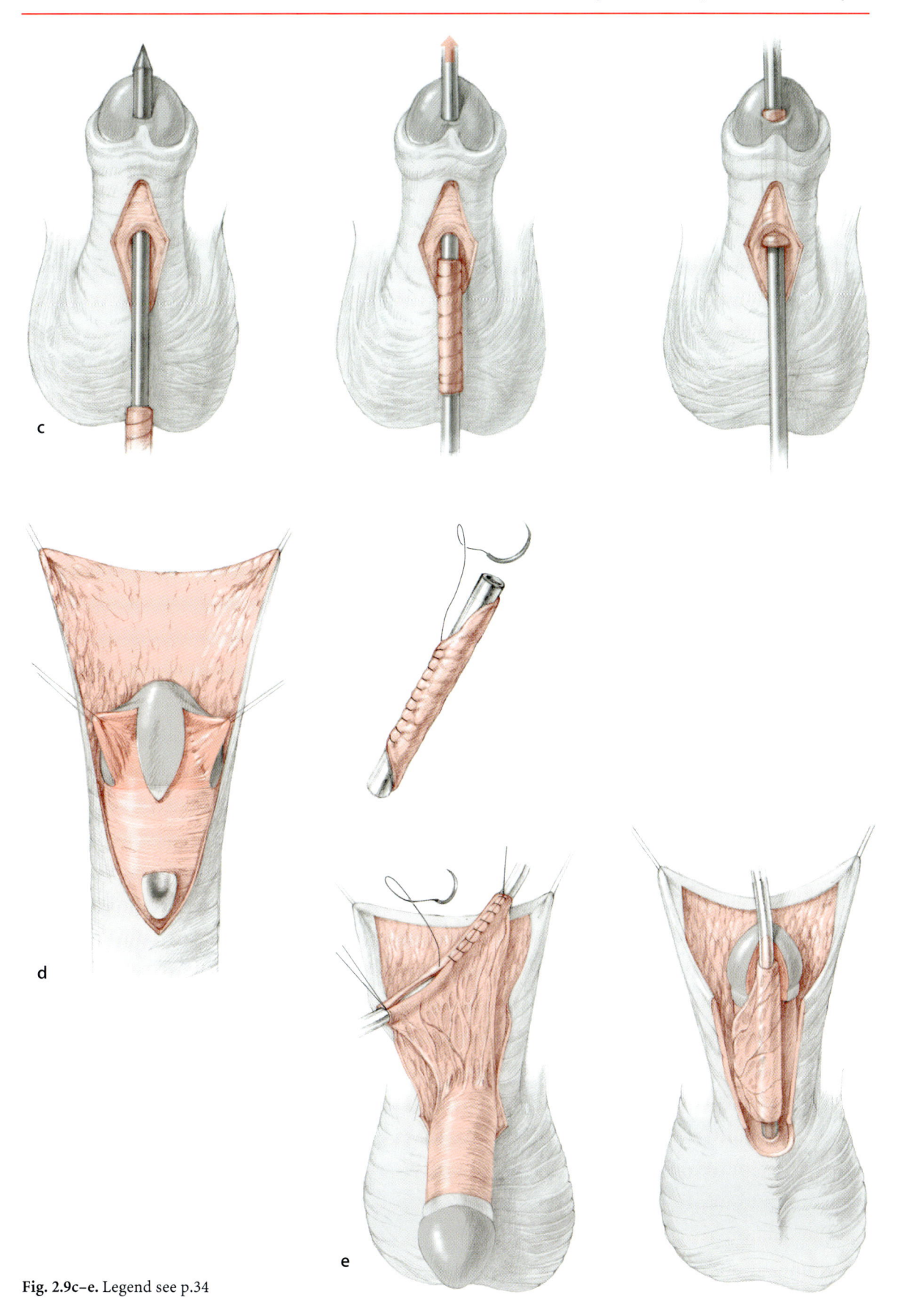

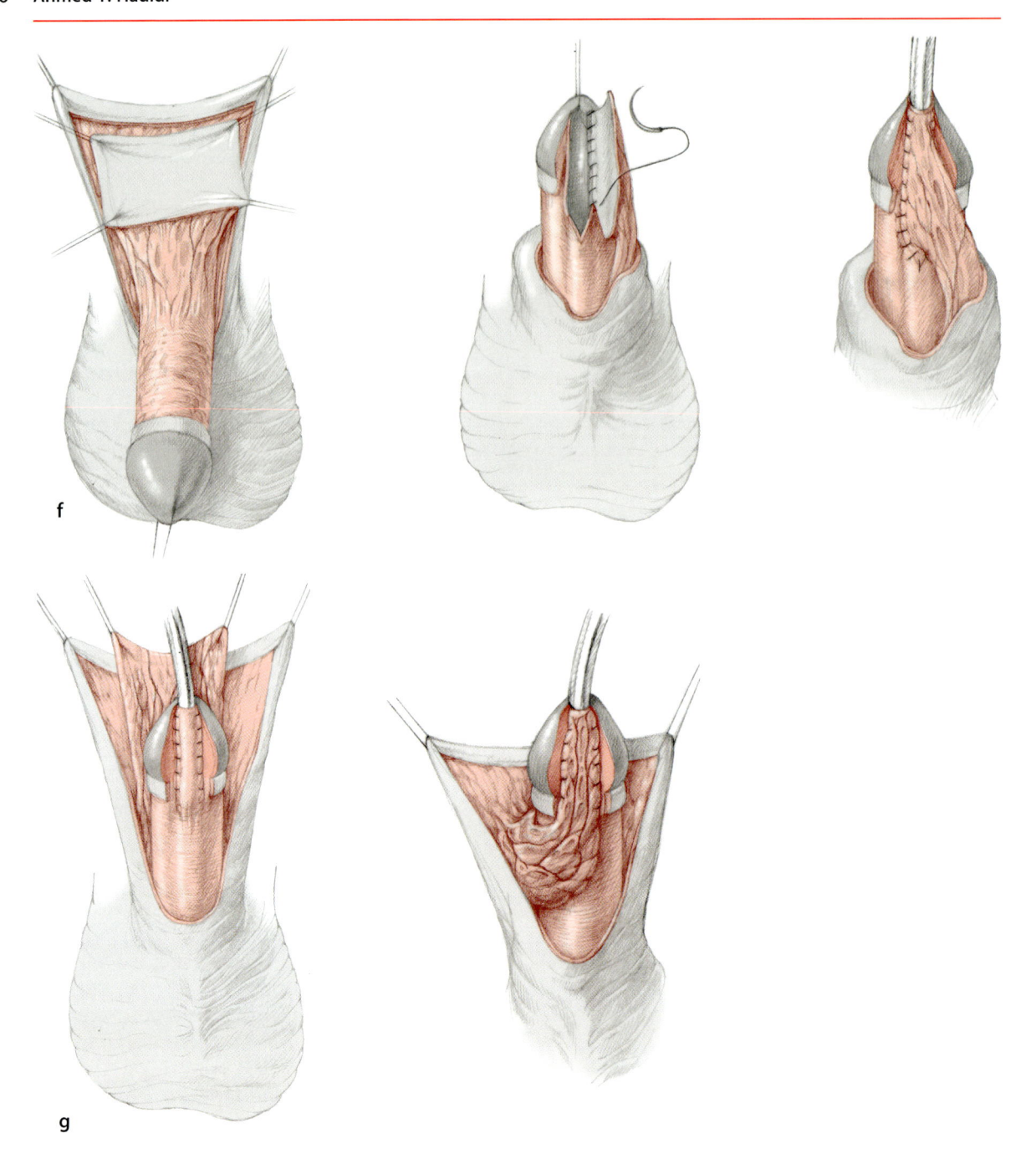

Fig. 2.9 (*continued*). **f** Onlay island flap as described by Elder et al. (1987). **g** Preputial vascular fascia as a second protective layer as described by Retik et al. (1988)

Combined Use of Prepuce and Skin Proximal to the Meatus

In proximal hypospadias, one needs to reconstruct a long neourethra. Another principle employs the combined use of parameatal skin and the prepuce. This was first suggested by van Hook (1896). Many authors, including Broadbent et al. (1961), DesPrez et al. (1961), Hinderer (1978), Koyanagi et al. (1983), Snow (1994) and Hadidi (2003), have described techniques using the same principle.

Van Hook (1896) suggested the use of a" lateral oblique flap" from the side of the penis. Broadbent et al. (1961), DesPrez et al. (1961) and Hinderer (1968) adopted the same principle and described a flap extending obliquely from the parameatal skin into the prepuce. Koyanagi et al. (1983) modified the technique by using two lateral flaps (from both sides). Snows (1994) described the yoke technique, which differed from Koyanagi in buttonholing the prepuce. Hadidi (2003) described the lateral-based flap technique using the same principle and combined it with Y-V glanuloplasty. The technique entails adequate mobilisation of the preputial vascular fascia with the flap. The lateral-based flap enjoys a double blood supply from the meatal base and the preputial vessels. The Y helps to bring the meatus to the tip, and the V excised from the tube helps to achieve a terminal slit-like meatus (Fig. 2.10).

Use of Scrotum

The scrotum may be used in four different ways in hypospadias reconstruction (Fig. 2.11):
1. The scrotal skin may be used to form a completely epithelialised neourethra. Bouisson (1861) was apparently the first to report the use of scrotal tissue to reconstruct the ventral wall of the neourethra. Rochet (1899) used a large scrotal flap for urethroplasty. This flap was buried in a tunnel on the ventral surface of the penis. Lowsley and Begg (1938) constructed the neourethra completely from the scrotum. This method fell into disuse because of the problem of hair growth into the neourethra.
2. The scrotal skin may be used to cover the neourethra. This was described by Beck in 1897.
3. The scrotal skin may be used to reconstruct the neourethra and at the same time the scrotum is used to protect the neourethra until healing is complete. Rosenberger (1891), Landerer (1891), Bidder (1892), used scrotal skin for urethroplasty. They described for the first time burying of the penis in the scrotum to obtain skin coverage. This was modified by Bucknall (1907).
4. The scrotum may be used as a bed for the neourethra, a technique that was popularised by Cecil (1946) and Culp in 1966.

Use of Dorsal Penile Skin

Davis, in 1940, tubed the dorsal penile skin with the base proximal in the direction of the circulation (Fig. 2.12). The detached distal end of this tube was passed through a channel in the glans and penis by angulating the penis acutely upward and backward. In the second stage, the proximal pedicle was cut and the penis returned to its normal position. The penile gymnastics required for the Davis procedure apparently seemed too demanding for most surgeons.

38   Ahmed T. Hadidi

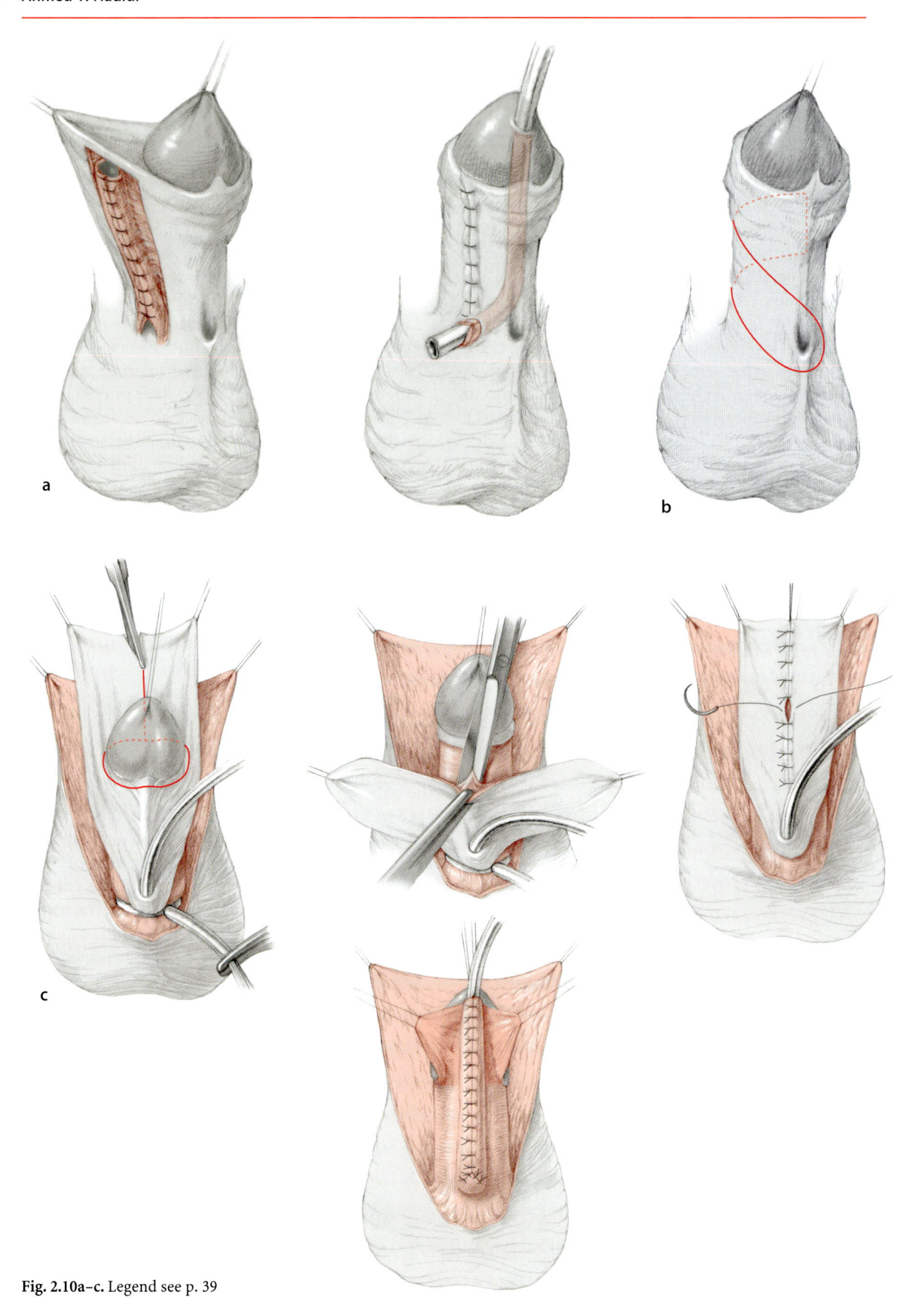

Fig. 2.10a–c. Legend see p. 39

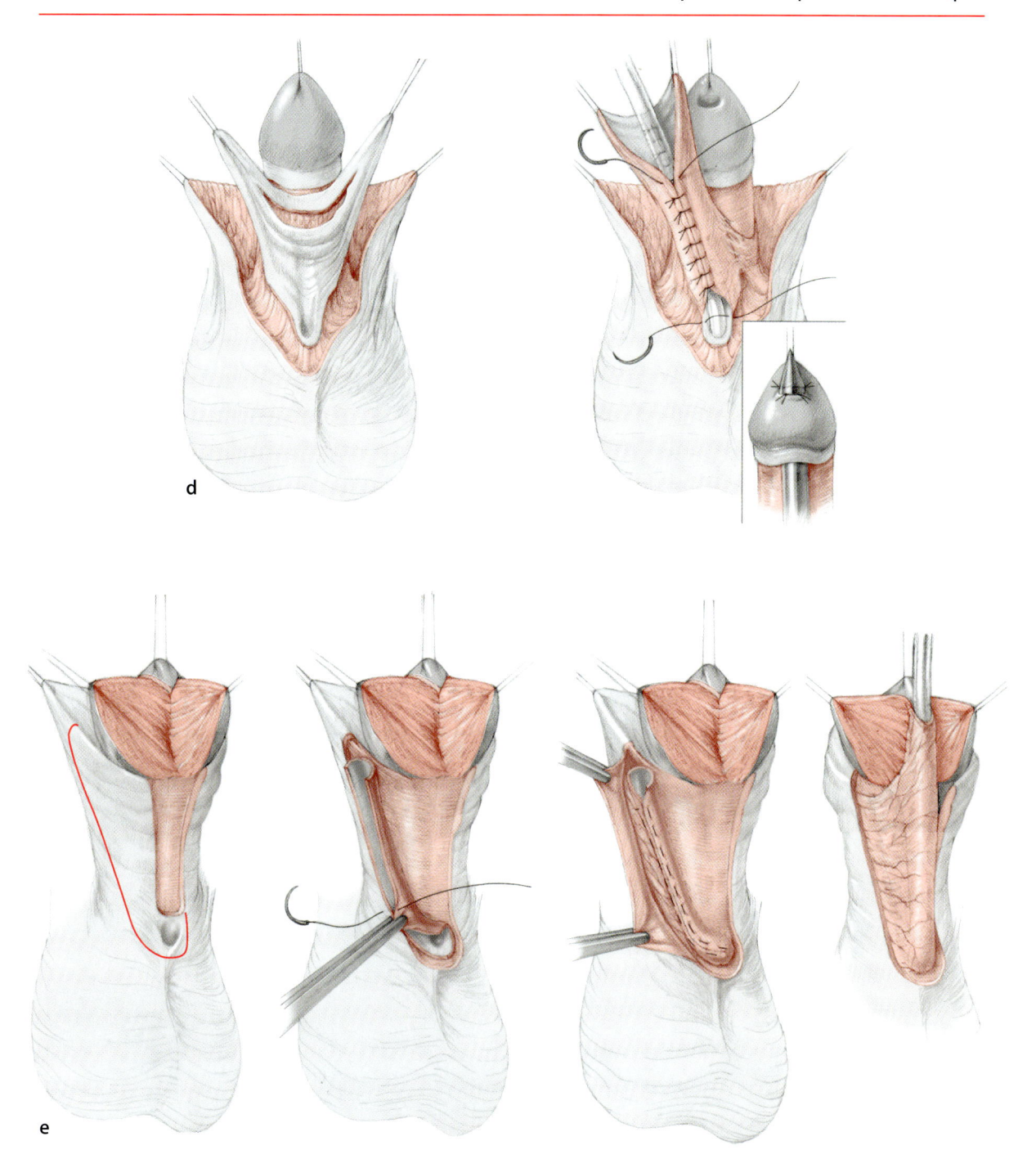

Fig. 2.10a–e. Combined use of prepuce and the skin proximal to the meatus. **a** Lateral oblique flap from the side of the penis suggested by Hook (1896). **b** One-stage repair for proximal hypospadias described by Broadbent et al. (1961). **c** Parameatal foreskin flap described by Koyanagi et al. (1983). **d** Yoke repair described by Snow (1994). **e** Lateral based flap combined with Y-V glanuloplasty described by Hadidi (2003)

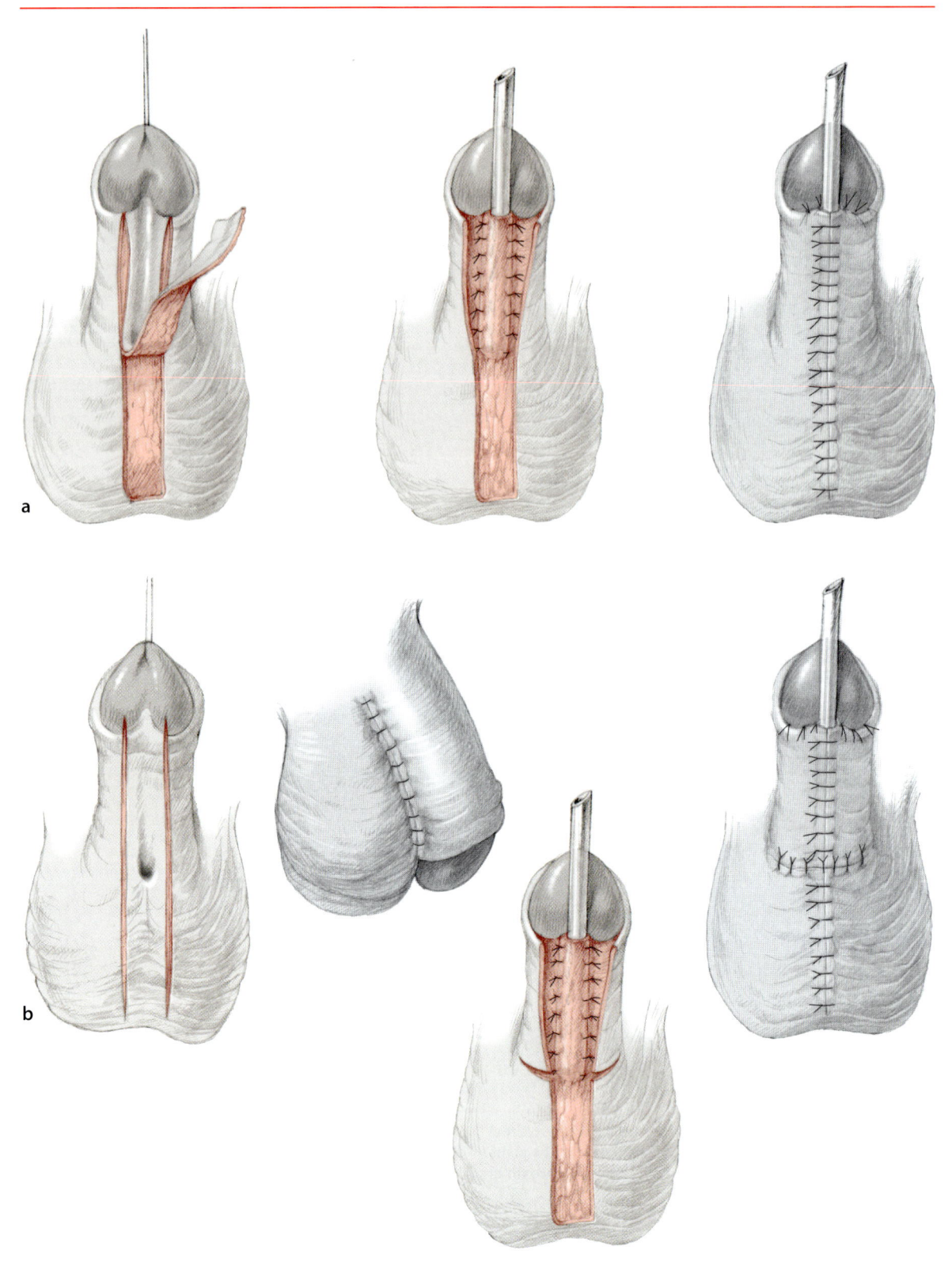

Fig. 2.11a–f. Use of scrotum in hypospadias repair. **a** Bouisson (1861) was the first to use scrotal skin for urethral reconstruction. **b** Rosenberger (1891) used scrotal tissue for urethroplasty and buried the penis in the scrotum. **c–f** see pp. 41, 42

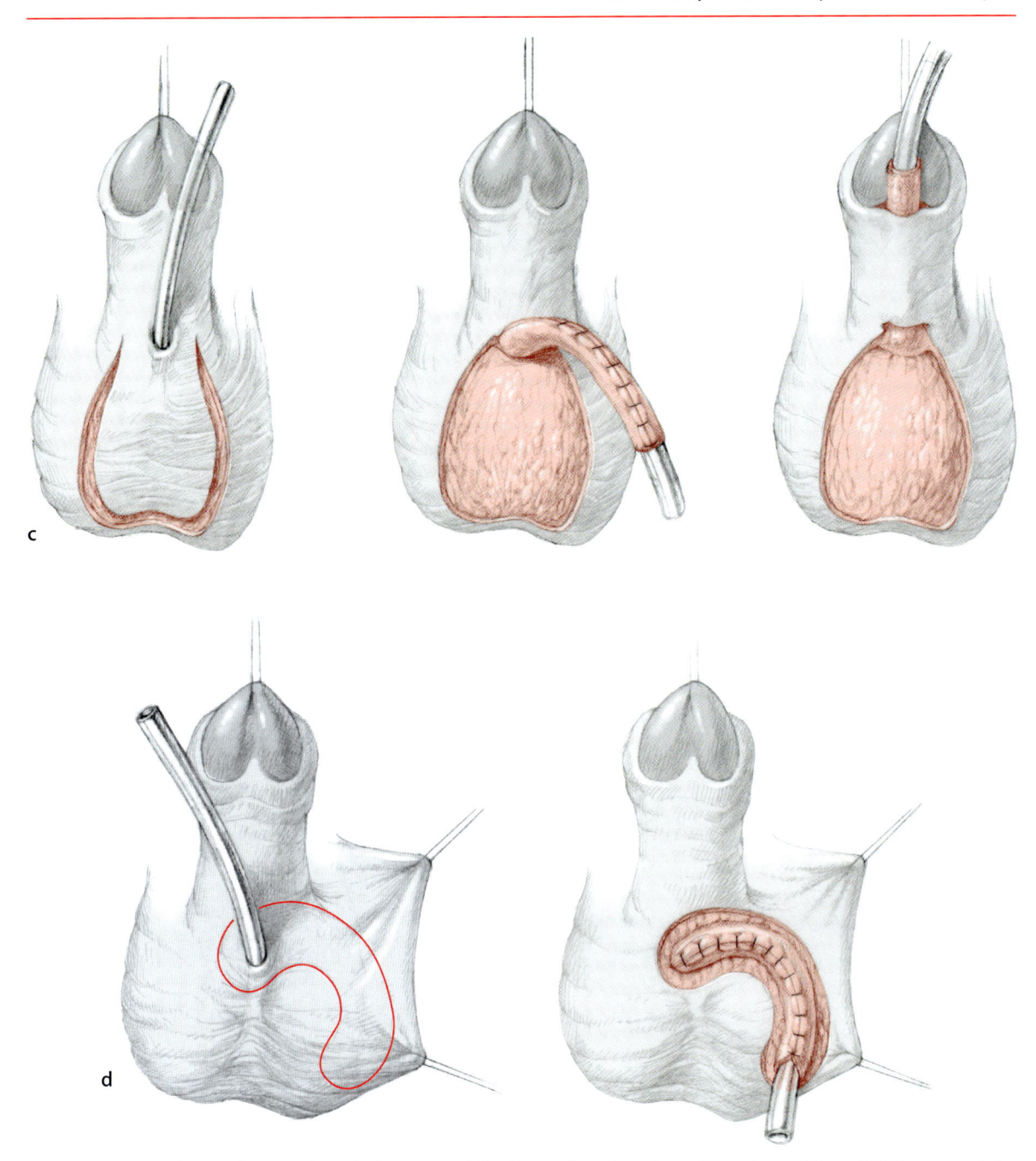

Fig. 2.11 (*continued*). **c** Rochet (1899) used a large scrotal flap for total urethroplasty. **d** Lowsley and Begg (1938) constructed a long urethral tube from scrotum. **e, f** see p. 42

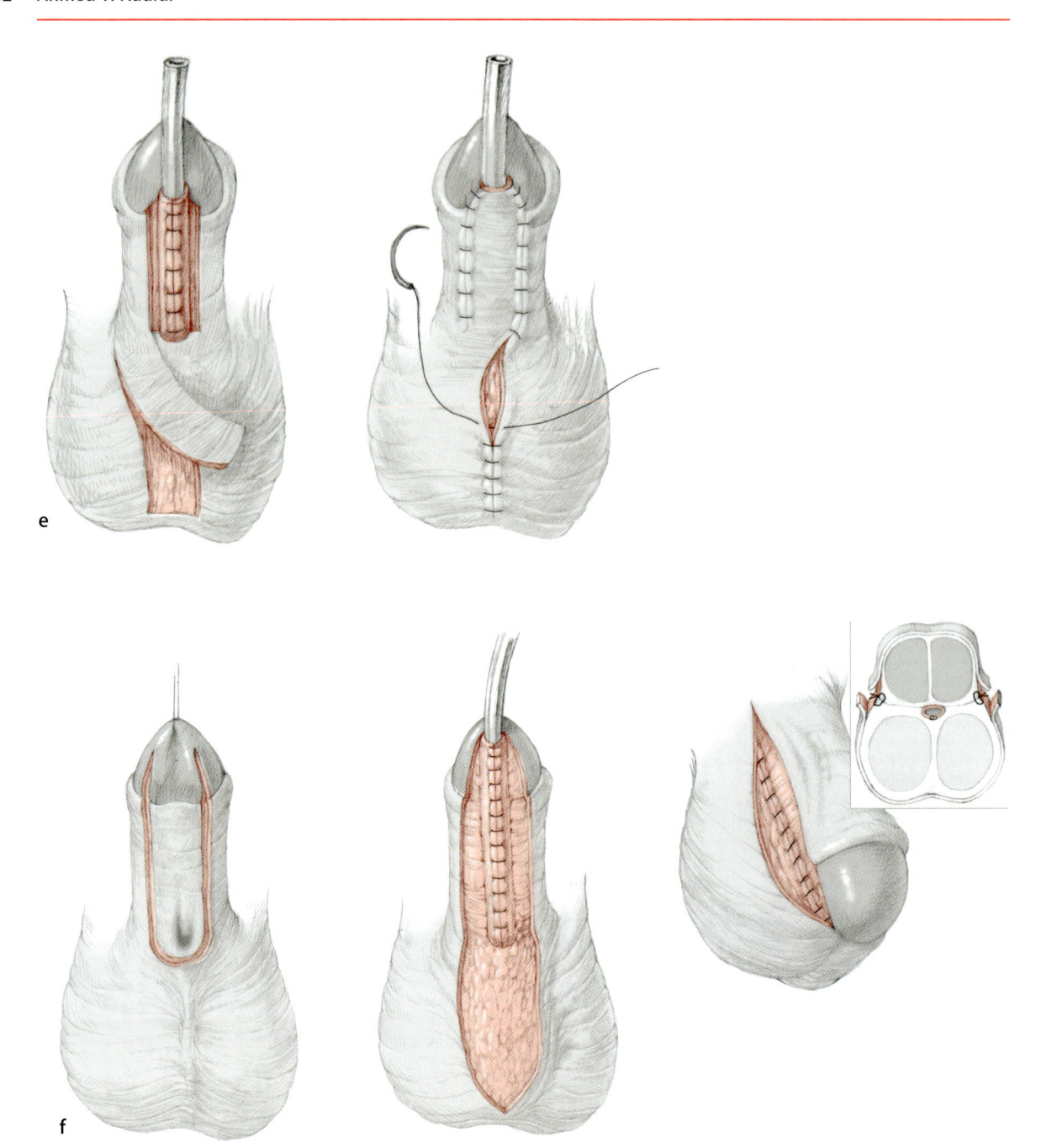

Fig. 2.11 (*continued*). **e** Beck (1897) suggested the Duplay type of urethroplasty and used a rotation flap from the scrotum for coverage. **f** Cecil (1946) used a modification of the Rosenberger operation following reconstruction of the urethra from ventral penile skin

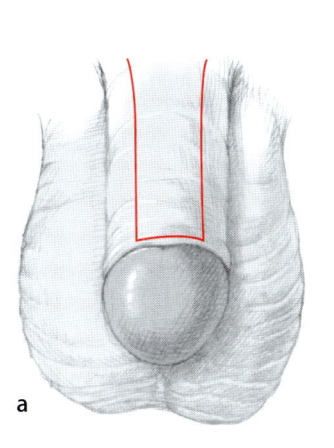

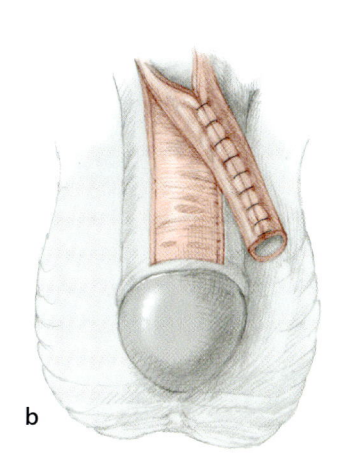

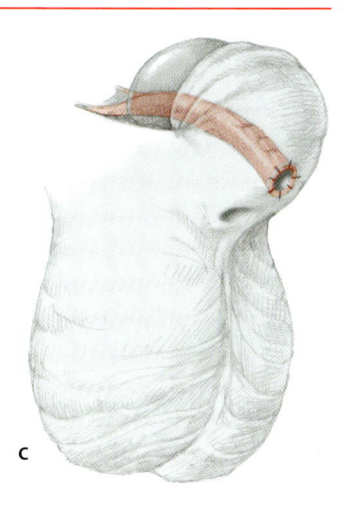

Fig. 2.12a–c. Davis operation (1940) using a dorsal tube pedicle flap to construct the neourethra

Use of Grafts

Nové-Josserand in 1897 started another school of urethroplasty which utilised the free inlay graft. He used a thin split-thickness free graft and applied the raw surface outward around a metal probe. Young and Benjamin (1948) used a split-thickness skin graft from the medial aspect of the upper arm. From 1909 to 1927 a whole series of homograft including vein, urethra, and appendix were attempted but never with any consistent success. Bracka (1995) used full-thickness skin graft from the prepuce. Memmelaar, in 1947, was the first to advocate the use of bladder mucosa. Although Humby (1941) first proposed and reported the use of buccal mucosa for hypospadias repair, Duckett in 1986 promoted the technique and is credited for the current enthusiasm and widespread acceptance of its use in complex hypospadias repairs (👁 Fig. 2.13).

Use of a Protective Intermediate Layer

Durham Smith (1973) was the first to describe the use of an intermediate or interposition layer between the neourethra and the cutaneous suture. Types of interposition waterproofing layer include Smith's (1973) de-epithelialised skin, Snow's (1986) tunica vaginalis wrap from the testicular coverings, Retik et al.'s (1988) dorsal subcutaneous flap from the foreskin, Motiwala's (1993) dartos flap from the scrotum and Yamataka et al.'s (1998) external spermatic fascia flap (👁 Fig. 2.14).

Abnormal Looking Glans Penis and Glanuloplasty and Meatoplasty

Thus, various tubes and patches were available to reconstruct the neourethra. The step was to bring the neourethra to the tip of the glans. The glans had always posed a challenge and had largely not been found amenable to tunnelling. Canalisation, tunnelling, and coring are essentially the same, with progressively larger channels. These are a testimony to glans stenosis.

There are several techniques employed to achieve an apical meatus (👁 Fig. 2.15):
a) Russell (1900) described the glans channel technique to deliver the urethra to the apex of the glans. Bevan (1917), Davis (1940), Ricketson (1958), Duckett (1980b) and Hendren (1981) used the same principle but different flaps or grafts.
b) Wing rotation is used in most recent techniques.
c) Devine and Horton (1961) and Mustarde (1965) popularised the glans channel procedure and included a dorsal V-flap with the glans channel.
d) The glans split has been used in various techniques to move the meatus to the apex (Beck 1917; Humby 1941; Barcat 1973; Mays 1951; Cronin and Guthrie 1973; Turner-Warwick 1979).
e) Duckett, in 1981, described the "meatal advancement and glanuloplasty incorporated" (MAGPI) procedure. Arap et al. (1984) modified the MAGPI technique by using two sutures instead of one. Decter, in 1991, described an "M inverted V" technique.
f) Rich et al. (1989) described incising the urethral plate in the midline (hinging). This helped to achieve a slit-like vertical meatus.

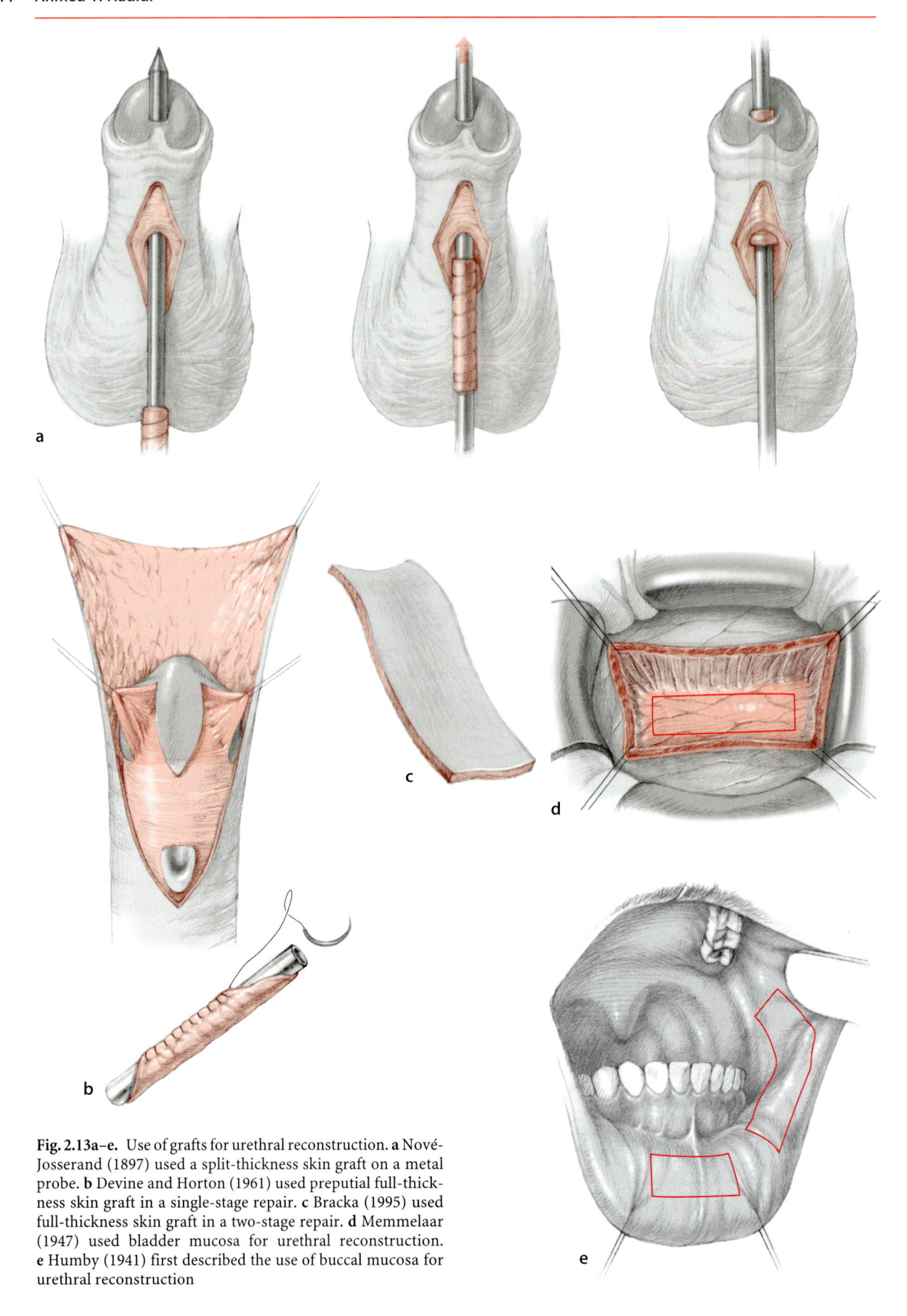

Fig. 2.13a–e. Use of grafts for urethral reconstruction. **a** Nové-Josserand (1897) used a split-thickness skin graft on a metal probe. **b** Devine and Horton (1961) used preputial full-thickness skin graft in a single-stage repair. **c** Bracka (1995) used full-thickness skin graft in a two-stage repair. **d** Memmelaar (1947) used bladder mucosa for urethral reconstruction. **e** Humby (1941) first described the use of buccal mucosa for urethral reconstruction

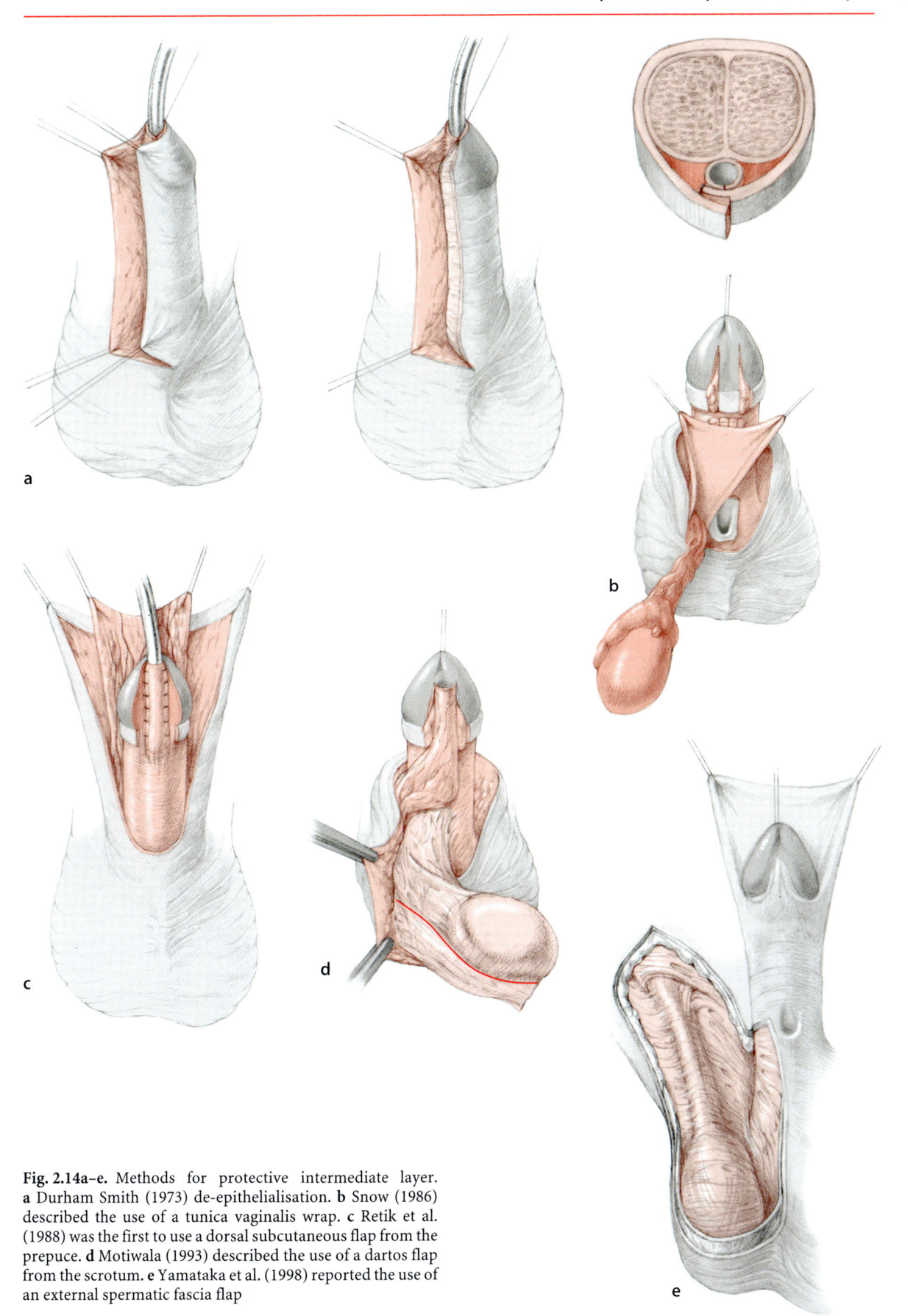

Fig. 2.14a–e. Methods for protective intermediate layer. **a** Durham Smith (1973) de-epithelialisation. **b** Snow (1986) described the use of a tunica vaginalis wrap. **c** Retik et al. (1988) was the first to use a dorsal subcutaneous flap from the prepuce. **d** Motiwala (1993) described the use of a dartos flap from the scrotum. **e** Yamataka et al. (1998) reported the use of an external spermatic fascia flap

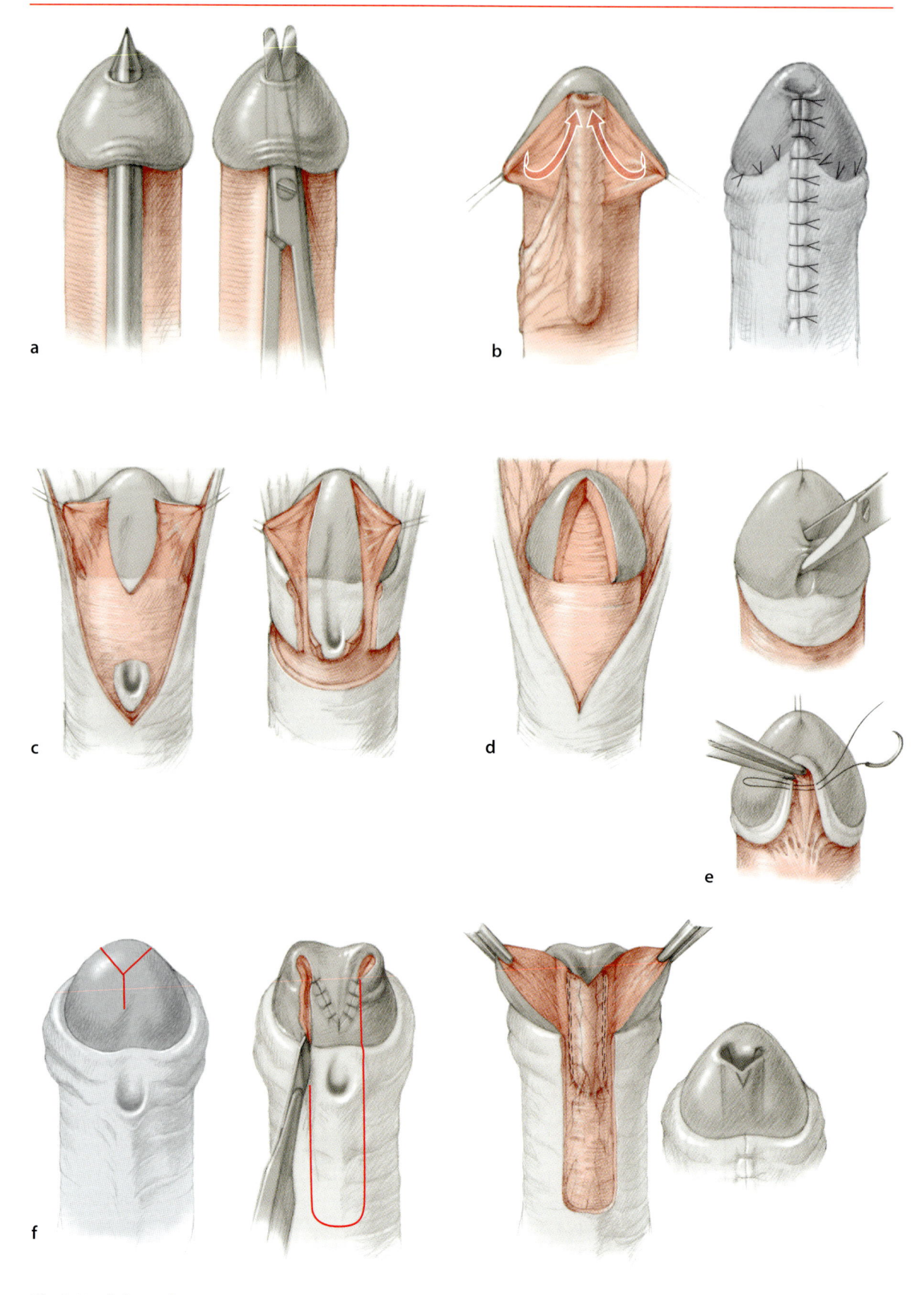

Fig. 2.15a–f. Legend see p.47

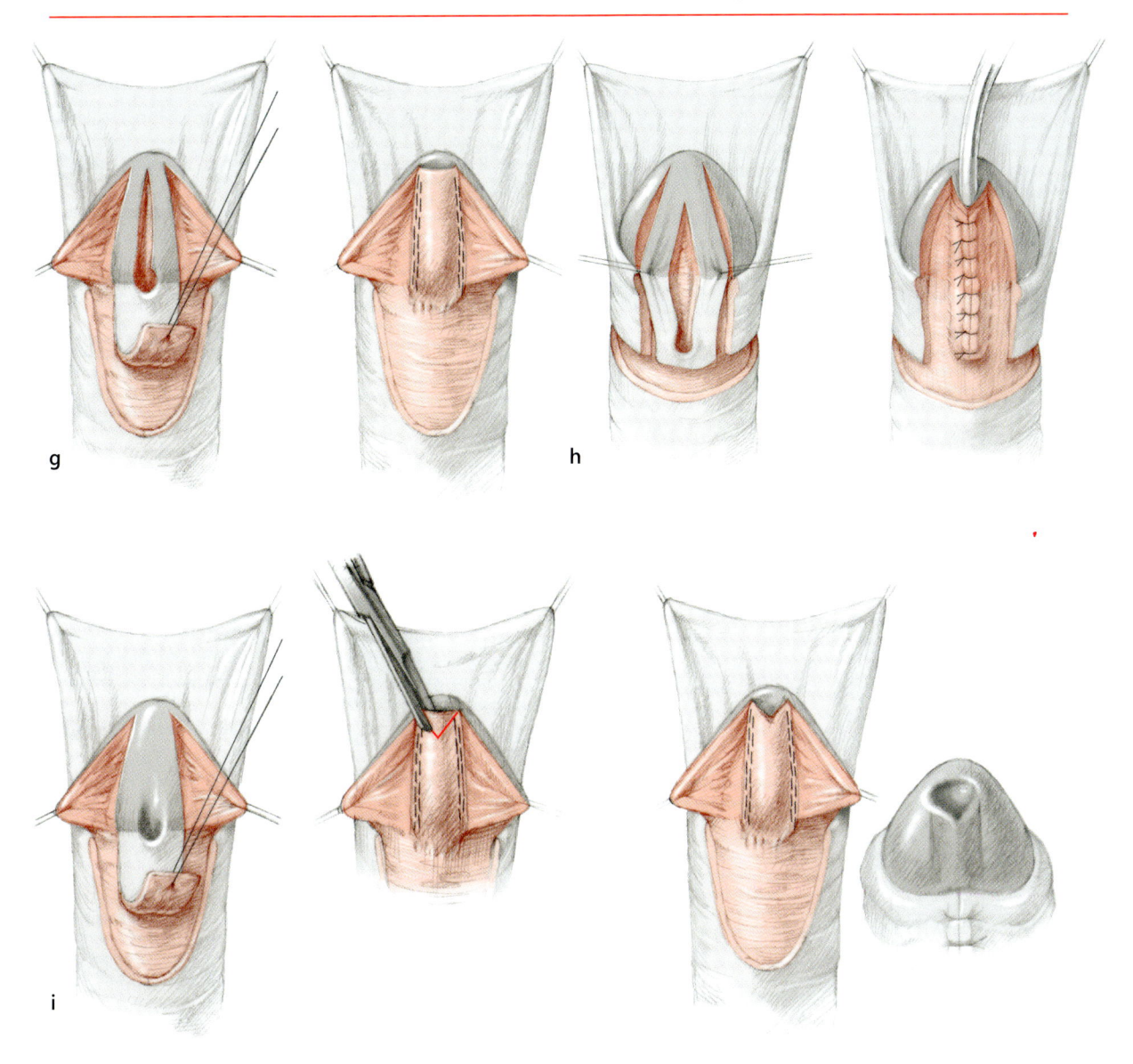

◄ **Fig. 2.15a–i.** Techniques of glanuloplasty. **a** Glans tunnelling, canalisation or coring. **b** Wing rotation. **c** Glans V in the posterior wall by Devine and Horton (1961), Mustarde (1965). **d** Glans splitting or kippering has been used for 1000 years. **e** MAGPI (Duckett 1981b). **f** Y-V glanuloplasty (Hadidi 1996). **g** Hinging of the urethral plate (Rich et al. 1989). **h** The tubularised incised plate (Snodgrass 1994) follows the same principle. **i** MAVIS (Boddy and Samuel 2000) a modification of the Mathieu technique, excises a triangle from the apex of the parameatal flap to create a slit-like meatus

g) Snodgrass (1994) extended the concept of urethral plate hinging by incising the whole urethral plate in the midline from the hypospadiac meatus distally. This helps in tabularisation of the plate.
h) Hadidi, in 1996, described the Y-V glanuloplasty. The centre of the Y is at the tip of the glans. Each limb is 0.5 cm long and the deep incision is closed as a V. The dog-ears created are widely opened to increase the circumference. A V is excised from the distal end of the neourethra to achieve a slit-like meatus. The Y-V glanuloplasty can be combined with most techniques of hypospadias repair, e.g. Mathieu, Onlay, Duplay, transverse preputial island flap urethroplasty and lateral-based flap.
i) Boddy and Samuel (2000), described the "Mathieu and V incision sutured" (MAVIS) technique, which results in a vertical slit meatus. In this technique a V incision is made and excised at the apex of the parameatal-based flap. Then each side of the V is sutured to the glanular wings.

References

Anger T: Hypospadias. Bull Soc Chir Paris. p. 32.

Anger MT: Hypospadias peno-scrotal, complique de coudure de la verge: redressement du penis et urethro-plastie par inclusion cutanee: guerison. Bull Soc Chir Paris. 1875; p 179.

Arap S, Mitre AI, DeGores GM: Modified meatal advancement and glanduloplasty repair of distal hypospadias. J Urol. 1984; 131:1140.

Asopa HS, Elhence EP, Atria SP, et al: One-stage correction of penile hypospadias using a foreskin tube. A preliminary report. Int Surg. 1971; 55:435.

Backus LH, de Felice CA: Hypospadias – then and now. Plast Reconstr Surg. 1960; 25:146

Barcat J: Symposium sur l'hypospadias. 16th meeting of the French Society of Children's Surgery. Ann Chir Infant. 1969; 10:287

Barcat J: Current concepts of treatment. In: Horton CE (ed): Plastic and reconstructive surgery of the genital area. Little Brown, Boston, pp 249–263; 1973.

Beck 1897: Cited by Horton CE, Devine CJ, Baran N: Pictorial history of hypospadias repair techniques. In: Horton CE (ed): Plastic and reconstructive surgery of the genital area. Little Brown, Boston, pp 237–248; 1973

Beck C: Hypospadias and its treatment. Surg Gynecol Obstet. 1917; 24:511.

Belman AB: Urethroplasty. Soc Pediatr Urol Newslett. December 1977; 1–2.

Bevan AD: A new operation for hypospadias. JAMA. 1917; 68:1032.

Bidder A: Eine Operation der Hypospadie mit Lappenbildung aus dem Scrotum. Dtsch Med Wochenschr. 1892; 10:208.

Boddy SA, Samuel M: A natural glanular meatus after "Mathieu and V incision sutured" MAVIS. BJU Int. 2000; 86:394–397.

Bouiisson MF: De l'Hypospadias et de son traitement chirurgical. Trib Chir. 1861; 2:484.

Bracka A: A versatile two-stage hypospadias repair. Br J Plast Surg. 1995a; 48:345–352.

Bracka A: Hypospadias repair: the two-stage alternative. Br J Urol. 1995b; 76 [Suppl 3]:31–41.

Broadbent TR, Woolf RM, Toksu E: Hypospadias: one-stage repair. Plast Reconstr Surg. 1961; 27:154.

Browne D: An operation for hypospadias. Proc R Soc Med. 1949; 41:466–468.

Bucknall RTH: A new operation for penile hypospadias. Lancet 1907; 2:887

Bussemaker UC, Daremberg CV: Oeuvres d'Oribase, texte Gre, en grande partie inedit collationnée sur les manuscrits (6 vols). Imprimerie National, Paris. p. 1851–1876.

Byars LT: Technique of consistently satisfactory repair of hypospadias. Surg Gynecol Obstet. 1955; 100:184.

Cecil AB: Repair of hypospadias and urethral fistula. J Urol. 1946; 56:237–242.

Cecil AB: Modern treatment of hypospadias. J Urol. 1952; 67:1006.

Cronin TD, Guthrie TH: Method of Cronin and Guthrie for hypospadias repair. In: Horton CE (ed): Plastic and reconstructive surgery of the genital area. Little Brown, Boston, pp 302–314; 1973.

Culp OS: Struggles and triumphs with hypospadias and associated anomalies. Review of 400 cases. J Urol. 1966; 96: 339–355.

Davis DM: The pedicle tube graft in the surgical treatment of hypospadias in the male. Surg Gynecol Obstet. 1940; 71: 790.

Decter RM: M inverted V glansplasty: a procedure for distal hypospadias. J Urol. 1991; 146:641

Decter RM: Chordee correction by corporal rotation, the split and roll technique. J Urol. 1999; 162:1152–1154

Des Prez JD, Persky L, Kiehn C: A one-stage repair of hypospadias by island-flap technique. Plast Reconstr Surg. 1961; 28:405.

De Sy WA, Oosterlinck W: Silicone foam elastomer: significant improvement in postoperative penile dressing. J Urol. 1982; 128:39–41.

Devine CJ Jr, Horton CE: A one-stage hypospadias repair. J Urol. 1961; 85:166.

Dieffenbach JF: Guérison des fentes congénitales de la verge, de l'hypospadias. Gaz Hebd Med. 1837; 5:156.

Duckett JW: Transverse preputial island-flap technique for repair of severe hypospadias. Urol Clin North Am. 1980a; 7:423.

Duckett JW: Hypospadias. Clin Plast Surg. 1980b; 7:149.

Duckett JW: Repair of hypospadias. In: Hendry WF (ed): Recent advances in urology/andrology, vol 3. Churchill-Livingstone, New York, pp 279–290; 1980c.

Duckett JW: The island-flap technique for hypospadias repair. Urol Clin North Am. 1981a; 8:503.

Duckett JW: MAGPI (meatal advancement and glanuloplasty): a procedure for subcoronal hypospadias. Urol Clin North Am. 1981b; 8:513.

Duckett JW: Hypospadias. In: Walsh PC, Gittes RF, Permutter AD et al (eds): Campbell's urology, 5th edn. Saunders, Philadelphia, pp 1969–1999; 1986.

Duckett JW, Baskin LS: Hypospadias. In: Gillenwater JY, Grayhack JT, Howards SS, Duckett JW (eds): Adult and pediatric urology, 3rd edn. Mosby-Year Book, St. Louis. 1996; pp 2549–2589.

Duckett JW, Keating MA: Technical challenge of the megameatus intact prepuce hypospadias variant: the pyramid procedure. J Urol. 1989; 141:1407.

Duplay S: Asselin, Paris; 1874. (Also in Arch Gen Med 1:513:1:657, 1874; and in Bull Soc Chir Paris. 49:157).

Duplay S: Sur le traitement chirurgical de l'hypospadias et de l'epispadias. Arch Gen Med. 1880; 5:527.

Edmunds A: An operation for hypospadias. Lancet. 1913; 1:447.

Elder JS, Duckett JW, Snyder HM: Onlay island flap in the repair of mid-and distal penile hypospadias without chordee. J Urol. 1987; 138:376.

Fevre M: Technique for anterior hypospadias. J Chir. 1961; 81:562

Galen (c. 130–201 A.D) In: Opera omnia, vol 10. Kühn, Leipzig, Cnobloch, p 1001

Glenister TW: The origin and fate of the urethral plate in man. J Anat. 1954; 288:413–418.

Gittes RF, McLaughlin AP III: Injection technique to produce penile erection. Urology. 1974; 4:473–475

Haberlick A, Schmidt B, Uray E, et al: Hypospadias repair using a modification of Beck's operation: followup. J Urol. 1997; 157:2308–2311.

Hadidi AT: Y-V Glanuloplasty a new modification in the surgery of hypospadias. Kasr El Aini Med J. 1996; 2:223–233.

Hadidi AT: Lateral based flap with dual blood supply: a single stage repair for proximal hypospadias. Egypt. J Plast Reconstr Surg. 2003; 27 (3)

Harrison DH; Grobbelaar AO: Urethral advancement and glanuloplasty (UGPI): a modification of the MAGPI procedure for distal hypospadias. Br J Plast Surg. 1997; 50:206.

Hendren WH: The Belt-Fuqua for repair of hypospadias. Urol Clin North Am. 1981; 8:431.

Hinderer U: Hypospadias repair in long-term results. In: Glodwyn RM (ed): Plastic and reconstructive surgery. Little Brown, Boston, pp 378–410; 1978.

Hodgson NB: A one-stage hypospadias repair. J Urol. 1970; 104:281.

Horton CE (ed): Plastic and reconstructive surgery of the genital area. Little Brown, Boston; 1973.

Humby G: A one stage operation for hypospadias. Br J Surg. 1941; 29:84.

Keramidas DC, Soutis ME: Urethral advancement, glanuloplasty and preputioplasty in distal hypospadias. Eur J Pediatr Surg. 1995; 5:348–351.

King LR: Hypospadias-a one-stage repair without skin graft based on a new principle: chordee is sometimes produced by skin alone. J Urol. 1970; 103:660.

King LR: Cutaneous chordee and its implications in hypospadias repair. Urol Clin North Am. 1981; 8:397.

Koff SA: Mobilization of the urethral in the surgical treatment of hypospadias. J Urol. 1981; 125:394.

Koff SA, Eakins M: The treatment of penile chordee using corporal rotation. J Urol. 1984; 131:931.

Koyanagi T, Matsuno T, Nonomura K, et al: Complete repair of severe penoscrotal hypospadias in 1 stage: experience with urethral mobilization, wing flap-flipping urethroplasty and "glanulomeatoplasty". J Urol. 1983; 130D:1150–1154.

Landerer: Dtsch Z Chir. 1891; p 32.

Lowsley OS, Begg CL: A three stage operation for the repair of hypospadias. Report of cases. JAMA. 1938; 110:487.

Mathieu P: Traitment en un temps de l'hypospadias balanique et juxta-blanique. J Chir (Paris). 1932; 39:481.

Mays HB: Hypospadias: a concept of treatment. J Urol. 1951; 65:279.

McCarthy JG: Introduction to plastic surgery. In: McCarthy JG (ed): Plastic surgery, vol 1. General principles. Saunders, Philadelphia, p 2; 1990.

McGowan AJ Jr, Waterhouse RK: Mobilization of the anterior urethra. Bull NY Acad Med. 1964; 40:776–782.

Memmelaar J: Use of bladder mucosa in a one-stage repair of hypospadias. J Urol. 1947; 58:68.

Mettauer JP: Practical observations on those malformations of the male urethra and penis, termed hypospadias and epispadias, with an anomalous case. Am J Med Sci. 1842; 4:43.

Monfort G, Lucas C: Dihydrotestosterone penile stimulation in hypospadias surgery. Eur Urol. 1982; 8:201–203.

Motiwala HG: Dartos flap: an aid to urethral reconstruction. Br J Urol. 1993; 72:260.

Mustarde JC: One-stage correction of distal hypospadias and other people's fistulae. Br J Plast Surg. 1965; 18:413.

Nesbit RM: Congenital curvature of the phallus: report of three cases with description of corrective operation. J Urol. 1965; 93:230.

Nové-Josserand G: Traitement de l'hypospadias: nouvelle method. Lyon Med. 1897; 85:198.

Ombrédanne L: Hypospadias penien chez l'infant. Bull Mem Soc Chir Paris. 1911; 37:1076

Ombrédanne L: Precis clinique et operation de chirurgie infantile. Masson, Paris, p 851; 1932.

Pancoast JA: Treatise on operative surgery. Carrey and Hart, Philadelphia, pp 317–318; 1844.

Paré A: The works of that famous chirurgion Ambroise Parey, translated out of Latin and compared with the French by Th Johnson. Cotes and Young, London, p 419; 1634 (2nd edn, p 655; 1649). Academy-HMB-L (Vault) WZ 250.

Physick: Cited by Pancoast JA: Treatise on operative surgery. Carrey and Hart, Philadelphia, pp 317–318; 1844.

Retik AB, Keating M, Mandell J: Complications of hypospadias repair. Urol Clin North Am. 1988; 15:223–236.

Rich MA, Keating MA, Snyder HM et al: "Hinging" the urethral plate in hypospadias meatoplasty. J Urol. 1989; 142:1551.

Ricketson G: A method of repair of hypospadias. Am J Surg. 1958; 95:279.

Rochet V: Nouveau procédé pour réfaire le canal pénien dans l'hypospadias. Gaz Hebd Med Chir. 1899; 4:673.

Rosenberger: Dtsch Med Wochenschr. 1891; 9:1250.

Russell RH: Operation for severe hypospadias. Br Med J. 1900; 2:1432.

Smith D: A de-epithelialized overlap flap technique in the repair of hypospadias. Br J Plast Surg. 1973; 26:106–114.

Snodgrass W: Tubularized incised plate urethroplasty for distal hypospadias. J Urol. 1994; 151:464–465.

Snow BW: Use of tunica vaginalis to prevent fistulas in hypospadias surgery. J Urol. 1986; 136:861–863.

Snow BW: Use of tunica vaginalis to prevent fistula in hypospadias surgery. J Urol. 1994; 151:464–465.

Standoli L: One-stage repair of hypospadias: preputial island-flap technique Ann Plast Surg. 1982; 9:81.

Stock J, Hanna MK: Distal urethoplasty and glanuloplasty procedure: results of 512 repairs. Urology. 1997; 49:449.

Thiersch C: Ueber die Entstehungsweise und operative Behandlung der Epispadie. Arch Heilkd. 1869; 10:20.

Toksu E: One stage repair. Plast Reconstr Surg. 1970; 45:365.

Turner-Warwick R: Observations upon techniques for reconstruction of the urethral meatus, the hypospadiac glans deformity and the penile urethra. Urol Clin North Am. 1979; 6:643.

Van Hook W: A new operation for hypospadias. Ann Surg. 1896; 23:378.

Waterhouse K, Glassberg KI: Mobilization of the anterior urethra as an aid in the one-stage repair of hypospadias. Urol Clin North Am. 1981; 8:521.

Wood J (1875): Cited by Mayo CH: JAMA. 1901 36:1157.

Young F, Benjamin JA: Repair of hypospadias with free inlay skin graft. Surg Gynecol Obstet. 1948; 86:439.

Yamataka A, Ando K, Lane G, et al: Pedicled external spermatic fascia for urethroplasty in hypospadias and closure of urethrocutaneous fistula. J Pediatric Surg. 1998; 33: 1788–1789.

Zaontz MR: The GAP (glans approximation procedure) for glanular/coronal hypospadias. J Urol. 1989; 141:359.

Epidemiology of Hypospadias

Helen Dolk

The Prevalence of Hypospadias

Most estimates of prevalence of hypospadias in Europe and the USA range up to a maximum of 3 per 1,000 births, with two-thirds to three-quarters of cases being glanular or coronal (Table 3.1).

It is highly likely that some of the differences in prevalence reported between countries and over time are artefacts of study methodology. Factors potentially affecting the estimation of prevalence and the proportion of distal cases include study population definition, exclusion or underascertainment of distal forms of hypospadias or cases not referred for surgery, definition of the boundary between "normal" and "abnormal" and other classification issues, underascertainment related to passive rather than active case ascertainment, and lack of validation of information by paediatric surgeons or urologists to avoid inclusion of false-positive diagnoses or cases with misclassified location.

A Dutch study reported a higher prevalence of 3.8 per 1,000 (Pierik et al. 2002), which may be in part related to sensitisation to diagnosis by special training of child health centre physicians for the survey, although it should be noted that the proportion of distal cases was not higher than usual. A study in Bristol (North et al. 2000) also reported a prevalence over 3 per 1,000, but cases were not confirmed by paediatric surgical records and may have included false-positive diagnoses or abnormalities of prepuce rather than hypospadias. The influential early Rochester study (Sweet et al. 1974) for the years 1940–1970, quoted in many paediatric urology and surgery textbooks, reported a high prevalence of 4 per 1,000 births but also a high proportion of glanular and coronal cases (87%), suggesting more complete diagnosis of the milder glanular cases and/or a shifted boundary between "normal" and "abnormal". A German study of 500 adult men (Fichtner et al. 1995) found that 13% had hypospadias (equivalent to a rate of 65 per 1,000 births) of whom 75% had glanular hypospadias, 98% coronal or glanular. It is probable that the high proportion of glanular hypospadias in this study was related to measurement and designation of the "normal/abnormal" boundary, possibly altered in adult men. Many of the men, including those assessed to have coronal hypospadias, had not previously been aware of any penile deformity.

A recent survey of regions of Europe with EUROCAT congenital anomaly registers found prevalence rates up to 3 per 1,000 (EUROCAT Working Group 2002a, b). Among the 26 registers in the survey, there was considerable variation in reported prevalence. One factor identified as underlying at least part of this variation was variation in the implementation of the EUROCAT guideline to exclude glanular cases: some registries included all glanular cases reported, some included glanular cases if surgical correction had been done/planned, some reported difficulty in making a reliable distinction between glanular and coronal cases, and some experienced difficulties in obtaining information about location or found that there was considerable disagreement between first reports of location (at diagnosis soon after birth) and later reports (in paediatric surgical records). For those registering glanular cases, a particular issue was the exclusion of incomplete prepuce incorrectly reported at birth as hypospadias.

The EUROCAT survey indicated that it was likely that reported prevalence estimates have been influenced by surgical policy. However, there are few reports in the literature indicating the proportion of children with hypospadias, particularly distal hypospadias, who undergo surgery, and many of the studies that exist (reviewed in Table 1) were not designed to give reliable estimates of the proportion with surgery. Some estimates suggest that less than half of reported cases were undergoing surgery in the 1970s in Hungary and Sweden, and in the 1970s and 1980s in Denmark. More recently in the Netherlands, in the years 1998–2000, it was reported (Pierik et al. 2002) that surgery was recommended for 78% of cases – 3 out of 12 glanular cases and virtually all other cases. A study in Southampton and Portsmouth

Table 3.1. Review of studies giving hypospadias prevalence estimates since 1970, distribution of location of meatus or proportion undergoing surgery

Type of study, place, time and reference	Prevalence estimate	Proportion glanular and coronal	Proportion with surgery	Comments
Thirty-two population-based congenital anomaly registers, Europe 1980–1999 (EUROCAT Working Group 2002a,b)	1–3 per 1,000 births	Glanular: 33%, 39% (two registries)	–	Many registers exclude glanular hypospadias or include only surgically corrected hypospadias
Population-based congenital anomaly register, Italy, 1978–1983 (Calzolari et al. 1986)	2 per 1,000 (168 cases)	Type 1 hypospadias in 75% of cases	–	Although "Type 1" has subsequently been used synonymously with "glanular", according to the diagram included in the paper, coronal cases may have been included in Type I
Hospital discharge and population based congenital anomaly register records, Denmark 1983–1993 (Weidner et al. 1998)	–	–	Of 1345 cases identified, 650 had record of surgical treatment (48%)	–
Military hospital discharge records from 15 military hospitals, USA (Gallentin et al. 2001)	3.5 per 1,000 (709 cases)	–	–	Not clear what discharge records refer to, or whether multiple episodes could be identified
Population-based congenital anomaly register, New York State 1983–1995 and hospital discharge data (Choi et al. 2001)	3.6 per 1,000	–	Surgical repair rate 0.6 per 1,000, suggesting only 17% have surgery	No trend in prevalence or surgical repair; no author comment on low surgical rate
Population based congenital anomaly register, Strasbourg 1979–87 (Stoll et al 1990)	1.5 per 1,000	69% glanular or coronal	–	–
Population-based surgical series, Southampton & Portsmouth 1992–1994 (Chambers and Malone 1999)	2.4 per 1,000 (84 cases)	31% glanular, 75% glanular or coronal	Policy to recommend surgery in virtually all cases of hypospadias	–
Population-based survey, Netherlands 1998–2000 (Pierik et al. 2002)	3.8 per 1,000 (53 cases)	25% glanular, 56% glanular or coronal	Surgery for 78%, 3/12 glanular, 14/15 coronal, all more severe anomalies	Special training of child health centre physicians for neonatal examinations and follow-up or referrals to paediatric urologist
Cohort study, Bristol 1991–1992 (North et al. 2000)	3.2 per 1,000 (51 cases)	No information	–	Enrolled women antenatally, hypospadias identified from annual questionnaires to mothers up to age 3, birth notifications and reports of neonatal examinations by paediatricians, cases not confirmed by paediatric surgery/urology records

Epidemiology of Hypospadias 53

Table 3.1 (continued)

Source	Rate	Severity	Associated findings	Comments
Hospital discharge database, Finland 1970–1994 (Aho et al. 2000)	1.4 per 1,000	No information	–	Surgery up to 8 years of age. Rate stable over time. PCR based rate in Finland over same time period starts much lower and increased to 1.4 per 1,000
Population and hospital based congenital anomaly registers, International, 1964–1997 (Paulozzi 1999)	Increase in prevalence during 1970s and 1980s in USA (up to 3.5 per 1,000), Scandinavia (up to <2 per 1,000) and Japan (up to <0.5 per 1,000). Little evidence of further increase anywhere after 1985	–	–	Limited detail on methodology for individual registries
Hospital series, excluding non-residents Rochester USA, 1940–1970 (Sweet et al. 1974)	4.1 per 1,000 (113 cases), no temporal trend, 0.5 per 1,000 excluding glanular/coronal	87% glanular or coronal hypospadias	24%, all either penile or with testicular associated anomalies	–
Survey of 500 hospitalised adult men, Germany, mean age 57 (Fichtner et al. 1995)	65 per 1,000 (13% of men)	75% glanular hypospadias, 98% coronal or glanular, 1 subcoronal	–	High proportion of glanular hypospadias in this study probably related to measurement and designation of "normal/abnormal" boundary, possibly altered in adult men; many of the men, including those assessed to have coronal hypospadias, had not previously been aware of any penile deformity
Population- and hospital-based congenital anomaly registers, International 1967–1982 (Kallen et al. 1986)	0.3 per 1,000 Mexico, 0.6 South America, 0.9 Denmark, 1.6–1.7 Spain, Hungary, Italy, 2.0 Sweden	69–85% of cases glanular or coronal	Surgery for 40% of case in Hungary in 1975, 31% Sweden 1974, 27% Denmark 1974–76	Proportion glanular/coronal did not correlate with prevalence; increasing trend in Denmark and Hungary; increasing trend up to 1973 in Sweden
Population-based congenital anomaly register, Atlanta 1968–1996 (Paulozzi et al. 1997)	Increase from 1.7 per 1,000 to 3.0 per 1,000	74% were first degree (meatus on ventral surface of glans penis)	–	No indication that proportion of first degree cases had increased during time period but location was unknown in majority of cases
Hospital-based congenital anomaly register, USA 1970–1993 (Paulozzi et al. 1997)	2.0 per 1,000 rising to 3.5 per 1,000	No information	–	Neonatal discharge summaries sole source of information
England and Wales National Congenital Anomaly System, 1964–1983 (Matlay and Beral 1985)	Rising from 0.7 to 1.8 per 1,000	–	–	–
Population-based congenital anomaly register, Victoria, Australia 1983–1995 (Riley et al. 1998)	1.7 per 1,000 rising to 2.9 per 1,000	–	–	–

(Chambers and Malone 1999) reported that policy was to recommend surgery for virtually all cases, including glanular, but as this study was based on surgery lists it may have missed some very mild cases. It is possible that the proportion of distal cases undergoing surgery has increased over the decades in some countries, encouraged by new surgical techniques. A Finnish study (Aho et al. 2000), however, commented for the period from 1970 to 1994 that "no major changes in the treatment policy have occurred ... since the 1960s or even earlier, even minor cases of hypospadias have been treated surgically before the children reached school age. More recently, modern operative techniques and equipment have enabled treatment at younger ages". In the 1970s and 1980s there was generally a trend towards earlier surgery (around 1 year of age), and this may in itself have increased reporting of hypospadias to congenital anomaly registers which are mainly geared to sources of information in early infancy.

Clearly there is much remaining variation in opinion on surgical policy. A recent German study (Fichtner et al. 1995) has questioned whether surgery for glanular and even many coronal cases is necessary, given the authors' survey of adult men which suggested no functional or psychological consequences for milder forms of abnormality. In a survey of four surgical centres in the UK (EUROCAT Working Group 2002a), one-quarter of cases were glanular in three of the surgery lists, while one centre operated on no glanular cases at all. Policy regarding age at surgery also varies, the EUROCAT survey finding that average age at operation varied from 13.6 months to 60.3 months in different European regions.

There is some evidence that the prevalence of hypospadias increased from the 1960s to the 1980s in Europe (Paulozzi 1999; Matlay and Beral 1985; Czeizel 1985; Kallen and Winberg 1982; Toppari et al. 1996) and in the USA (Paulozzi et al. 1997), although recent reports suggests that these trends might not be continuing (Paulozzi 1999; Toppari et al. 1996) (Table 3.1). It could be that any reported rising trend simply reflects a more frequent or early diagnosis of more distal forms of hypospadias over time, or an increasing tendency to report them to congenital anomaly registers. One US report of rising prevalence (Paulozzi et al. 1997) therefore looked also at the trend in prevalence of severe (proximal) cases. They found a parallel trend in severe cases, suggesting that the trend was not an artefact of reporting changes, but a majority of cases in the survey were of unspecified severity. A Finnish study found that a previously reported increase in the prevalence of hypospadias in Finland was probably due to general improvement of ascertainment by the congenital anomaly register, since surgical discharge records showed a stable prevalence (Aho et al. 2000). Paulozzi (1999) has proposed that, since the foreskin is used in some surgical repair procedures and therefore circumcision must be deferred if hypospadias is present, medicolegal considerations may increasingly cause physicians to examine the penis carefully before circumcision, i.e. there is a change in the detection of mild hypospadias rather than in surgical policy per se. It is probable that we will never be able to retrospectively resolve exactly what the true changes in prevalence of hypospadias have been in any one region. What gives the evidence relating to increasing prevalence over time some weight is the fact that prevalence has been observed to increase in a number of regions/countries, with prevalence studies using different data collection methods, and that the increase in prevalence seems to be mirrored in other possibly aetiologically related conditions.

Endocrine-Disrupting Chemicals and Hormonal Aetiological Factors

At the same time as hypospadias prevalence has appeared to be rising, increases in the frequency of new cases of related abnormalities such as cryptorchidism (undescended testes) and testicular cancer have been reported, as well as a fall in male fertility (Sharpe and Skakkeback 1993). While there are problems with the interpretation of the changes in frequency of the various disorders, the concomitant increase in apparently aetiologically related disorders in the absence of increases in other congenital anomalies or cancers has tended to strengthen the interpretation of these changes as real phenomena. In addition, there have been some geographical correlations. For example, the hypospadias rate in Finland seems low (Table 3.1) and Finland also has a low rate of testicular cancer and high semen quality compared to other Scandinavian countries (Sharpe and Skakkeback 1993), although comparisons are no longer clear in light of the revised Finnish hypospadias rate (Aho et al. 2000).

It has been hypothesised that the underlying cause of the change in frequency of all these conditions, as well as reproductive abnormalities observed in fish and other animals, may be exposure to endocrine-disrupting chemicals (including xeno-oestrogens) (Toppari et al. 1996; Colborn 1995; Burdorf and Nieuwenhuisen 1999; Joffe 2001). Endocrine-disrupting chemicals are exogenous substances that cause adverse health effects through interference with the endocrine system, either by mimicking hormones (agonists); binding to receptor sites without activation, thereby antagonising endogenous hormones; interfering with the synthesis or degradation of hormones; or in some other way (in)directly interfering with the functioning of hormones. In relation to hypospadias, evidence suggests that an antiandrogen mechanism (one that hampers the activity of male hormones) is most likely (Baskin et al. 2001). Potential endocrine-disrupting chemicals include dioxins and furans, PCBs and organochlorine pesticides, and also dietary phyto-oestrogens (such as in soy products) (Colborn 1995; Burdorf and Nieuwenhuisen 1999; Joffe 2001). Exposure to these substances may occur particularly in the occupational setting but also through more general environmental exposure, exposure in the home, food packaging, and diet (Burdorf and Nieuwenhuisen 1999).

There has been very little research directly investigating the hypothesised relationship between exposure to endocrine-disrupting chemicals in the environment and risk of hypospadias. Research to date, both animal and human, has been recently reviewed (Baskin et al. 2001). The ALSPAC cohort study (North et al. 2000) found vegetarian diet to be a risk factor for hypospadias, with the implication that high soy (a phyto-oestrogen) intake or pesticide intake might be causal factors, although numbers were too small for detailed analysis. To date, no further published studies have looked at vegetarian diet. A study of residents near hazardous waste landfills found an increased risk of hypospadias and some other congenital anomalies, but no specific chemical exposures could be characterised in that study (Dolk et al. 1998).

Since the development of the male genital tract is under hormonal influence, indicators for both endogenous and exogenous endocrine factors have been suggested to play a role in the aetiology of hypospadias (Dolk 1998; Moller and Weidner 1999). Several epidemiological case-control studies of hypospadias have looked at a range of possible indicators of "fertility" or maternal endocrine function in its broadest sense, including age at menarche, menstrual cycle irregularities, parity, age, previous spontaneous or induced abortions, time to pregnancy, strength of contractions and other characteristics of delivery. Possibly the most consistent findings have been associations with threatened abortion. Low birthweight or intrauterine growth retardation have also been found to be associated with hypospadias (Moller and Weidner 1999) consistent with some explanations involving fetal androgen production. Testicular abnormalities and subfertility have been reported to be more prevalent among fathers of children with hypospadias than other fathers (Baskin et al. 2001; Kallen et al. 1991; Fritz and Czeizel 1996). An international ecological study suggested that differences in prevalence rates between countries might be associated with the proportion of subfertile couples among parents (Kallen et al. 1991). It has similarly been suggested that rising prevalence may be a result of improving fertility treatment increasing the number of children born to subfertile men (Fritz and Czeizel 1996).

The main exogenous hormones investigated have been oral contraceptive use in early pregnancy, hormones used in pregnancy tests, and progestagens used on indication of threatened abortion or previous miscarriages. The evidence is not strong for a risk of hypospadias associated with these exposures (Raman-Wilms et al. 1995). It has also been pointed out that oral contraceptive use is not a frequent enough exposure in early pregnancy for any small excess use to explain such a large increase in prevalence of hypospadias (Matlay and Beral 1985).

A follow-up of diethylstilboestrol (DES)-exposed offspring has not given strong evidence of a risk of hypospadias (Baskin et al. 2001). However, a higher risk of hypospadias has been found in sons of women exposed in utero to DES (Henderson et al. 1976; Klip et al. 2001). A consistent picture regarding risk after IVF and other assisted conception techniques has not yet emerged (Baskin et al. 2001; Silver et al. 1999; Schwartz et al. 1986), and interpretation is complicated by confounding by subfertility, multiple births, low birthweight and maternal age.

Studies of occupational exposures in relation to hypospadias are few. Farmers and gardeners have been one occupational group of concern because of their work with pesticides, many of which have potential endocrine-disrupting properties. Studies have suggested both no relationship between hypospadias risk and parental work in agriculture or gardening (Schwartz et al. 1986; Weinder et al. 1998; Garcia et al. 1999) and a positive relationship (Kristensen et al. 1997). More general studies of occupation and birth defects have identified several occupations with increased risks of hypospadias [paternal work as vehicle mechanics (Irgens et al. 2000) and paternal work in forestry and logging, carpentry and woodwork, and as service station attendants (Olshan et al. 1991)], but these associations are detected in many combinations of occupation and birth defects tested, and thus some spuriously significant results can be expected.

A study based on the England and Wales National Congenital Anomaly Notification System looked at the relation between potential endocrine-disruptor exposure based on job title and risk of hypospadias (EUROCAT Working Group 2002a; Vrijheid et al. 2002). There was little evidence of any increased risk of hypospadias, although further surveillance of hairdressers as a relatively large potentially exposed group was recommended.

Conclusion

Interest in hypospadias, its prevalence and aetiology, has been rekindled in recent years by fears that hypospadias might be one outcome of increasing population exposure to endocrine-disrupting chemicals. To respond to this public health concern, we need to keep accurate records of hypospadias cases in the population for surveillance, and mount further case-control studies of aetiological factors taking into account the huge advances now being made in identifying and quantifying potential endocrine disrupting exposures and addressing the pathways by which parental subfertility may influence hypospadias risk.

References

Aho M, Koivisto A-M, Tammela TLJ, et al: Is the incidence of hypospadias increasing? Analysis of Finnish Hospital Discharge Data 1970–1994. Environ Health Perspect. 2000; 108:463–465.
Baskin LS, Himes K, Colborn T: Hypospadias and endocrine disruption: is there a connection? Environ Health Perspect. 2001; 109:1175–1183.
Burdorf A, Nieuwenhuisen MJ: Endocrine disrupting chemicals and human reproduction: fact or fiction? Ann Occup Hyg. 1999; 43:435–437.
Calzolari E, Contiero MR, Roncarati E, et al: Aetiological factors in hypospadias. J Med Genet. 1986; 23:333–337.
Chambers EL, Malone PSJ: The incidence of hypospadias in two English cities: a case-control comparison of possible causal factors. BJU Int. 1999; 84:95–98.
Choi J, Cooper KL, Hensle TW, et al: Incidence and surgical repair rates of hypospadias in New York State. Pediatr Urol. 2001; 57:151–153.
Colborn T: Environmental estrogens: health implications for humans and wildlife. Environ Health Perspect. 1995; 103 [Suppl 7]:135–136.
Czeizel A: Increasing morbidity in the male reproductive system. Lancet. 1985; 1:462–463.
Dolk H: Rise in prevalence of hypospadias. Lancet. 1998; 351:770.
Dolk H, Vrijheid M, Armstrong B, et al: Risk of congenital anomalies near hazardous-waste landfill sites in Europe: The EUROHAZCON Study. Lancet. 1998; 352:423–427.
EUROCAT Working Group: EUROCAT Special Report, an assessment and analysis of existing surveillance data on hypospadias in UK and Europe, University of Ulster, 2002a.
EUROCAT Working Group: EUROCAT Report 8. Surveillance of congenital anomalies in Europe 1980–1999, University of Ulster, 2002b.
Fichtner J, Filipas D, Mottrie AM, et al: Analysis of meatal location in 500 men: wide variation questions the need for meatal advancement in all pediatric anterior hypospadias cases. J Urol. 1995; 154:833–834.
Fritz G, Czeizel AE: Abnormal sperm morphology and function in the fathers of hypospadias. J Reprod Fertil. 1996; 106:63–66.
Gallentin ML, Moreu AF, Thompson IM Jr: Hypospadias: a contemporary epidemiologic assessment. Pediatr Urol. 2001; 57:788–790.
Garcia AM, Fletcher T, Benafvides FG, et al: Parental agricultural work and selected congenital malformations. Am J Epidemiol. 1999; 149:64–74.
Henderson BE, Benton B, Cosgrove M, et al: Urogenital tract abnormalities in sons of women treated with diethylstilbestrol. Pediatrics. 1976; 58:505–507.
Irgens A, Kruger K, Skorve AH, et al: Birth defects and paternal occupational exposure. Hypotheses tested in a record linkage based dataset. Acta Obstet Gynecol Scand. 2000; 79(6):465–470.
Joffe M: Are problems with male reproductive health caused by endocrine disruption? Occup Environ Med. 2001; 58: 281–288.
Kallen B, Winberg J: An Epidemiological study of hypospadias in Sweden. Acta Paediatr Scand. 1982; 293 [Suppl]: 1–21.
Kallen B, Bertollin R, Castilla E, et al: A joint international study on the epidemiology of hypospadias. Acta Paediatr Scand. 1986; 324 [Suppl]:5–52.
Kallen B, Castilla EE, Kringelbach M, et al: Parental fertility and infant hypospadias: an international case-control study. Teratology. 1991; 44:629–634.
Klip H, Verloop J, Van Gool J, et al: Increased risk of hypospadias in male offspring of women exposed to diethylstilbestrol in utero. Paediatr Perinatal Epidemiol. 2001; 15:A1-A38.
Kristensen P, Irgens LM, Andersen A, et al: Birth defects among offspring of norwegian farmers, 1967–1991. Epidemiology. 1997; 8:537–544.
Matlay P, Beral V: Trends in congenital malformations of external genitalia. Lancet. 1985; 1:108.
McDowell ME: Occupational reproductive epidemiology: the use of routinely collected statistics in England & Wales, 1980–1982. Stud Med Popul Subj no 50, HMSO, 1985.
Moller H, Weidner IS: Epidemiology of cryptorchidism and hypospadias. Epidemiology. 1999; 10:352–354.
North K, Golding J, The ALSPAC Study Team: A maternal vegetarian diet in pregnancy is associated with hypospadias. BJU Int. 2000; 85:107–113.
Olshan AF, Teschke K, Baird PA: Paternal occupation and congenital anomalies in offspring. Am J Ind Med. 1991; 20:447–475.
Paulozzi LJ: International trends in rates of hypospadias and cryptorchidism. Environ Health Perspect. 1999; 107:297–302.
Paulozzi LJ, Erickson JD, Jackson RJ: Hypospadias trends in two US surveillance systems. Pediatrics. 1997; 100:831–834.
Pierik FH, Burdorf A, Nijman JMR, et al: A high hypospadias rate in the Netherlands. Hum Reprod. 2002; 17:1112–1115.
Raman-Wilms L, Lin-in Tseng A, Wignardt S, et al: Fetal genital effects of first-trimester sex hormone exposure: a meta-analysis. Obstet Gynecol. 1995; 85:141–149.
Riley MM, Halliday JL, Lumley JM: Congenital malformations in Victoria, Australia 1983–1995: an overview of infant characteristics. J Paediatr Child Health. 1998; 34:233–240.

Schwartz DA, Newsum LA, Markowitz Heifetz R: Parental occupation and birth outcome in an agricultural community. Scand J Work Environ Health. 1986; 12:51–54.

Sharpe RM, Skakkebaek NE: Are oestrogens involved in falling sperm counts and disorders of the male reproductive tract? Lancet. 1993; 341:1392–1395.

Silver RI, Rodriguez R, Chang TS, et al: In Vitro fertilization is associated with an increased risk of hypospadias. J Urol. 1999; 161:1954–1957.

Stoll C, Alembik Y, Roth MP, et al: Genetic and environmental factors in hypospadias. J Med Genet. 1990; 27:559–563.

Sweet RA, Schrott HG, Kurland R, et al: Study of the incidence of hypospadias in Rochester, Minnesota, 1940–1970, and a case-control comparison of possible aetiological factors. Mayo Clin Proc. 1974; 49:52–58.

Toppari J, Larsen JC, Chrostiansen P, et al: Male reproductive health and environmental xenoestrogens. Environ Health Perspect. 1996; 104 [Suppl 4]:741–803.

Vrijheid M, Dolk H, Armstrong B, et al: Hazard potential ranking of landfill sites and risk of congenital anomalies. Occup Environ Epidemiol. 2002; 59:768–776.

Weidner IS, Moller H, Jensen TK, et al: Cryptorchidism and hypospadias in sons of gardeners and farmers. Environ Health Perspect. 1998; 106:793–796.

Genetic Aspects of Hypospadias

Margo Whiteford

Hypospadias is one of the most common urogenital anomalies, occurring in about 3 per 1,000 male births. The heritability of the condition is well recognised, and empiric recurrence risks suggest that brothers of an affected individual have a 6–17% chance of also being affected (Angerpointer 1984; Stoll et al. 1990). Data regarding the offspring risk for an affected father are scanty but one study has indicated that the incidence of hypospadias among fathers of affected boys is increased fivefold (Angerpointer 1984).

Isolated hypospadias is heterogeneous and various patterns of inheritance have been proposed. There have been reports of several affected males in large consanguineous families (Frydmen et al. 1985; Tsur et al. 1987), suggesting autosomal recessive inheritance, and also reports of hypospadias occurring in several generations of non-consanguineous families, such as the three-generation family described by Cote et al. (1979), in which male-to-male transmission was also observed, thus indicating autosomal dominant inheritance to be the most likely explanation. In 1953 Sorensen reviewed the families of 103 probands attending departments of surgery in Denmark and proposed an autosomal recessive pattern of inheritance to explain the familial clusterings (Sorensen 1953). The same families were revisited in 1993, by Harris, and using two different methods of segregation analysis it was felt that autosomal dominant and codominant models or non-mendelian sibship clustering were more likely than autosomal recessive inheritance (Harris and Beaty 1993). A recent study of 2005 families in Sweden has further suggested that inherited hypospadias is due to monogenetic factors in only a small proportion of families and that in the majority of families a multifactorial cause is more likely (Fredell et al. 2002).

Several of the epidemiological studies cited above have emphasised the importance of trying to separate cases of uncomplicated hypospadias, when calculating empiric recurrence risks, from that occurring as a feature of recognised genetically inherited syndromes and from hypospadias due to other known aetiological factors. Boehmer studied 63 unselected males with severe hypospadias attending a single centre and found that in 31% of cases aetiological factors could be identified, including 17% who had complex genetic syndromes and 9.5% who had chromosomal anomalies (Boehmer et al. 2001).

There have been numerous reports of males with chromosomal anomalies who have hypospadias as a feature. Such chromosomal anomalies may provide clues to the chromosomal location of genes important for the occurrence of hypospadias. In 1998 Brewer et al. searched the Human Cytogenetics Database (Schinzel 1994) for patients with pure chromosomal deletions or duplications and, using 47 specific congenital malformations, checked for significant associations between particular chromosomal regions and the malformations (Brewer et al. 1998, 1999). Hypospadias was found to be significantly associated with deletions of the chromosomal bands 1q42–44, 4p16–13, 7q34 and 11p13 and duplications of bands 2q35–37, 8q12 and 16q21–24. This information may, in time, help in the identification of candidate genes important for the normal development of male genitalia.

Hypospadias is usually an isolated anomaly but it is estimated that 10–15% of patients with this condition have additional congenital malformations, particularly affecting the urogenital system. Some of these patients will have a pattern of malformations suggestive of recognisable and detectable chromosomal abnormalities, of which some are summarised in Table 4.1. Karyotyping should therefore be considered in children who have hypospadias in addition to other anomalies.

Table 4.1. Syndromes due to chromosomal anomalies in which hypospadias is a recognised feature

45X0/46XY mosaic Turner syndrome
Wolf-Hirschhorn syndrome (4p deletion)
Cat-eye syndrome (5p deletion)
Mosaic trisomy 22
Uniparental disomy chromosome 16

The Online Mendelian Inheritance in Man database lists 50 syndromes in which hypospadias may be a feature and the London Dysmorphology Database (Winter and Baraitser) lists 186, so it is obviously not practical to discuss all of these in detail in this text. It would, however, be pertinent to mention some of these in a bit more detail as they may have high recurrence risks or have implications for other relatives.

Hypertelorism with Oesophageal Abnormality and Hypospadias

This condition has variously been called G syndrome, Opitz G syndrome, Opitz BBB syndrome and a number of other synonyms. It was initially thought to be an X-linked condition, as females tend to be more mildly affected, but it is now known to be heterogeneous with an autosomal dominant form mapping to chromosome 22q11.2 and an X-linked form mapping to Xp22. The clinical features consist of hypertelorism or telecanthus (89%), laryngotracheo-oesophageal clefts (44%), clefts of the lip, palate or uvula (34%), genitourinary defects [particularly hypospadias in males (100%) but also splayed labia in females] and mental retardation (38%) (Wilson and Oliver 1988). Other midline defects such as anal anomalies and congenital heart defects have also been described.

This condition should be considered in males with hypospadias who present with a hoarse cry or swallowing difficulties in the neonatal period. As affected mothers may have only telecanthus, this should be borne in mind when counselling the parents regarding the recurrence risk.

McKusick–Kaufman Syndrome

McKusick–Kaufman syndrome is an autosomal recessively inherited condition first described in 1964 (McKusick et al. 1964). Its features consist of varying combinations of hydrometrocolpos, post-axial polydactyly and congenital heart defects. However, it is important to note that hypospadias may be the only feature in affected males and therefore detailed family histories should always be sought.

This syndrome is very rare but occurs more frequently in certain inbred populations, such as the Amish, and in some Arab communities. This is most likely to be a heterogeneous condition but mutations in a gene on chromosome 20p12 have been shown to be responsible for both McKusick–Kaufman syndrome and Bardet–Biedl syndrome (BBS6) (Stone et al. 2000). Therefore, in some cases, molecular confirmation of the diagnosis and prenatal diagnosis may be possible.

Pallister–Hall Syndrome

Pallister–Hall syndrome can be of variable severity, but is often lethal in the neonatal period. It is of autosomal dominant inheritance, with the majority of cases representing new mutations, and is known to be due to mutations in the GLI3 gene on chromosome 7 (Kang et al. 1997). The hallmark of this condition is a hypothalamic hamartoma, but other features include: dysmorphic facies (flat nasal bridge, short upturned nose, posteriorly rotated ears and a small tongue), laryngeal cleft, pituitary dysfunction, polydactyly and syndactyly, dysplastic nails, hydrocephalus, anal anomalies and genitourinary anomalies including hypospadias. Cranial MRI should be considered in infants with hypospadias who exhibit these dysmorphic features or other anomalies.

Mildly affected parents have been shown to have asymptomatic hypothalamic hamartomata, and MRI scanning of the parents should also be considered when discussing the recurrence risk.

Smith–Lemli–Opitz Syndrome

The features of Smith–Lemli–Opitz syndrome (SLO) overlap with those of other syndromes already described and include growth retardation, cleft palate, polydactyly, syndactyly, microcephaly, small upturned nose, cataracts, blepharoptosis, congenital heart defects, genital anomalies and mental retardation. This condition was also first described in 1964 (Smith et al. 1964), but 30 years elapsed before the discovery that it was due to a defect of cholesterol biosynthesis (Tint et al. 1994). SLO is thought to affect approximately 1:20,000–30,000 births in European populations. More cases have been described in males than in females, but this is probably ascertainment bias due to the high frequency of hypospadias in affected males. Some affected children have only one or two of the associated anomalies, but if there is any suspicion that SLO may be the cause of hypospadias the condition can be diagnosed by means of a biochemical test looking for elevated levels of 7-dehydrocholesterol in plasma. It is important to recognise patients with SLO as treatment with cholesterol supplementation has been shown to result in improved growth and more rapid developmental progress (Elias et al. 1997).

SLO is an autosomal recessive condition with a 25% recurrence risk. Prenatal diagnosis is possible by means of biochemical analysis of a chorionic villus sample. In addition some children with SLO have been shown to have mutations in the gene responsible for the production of the enzyme sterol delta-7-reductase, so molecular confirmation of the diagnosis and prenatal diagnosis may be possible.

Other Associations

Hypospadias, especially in its most severe form, can occur as part of the spectrum of ambiguous genitalia, and genetically inherited conditions resulting in ambiguous genitalia should also be considered within the differential diagnosis of hypospadias. A knowledge of the embryological development of male genitalia is essential for understanding the conditions that result in ambiguous genitalia. All foetuses, whether genetically male or female, start life with the capacity to develop either a male or a female reproductive system. Every foetus has non-specific genitals (a genital tubercle, urethral folds and labioscrotal swellings) for the first 8 weeks after conception. In male foetuses the presence of a Y chromosome initiates the formation of the testes and suppression of female internal organ development. Androgens produced by the testes then act on androgen receptors to produce male external genitalia. With androgen insensitivity syndrome the sex chromosome complement is XY so female internal organ development is suppressed. However, the tissues are not able to respond to the androgens produced by the testes and the external genitalia remain female. Complete androgen insensitivity syndrome results in a completely normal female phenotype, but partial androgen insensitivity syndrome can result in a phenotype anywhere between normal female and normal male, including hypospadias as the only abnormal feature. Nevertheless, studies have suggested that androgen receptor defects are a rare cause of hypospadias[9]. Androgen insensitivity syndrome is inherited in an X-linked pattern and there may be a family history of ambiguous genitalia or infertility in females.

Similarly, partial deficiency of the enzymes required for testosterone biosynthesis (e.g. 17-ketosteroid reductase, 17-alpha-hydroxylase, 3-beta-hydroxysteroid dehydrogenase, 17-beta-hydroxysteroid dehydrogenase) result in varying degrees of failure of masculinisation and may present with hypospadias. These enzyme defects are inherited in an autosomal recessive fashion and are diagnosed by biochemical analysis.

References

Angerpointer TA: Hypospadias – genetics, epidemiology and other possible aetiological influences. Z Kinderchir. 1984; 39:112–118.

Boehmer AL, Nijman RJ, Lammers BA, et al: Etiological studies of severe or familial hypospadias. J Urol. 2001; 165: 1246–1254.

Brewer C, Holloway S, Zawalnyski P, et al: A chromosomal deletion map of human malformations. Am J Hum Genet. 1998; 63:1153–1159.

Brewer C, Holloway S, Zawalnyski P, et al: A chromosomal duplication map of malformations: Regions of suspected haplo and triplolethality – and tolerance of segmental aneuploidy – in humans. Am J Hum Genet. 1999; 64: 1702–1708.

Cote GB, Petmezaki S, Bastakis N: A gene for hypospadias in a child with presumed tetrasomy 18p. Am J Med Genet. 1979; 4:141–146.

Elias ER, Irons MB, Hurley AD, et al: Clinical effects of cholesterol supplementation in six patients with the Smith–Lemli–Opitz syndrome (SLOS). Am J Med Genet. 1997; 68:305–310.

Fredell L, Iselius L, Collins A, et al: Complex segregation analysis of hypospadias. Hum Genet. 2002; 111:231–234.

Frydmen M, Greiber C, Cohen HA: Uncomplicated familial hypospadias: evidence for autosomal recessive inheritance. Am J Med Genet. 1985; 21:51–55.

Harris EL, Beaty TH.: Segregation analysis of hypospadias: a reanalysis of published pedigree data. Am J Med Genet. 1993; 45:420–425.

Kang S, Graham JM, Olney AH, et al: GLI3 frameshift mutations cause autosomal dominant Pallister-Hall syndrome. Nat Genet. 1997; 15:266–268.

McKusick VA, Bauer RL, Koop CE, et al: Hydrometrocolpos as a simply inherited malformation. JAMA. 1964; 189:816.

Online Mendelian Inheritance in Man (OMIM) http://www.ncbi.nlm.nih.gov/Omim

Schinzel A: Human Cytogenetics Database. Oxford University Press, Oxford, 1994.

Smith DW, Lemli L, Opitz JM: A newly recognized syndrome of multiple congenital anomalies. J. Pediat. 1964; 64: 210–217.

Sorensen HR: Hypospadias with special reference to aetiology. Munksgaard, Copenhagen, 1953.

Stoll C, Alembik Y, Roth MP, et al: Genetic and environmental factors in hypospadias. J Med Genet. 1990; 27:559–563.

Stone DL, Slavotinek A, Bouffard GG, et al: Mutation of a gene encoding a putative chaperonin causes McKusick-Kaufman syndrome. Nat Genet. 2000; 25:79–82.

Tint GS, Irons M, Elias ER, et al: Defective cholesterol biosynthesis associated with the Smith-Lemli-Opitz syndrome. N Engl J Med. 1994; 330:107–113.

Tsur M, Linder N, Cappis S: Hypospadias in a consanguineous family (letter). Am J Med Genet. 1987; 27:487–489.

Wilson GN, Oliver WJ: Further delineation of the G syndrome; a manageable genetic cause of infantile dysphagia. J Med Genet. 1988; 25:157–163.

Winter R, Baraitser M: London Dysmorphology Database. Oxford University Press, Oxford.

Embryology and Anatomy of Hypospadias

John M. Hutson, E.C. Penington

5.1

Normal Embryology of External Genitalia

The embryology of the urogenital region remains controversial and confusing, in part related to the fact that observations have been extrapolated to the human from many different species. There are reports in the literature describing mice (van der Werff et al. 2000), rats (Forsberg 1961; Kluth et al. 1988), red squirrels (Barnstein and Mossman 1938), sheep (Tourneux 1888), pigs (van der Putte and Neeteson 1983), dogs (Kanagasuntheram and Anandaraja 1960) and humans (Nievelstein et al. 1998; de Vries and Friedland 1987).

The description in this chapter is based on a comparative study of 57 human embryos (crown-rump length 3–65 mm) and over 140 rat embryos (between 11 and 21 days' gestation) (Penington and Hutson 2003a, b). The observations have been correlated with the published findings in the literature in all species in an attempt to distil the common developmental steps in the development of mammalian genitalia. Histological sections of the human embryos are housed at the Anatomy and Developmental Biology Department, St. George's Hospital, London; the Department of Anatomy, University of Cambridge; Department of Plastic and Reconstructive Surgery, University Hospital, Rotterdam; and the Institute of Anatomy, UFR Biomedicale des Sts Pères, Paris. The rat embryos were prepared, sectioned and stained in our own laboratory. The observations form part of a thesis for a Doctorate of Medicine, University of Melbourne (E.C.P.) (Penington 2002).

The Cloacal Cavity and the Cloacal Plate

The cloacal cavity is the most caudal part of the definitive endodermal gut tube in the developing embryo. Cranially it is in continuity with the more caudal part of the gut tube (the hindgut) posteriorly and (in the human) with the allantoic diverticulum anteriorly. The tail gut exits the cloacal cavity caudally (Fig. 5.1.1). The cloacal membrane limits the cloaca ventrally at first, but proliferation of the infraumbilical mesenchyme in the midline leads to the formation of the early genital tubercle and displaces the cloacal cavity caudally within the tubercle (Fig. 5.1.2).

In addition, the endodermal lining of the cloaca becomes thickened and apposed side-to-side in the sagittal plane (Fig. 5.1.3). This results in an endodermal plate of cells orientated in the midsagittal plane extending from the tail fold to the tip of the genital tubercle which then forms the floor of the cloacal cavity over the whole length of what had been the cloacal membrane (Penington and Hutson 2003a) (Fig. 5.1.4). This nearly solid plate of cells, which

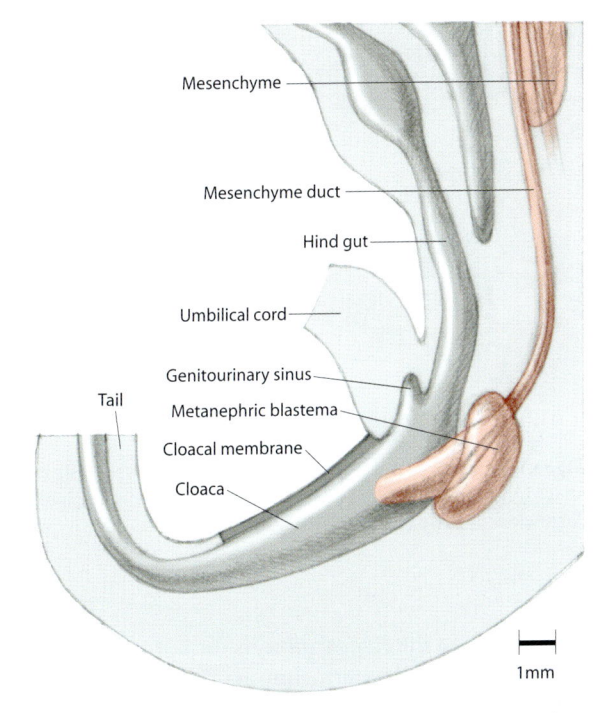

Fig. 5.1.1. Midsagittal reconstruction with mesenchyme duct and metanephric blastema (lying in lateral plane) overlaid in *red* (reconstruction of 17 serial sections of day 12 rat embryos). Tailgut is caudal to cloaca, and cloacal membrane in tail

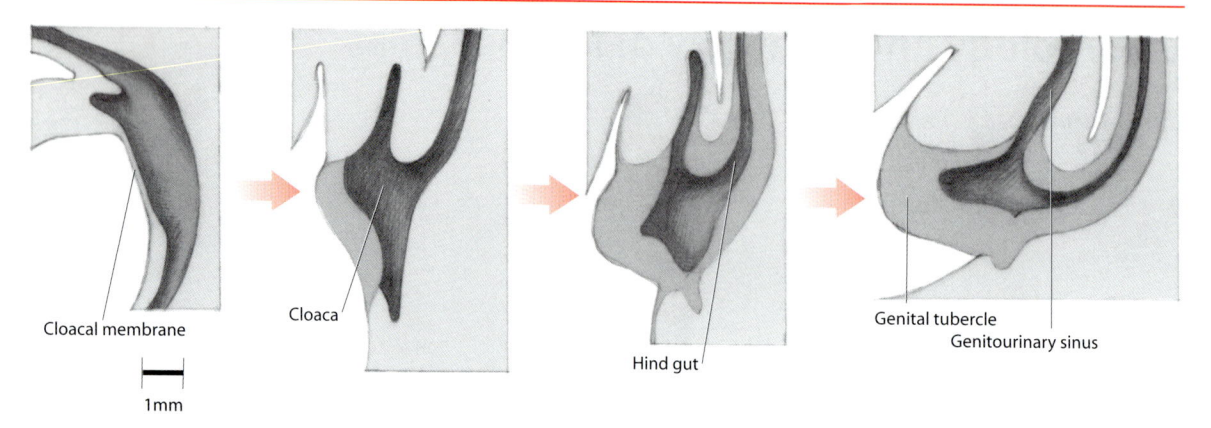

Fig. 5.1.2. Composite diagrams of midsagittal sections of day 12–13 rat embryos showing formation of genital tubercle

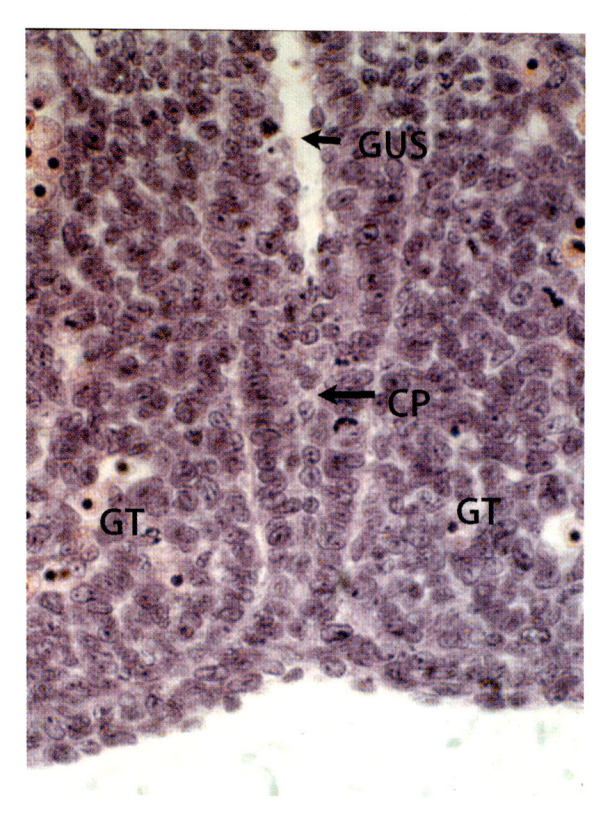

Fig. 5.1.3. Section of day 14 rat embryo, transverse with respect to genital tubercle (*GT*). Inner apposed walls of cloaca form cloacal plate (*CP*). *GUS* Genitourinary sinus

can be termed the *cloacal plate*, is the key structure in development of the perineum. Its complete description allows the development of the urethral plate to be more clearly understood (Penington and Hutson 2003b).

The Fate of the Cloacal Plate

In both rat and human embryos the cloacal plate gradually loses height posteriorly as the urorectal septum and the perineum approximate and the hindgut gains an outlet onto the perineum. The timing of the changes in the cloacal plate compared with growth and apoptosis in the structures adjacent to it varies across species (Penington 2002). In human embryos (and pigs) the cloacal plate reverts to a two-layer membrane posteriorly, breaking down soon afterwards to expose both the anorectal and urogenital tracts, as reported by Nievelstein et al. (1998) and others (Paidas et al. 1999; Arey 1965). Rupture of the cloacal membrane creates a midline groove in the perineum lined by endoderm.

In rats, on the other hand, the urorectal septum meets the top of the cloacal plate (which maintains a vertical height along its entire length), giving the appearance of fusion between the septum and the plate (◉ Fig. 5.1.5) (often described as fusion between the urorectal septum and the cloacal membrane). The anal canal forms by a process of apoptosis through the epithelial plate, and by the time the canal is patent, the urorectal septum mesenchyme forms the perineum as it does in humans, and the posterior part of the cloacal plate is no longer present (◉ Fig. 5.1.6).

A review of the key embryology papers by Tourneux (1888) and van der Putte and Neeteson (1983) show that the same pattern of development is followed in sheep and pigs. In Tourneux's drawings from sheep embryos the cloacal plate is shown to revert to a membrane over a very short distance posteriorly such that the urorectal septum appears to meet the *back* of the cloacal plate. Tourneux himself, however, noted that the midline of the perineum was initially formed by the endoderm covering the leading edge of the

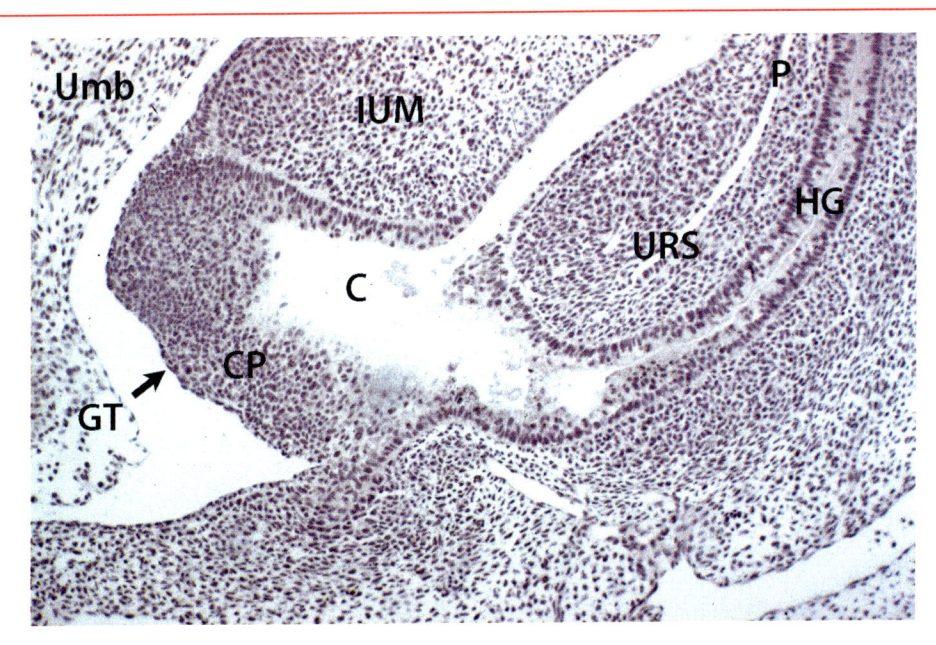

Fig. 5.1.4. Midsagittal section of day 13.5 rat embryo showing cloacal plate (*CP*) forming floor of cloaca (*C*) to tip of genital tubercle (*GT*). *HG* Hindgut, *IUM* infraumbilical mesenchyme, *P* prostate, *UM* umbilicus, *URS* urorectal septum

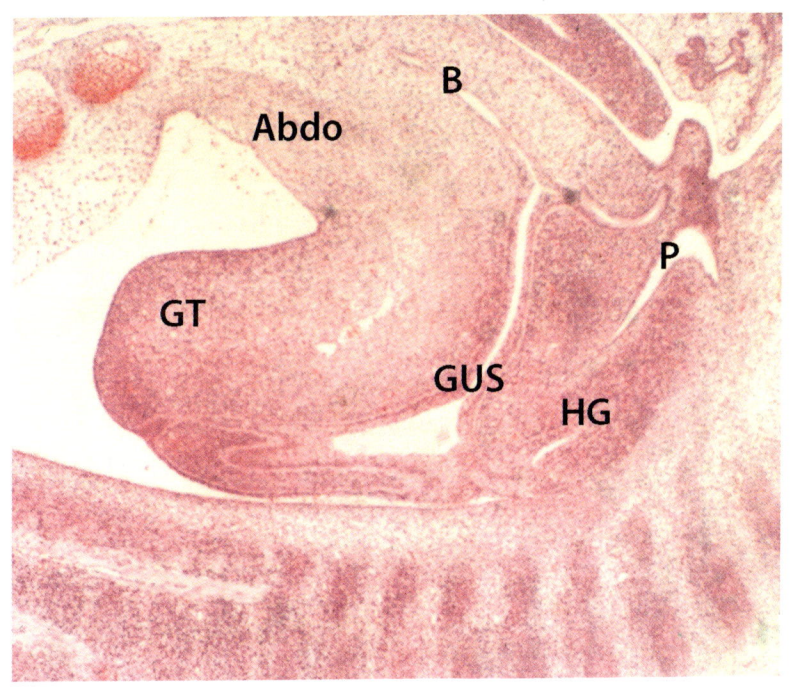

Fig. 5.1.5. Sagittal section of day 15 rat embryo, showing urorectal septum abutting cloacal plate to divide cloaca into genitourinary sinus (*GUS*) and hindgut (*HG*). *Abdo* Abdomen, *B* bladder, *GT* genital tubercle, *P* prostate

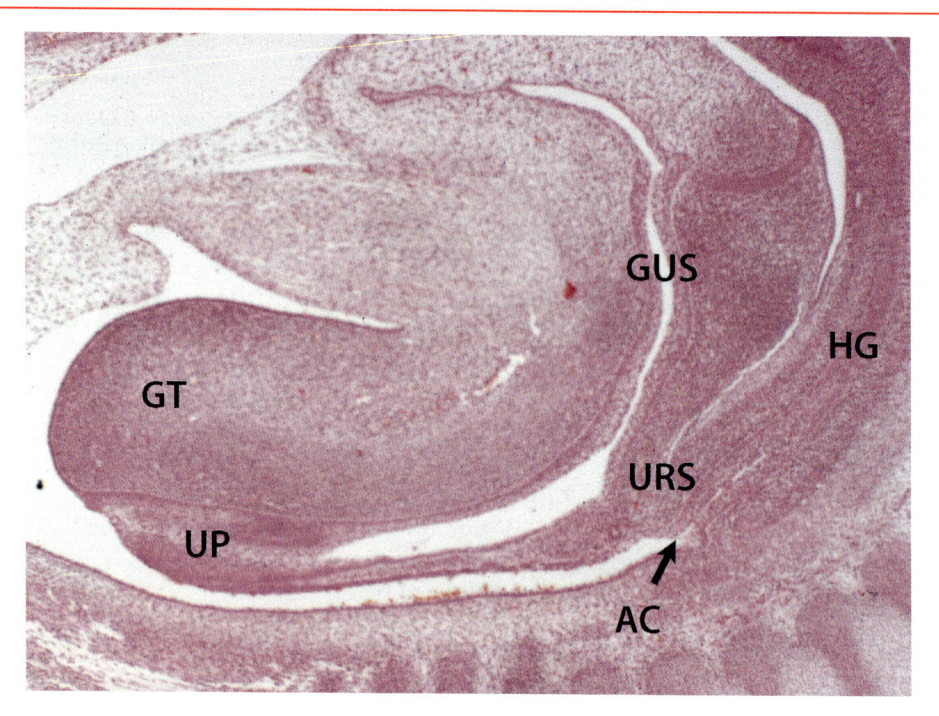

Fig. 5.1.6. Sagittal section of day 15.5 rat embryo showing patent anal canal (*AC*) and urethral plate (*UP*) extending to tip of genital tubercle (*GT*). *HG* Hindgut, *GUS* genitourinary sinus, *URS* urorectal septum

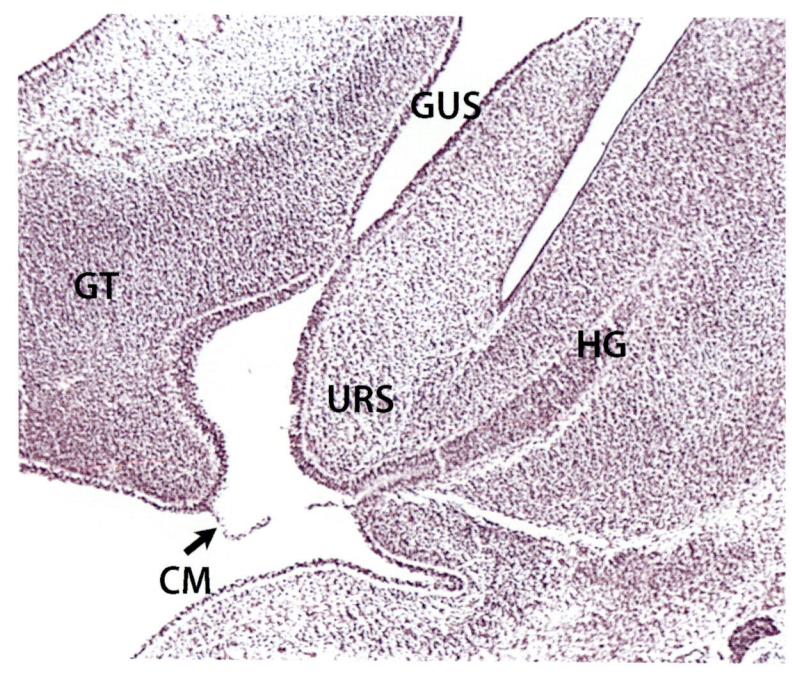

Fig. 5.1.7. Oblique sagittal section of 18-mm human embryo showing reformed cloacal membrane (*CM*) just caudal to urorectal septum (*URS*). Cloacal plate is out of plane of section ventrally. *GT* Genital tubercle, *HG* hindgut, *GUS* genitourinary sinus

urorectal septum. Van der Putte found a sequence of development in pigs similar to that described for humans (van der Putte and Neeteson 1983).

The ventral part of the cloacal plate persists as the *urethral plate* in both species, but from the time of rupture of the reformed posterior cloacal membrane in the human (and in pigs), the urogenital sinus and the hindgut are open to the amnion (Fig. 5.1.7), whereas in the rat there is no definite urogenital opening on the perineum until later in development (Qi et al. 2000).

The Urethral Plate and Formation of the Urethra

The origin of the urethral mucosa has been variously described as endodermal (van der Werff et al. 2000; Barnstein and Mossman 1938), ectodermal (Moore and Persaud 1993) or mixed (Wood-Jones 1904). In the 1950s Glenister proposed that the male urethra develops by a process of tubularisation of a sagittally oriented epithelial plate, which grows as an anterior extension of the endodermal lining of the genitourinary sinus into the perineal surface of the genital tubercle (Glenister 1954, 1958). He proposed that the plate and its contained urethra finally meet up with an ingrowth of epithelium at the tip of the glans to form the fossa navicularis.

Although Glenister's description of urethral development gained wide acceptance, his own study included photographs of the cloacal/urethral plate extending to the tip of the very early genital tubercle as discussed above. Several other authors have described the presence of the urethral plate throughout the length of the genital tubercle (Barnstein and Mossman 1938; Kanagasuntheram and Anandaraja 1960; Anderson and Clark 1990; Altemus and Hutchins 1991; Baskin 2000).

The formation of the urethra from the urethral plate is still a matter of speculation. The long-accepted assumption that the urethra forms by infolding of urogenital folds with midline fusion of the opposing sides has been challenged in recent times. Van der Putte's study in pigs (van der Putte and Neeteson 1983) failed to find evidence of midline urethral fusion on morphological grounds, and studies looking for evidence of epithelium to mesenchyme transformation, the hallmark of epithelial fusion, also failed to find evidence to prove that fusion plays a role in the formation of the urethra (Baskin 2000).

The presence of the perineal raphe is often cited as evidence for fusion playing a role in the formation of the urethra. It is worth noting, however, that other sites of skin fusion, such as the midline posteriorly over the vertebrae, are not marked by a skin "raphe". In hypospadias, the raphe can be seen to split at the distal limit of the spongiosus, with a "branch" extending to each corner of the dog-ears. Such a bifurcation belies the notion that the skin marking and the urethra form exclusively by a process of fusion.

Within the genital tubercle the urethral plate is hourglass in cross section, resembling urethral duplication. In female rat embryos the urethral plate undergoes massive apoptosis around day 19, exposing the internal surface of the urogenital sinus to the amnion and causing the genital tubercle to become folded down onto the perineum. Unopposed growth of the superior aspect of the genital tubercle accentuates the chordee resulting from involution of the urethral plate (Penington and Hutson 2003b).

In the male rat embryo the urethral plate becomes canalised progressively until the lumen finally reaches the tip of the genital tubercle. As also reported by van der Werff et al. (2000), canalisation results from apoptosis within the urethral plate. At the same time, the developing urethra becomes gradually separated from the external surface of the genital tubercle by growth of mesenchyme between the plate and the surface skin. There is no evidence of an ectodermal ingrowth from the tip of the phallus joining with the urethral plate.

The urethral plate similarly extends to the tip of the genital tubercle throughout development in human embryos. The urogenital sinus is open to the amniotic cavity from the time of breakdown of the cloacal membrane, but in other respects the anatomy is as described above for the rat. In particular, no significant ingrowth of ectoderm is seen in the developing glans.

It is possible that Glenister formed his opinion that ectoderm may be involved in male urethral development because of the stratified squamous epithelium of the urethral plate. The evidence, however, supports the view that this is entirely endodermal in origin, as is the oesophageal mucosa and the female urethra (Sadler 1990).

Some authors have proposed that the urethral plate is derived from an ectodermal fusion of the inner surfaces of paired genital swellings (van der Werff et al. 2000; Forsberg 1961; Barnstein and Mossman 1938; Pohlman 1911). However, careful study of both the rat and the human embryo failed to show any ectodermal contribution to the urethral plate. In addition, we failed to observe paired genital swellings in formation of the genital tubercle.

Phallus and Prepuce

Enlargement of the genital tubercle occurs by growth of the infraumbilical mesenchyme (Vermeij-Keers et al. 1996). Simultaneously the opening of the urogenital sinus is carried forward onto the shaft of the phallus by growth of mesenchyme from the urorectal septum and the developing perineal body. As the urethral plate is canalising by apoptosis, forward growth of the mesenchyme possibly contributes to development of the corpus spongiosum.

The prepuce begins to form as solid lamellae of epithelial cells (the glans lamellae) that dip into the genital tubercle dorsally and laterally, their proximal extent defining the floor of the coronal groove. The glans lamellae extend laterally and ventrally and become confluent with the margin of the urethral plate, and dorsally with its opposite fellow. Epithelial proliferation and desquamation causes a split in the lamella and raises a fold of skin, which then grows distally as a sleeve that covers the dorsum and sides of the glans. The frenulum and midventral foreskin form last as growth of the ventral penile mesenchyme reaches the tip of the penis.

Abnormal Development in Hypospadias

Abnormal morphogenesis in hypospadias affects three main anatomical features: (1) the ectopic urethral orifice, (2) the abnormal foreskin, including irregular penile raphe and dorsal hood, and (3) the chordee, or congenital bend in the penis observed on erection (Stephens et al. 2002) (Fig. 5.1.8).

Ectopic Orifice

The primary anomaly in nearly all cases of hypospadias is failure of the midline perineal mesenchyme to grow ventrally to cover the urethral plate as it canalises. Incomplete morphogenesis is the commonest embryological defect, and in hypospadias the opening of the urethra is commonly arrested at or near the coronal groove of the glans. This position is normal in 9- and 10-week human embryos (Fig. 5.1.9) (Clarnette et al. 1997). Where the opening is more proximal on the penile shaft or in the perineum, it suggests a more severe local anatomical anomaly or a defect in androgenic action. The most proximal opening in the perineum, representing the original opening of the urogenital sinus and the normal site of the urethra in females, is seen in complex anatomical defects of perineal morphogenesis (often with imperforate anus) or in forms of intersex.

Fig. 5.1.8. Diagrams of clinical forms of hypospadias and corresponding embryological stages of development/gestation time and corresponding crown-rump length. *A* Perineal, urethral plate (*arrow*). *A′* Open urogenital sinus, inner and outer genital folds, proximal urethral orifice. *B* Scrotal, perineal raphe (*bottom arrow*), bifurcated raphe (*middle arrow*), distal urethral plate (*top arrow*). *B′* Partly covered urethral plate with scrotal raphe. *C* Mid-penile orifice, Littre gland orifice (*lower arrow*), dog-ear (*upper arrow*). *C′* Urethral plate (*arrow*) in urethral groove. *D* Distal penile orifice, bifurcation of raphe hypoplastic triangle of skin (*arrow*). *D′* Urethral plate open on glans. *E, E′* Coronal orifice, deficient ventral prepuce. *F, F′* Navicular orifice. *G* Mid-glanular orifice. *G′* Frenular attachment to glans (*arrow*). *H, H′* Sub-apical orifice (stenotic), deviated raphe. (Reproduced with permission from Stephen et al. 2002, Martin Dunitz)

Failure of the urethral plate to be covered by mesenchyme (and skin) leaves the outer genital folds separated as two hemiscrota. An open midline gutter with pin-point orifices of presumed Littre's glands distal to the ectopic orifice indicates the persisting urethral plate.

Dorsal Hood and Raphe

The dorsal hooded prepuce is characteristic of hypospadias and may be explained by failure of androgen-dependent growth of the ventral penile mesenchyme. This leaves a wedge-shaped defect in the ventral prepuce, including an absent frenulum. At each corner of the dorsal hood, the bifurcated penile raphe ends in a "dog-ear" (Fig. 5.1.10). The dog-ears represent the most distal points of external preputial skin that would normally be joined together. In the more severe forms of hypospadias where the dorsal skin of the penis remains fused with the scrotal folds, there are no dog-ears.

The median raphe of the phallus is abnormal in hypospadias (Fig. 5.1.11). Deficiency of mesenchymal growth along the shaft may lead to a zigzag course of the raphe. Just proximal to the ectopic orifice the raphe bifurcates, with each branch continuing distally to the dog-ears on the prepuce. These raphe branches indicate the distal edge of migration of the mesenchyme that forms the Buck's fascia and subcutaneous tissue, which are lacking in the triangular area between the branches. In cases where the raphe bifurcates some distance proximal to the orifice, the urethra is very superficial and lacks adequate supporting tissue and corpus spongiosum.

Embryology and Anatomy of Hypospadias 69

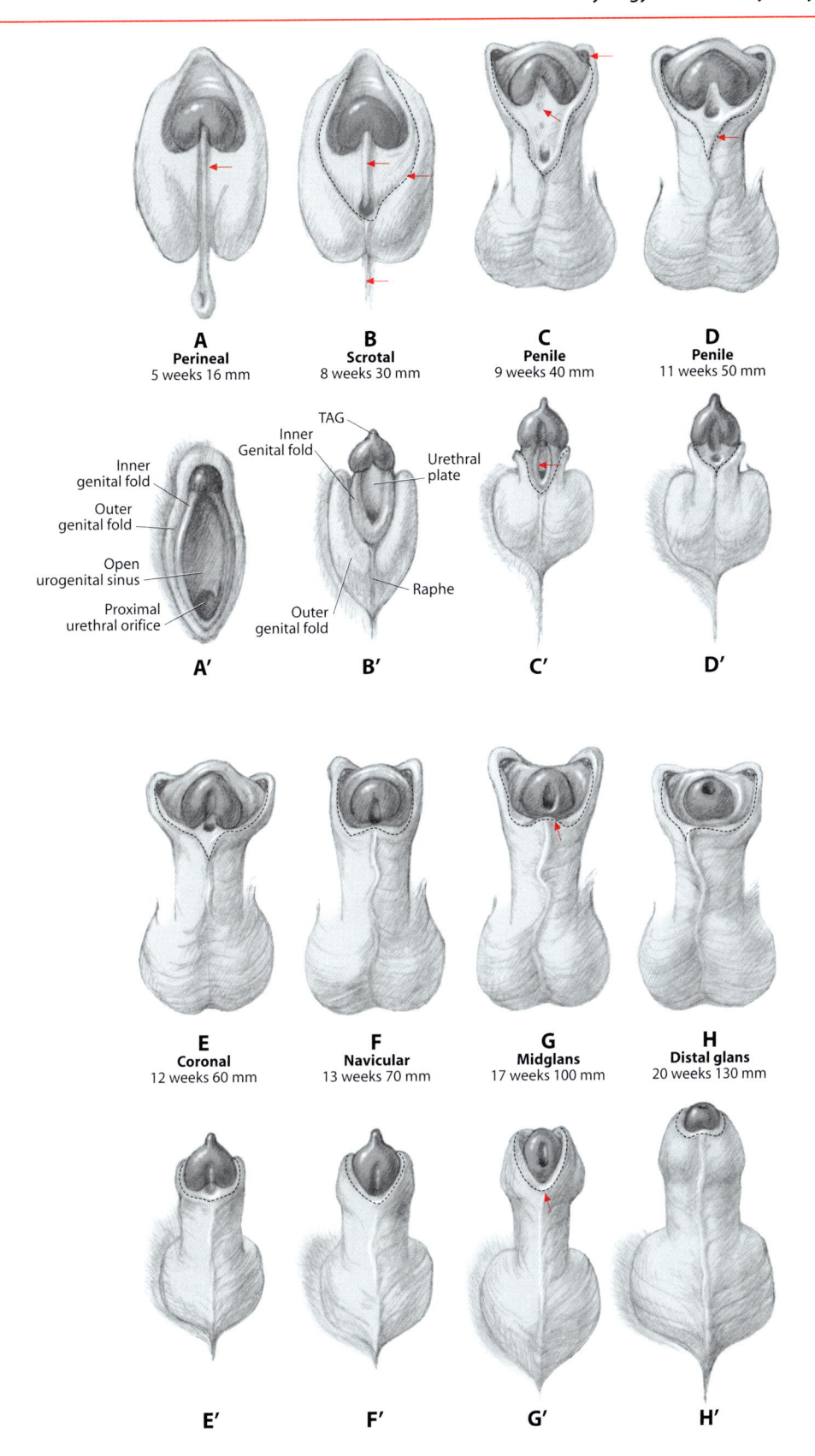

A Perineal 5 weeks 16 mm
B Scrotal 8 weeks 30 mm
C Penile 9 weeks 40 mm
D Penile 11 weeks 50 mm

A′ — Inner genital fold, Outer genital fold, Open urogenital sinus, Proximal urethral orifice
B′ — TAG, Inner Genital fold, Urethral plate, Outer genital fold, Raphe
C′
D′

E Coronal 12 weeks 60 mm
F Navicular 13 weeks 70 mm
G Midglans 17 weeks 100 mm
H Distal glans 20 weeks 130 mm

E′
F′
G′
H′

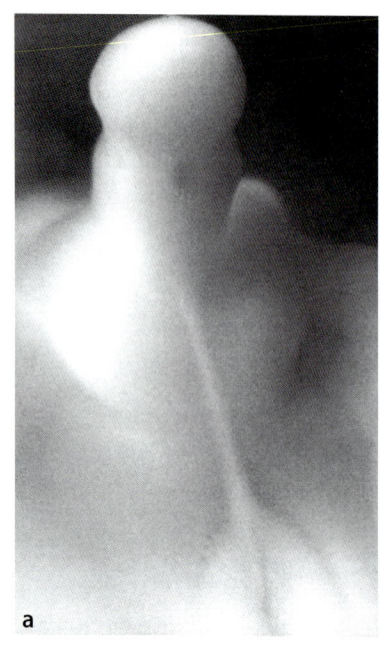

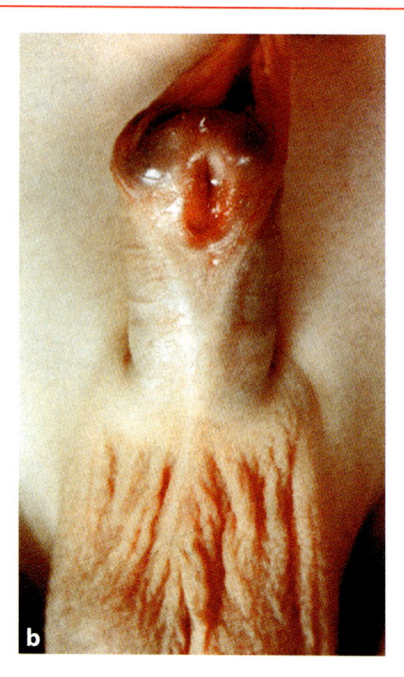

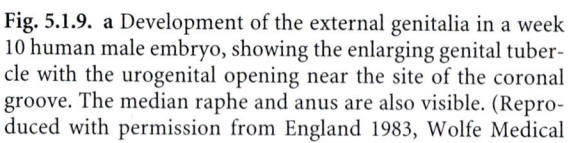

Fig. 5.1.9. a Development of the external genitalia in a week 10 human male embryo, showing the enlarging genital tubercle with the urogenital opening near the site of the coronal groove. The median raphe and anus are also visible. (Reproduced with permission from England 1983, Wolfe Medical Publications). **b** Opening of the urethra at the coronal groove in a boy with hypospadias. Note that the urethral plate has broken down distally to form a groove, but the urethral orifice remains proximal

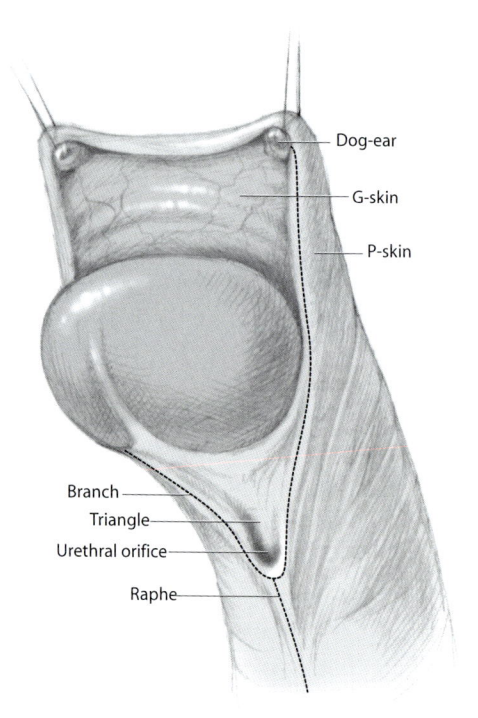

Fig. 5.1.10. Features of hypospadias with chordee. Ectopic urethral orifice triangle between branches of raphe and glans; penile skin of outer genital folds (*P-skin*); inner skin of prepuce (*G-skin*) and the two skin tufts (dog-ears of prepuce). (Reproduced with permission from Stephens et al. 2002; Martin Dunitz)

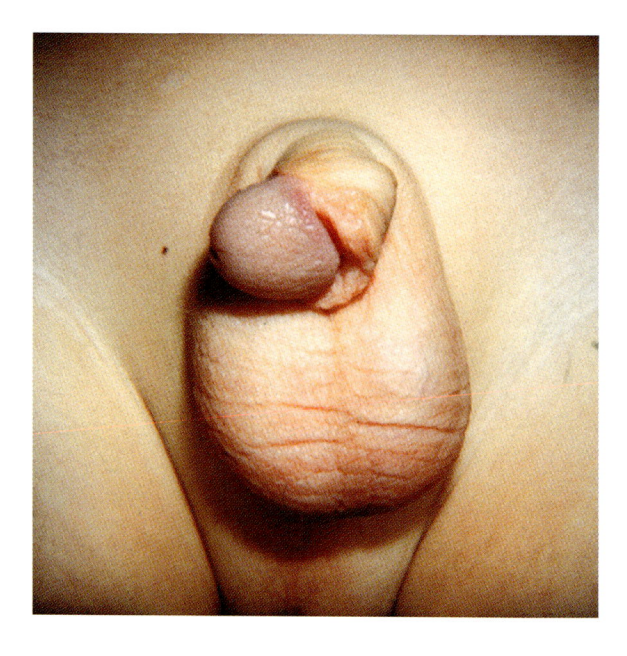

Fig. 5.1.11. Penile torsion with 90° rotation

Chordee

Chordee is present in most patients with hypospadias, but is related to the severity of the underlying anomaly. In a group of 46 patients with hypospadias, chordee was present in all perineal or scrotal anomalies (7/7), 15 of 16 cases with penile or coronal hypospadias, and in 11 of 23 of those with glanular hypospadias (Cook and Stephens 1998).

The perineal and scrotal anomalies showed feminine development of the phallus consistent with possible testicular dysplasia and/or abnormal function of androgens (Rowsell and Morgan 1987). The phallus showed a hairpin bend of the corpora cavernosa similar to the clitoris, which is known to be produced by apoptosis of the urethral plate in the absence of androgenic stimulation (Penington and Hutson 2003b).

In more distal variants, the arrest of mesenchymal growth and/or the initiation of apoptosis occurs later, leading to progressively less severe chordee, with most of the chordee caused by deficient periurethral growth rather than a bend in the corpora. In glanular hypospadias, chordee also may result from deficient growth of the distal urethral plate (Ben-Ari et al. 1985), although the appearance of a short urethral plate may simply result from relatively greater growth of the dorsal side of the developing glans.

References

Altemus AR, Hutchins GM: Development of the human anterior urethra. J Urol. 1991; 146:1085–1093.
Anderson CA, Clark RL: External genitalia of the rat: normal development and the histogenesis of 5-alpha-reductase inhibitor-induced abnormalities. Teratology. 1990; 42: 483–496.
Arey LB: Developmental anatomy, 7th edn. Saunders, Philadelphia, 1965.
Barnstein NJ, Mossman HW: The origin of the penile urethra and bulbo-urethral glands with particular reference to the red squirrel (*Tamiasciurus hudsonicus*). Anat Rec. 1938; 72:67–85.
Baskin LS: Hypospadias and urethral development. J Urol. 2000; 163:951–956.
Ben-Ari J, Merlob P, Mimouni F, et al: Characteristics of the male urethra in the newborn penis. J Urol. 1985; 134:521–522.
Clarnette TD, Sugita Y, Hutson JM: Genital anomalies in human and animal models reveal the mechanisms and hormones governing testicular descent. Br J Urol. 1997; 79:99–112.
Cook WA, Stephens FD: Pathoembryology of the urinary tract. In: King LR (ed) Urological surgery in neonates and young infants. Saunders, Philadelphia, 1988; pp 1–23.
de Vries PA, Friedland GW: The staged sequential development of the anus and rectum in human embryos and fetuses. J Pediatr Surg. 1987; 9:755–769.
England MA: A colour atlas of life before birth. Normal fetal development. Wolfe Medical Publications, Weert, Netherlands; 1983.
Forsberg JG: On the development of the cloaca and the perineum and the formation of the urethral plate in female rat embryos. J Anat. 1961; 95:423–435.
Glenister TW: The origin and fate of the urethral plate in man. J Anat. 1954; 88:413–425.
Glenister TW: A correlation of the normal and abnormal development of the penile urethra and of the infra-umbilical abdominal wall. Br J Urol. 1958; 30:117–126.
Kanagasuntheram R, Anandaraja S: Development of the terminal urethra and prepuce in the dog. J Anat. 1960; 94: 121–129.
Kluth D, Lambrecht W, Reich P: Pathogenesis of hypospadias – more questions than answers. J Pediatr Surg. 1988; 23: 1095–1101.
Moore KL, Persaud TVN: The developing human, 5th edn. Saunders, Philadelphia, 1993.
Nievelstein RAJ, van der Werff JFA, Verbeek FJ, et al: Normal and abnormal embryonic development of the anorectum in human embryos. Teratology. 1998; 57:70–78.
Paidas CN, Morreale RF, Holoski KM, et al: Septation and differentiation of the embryonic human cloaca. J Pediatr Surg. 1999; 34:877–884.
Penington EC, Hutson JM: The cloacal plate – the missing link in anorectal and urogenital development. BJU Int. 2002; 89:726–732.
Penington EC, Hutson JM: The urethral plate – does it grow into the genital tubercle or with it? BJU. Int. 2002; 89:733–739.
Penington EC: MD Thesis, University of Melbourne, 2002.
Pohlman AG: The development of the cloaca in human embryos. Am J Anat. 1911; 12:1–26.
Qi BQ, Williams A, Beasley S, et al: Clarification of the process of separation of the cloaca into rectum and urogenital sinus in the rat embryo. J Pediatr Surg. 2000; 35:1810–1816.
Rowsell AR, Morgan BDE: Hypospadias and the embryogenesis of the penile urethra. Br J Plastic Surg. 1987; 40: 201–206.
Sadler TW: Langman's medical embryology, 6th edn. Williams and Wilkins, Baltimore, 1990, pp 237–259.
Setchell BP: Reproduction in male marsupials. In: Stonehouse B, Gilmore G (eds): The biology of marsupials. Macmillan, London, 1977; pp 411–455.
Stephens FD, Smith ED, Hutson JM: Congenital anomalies of the kidney, urinary and genital tracts, 2nd edn. Dunitz, London, 2002.
Tourneux F: Sur les premiers développements du cloaque du tubercule génital et de l'anus chez l'embryon de mouton. Anat Physiol. 1888; 24:503–517.
Van der Putte SCJ, Neeteson FA: The normal development of the anorectum in the pig. Acta Morphol Neerl Scand. 1983; 21:107–132.
van der Werff JFA, Nievelstein RAJ, Brands E, et al: Normal development of the male anterior urethra. Teratology 2000; 61:172–183.
Vermeij-Keers C, Hartwig NG, vander Werff, JFA: Embryonic development of the ventral body wall and its congenital malformations. Semin Pediatr Surg. 1996; 5:82–89.
Wood-Jones F: The nature of the malformations of the rectum and urogenital passages. BMJ. 1904; 2:1630–1634.

Blood Supply of the Penile Skin

Zacharias Zachariou

Introduction

Most cases of hypospadias, regardless of severity, are associated with a prepuce that could be sufficient to create a neourethra to bridge the existing gap and cover the repair with skin. Success is in a major part dependent on three preconditions:
- The inner layer of the prepuce has to be long enough.
- The epithelial surface of the prepuce has to be adequate.
- The subcutaneous tissue between the outer and inner layer of the prepuce has to be sufficient and carry enough blood vessels for vascularisation of the two layers.

However, any technique using the prepuce for the repair jeopardises the blood supply, endangering the result. Knowledge of the blood supply of the prepuce is essential so that preservation of the preputial vascularisation is not merely fortuitous.

Embryology

At approximately 8 weeks of gestation the penis and the glans develop from the genital tubercle. At this point the prepuce has not yet developed. At the beginning of the 10th week symmetrical low ridges arise just proximal to the coronal sulcus, progressing dorsally until they form a fold surrounding the glans, leaving the ventral midline uncovered, where they are blocked by the incompletely developed urethra (Fig. 5.2.1a) (Hunter 1936). This nascent prepuce rolls over the base of the glans, leaving a groove between it and the coronal sulcus. This groove is filled simultaneously with actively proliferating glanular lamella, an ingrowth of epithelium many cells thick (Fig. 5.2.1b) (Glenister 1954, 1956). Due to an enormous active proliferation of the epithelium at the apex (proximal end) of the groove, the ridge of the preputial fold is pulled towards the summit of the glans, which is then overtopped owing to proliferation of the mesenchyme of the epithelial layers (Fig. 5.2.1c). By the 30th week of gestation the single epithelial layer between the developed prepuce and the glans begins to split into two layers from the distal ridge (Deibert 1933). This procedure continues till birth when the two layers have been formed (Fig. 5.2.1d). They are still connected with the glans by desquamated epithelium.

In summary the prepuce is formed by three processes:
- The skin is folded at the base of the glans, creating a groove.
- A shelf is formed by epithelial cells which proliferate in the groove and carry the prepuce to the summit of the glans. Mesenchymal growth within the prepuce supports the development.
- Two prepuce layers are formed due to separation of the epithelial layer between the prepuce and the glans.

The preputial skin with its accompanying superficial fascia and vessels is ideal for the constructions of flaps for hypospadias repair. It is relatively thin and pliable, and especially the thin epithelialised layer on the inside of the prepuce tolerates prolonged contact with urine better than any other tissue except the bladder urothelium.

Preputial Arterial Supply and Venous Drainage

The blood supply of the penile skin is symmetrical (Juskiewenski et al. 1982). The superior and inferior external pudendal arteries arise from the femoral artery. They are attached to the Scarpa fascia, which extends to the base of the penis. At this point they divide into four branches as superficial penile arteries. Two enter the superficial penile fascia (Colles fascia) dorsolaterally and two enter it ventrolaterally (Fig. 5.2.2). Numerous collaterals between these four arteries create a fine subcutaneous arterial plexus

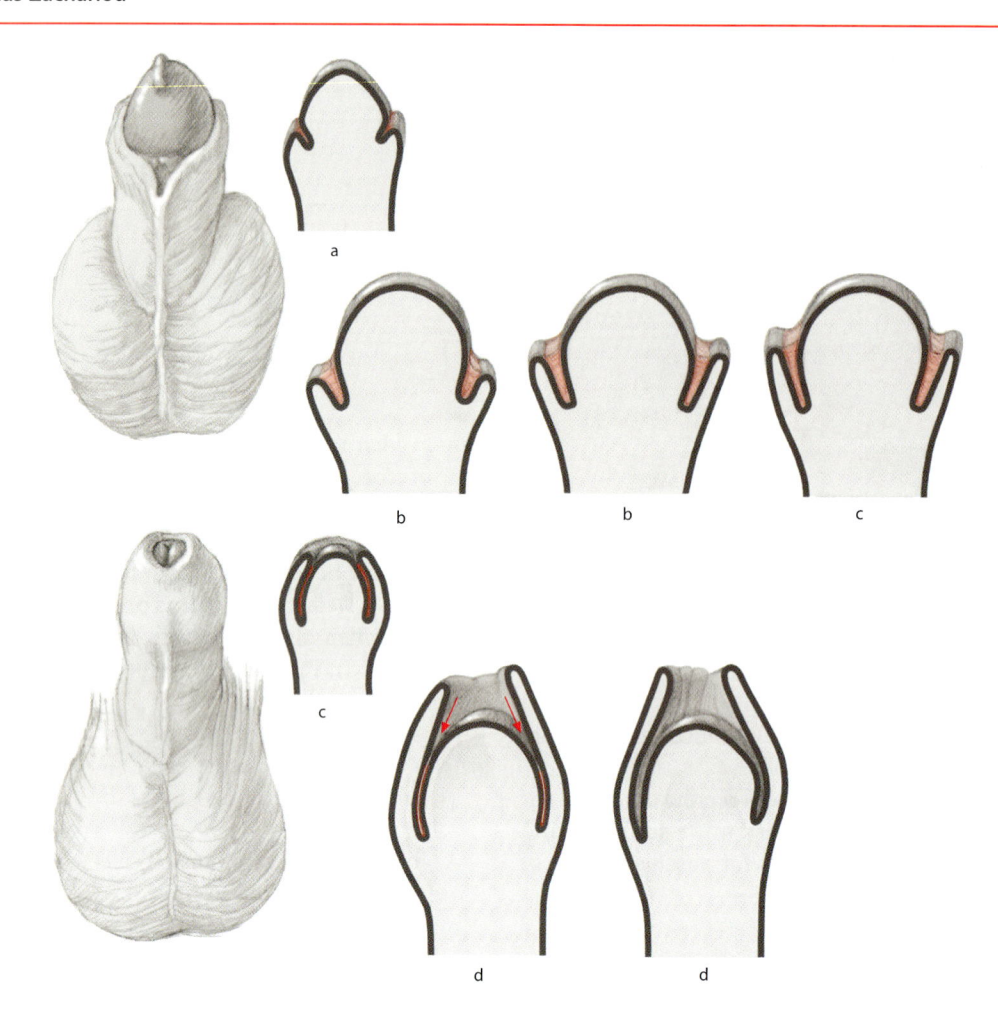

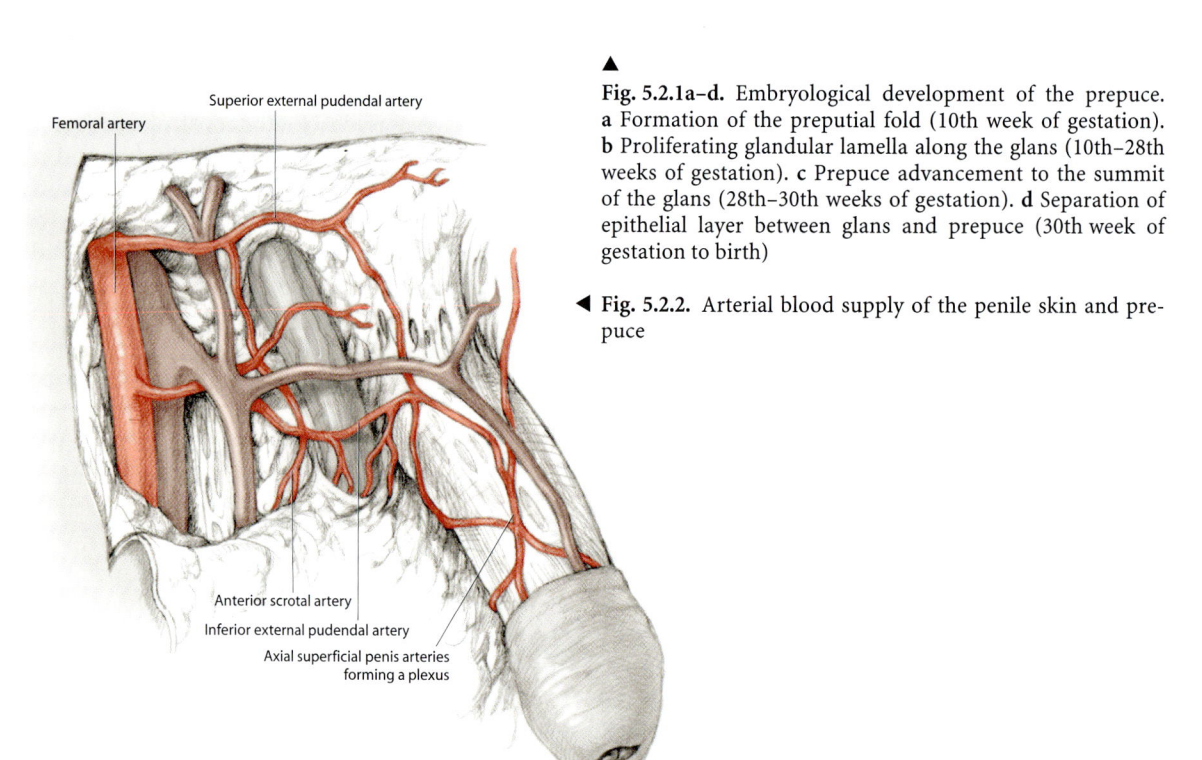

Fig. 5.2.1a–d. Embryological development of the prepuce. **a** Formation of the preputial fold (10th week of gestation). **b** Proliferating glandular lamella along the glans (10th–28th weeks of gestation). **c** Prepuce advancement to the summit of the glans (28th–30th weeks of gestation). **d** Separation of epithelial layer between glans and prepuce (30th week of gestation to birth)

Fig. 5.2.2. Arterial blood supply of the penile skin and prepuce

up to the preputial ring (Fig. 5.2.3) (Quartey 1997). Behind the sulcus in the distal part of the penile shaft, small vessels penetrate the Buck's fascia, making an anastomosis with the dorsal penile artery. Beyond the preputial ring on the inner surface the terminal branches become minute (Fig. 5.2.4). Variations of the superficial penile arteries are possible with dominance of one side pair.

The blood supply to the frenulum is also symmetrical and arises from the dorsal penile artery, which branches at the level of the sulcus with small arteries that curve around each side of the distal shaft to enter the glans and the frenulum ventrally (Fig. 5.2.5).

The venous drainage of the penile skin and prepuce is less well organised (Fig. 5.2.6). Multiple minute veins in the prepuce form a plexus without particular orientation joining the superficial dorsal penile vein, which drains into the external pudendal vein, which in turn empties into the saphenous or femoral vein.

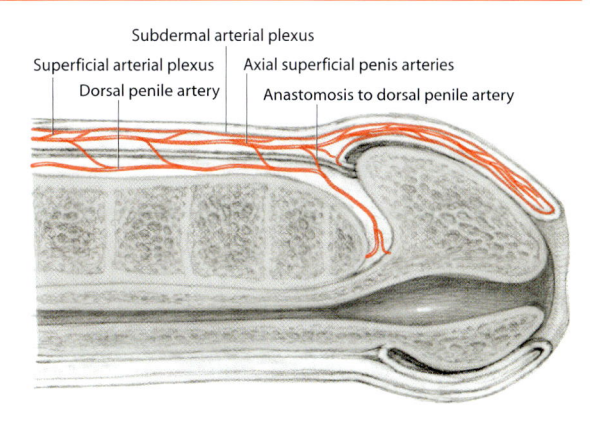

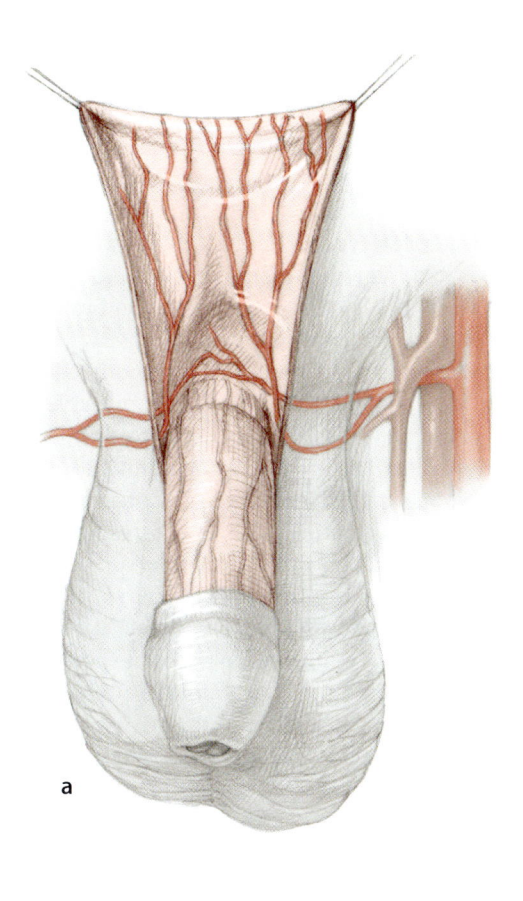

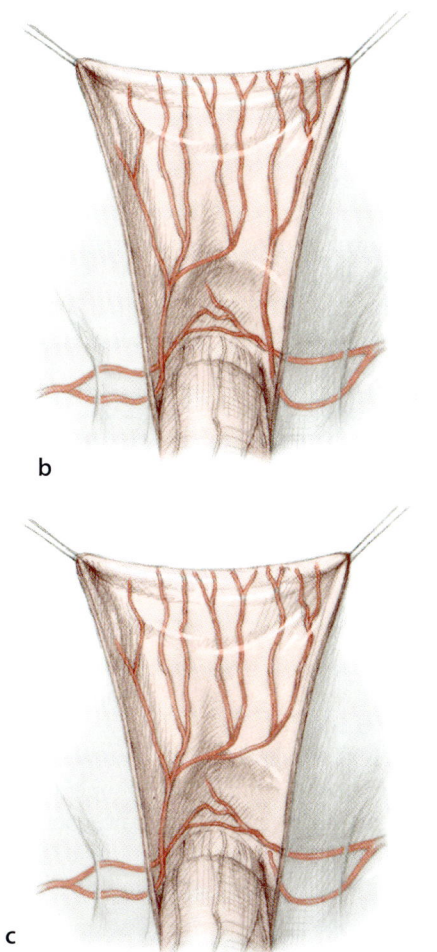

Fig. 5.2.3. Peripheral arterial blood supply of the penis

Fig. 5.2.4a–c. End arteries to the prepuce: **a** normal blood supply, equal distribution from both sides; **b, c** dominant right-sided distribution

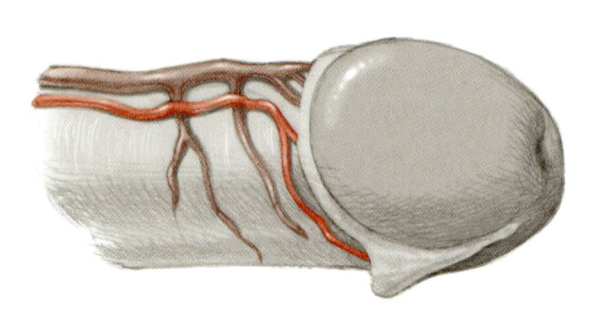

Fig. 5.2.5. Arterial blood supply of the frenulum

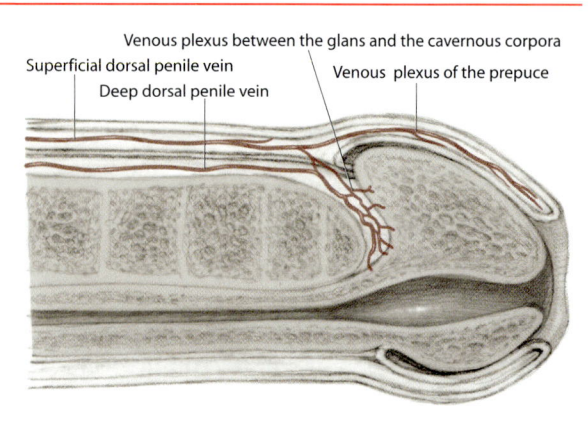

Fig. 5.2.6. Peripheral venous drainage of the penis

Surgical Considerations

According to the anatomical studies of Hinman (1991), the prepuce develops over a mesodermal core that is later split, and not by distal shaft skin sliding to cover the glans. Although its arterial blood supply would be expected to run distally in the connective core terminating at the preputial ring, this is not the case. The arterial supply of the prepuce origins from the dorsal aspect of the penis, and the minute arteries supplying the outer prepuce layer fold by 180° to terminate at the corona (Fig. 5.2.3). The reason is that the prepuce must form a one-layer skin sheet during erection and the terminal vessels become straightened when erection and preputial retraction begin. When erection terminates the prepuce vessels loop back upon themselves, terminating at the corona and not at the preputial ring (Fig. 5.2.7).

Taking into consideration the above-mentioned anatomy, an incision along the coronal sulcus would not damage the arterial supply of the prepuce in any way as the vessels terminate at this site (Fig. 5.2.8a). The inner layer of the prepuce can be dissected without jeopardising the vascular pedicle (Fig. 5.2.8b). After separation of the outer layer of the prepuce and careful dissection of the vascular pedicle the flap may be rolled into a tube for construction of the neourethra (Fig. 5.2.8c).

However, the clinical experience of a number of authors that have widely published their operative results as well as the follow-up of a great number of patients has not encountered the limitations of the above-mentioned embryoanatomical premises.

Conclusions

The surgeon performing hypospadias repair using a pedicle flap has to be aware of the normal vascularisation of the prepuce. Although it is very difficult to identify individual arterial variations, especially during surgery, it is of great importance to look for them. These vessels can be then used individually, selectively or collectively, according to the anatomical variation present and the choice of flap to be performed. In the majority of cases the desired success should be guaranteed. However, in addition, some rules have to be kept in mind when operating:

- Keep intact at least one of the two branches of the right or left external pudendal artery.
- Perform only longitudinal incisions in the superficial penile fascia in order to preserve the axial arrangement of the superficial plexus.
- Consider the prepuce as one unit with a common blood supply to the inner and outer prepuce layers.
- The inner epithelial layer, corresponding to the more distal part of the unfolded prepuce, must be left generously attached to the superficial fascia supplying it with blood.
- The outer epithelial layer, corresponding to the proximal part of the unfolded prepuce, is to be used to cover the neourethra. The preservation of its arterial blood supply is essential.
- The use of magnification for identifying the terminal, minute arterial vessels is in my opinion a prerequisite for every hypospadias repair.

Blood Supply of the Penile Skin 77

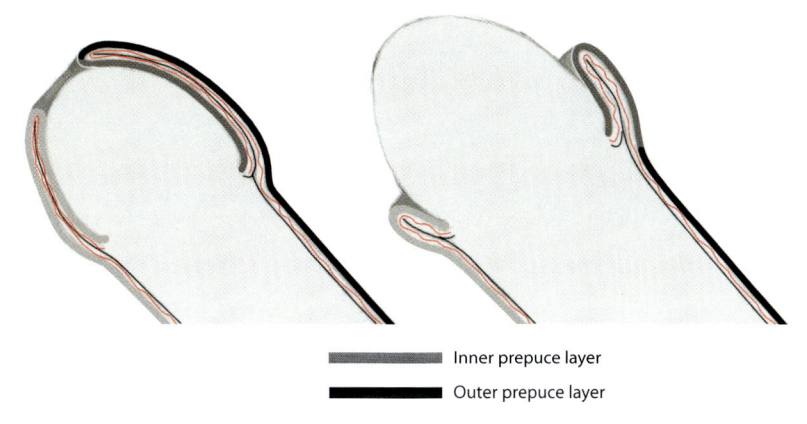

Fig. 5.2.7. One-layer skin sheet of the prepuce during erection

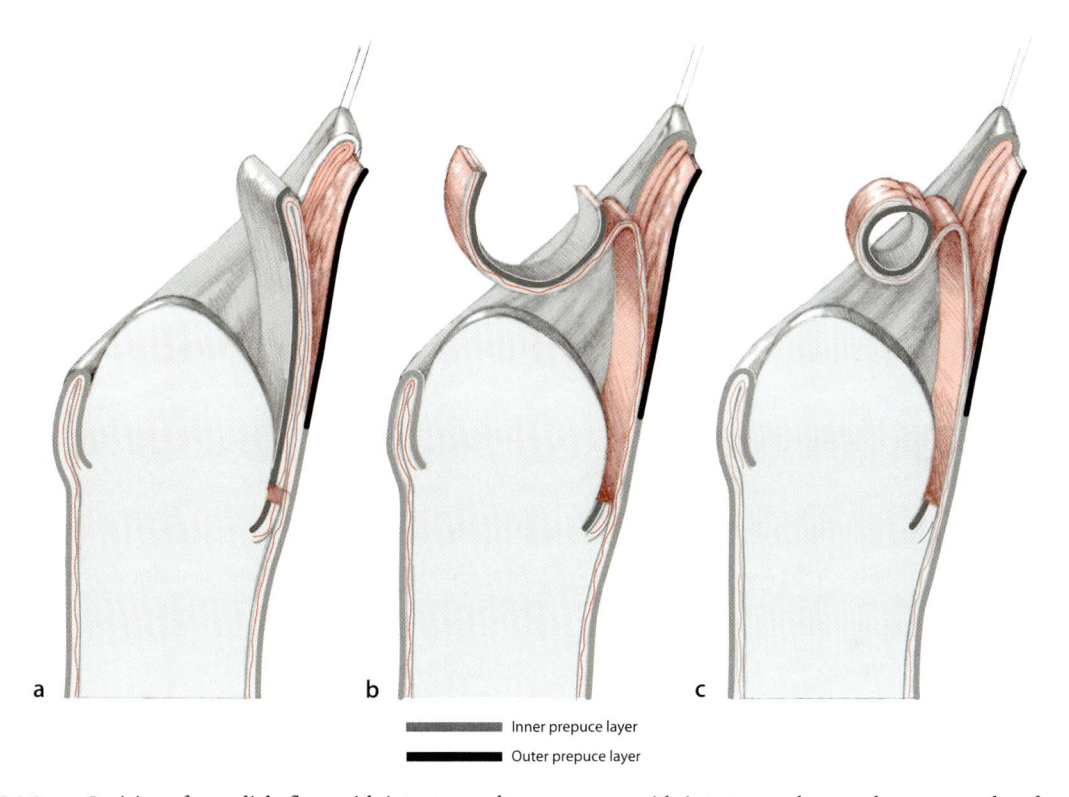

Fig. 5.2.8a–c. Incisions for pedicle flaps with intact vascular blood supply: **a** incision at the coronal sulcus where the vessels terminate; **b** dissection of the inner and outer layer of the prepuce with intact vascular supply; **c** neourethra from the inner prepuce layer and well-vascularised outer prepuce layer to cover the defect

References

Deibert GA: The separation of the prepuce in the human penis. Anat Rec. 1933; 57:387.
Glenister TW: The origin and fate of the urethral plate in man. J Anat. 1954; 88:413.
Glenister TW: A consideration of the processes involved in the development of the prepuce in man. Br J Urol. 1956; 28:243.
Hinman F: The blood supply to preputial island flaps. J Urol. 1991; 145:1232–1235.
Hunter RH: Notes on the development of the prepuce. J Anat. 1936; 70:68.
Juskiewenski S, Vaysse P, Moscovici J: A study of the arterial blood supply to the penis. Anat Clin. 1982; 4:101.
Quartey JKM: Microcirculation of penile and scrotal skin. Atlas Urol Clin North Am. 1997; 5:1

Classification of Hypospadias

Ahmed T. Hadidi

5.3

The anatomic classification of hypospadias recognizes the level of the meatus without taking into account curvature. In Smith's classification, the first degree locates the meatus from the corona to the distal shaft, the second degree from the distal shaft to the penoscrotal junction, and the third degree is from the penoscrotal junction to the perineum (Smith 1938). Schaefer and Erbes (1950) classified the location as glanular from the subcorona out, penile from the corona to the penoscrotal junction, and perineal from there down. The system of Browne (1936) was more specific, with subcoronal, penile, midshaft, penoscrotal, scrotal and perineal varieties. Duckett (1966) classified hypospadias according to meatal location after release of curvature into anterior, middle and posterior hypospadias.

Confusion stems from the methods of classification of hypospadias in general use. The deformity is usually described according to the site of meatus. The degree of chordee is not usually remarked upon and may go unnoticed except by urologists with wide experience in these diseases. Therefore, many authors prefer the classification specifying the new location of the meatus after the curvature has been released (Barcat 1973).

Welch (1979) collected more than 1000 cases of hypospadias from seven separate reports and estimated that 62% of the openings were subcoronal or penile, 22% were at the penoscrotal angle, and 16% opened in the scrotum or perineum. Juskiewenski and colleagues (1983) reported a study of 536 patients with hypospadias. Anterior hypospadias comprised 71%, middle 16%, and posterior 13%. Juskiewenski subdivided the hypospadias of the anterior group of 383 patients into 13% balanic, 43% subcoronal, 38% distal shaft and 6% with prepuce intact. Out of 1286 cases over 5 years at the Children's Hospital of Philadelphia, Duckett (1996) reported that 49% were anterior, 21% were middle, and 30% were in a posterior location (Fig. 5.3.1).

However, from a practical clinical point of view the detailed subclassifications may seem rather theoretical. Moreover, there are no specific operations designed for midpenile hypospadias. Depending on the actual position of the meatus after curvature correction, one uses either techniques designed for distal or proximal hypospadias. Also, most surgeons use the same techniques for proximal, penoscrotal and perineal hypospadias.

In order to achieve a universal, comparable classification, two assessments are recommended: (1) A preoperative assessment, based on the clinical site of the meatus, should indicate the presence or absence of visible chordee (2) An intraoperative assessment based on the position of the meatus after correction of chordee or penile curvature. Ideally, the classification should embrace condition of prepuce, chordee, rotation and scrotal transposition (if present).

Thus, the proposed classification should indicate:
1. Site of urethral meatus (before chordee correction):
   a) Glanular hypospadias
   b) Distal penile hypospadias
   c) Proximal hypospadias
2. Site of urethral meatus (after chordee correction):
   a) Glanular hypospadias
   b) Distal penile hypospadias
   c) Proximal hypospadias
3. Prepuce (complete or incomplete)
4. Glans, (cleft, incomplete cleft or flat; Fig. 5.3.2) (see Chap. 27)
5. Chordee (present or absent)
6. Urethral plate width (<1 cm, ≥1 cm)
7. Penile rotation (present or absent)
8. Scrotal transposition (present or absent)

Such a classification (Fig. 5.3.3) should help to standardise the description of the different types of hypospadias and associated malformations all over the world. This should make it easier to conduct multicentre prospective studies and also facilitate objective evaluation and comparison of the results of different surgical techniques in different centres.

80 Ahmed T. Hadidi

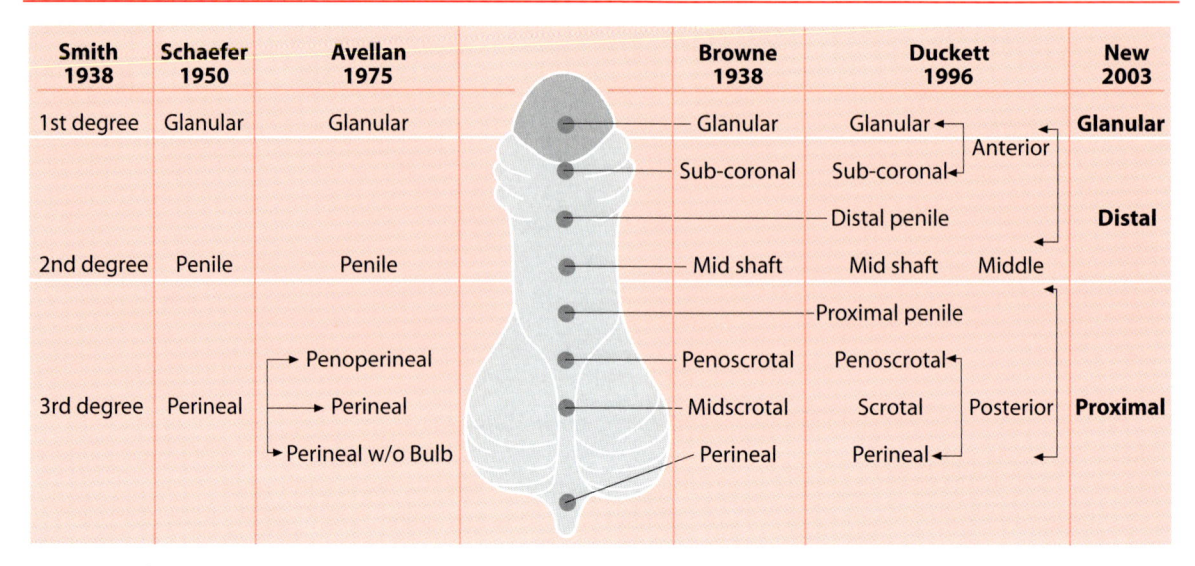

Smith 1938	Schaefer 1950	Avellan 1975		Browne 1938	Duckett 1996		New 2003
1st degree	Glanular	Glanular		Glanular	Glanular ← Anterior		**Glanular**
				Sub-coronal	Sub-coronal ←		
				Distal penile			**Distal**
2nd degree	Penile	Penile		Mid shaft	Mid shaft	Middle	
					Proximal penile		
		→ Penoperineal		Penoscrotal	Penoscrotal ←		
3rd degree	Perineal	→ Perineal		Midscrotal	Scrotal	Posterior	**Proximal**
		→ Perineal w/o Bulb		Perineal	Perineal ←		

Fig. 5.3.1. Different classifications of hypospadias, according to location of meatus. (Modified from Sheldon and Duckett 1987)

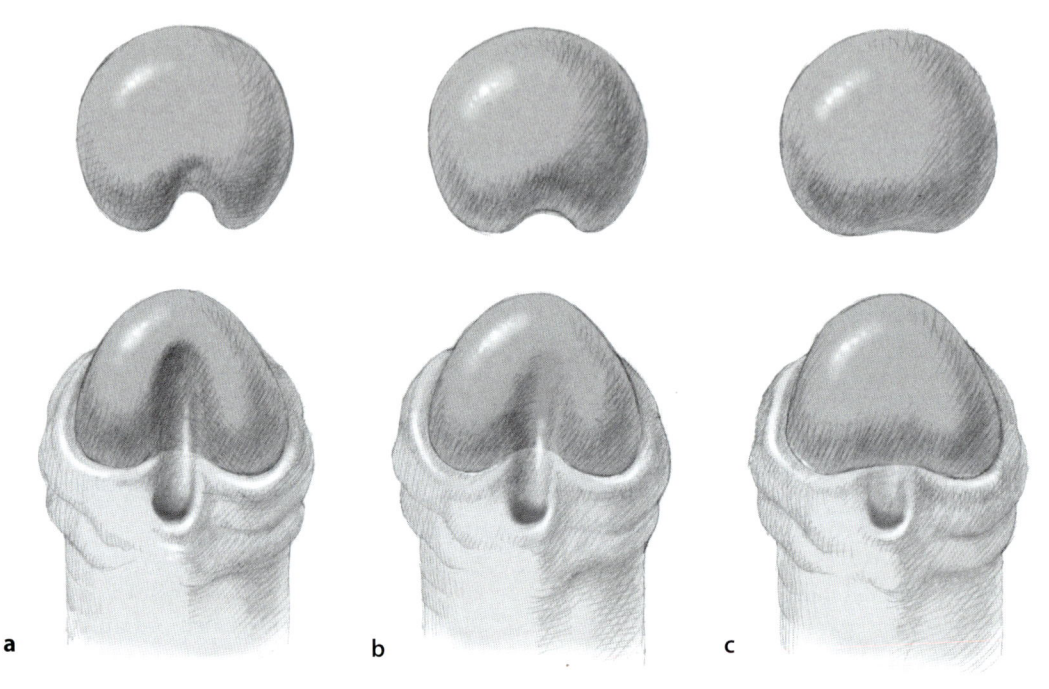

Fig. 5.3.2a–c. Classification of glans configuration in hypospadias. **a** *Cleft glans.* There is a deep groove in the middle of the glans with proper clefting; the urethral plate is narrow and projects to the tip of the glans. **b** *Incomplete cleft glans.* There is a variable degree of glans split, a shallow glanular groove and a variable degree of urethral plate projection. **c** *Flat glans.* The urethral plate ends short of the glans penis, no glanular groove. There may be a variable degree of chordee, especially in proximal forms of hypospadias

Classification of Hypospadias

1. Site of urethral meatus (before chordee correction): Glanular Hypospadias ☐ Distal Penile Hypospadias ☐ Proximal Hypospadias ☐

2. Site of urethral meatus (after chordee correction): Glanular Hypospadias ☐ Distal Penile Hypospadias ☐ Proximal Hypospadias ☐

3. Prepuce: Complete ☐ Incomplete ☐

4. Glans: Cleft ☐ Incomplete cleft ☐ Flat ☐

5. Chordee: No chordee ☐ Superficial chordee ☐ Deep chordee ☐

6. Urethral plate width: <1cm ☐ ≥1cm ☐

7. Penile torsion: No torsion ☐ Present ☐

8. Scrotal transposition: No transposition ☐ Present ☐

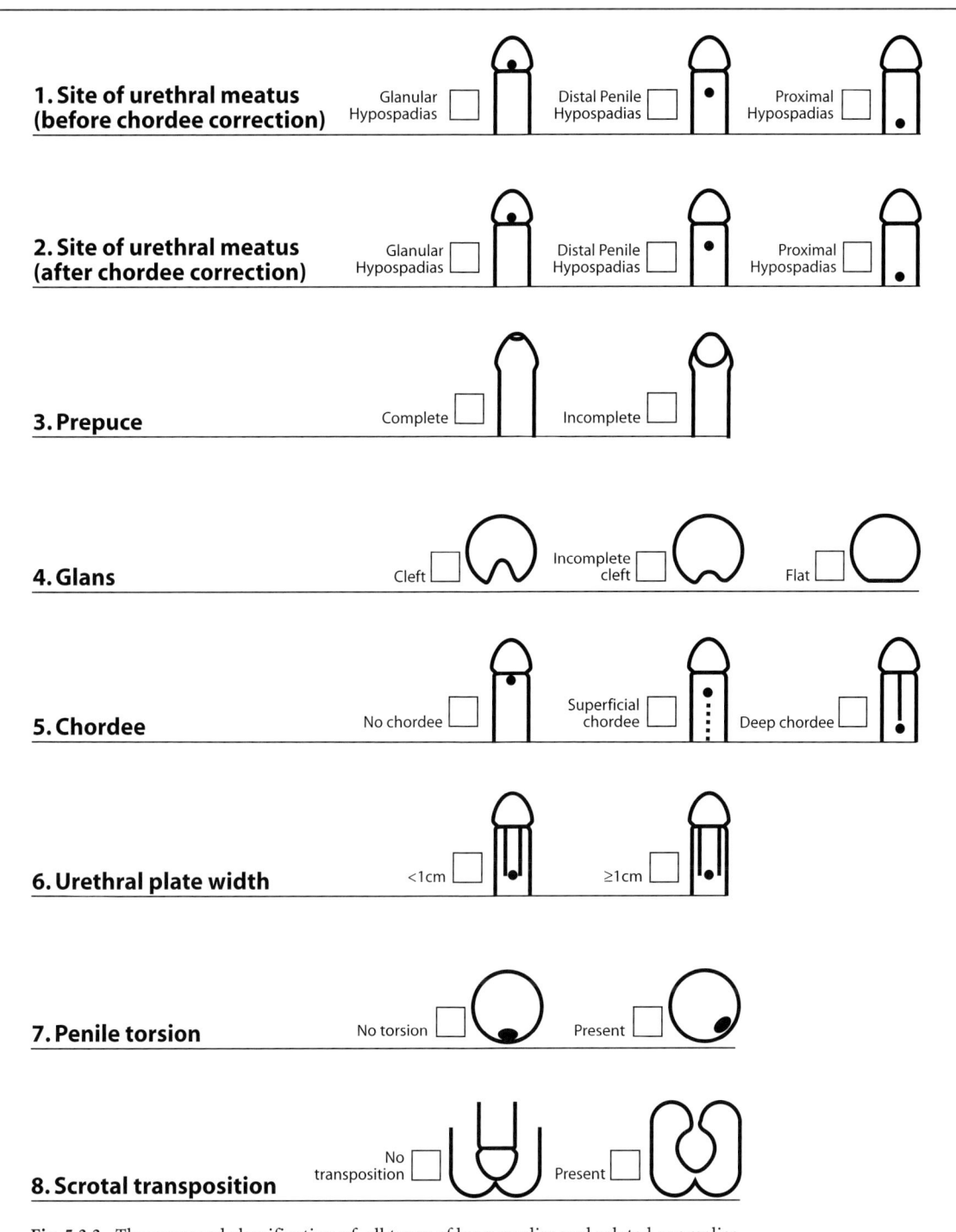

Fig. 5.3.3. The proposed classification of all types of hypospadias and related anomalies

References

Avellan L: The incidence of hypospadias in Sweden. Scand J Plast Reconstr Surg. 1975; 9:129.

Barcat J: Current concepts of treatment of hypospadias. In: Horton CE (ed): Plastic and reconstructive surgery of the genital area. Little Brown, Boston. 1973; pp 249–263.

Browne D: An operation for hypospadias. Lancet 1936; 1:141.

Duckett JW: Hypospadias. In: Gillenwater JY, Grayhack JT, Howards SS, Duckett JW (eds): Adult and pediatric urology, 3rd edn. Mosby Year Book, St Louis, 1996, pp 2550.

Juskiewenski S, Vaysse P, Guitard J, et al: Traitement des hypospadias anterieurs. Chir Pediatr. 1983; 24:75.

Schaeffer DD, Erbes J: Hypospadias. Am J Surg 1950; 80:183.

Sheldon CA, Duckett JW: Hypospadias. Pediatr Clin North Am 1987; 34:1259.

Smith CK: Surgical procedures for correction of hypospadias. J Urol 1938; 40:239.

Welch KJ: Hypospadias. In: Ravitch MM, Welch KJ, Benson CD et al (eds): Pediatric surgery, 3rd edn. Year Book Medical Publishers, Chicago, 1979; pp 1353–1376.

Timing of Elective Hypospadias Repair

Athanasios Zavitsanakis, Ewagelia Gougoudi

6.1

Several factors influence, directly or indirectly, the timing of elective repair of hypospadias in childhood. The most important of them are the age-related anaesthetic and surgical risks and benefits, in relation to the psychological impact of the procedure, during the various stages of the child's development (Kelalis et al. 1975).

The American Academy of Pediatrics, in 1975, concluded that hypospadias surgery was best performed after a child's 3rd birthday. Since that time the operative strategy has been modified as a result of factors such as: (1) the understanding of the psychological implications of genital surgery in children, (2) the improvement in the technical aspects of surgery for hypospadias and (3) the advances in paediatric anaesthesia (Kelalis et al. 1975).

The psychological factors include the child's emotional development, its sexual development and the psychological effects of surgery and anaesthesia.

Emotional Development

During the first year of life, a strong and stable mother–father–child relationship is established. This attachment may be affected by the presence of a congenital birth defect. From this point of view the period from 6 months to approximately 15 months of age, may be a relatively less difficult emotional developmental period for surgery, if parental separation is kept to the minimum. In that way a non-life-threatening congenital defect such as hypospadias can be corrected as early as possible and the family relationships are not irreparably disturbed. The next most appropriate time for operative procedure is the period from 24 to 36 months, in which the trauma of an operation is less difficult. However, that period has the disadvantage of prolonging the child's defective status and crystallizing any disruption in family relationships (Brazelton and Als 1979; Stern 1985).

Another important factor in determining the impact of hospitalisation is the family situation. This variable is also the most difficult to change. Normal postoperative and posthospitalisation reactions have been noted in children from families with good relationships among the individual members. Children from families with no or less communication face anxiety about separation and surgery and show an adverse emotional reaction postoperatively (Kelalis et al. 1975).

The psychological preparation for hospitalisation and operation is of great importance for a normal reaction. Both the parents and the child feel insecure and are not sure what is going to be done. Diagrams, slides or a movie with details of hospitalisation and surgery may be helpful for parents and for the child and may reduce the postoperative psychological disturbance. Parents' presence beside their child before anaesthesia and during recovery is also important (Kelalis et al. 1975).

Sexual Development

A child with a birth defect of the external genitalia such as hypospadias may develop distortions of body image. The defect per se may reflect other people's communicative evaluations of the child's body, and it is also important for paternal response. The repair of hypospadias as early as possible will help achieve a psychologically healthy body image. On the other hand, a person's sexual body image is largely a function of socialization (Money and Ehrhardt 1972; Money and Norman 1987). Boys with hypospadias at school age more frequently have gender-atypical behaviour than boys with normal external genitalia (Sandberg et al. 1989). The repair of hypospadias before 30 months of age seems to be important because the awareness of the deformity begins at that time. Furthermore, boys' socialization at that age includes comparison of genitalia, and a boy who sits to urinate or who has a visible penile defect will be exposed to the social response of his peers. Moreover, from the age of 30 months to 5.5 years the fear of physical harm is significant. Boys who undergo hypospadias repair before the age of 30 months do not suffer from anxiety that their sex may be changed or their genitalia mutilated (Schneider 1960; Lane 1966).

Psychological Effects of Surgery and Anaesthesia

The psychological effects of surgery and anaesthesia in children depends on the age of the patient, the duration of hospitalisation and the behaviour of the anaesthesiologist. Factors that are considered less significant include birth order, prior hospitalisation, preoperative behaviour of the child, characteristics of the illness or the treatment, degree of pain during hospitalisation and presence or absence of the mother during anaesthesia (Vernon et al. 1967). The highest incidence of postoperative emotional disturbance has been noted at the ages of 1–3 years. The most common problems are prolonged night terrors, negativism and various fears including hysterical reactions, phobias and anxiety reactions. Children at that age are strongly dependent on their mother, do not have extensive social contacts outside the home, and show a decreased facility to handle anxiety. Because of that they represent postoperatively a greater emotional hazard and develop behavioural changes due to emotional trauma in 10% of cases (Levy 1945; Jackson 1951). Inadequate preoperative sedation in young children may result in excessive preoperative fear and anxiety in addition to postoperative emotional disturbances (Garfield 1974). Brief hospitalisation, minor surgical pain and skilful anaesthesia result in no residual behavioural effects in the majority of children (Davenport and Werry 1970).

Improvement in Technical Aspects of Surgery and Advances in Paediatric Anaesthesia

Technical considerations used to be limiting factors in determining the time for hypospadias surgery in the past. At that time the reconstructive techniques were multistage, with correction of the chordee and urethral reconstruction separated by an interval of 6–12 months. The duration of hospitalisation was 5–14 days each time, mostly without parental rooming-in. Today, increased surgical experience has changed the operative rules. Single-stage hypospadias repair is performed in almost all cases, with the multistage procedure reserved for the most complicated malformations (Duckett 1981; Belman 1982; Kass and Bolong 1990; Retik et al. 1988). The use of microinstrumentation and delicate suture material and also the routine use of optical magnification have made the operative procedure technically feasible in small infants (Manley and Epstein 1981; Belman and Kass 1982). Experienced paediatric urology surgeons can perform early reconstructive surgery with cosmetic and functional results equal to those achieved in older children (Culp 1959; Hodgson 1970). Furthermore, parental rooming-in is possible in almost all centres and in that way the psychological effects can be decreased even more. On the other hand, children are hospitalised for shorter times despite the fact that the operative techniques have become more complex and the children are younger at the time of operation. Hypospadias is performed as an outpatient procedure or with only overnight hospitalisation in some centres. The most important positive outcome is the lessening of emotional trauma from parent–child separation (Vernon et al. 1965).

On the other hand the dramatic improvements in paediatric anaesthesia, including pharmacological advances, safer perioperative monitoring and increased understanding of the physiologic response of neonates, infants and children to anaesthesia, has improved the management of respiratory problems and cardiovascular response. Furthermore, paediatric anaesthesiologists have acquired an improved understanding of the importance of minimizing the period of parent-child separation (Tiret et al. 1988; Smith 1980; Mayhew and Guiness 1986; Patel and Hanallah 1988).

In conclusion, in centres where the above-mentioned criteria can be met, surgery for hypospadias can successfully be achieved in children between 6 and 12 months of age.

Editorial Comment

Because a normal penis grows only about 0.8 cm between the ages of 1 and 3 years (Schonfeld and Beebe 1942), the size of the phallus is not an important technical consideration. There can be considerable variation in phallic size, but a penis that is small at 6 months will still be a small penis at the age of 3 years. One excellent study compared the emotional, psychosexual, cognitive and surgical risks for hypospadias (Schulz et al. 1983). The optimal window recommended for repair was about 6–15 months of age (Fig. 6.1.1 and Table 6.1.1). Delicate surgical techniques, optical magnification and careful haemostasis have encouraged many surgeons (including myself) to operate when the patient is between the ages of 3 and 9 month, with very satisfactory results (Duckett and Baskin 1996).

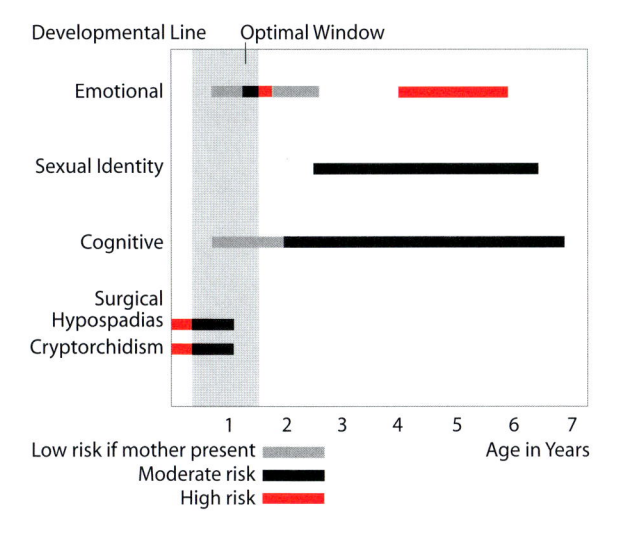

Fig. 6.1.1. Evaluation of risk for hypospadias repair from birth to age 7 years. The optimal window is from 3 to 15 months of age. (Modified from Schulz et al. 1983)

Table 6.1.1. Stretched penile length (centimetres)

Age	Mean ± SD	Mean ± 2.5 SD
Newborn, 30 weeks' gestation	2.5 ± 0.4	1.5
Newborn, 34 weeks' gestation	3.0 ± 0.4	2.0
0–5 months	3.9 ± 0.8	1.9
6–12 months	4.3 ± 0.8	2.3
1–2 years	4.7 ± 0.8	2.6
2–3 years	5.1 ± 0.9	2.9
3–4 years	5.5 ± 0.9	3.3
4–5 years	5.7 ± 0.9	3.5
5–6 years	6.0 ± 0.9	3.8
6–7 years	6.1 ± 0.9	3.9
7–8 years	6.2 ± 1.0	3.7
8–9 years	6.3 ± 1.0	3.8
9–10 years	6.3 ± 1.0	3.8
10–11 years	6.4 ± 1.1	3.7
Adult	13.3 ± 1.6	9.3

Reproduced from Elder (1996) with permission.

References

Belman AB, Kass EJ: Hypospadias repair in children less than 1 year old. J Urol. 1982; 128:1273–1274.
Belman AB: The modified Mustarde hypospadias repair. J Urol. 1982; 127:88–90.
Brazelton B, Als H: Four early stages in the development of mother-infant interaction. Psychoanal Study Child. 1979; 34:349–369.
Culp OS: Experiences with 200 hypospadiacs: evolution of a therapeutic plan. Surg Clin North Am. 1959; 39:1007–1013.
Davenport H, Werry J: The effect of general anesthesia, surgery, and hospitalization upon the behavior of children. Am J Orthopsychiatry. 1970; 40:806–824.
Duckett JW: The island flap technique for hypospadias repair. Urol Clin North Am. 1981; 8:503–511.
Duckett JW, Baskin LS: Hypospadias. In: Gillenwater JY, Grayhack JT, Howards SS, Duckett JW (eds): Adult and pediatric urology, 3rd edn. Mosby-Year Book, St Louis, p 2580; 1996.
Elder JS: Abnormalities of the genitalia in boys and their surgical management. In: Walsh PC (ed) Campell's urology. Saunders, Philadelphia, p 2326; 2002.
Garfield JM: Psychologic problems in anesthesia. Am Fam Physician. 1974; 10:60–67.
Hodgson NB: A one stage hypospadias repair. J Urol 1970; 104:281–287.
Jackson K: Psychological preparation as a method of reducing the emotional trauma of anesthesia in children. Anesthesiology. 1951; 12:293–300.
Kass EJ, Bolong D: Single stage hypospadias reconstruction without fistula. J Urol. 1990; 144:520–522.
Kelalis P, Bunge R, Barkin M, et al: The timing of elective surgery on the genitalia of male children with particular reference to undescended testes and hypospadias. Pediatrics. 1975; 56:479–483.
Lane RW: The effect of pre-operative stress on dreams. Doctoral dissertation, University of Oregon, Eugene, OR; 1966.
Levy D: Psychic trauma of operations in children. Am J Dis Child. 1945; 69:7–25.
Manley CB, Epstein ES: Early hypospadias repair. J Urol. 1981; 125:698–700.
Mayhew JF, Guiness WS: Cardiac arrest due to anesthesia in children. JAMA. 1986; 256:216. Letter.
Money J, Ehrhardt A: Man and woman, boy and girl. Johns Hopkins University Press, Baltimore, MD; 1972.
Money J, Norman BF: Gender identity and gender transposition: longitudinal outcome study of 24 male hermaphrodites assigned as boys. J Sex Marital Ther. 1987; 13:75–92.
Patel RI, Hanallah RS: Anesthetic complications following pediatric ambulatory surgery: a 3-year study. Anesthesiology. 1988; 69:1009–1012.
Retik AB, Keating M, Mandell J: Complications of hypospadias repair. Urol Clin North Am. 1988; 15:223–236.
Sandberg DE, Meyer-Bahlburg MFL, et al: Boys with hypospadias: a survey of behavioral difficulties. J Pediatr Psychol. 1989; 14:491–514.
Schneider CS: An analysis of presurgical anxiety in boys and girls. University of Michigan, Ann Arbor MI, 1960. Doctoral dissertation.
Schonfeld WA, Beebe CW: Normal growth and variation in the male genitalia from birth to maturity. J Urol. 1942; 48:759
Schulz JR, Klykylo WM, Wacksman J: Timing of elective hypospadias repair in children. Pediatrics. 1983; 71:342–351
Smith RM: Anesthesia for infants and children, 4th edn. Mosby, St Louis. 1980; pp 653–661.
Stern DN: The interpersonal world of the infant. Basic Books, New York; 1985.
Tiret L, Nivoche TY, Hatton R, et al: Complications related to anesthesia in infants and children: prospective survey of 40240 anaesthetics. Br J Anaesth. 1988; 61:263–269.
Vernon D, Foley JM, Schulman JL: Effect of mother-child separation and birth order on young children's responses to two potentially stressful experiences. J Pers Soc Psychol. 1967; 5:162–174.
Vernon DTA, Foley JM, Sipowics RR, et al: The psychological responses of children to hospitalization and illness. Thomas, Springfield, Illinois; 1965.

General Principles

Amir F. Azmy

The estimated incidence of hypospadias is 3.2 in 1,000 live male births or 1 in every 300 male children. Incomplete formation of the prepuce and excess dorsal hood lead to recognition of the defect soon after birth. Prenatal ultrasound may detect a genital abnormality; a wide distal end of the penis corresponds to the excess dorsal prepuce. Sonography can be performed with a vaginal probe in early gestation and an abdominal sector scanner in advanced pregnancy. Other genital anomalies can be detected, such as epispadias, ambiguous genitalia, testicular feminisation syndrome and Smith–Lemli–Opitz syndrome (Bronshtein et al. 1995).

Prenatal detection of anomalies can be helpful in evaluation of fetuses with severe multi system anomalies, as well as lesions more amenable to correction in the neonatal period. Detection is particularly important in neonates with endocrine disorders and in those with complex genitourinary and anorectal malformations (Mandell et al. 1995).

History

Detailed family history should be obtained. Previous members of the family with hypospadias should be recorded. Fourteen per cent of male siblings of an index child have hypospadias. If two members of the family have hypospadias, then the risk is 21% in subsequent male children. Maternal ingestion of hormone medications during pregnancy must be ascertained.

Examination

The position of the meatus, its configuration and diameter must be documented clearly as a megameatus may be present, particularly in the presence of intact and complete foreskin (megameatus intact foreskin variant). Ventral chordee may be present and it may vary; the best way to assess the degree of chordee and its nature is by performing an intraoperative erection test. One should assess the elasticity and/or agility of the ventral skin and the urethral plate and the adequacy of the foreskin. The glans is carefully inspected to assess the presence of ventral groove or shallow glans because this affects the operative correction. Careful palpation of the testes in the scrotum is recommended, and any associated penoscrotal abnormalities or penile torsion should be recorded.

The Role of Imaging

To assess the role of routine radiographic screening of boys with hypospadias, in 1990 Moore conducted a prospective study of 153 boys with hypospadias. They were screened by intravenous urography and voiding cystourography; urinary tract anomalies were found in 23.5% of cases and significant anomalies in 11% on the initial examination and a further 4.5% on follow-up requiring later surgery. The overall incidence of surgical intervention, not including hypospadias repair, was 11.7% and Moore recommended routine screening in boys with hypospadias. However, similar studies show a low incidence of anomalies, most not requiring intervention. In view of this, ultrasound has been suggested as a screening procedure for boys with hypospadias and should be considered in severe types of hypospadias as there is a low incidence of upper urinary tract anomalies in mild hypospadias. Vesicoureteric reflux was found in 17% of 305 boys, in the majority low grade and not associated with renal damage.

It is generally agreed that upper renal and ureteric anomalies with hypospadias are extremely rare. Only seven significant renal anomalies were found in 360 patients, in 3 of whom renal investigation would have been performed anyway because of anorectal malformation (Kelly et al. 1984; Cerasaro et al. 1986; Davenport and MacKinnon 1988).

Micturating cystourethrography has been suggested only if there is a history of recurrent urinary tract infection and in cases of true ambiguous genitalia to assess the presence of müllerian duct remnants. Such remnants are usually asymptomatic and do not require routine surgical resection. Cystoscopy does not add much to our knowledge of the child with hypospadias, except in severe forms, where it may show utricular enlargement. Enlargement of utricle may be noted in 57% of boys with perineal hypospadias, the incidence and severity correlated directly with the degree of hypospadias (Icoma et al. 1986). Occasionally resection of the utricle may be necessary because of recurrent urinary tract infection, urinary dribbling or stone formation. A uterus and tubes may be present, suggesting a greater degree of intersex.

Associated Anomalies

Undescended testicle and hernia are the most common associated anomalies. Urinary tract anomalies are infrequent as the external genitalia are formed much later. The penile skin may be very thin and this prevents the use of perimeatal skin flaps for repair urethral plate. The penile skin may be well developed, elastic and nontethering; however, it may equally be underdeveloped and act as a tethering fibrous band that bends the penis during micturition or erection. Desautel et al. in 1999 studied 26 patients ranging from 1 month to 19 years of age with müllerian duct remnant; between 1984 and 1998 ten of these had associated penoscrotal hypospadias and were treated conservatively. However, five patients developed recurrent urinary tract infections and were maintained on long-term prophylactic antibiotics. Utriculus masculinus may be mild, but in severe cases it causes recurrent urinary tract infection and difficulty in passing a urethral catheter.

Hypoplasia of the Penis

The normal penile stretch length in the newborn is 3.9 cm, range 3.1–4.7 cm. The response to testosterone stimulation should be tested.

Reports of long-term testosterone treatment of congenital hypoplasia of the penis are scarce. Among 66 children with penile hypoplasia of whom 35 had associated hypospadias, the effect of testosterone intramuscularly was evaluated in 40 children treated under the age of 10 years. The increase in penis length was greater in children with isolated micropenis than when associated with hypospadias and greater when treatment started in the neonatal period. The penile length at the last follow-up was related not to the total dose of testosterone, but to the length at the time of first evaluation (Velasquez-Uzzola et al. 1998).

Preoperative Evaluation

Early diagnosis is recommended. This is usually done at the maternity unit soon after birth and the boys are then referred for early surgical consultation to detect any anomalies requiring early intervention, such as meatal stenosis requiring meatotomy at an early age, and to decide on the timing of the definitive surgery. The degree of hypospadias should be documented, the condition of the meatus and the presence of chordee. Explanation and assurance should be given to the parents about the potential treatment and possible outcome.

Preoperative Preparation

The child is admitted and confirmed fit for general anaesthesia. An enema is given the evening before the operation to clear the bowel as most urinary leakage occurs within a few days of the operation. It may also be useful to start the child on lactulose for the first few days to avoid constipation and allow soft stooling. Cleanliness of the penile and scrotal area may not be necessary, however. Local application of mercurochrome over the genital skin before surgery in addition to soap and water scrubs has been shown to decrease the incidence of infection in patients undergoing hypospadias surgery and thereby the incidence of fistula formation (Ratan et al. 2001).

Preoperative Hormonal Stimulation

The repair of hypospadias in a child with microphallus is technically difficult. To enhance the size of the penis and to achieve satisfactory repair, preoperative androgen therapy has been suggested before reconstruction. This allows early surgical correction, thereby avoiding the psychological problems that may occur in cases where surgery is delayed to allow sufficient growth of the penis.

Gonadotrophin or testosterone may be used. Preoperative treatment with gonadotrophins has not been well supported because of lack of treatment protocols. Further problems are the wide variation in response to treatment with human chorionic gonadotrophin (HCG), the failure to assess androgen receptors or 5-α reductase status, and the lack of measurement of testosterone levels before and after treatment. However, treatment with HCG showed decrease in the degree of the severity of proximal hypospadias and improved chordee (Koff and Jayanthi 1999; Husmann 1999).

Defects in androgen receptors and 5-α reductase function and testicular steroidogenesis can result in hypospadias. However, gonadotrophin stimulation of testes in patients with defective testicular steroidogenesis and partial receptor abnormality may not be able to increase serum testosterone level enough to overcome the physiological defect, and gonadotrophin alone cannot enhance penile size, as in cases of hypergonadotrophic hypogonadism.

Testosterone has been shown to be more beneficial than HCG in stimulating the growth of the hypospadiac micropenis; the testosterone may be applied locally as testosterone propionate cream 2% to the penis three times daily for 3 weeks, preferably by the father, or by the mother wearing gloves to avoid absorption of testosterone. The advantages of local application of testosterone propionate cream are: good response of increased size of penis; easy application; lack of pain. However, there has been great variability of response depending on the degree of absorption and the amount of cream applied.

The advantage of intramuscular application is that it ensures an increase in serum testosterone level. Koff and Jayanthi conducted a study of 12 boys with proximal hypospadias treated preoperatively with HCG for 5 weeks immediately preceding the repair and concluded that pretreatment with HCG resulted in disproportional penile enlargement which advances the meatus distally to decrease the severity of hypospadias and chordee. The penile shaft proximal to the urethral meatus shows greater growth than the proximal shaft and causes the meatus to move distally away from the penoscrotal junction.

The most reliable method of administration is parenteral injections; however, topical testosterone cream may be applied directly to the penis (Sakakibara et al. 1991). Davits et al. (1993) found that a dose of 2 mg/kg given 5 weeks and again 2 weeks preoperatively was effective. Belman uses 25 mg testosterone enanthate 6 and 3 weeks before repair. Koff and Jayanthi (1999) used HCG stimulation 6–8 weeks prior to repair in 12 boys aged 6–12 months; after a 5-week course, there was significant reduction in chordee and an increase in penile length.

Consent

Consent, i.e. the agreement of a person (the patient or legal guardian) to go ahead with an examination, investigation or treatment, is valid only if the following conditions are fulfilled:

- Consent is given after appropriate information
  - Enough information is given
  - Information is timely, provided well before a planned procedure
  - Information is appropriate to the individual
- Consent is voluntary
  - Own decision
  - No pressure
  - Sufficient time to decide
- The patient or guardian must be capable
  - Able to understand and retain relevant information
  - Believes the information
  - Uses it when reaching a decision

Consent for hypospadias surgery is given by parents on behalf of their child and should be in the best interest of the child.

The surgeon who will perform the proposed procedure should obtain the consent; however, he or she may delegate this to another clinician as long as the latter is suitably trained and qualified, has sufficient knowledge of the proposed procedure and understands the risks involved. It is no longer acceptable for a junior house officer to obtain a patient's consent for major or complex surgery, especially if they do not know the exact nature and risks of the procedure. A child under the age of consent who has achieved sufficient understanding to enable him to comprehend and evaluate what is proposed will be able to give consent himself, although the parental right to give consent to their child's treatment still exists and would be relevant if there were any doubt about the child's capacity. It is for the clinician, when dealing with individual minors, to decide whether or not they have sufficient understanding of the treatment proposed. As the majority of hypospadias surgery is performed in the first few years of life, the consent is usually given by parents on behalf of their child. The doctor has a duty to inform the parents of the possible risks and benefits of the proposed procedure in order to obtain valid consent; however, the amount of information given has to be weighed up so that the parents do not reject an operation that would clearly benefit their child.

Written consent should be obtained when the proposed surgery is complex or involves significant risk.

Changing to a procedure other than the one consented to on the day of surgery is unacceptable. However, in the case of hypospadias surgery, examination under anaesthesia often shows that a different procedure may be more suitable. Parents should be aware that the best procedure may be better judged when the child is under anaesthesia, and the surgeon may need to explain the possible alternatives in advance.

Informed consent should be obtained from the parents after full explanation of the anomaly, its degree and any associated malformation requiring correction at the time of hypospadias surgery or at a later date. A brief but clear outline of the outcome, cosmetic results and possible complications, particularly in relation to fistula formation, stricture or dehiscence, must be given. Also the parents should be aware that their child may require a multistage procedure, a "redo" operation or a minor corrective procedure to trim the foreskin or dilate the meatus. There may be a need to repeat the explanation on admission, after previous discussion during an outpatient consultation.

Penoscrotal Transposition

Penoscrotal transposition is an infrequent congenital malformation due to a defect in the caudal migration of the scrotum during foetal life. The anomaly has been classified into a bifid scrotum, incomplete or partial penoscrotal transposition, complete penoscrotal transposition or prepenile scrotum, and lastly ectopic scrotum.

Ambiguous Genitalia

Patients with severe hypospadias, either penoscrotal or perineal, with impalpable gonads should be investigated for intersex, as should girls with severe masculinisation with adrenogenital syndrome. The presence of a testicle in the scrotal sac indicates male gender. Chromosome abnormalities may be suspected in hypospadias with a palpable single testicle, particularly if this is associated with dysmorphic features. Buccal smear and karyotyping should be performed and the internal genitourinary structures should be assessed by micturating cystourethrography, genitography, cystoscopy and examination under anaesthesia.

Incidence of Intersexuality in Children with Cryptorchidism and Hypospadias

The combined presence of cryptorchidism and hypospadias often indicates the existence of an intersex state. Testicular maldescent and incomplete tubularisation of the urethral plate occur in a spectrum, with the severity of the two processes probably dependent on the degree of pathophysiology in the adrenogenic hormonal access. The incidence of intersexuality of children with undescended testicle, hypospadias and otherwise unambiguous genitalia has been reported to be 27%. A total of 2,105 cases of undescended testicle and 1,057 cases of hypospadias were studies between 1982 and 1986. Seventy-nine patients presented with both undescended testicle and hypospadias, and a phallus was believed to be a possible penis; intersex conditions were identified with nearly equal frequency in 44 cases of unilateral and 35 cases of bilateral cryptorchidism. In the unilateral undescended testicle group, patients with an impalpable testis were at least three times more likely to have intersex (Kaefer et al. 1999).

A case-control study of 6,177 boys with cryptorchidism, 1,345 cases with hypospadias and 23,273 male controls from 1983 to 1992 was carried out to determine the relationship between cryptorchidism and hypospadias and the presence of other anomalies, abnormalities in an older brother, birthweight, weeks of gestation, maternal history of stillbirth, parity, twin birth, parental age, nationality and professional status. They found that simultaneous cryptorchidism and hypospadias were more common than expected, that there was an increased risk of both entities when the same abnormality was present in an older brother, and that the risk of cryptorchidism and hypospadias increased with decreasing birthweight independent of weeks of gestation. Twins were at a lower risk than singletons of both entities in all lower birthweight groups. An increased risk of hypospadias was noted in the sons of women with a previous stillbirth. The risk of cryptorchidism and hypospadias slightly increased with decreasing parity (Weinder et al. 1999). Both cryptorchidism and hypospadias were positively associated with other congenital malformations and inversely with maternal parity. There is evidence that being born small for age and before 33 weeks of gestation have a greater than additive effect with respect to both cryptorchidism and hypospadias (Akre et al. 1999). McAleer and Kaplan (2001) set out to determine whether association of hypospadias and cryptorchidism is associated with a high incidence of chromosomal abnormalities and whether they warrant routine karyotype screening. Complete anatomical, karyotypic, pathological and radiological information was available for 48 patients: 8 had chromosomal abnormalities, 2 had karyotypic intersex disorder, 6 had autosomal chromosomal abnormality. The authors concluded that most patients who present for evaluation of hypospadias, chordee and undescended testicle have normal karyotype and routine karyotyping does not seem necessary. If karyotypic intersex abnormalities are identified, these patients are more likely to have ambiguous genitalia, especially those with perineal hypospadias and cryptorchidism.

The following genital phenotypes are considered ambiguous:
- Hypospadias with impalpable gonads
- Hypospadias with micropenis and either one or no palpable gonads
- Newborn with female external genitalia and a gonadal mass in the labia or labial fusion and/or clitoral enlargement

The diagnostic evaluation should include history, physical examination, serum electrolytes, plasma 17-hydroxyprogesterone, chromosome analysis, lymphocyte culture, ultrasound of the abdomen and pelvis, genitography and, whenever necessary, measurement of plasma concentration of testosterone as baseline and after stimulation with HCG. Laparotomy may be necessary for definitive histological examination of the gonads. In all children with male pseudohermaphroditism or incomplete masculinisation consisting of hypospadias, mostly of the perineal type, with micropenis and/or bilateral or unilateral cryptorchidism, the male sex is assigned. The most common cause of ambiguous genitalia is congenital adrenal hyperplasia due to 21-hydroxy deficiency in 46XX cases presenting with ambiguous genitalia; those with 46XY have a wider range of diagnoses (androgen sensitivity syndrome, gonadal dysgenesis). Despite thorough investigation, 23.5% of children studied had no definite final diagnosis of genital ambiguity.

Gender assignment is a neonatal surgical emergency; early evaluation and the treatment of intersexuality require a team approach. Early reconstruction of most anomalies is feasible, avoiding social disaster and the associated emotional problems. Incomplete masculinisation has been found to be due to a defect in the androgen receptors, 5-alpha reductase or enzymes in the pathway from steroid cholesterol to testosterone. Point mutations have been implicated in 46XY pure gonadal agenesis; retained müllerian ducts have been attributed to point mutations in the müllerian inhibiting syndrome gene. If patients are to be raised as males, various types of hypospadias repair can be done, gonads can be replaced with prosthesis later on, a prepenile scrotum can be reconstructed and the müllerian duct structures can be removed with preservation of the vas deferens. Replacement therapy with glucocorticoids and mineralocorticoids must be precisely administered to promote proper growth. Testosterone, oestrogen and progesterone replacement must be considered and carefully managed.

Assessment of Results of Hypospadias Surgery

The objective of the hypospadias repair is to enable the young boy to micturate in a normal manner and to allow normal development of the penis. Assessment of the results of the urethroplasty will be based on the observation of the pattern of micturition, the stream should be straight and strong, but it may be deviated or there is a spraying of urine, the stream may be interrupted or the presence of post micturition dribbling or hesitancy. Cosmetic appearance is judged by the location of the meatus and the skin cover and the absence of any residual chordee. The condition of the ventral skin and the presence of any excess dorsal skin.

Meatal and Urethral Calibration

Meatal or urethral calibration can be performed at an outpatient attendance, simply by calibrating the urethral meatus according to the age of the child. The meatus of a boy under 1 year of age should accept a 5-Fr feeding tube; between 1 and 6 years this increases to 8 Fr.

Assessment Using Uroflowmetry

To determine the role of uroflowmetry in the evaluation of the functional results of hypospadias repair, a retrospective review of children who underwent hypospadias repair and urethral reconstruction was conducted (Garibay et al. 1995). Patients with a plateau pattern and a maximum flow rate two standard deviations below the mean for age, body surface and voided volume in more than one determination were considered to have urethral obstruction. Meatal dilatation or meatoplasty corrected the urethral restriction and improved urinary flow.

Marte et al. (2001) reported on the functional evaluation of tubularised incised urethral plate repair of midshaft to proximal hypospadias using uroflowmetry. Patients were assessed when they could void on volition and had no fistula. The investigators measured the flow pattern and the maximum and mean flow rate, and the results were expressed in centiles and compared with values in normal children. Maximum and mean flow rate were considered normal if above the 25th percentile, equivocally obstructed from the 5th to the 25th percentile and obstructed if below the 5th percentile. Patients with obstructed flow responded to meatal dilatation or meatoplasty.

Objective Scoring System for Results of Hypospadias Surgery

Holland et al. (2001) presented an objective scoring system (HOSE) for evaluating the results of hypospadias surgery. The HOSE system was designed to provide an objective appraisal of the outcome of the repair, based on meatal position, meatal shape, urinary stream, straightness of erection and complexity of any complicating urethral fistula. The patients were randomly selected and independently reviewed, and the authors concluded that interobserver evaluation using HOSE was minimal, supporting its use as an objective outcome measure after hypospadias surgery (Holland et al. 2001).

Analysis of Cosmetic Outcome Using Photography

Baskin (2001) analysed the cosmetic outcomes after hypospadias surgery using photography rather than the classical assessment on the basis of rates of reoperation for fistula, diverticulum, stenosis or residual penile curvature. Photographs were taken before and immediately after surgery and 3–12 months later. One hundred and fifty-three patients were followed up. After critical analysis, the author concluded that photography is an objective means to document the cosmetic results. Patients who had undergone previous surgery had the least satisfactory results.

References

Akre O, Lipworth L, Criattingius S, et al: Risk factor pattern for cryptorchidism and hypospadias. Epidemiology. 1999; 10:364–369.

Baskin L.: Hypospadias, critical analysis of cosmetic outcomes using photography. BJU Int 2001; 87:534–539.

Bronshtein M, Riechler A, Zimmier GZ: Prenatal diagnosis. 1995; 15:212–219.

Cerasaro TS, Brock WA, Kaplan GW: Upper urinary tract anomalies with congenital hypospadias: is screening necessary? J Urol. 1986; 135:537–538.

Davenport M, MacKinnon AE: The value of ultrasound screening for the upper urinary tract in hypospadias. Br J Urol. 1988; 62:595–596.

Davits RJ, Vanden Aker ES, Scholineijer RJ, et al: Effect of parenteral testosterone therapy on penile development in boys with hypospadias. Br J Urol. 1993; 71:593.

Desautel MG, Stock J, Hanna MK: Mullerian duct remnants: surgical management and fertility issues. J Urol. 1999; 162:1008–1013.

Garibay JT, Reid C, Gonzalez R: Functional evaluation of the results of hypospadias surgery with uroflowmetry. J Urol. 1995; 154:835–836.

Holland AJ, Smith GH, Ross FI, et al: HOSE: an objective scoring system for evaluating the results of hypospadias surgery. BJU Int. 2001; 88:255–258.

Husmann DA: Microphallic hypospadias: the use of human chorionic gonadotropin and testosterone before surgical repair [editorial; comment]. J Urol. 1999; 162:1440–1441.

Icoma F, Shima H, Yabumoto H, et al: Surgical management for enlarged prostatic utricle vagina masculina in patients with hypospadias. Br J Urol. 1986; 58:423.

Kaefer M, Diamond D, Hendren WH, et al: The incidence of inter-sexuality in children with cryptorchidism and hypospadias. Stratification based on gonadal palpability and meatal position. J Urol. 1999; 162: 1003–1006.

Kelly D, Harte FB, Rose P: Urinary tract anomalies in patients with hypospadias. Br J Urol. 1984; 56:316–318.

Koff SA, Jayanthi VR: Preoperative treatment with human chorionic gonadotrophin in infancy decreases the severity of proximal hypospadias and chordee. J Urol. 1999; 162: 1435–1439

Mandell J, Bromley B, Peters CA, et al: Prenatal sonographic detection of genital malformations. J Urol. 1995; 153: 1994–1996.

Marte A, Di Iorio G, De Pasquale M, et al: Functional evaluation of tubularised incised plate repair of mid shaft – proximal hypospadias using uroflowmetry. BJU Int. 2001; 87: 540–543.

McAleer IM, Kaplan GW: Is routine karyotyping necessary in the evaluation of hypospadias and cryptorchidism? J Urol. 2001; 165:2029–2031.

Moore CC: The role of routine radiographic screening of boys with hypospadias: a prospective study. J Paediatr Surg. 1990; 25:339–341.

Ratan SK, Sen A, Ratan J, et al: Mercurochrome as a adjunct to local preoperative preparation in children undergoing hypospadias repair. BJU Int. 2001; 88:259–262.

Sakakibara N, Nonomura K, Koyanagi T, et al: Use of testosterone ointment before hypospadias repair. Urol Int. 1991; 47:40.

Velasquez-Uzola A, Leger J, Aigrain Y, et al: Hypoplasia of the penis: etiologic diagnosis and results of treatment with delayed-action testosterone. Arch Pediatr. 1998; 5:844–850.

Weinder IS, Moller H, Jensen TK, et al: Risk factors for cryptorchidism and hypospadias. J Urol. 1999; 161:1606.

Plastic Surgery Principles

Ahmed T. Hadidi

Plastic surgery, although thought of as a technique-oriented specialty, is in fact a problem-solving field. The plastic surgery training allows the surgeon to see surgical problems in a different light and select from a variety of options to solve surgical problems. In order to achieve optimum results in hypospadias surgery, one must have full command of the basic principles of plastic surgery and the potential flaps for use in the reconstruction of the neourethra.

The basic principles of plastic surgery are careful analysis of the surgical problem, careful planning of procedures, precise technique, and atraumatic handling of tissues. This chapter discusses specific issues of skin grafts and flaps. Other relevant factors, including tissue handling and viability, instruments and magnification, suture material and knots, suturing techniques, diversion and dressings, are discussed in detail in Chap. 8.

Skin is a compound organ. The two layers of the skin are derived from different embryologic layers and differ in character. The outermost thinner layer is the epidermis; the innermost thicker layer is the dermis, which consists of connective tissue. The two layers are intimately connected by means of fine protoplasmic processes and elastic fibers. The epidermis contains no blood vessels; the dermis, acting as the nutrient base of the epidermis, is thus indispensable.

Skin Grafts

A skin graft is skin that has been completely detached from its original donor site and transferred to another site, where it will develop a new blood supply. The first recorded successful skin graft was by Sir Astley Cooper in 1817 (McCarthy 1990). Grafts may be classified according to species or to thickness:

- According to origin, grafts may be classified as autografts, isografts, homografts, or xenografts:
    - An autograft is taken from one site and placed on a different site in the same individual.
    - An isograft is taken from one individual and placed on another individual with the same genotype, e.g. an identical twin.
    - A homograft, or allograft, is taken from one individual and grafted to another individual of the same species but of a different genotype.
    - A xenograft, or heterograft, is grafted to an individual of a different species.
- Skin grafts may either be full thickness or split (Fig. 7.1):
    - A full-thickness skin graft consists of epidermis and the full thickness of the dermis.
    - Split skin grafts consist of epidermis and a variable thickness of the dermis. They are described as thin (10–12 thousands of an inch) intermediate (13–17 thousands of an inch) or thick (18–20 thousands of an inch).

However, these various categories of graft are not really completely distinct from one another. The real difference in practice is that the full-thickness skin graft is cut with a scalpel while the split skin graft of whatever thickness is usually cut with razor blades, skin grafting knives (Blair, Ferris Smith, Humby, Goulian), manual drum dermatomes (Padgett, Reese), and electric or air-powered dermatomes (Brown, Padgett, Hall). The electric and air-powered dermatomes are the most widely used because of their reliability and ease of operation.

Split Skin Grafts

Split grafts include the complete epidermis with a variable thickness of dermis. The grafts may be thin, medium, or thick. Donor skin for grafting may be obtained with a knife or with a mechanical dermatome. Some dermal appendages remain in the original donor bed, including sweat glands, sebaceous glands, and hair follicles. From these remaining skin appendages and from the wound edges, the donor site heals by epithelialisation. The thicker the graft, the longer

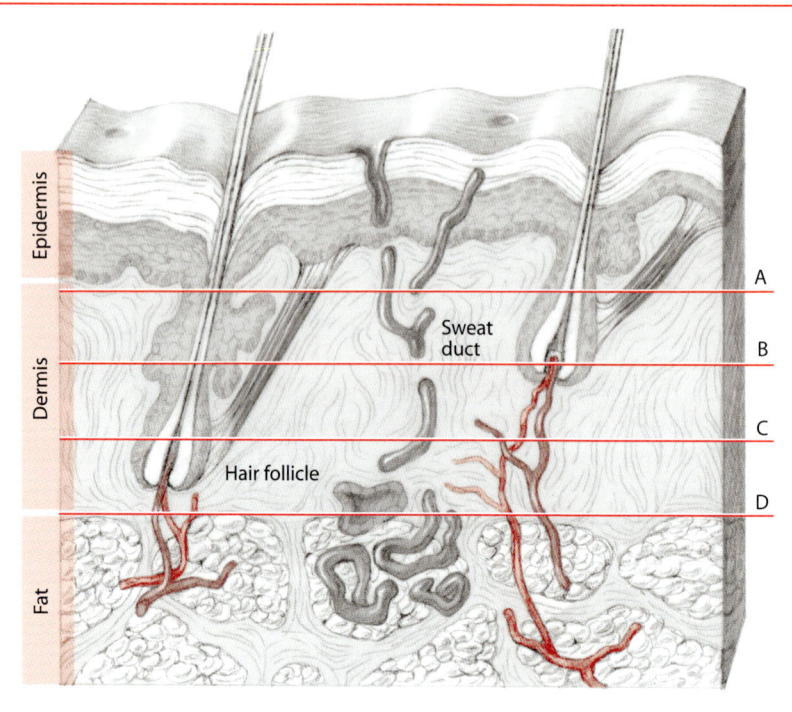

Fig. 7.1. Section of skin to illustrate the comparative thickness of skin grafts. *A* Line of section of the thin split-thickness (Thiersch) graft. *B* Line of section of the split-thickness graft. *C* Line of section of the thick split-thickness or three-quarter thickness graft. *D* Line of section of the full-thickness graft. Note that the junction between the dermis and the subcutaneous tissue is irregular. The protrusions of the subcutaneous fat into the dermis are known as the columnae adiposae

the time required for complete donor site healing. Most split-thickness graft donor areas heal in approximately 2–3 weeks. With thin grafts, the donor site may heal within 10–14 days and may be used for grafting again if necessary.

Thin split skin grafts more easily survive grafting, and the donor site heals faster than with thick grafts. However, thick grafts contract less, are more like normal skin, resist trauma, and aesthetically are more acceptable than thin grafts. Thick graft donor sites heal more slowly with more scarring than thin graft donor sites. The most common donor sites are the thigh, buttock, and abdomen.

Meshed grafts are usually thin or intermediate split-thickness grafts that have been rolled under a special cutting machine to create a mesh pattern. Although grafts with these perforations can be expanded from one and a half to nine times their original size, expansion to one and a half times the unmeshed size is the most useful.

Full-Thickness Skin Grafts

Full-thickness skin grafts include the epidermis and the entire dermis. These grafts provide good coverage because they are full-thickness skin. They resist trauma better, are aesthetically more pleasing, and contract less than split-thickness skin grafts. Full-thickness grafts vascularise more slowly and are less likely to survive than split-thickness skin grafts because of their greater thickness.

Donor sites for full-thickness grafts must be closed primarily or with split-thickness grafts. Donor sites are usually areas of thin skin such as the postauricular, supraclavicular and inguinal areas. In addition to graft durability and donor site morbidity, colour matching is very important, especially on the face.

Cultured Epithelial and Dermal Grafts ▶ Epithelial cells were the first to be cultured in vitro and made to coalesce into sheets that could be used to cover full-thickness wounds. Although these culture epithelial sheets were used in the treatment of burns, the result was unsatisfactory because the coverage was very fragile. More recently, success has been obtained with artificial dermis which, when placed in an appropriate bed, will revascularise and can then be covered by a very thin (0.05 cm) split-thickness skin graft. This artificial dermis is increasingly being used in the treatment of burns. Modifications of this concept have also been

Table 7.1. Advantages and disadvantages of various types of skin grafts

Type of graft	Advantages	Disadvantages
Thin split-thickness	Survives transplantation most easily; donor sites heal most rapidly	Fewest qualities of normal skin; maximum contraction; least resistance to trauma; sensation poor; aesthetically poor
Thick split-thickness	More qualities of normal skin; less contraction; more resistant to trauma; sensation fair; aesthetically more acceptable	Survives transplantation less well; donor site heals slowly
Full thickness	Nearly all qualities of normal skin; minimal contraction; very resistant to trauma; sensation good; aesthetically good	Survives transplantation least well; donor site must be closed surgically; donor sites are limited

applied to the care of chronic ulcers, particularly in the leg. The artificial dermis is made out of a collagen matrix and has very low or no antigenicity (Vasconez and Vasconez 2003).

Table 7.1 summarises the characters of different types of skin grafts.

Skin Graft Survival

The conditions necessary to ensure free graft survival include (1) a well-vascularised host bed, (2) rapid onset of imbibition, (3) close apposition of the graft to the host bed, (4) immobilisation of the graft and (5) rapid onset of inosculation. Movement of the graft on its bed is likely to interfere with graft survival; consequently, immobilisation is an important factor for success.

Initially, both split-thickness and full-thickness grafts adhere to the recipient bed by fibrin bonding. This usually lasts approximately 72 h. If fibrin is absent or dissolves, the graft fails. During the first 2 days, the graft is nourished by fluid from the recipient bed. This is the phase of plasma imbibition. The graft initially gains weight from the diffusion, absorption, and capillary action of fluid movement. Revascularisation of the graft takes place between the 3rd and 5th days (inosculation). The revascularisation may occur by reanastomosis of vessels between the recipient bed and the graft or by the growth of new vessels into the graft. The circulation in the graft is usually restored by 4–7 days. Lymphatic circulation usually parallels the restoration of the blood supply.

In grafted skin, the epidermis initially undergoes a period of depressed epidermal cellular function until vascular ingrowth occurs. By 4–8 days, proliferation and thickening of the epithelial cell layers with gross desquamation occur. Fibroblasts migrate into the dermis by the 3rd day and outnumber those of normal skin by 8 days. Most of the collagen in the graft is replaced; a split-thickness skin graft replaces less collagen than a full-thickness skin graft.

Both split-thickness and full-thickness grafts assume the sensory innervation pattern of the recipient site. Split-thickness grafts usually have less return of innervation than full-thickness grafts. Reinnervation follows the neurolemmal sheaths of the graft. Sensory recovery usually takes 1–2 years; the sense of pain returns first, followed by light touch and temperature.

Skin grafts undergo both primary and secondary contraction. Primary contraction occurs immediately on harvesting of the graft. Full-thickness grafts contract by about 40%, split-thickness grafts by about 10–20% of their original volumes. Secondary contraction occurs after the graft is vascularised and is related to the amount of dermis in the graft. Full-thickness grafts undergo very little secondary contraction, whereas split-thickness grafts tend to contract more.

Skin grafts may undergo variable pigmentation changes. Thinner grafts usually exhibit greater colour changes. Ultraviolet light induces hyperpigmentation in immature grafts. Grafts in darker-haired individuals may progressively darken, while in lighter-haired subjects they may lighten.

Several dressings for the donor site have been described. These include scarlet red ointment, petroleum jelly gauze, pigskin heterograft, Op-Site, and exposure techniques. Op-Site is probably associated with less pain, whereas a heterograft has increased infection and scarring.

The most common cause of skin graft failure is haematoma or seroma under the graft. This inhibits adherence and vascularisation of the graft. Another cause of graft failure is inadequate immobilisation of the graft. After the graft is transferred to the recipient site, it should be completely in contact with the bed and adequately immobilised and covered with a pressure stent dressing to decrease shearing forces. If the wound has a large amount of serous drainage, the graft may be treated open. Infection is another cause

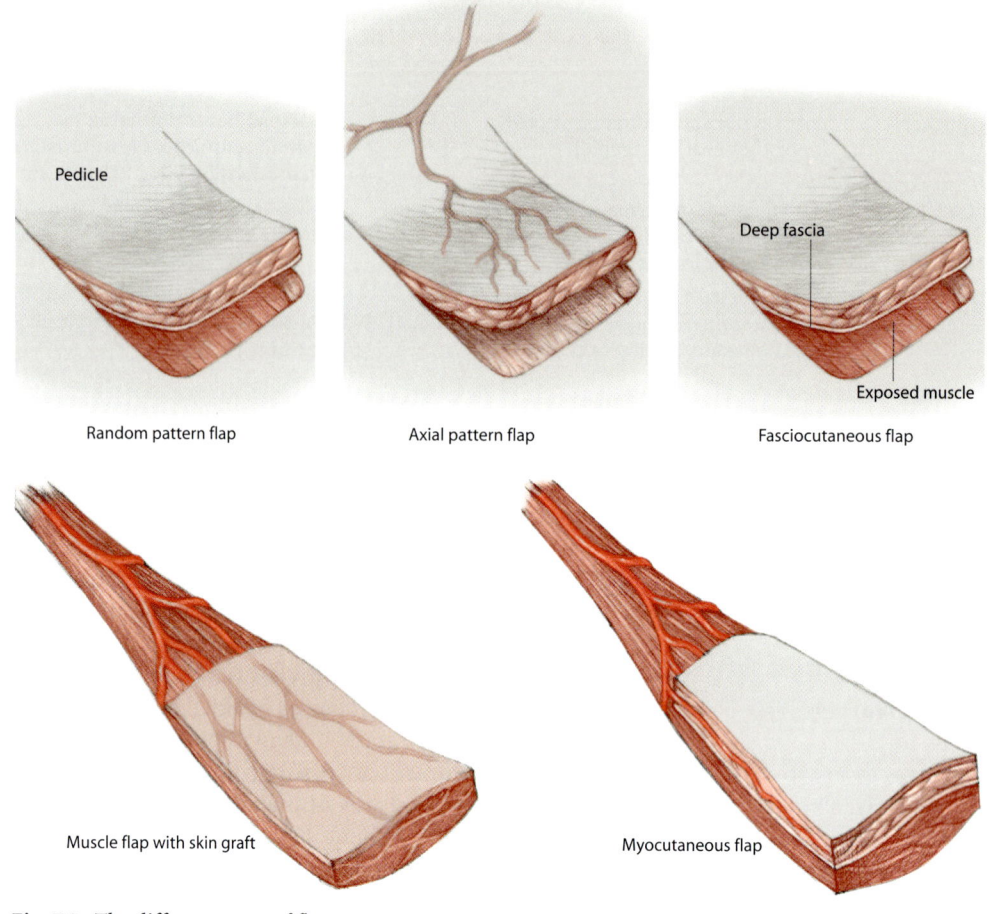

Fig. 7.2. The different types of flaps

of graft failure. The bed should be debrided and well vascularised and should have a bacterial count of fewer than 10^5 organisms per gram of tissue. If the wound bed is poorly vascularised, the wound must be debrided until vascularised tissue is obtained or it must be covered with a flap.

Flaps

> Grafts are dead tissues that you try to bring to life, flaps are living tissue that you try not to bring to death.

A flap is a tissue that is transferred from one area of the body to another with its original blood supply intact. Flaps may consist of skin, subcutaneous tissue, muscle, fascia, bone, nerve, omentum, or other tissues (such as intestine). Flaps may be classified according to their blood supply or to the tissue transferred (Fig. 7.2):

- A flap which consists of skin and superficial fascia is referred to as a *skin flap*.
- When the investing layer of deep fascia is included, the flap becomes *fasciocutaneous*.
- A flap may consist of a muscle: a *muscle flap*.
- If the skin overlying the muscle is included, or the bone to which the muscle is attached, a composite flap results, *myocutaneous* or *osteomyocutaneous*.

Before the development of microvascular techniques, flaps had to retain a vascular attachment to the body throughout their transfer, but it is now possible to transfer a flap en bloc to a distant site in a single stage, as a free flap.

Blood supply to flaps may arise from segmental, anastomotic and axial vessels that have perpendicular muscle perforations terminating in the dermal–subdermal plexus of the skin. Random flaps are based on this blood supply. Random cutaneous flaps are perfused through this dermal–subdermal plexus in the dermal and perifollicular layers of the skin. Myocutaneous flaps have these perforating musculocutaneous vessels that enter the base of the flap, supplying a small skin area.

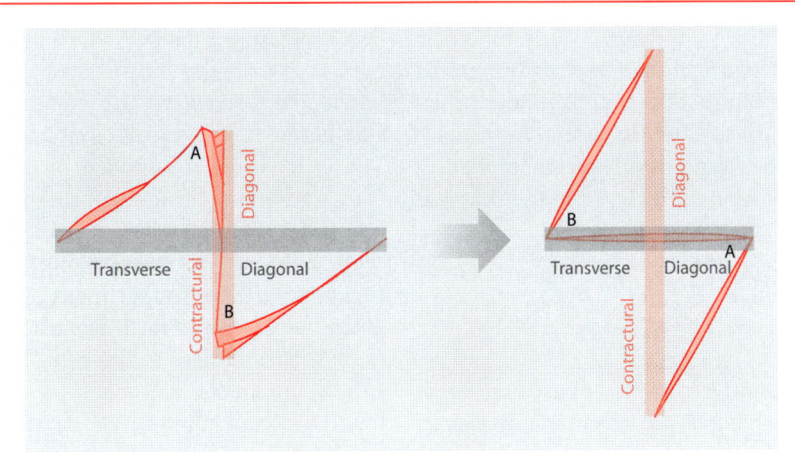

Fig. 7.3. The diagonals of the Z-plasty, showing how, with transposition of the Z-plasty flaps, the contractural diagonal is lengthened and the transverse diagonal is shortened

Flap blood may also be supplied by vessels that penetrate the underlying muscle fascia and lie in the subcutaneous tissue. These longitudinally oriented vessels supply the dermal–subdermal plexus directly. Axial flaps are based on this blood supply. Axial flaps not only have an arterial pedicle portion but also distally have a random-pattern portion of the flap.

Random Flaps

Random flaps are based on perforating vessels. They have a limited length-to-width ratio because of their blood supply. In the head and neck area, random flaps may have a length-width ratio of 2:1 or 3:1. In the rest of the body, length-width ratios of 1.5:1 or 1:1 may be safely designed. The dermal–subdermal plexus should be maintained when designing these flaps.

Random cutaneous flaps may be divided according to their design and positioning. Two types of random flap used to close local defects are rotation flaps, which rotate around a pivot, and advancement flaps.

Flaps that rotate are divided into true rotation flaps and transposition flaps, both of which are positioned into a defect. They are generally rotated from an area that has enough laxity to allow primary closure of the donor site (secondary defect). The donor site may require the use of a back cut (relaxing incision) or skin graft for closure. Secondary defects should not be closed under tension.

True rotation flaps are semicircular and rotate around an axis into the defect for local closure.

Transposition flaps are advanced laterally along an axis that is at an angle to the original axis of the flap. These flaps are generally rectangular. They are usually used for local coverage of a triangular defect. The flap should be made longer than the side of the defect so that the actual diagonal length from the pivot before transfer and the estimated length after transfer are similar. This flap may also require a short back cut across part of the base to reduce tension. The secondary defect must be closed, and therefore a graft may be necessary. The flap donor site may also be closed by transposition of a secondary flap from the most lax skin at right angles to the primary flap. This technique is known as a bilobed flap.

Another transposition flap is the Z-plasty (Fig. 7.3), where two triangular flaps are raised (undermined) and transposed. The transposition achieves a gain in length along the direction of the common limb of the Z, and the direction of the common limb of the Z is changed (McGregor and McGregor 1995). A Z-plasty has one central member or limb and two angled limbs, which together resemble a Z. The angled limbs, are equal in length to the central limb and are usually angled at 60. A greater angle may be selected in a series when not enough tissue is available for one large Z-plasty and when the aesthetic result is of primary concern. Other transposition flaps include a Limberg flap and an interpolation flap. The Limberg flap is useful for closure of rhomboid defects with angles of 60° and 120°. The sides are the same length as the short axis of the rhomboid defect.

An interpolation flap is a skin and subcutaneous flap that is transposed into a local but not immediately adjacent defect. The pedicle must pass over or under adjacent tissue to be placed into the defect. A common interpolation flap is a deltopectoral flap.

Advancement flaps are designed and moved directly forward to close a defect. In a single-pedicle advancement flap, a rectangle of skin is incised on three sides, undermined, and moved forward. With bipedicle advancement flaps, two incisions are made parallel to the defect to create a flap that is undermined and advanced forward to close the defect. In the case of V-Y flaps, another type of advancement flap, a V-shaped incision is made and closed in the shape of a Y (Slate 1999).

Axial Flaps

Axial pattern flaps or arterial flaps are based on direct longitudinal vessels lying in the subcutaneous tissue. These flaps carry their own direct artery and vein, which branch into the dermal–subdermal plexus. Because these flaps include their own major blood vessels, they can have large length-width ratios, with long, narrow flaps created. If the flap has its artery, veins and skin intact in its pedicle, it is called a peninsular flap. If the skin in the pedicle is cut and the flap is connected to the body by only its intact vessels, it is called an island flap. An island flap in which the artery and veins are divided, the flap transferred to a new site, and the vessels reanastomosed to the recipient vessels is called a free flap.

Microsurgical techniques allow for large segments of tissue to be detached and transferred to a recipient site. Using microsurgery, the arterial and venous axial vessels are anastomosed to the recipient vessels. Anastomosis of vessels 0.5–2.0 mm in diameter can routinely be successfully performed. With vessels in the 2.0–4.0 mm range, the vessel can be anastomosed using a coupling device. Cutaneous, muscle, musculocutaneous, fascial, fasciocutaneous, osteocutaneous, and osteomusculocutaneous flaps and free vascularised bone grafts are some of the free flaps that have been successfully constructed and transferred. Sensory and motor flaps can restore sensation and function. These microtechniques have also allowed for successful reattachment.

Fasciocutaneous Flaps

Fasciocutaneous flaps are composed of fascia and skin based on the vascular systems of the deep fascia. The deep fascia is supplied by perforating arteries from underlying muscle, subcutaneous arteries in the fat, and subfascial arteries from the intermuscular septa. Blood vessels extend along the fibrous septa between muscles or compartments and then branch out at the deep fascia to form plexuses. From the plexuses, branches radiate to the skin. Based on the blood supply, fasciocutaneous flaps may be either pedicle or free flaps, depending on the fasciocutaneous system involved. Some flaps such as forearm free flaps may also include tendons, muscle and vascularised bone. Fasciocutaneous flaps are generally very simple and quick to raise and are highly reliable.

References and Suggested Reading

McCarthy JG: Introduction to plastic surgery. In: McCarthy JG (ed): Plastic surgery, vol 1: general principles. Saunders, Philadelphia, pp 48–66, 1990.

McGregor IA, McGregor AD (eds): Fundamental techniques of plastic surgery and their surgical applications. Churchill Livingstone, Edinburgh, pp 21–121, 1995.

Slate RK: Principles of plastic surgery. In: Ehrlich RM, Alter GJ (eds): Reconstructive and plastic surgery of the external genitalia, adult and pediatric. Saunders, Philadelphia, pp 1–5, 1999.

Vasconez LO, Vasconez HC: Plastic and reconstructive surgery. In: Way LW, Doherty GM (eds): Current surgical diagnosis and treatment, 11th edn. McGraw-Hill, USA, pp 1230–1242, 2003.

Principles of Hypospadias Surgery

Ahmed T. Hadidi

The majority of hypospadias surgery is performed in children. The ideal age is from 3 to 9 months (Duckett and Baskin 1996). Although a normal penis grows only about 0.8 cm between the ages of 1 and 3 years (Schonfeld and Beebe 1942), hypospadias surgeons should use magnification and fine plastic surgery instruments. Just as the best golf clubs do not make a professional out of a duffer, however, neither does specialised equipment ensure good operative results.

This chapter deals with general operative principles of hypospadias surgery under the following categories: positioning; magnification; traction and retraction; tissue handling and viability; instruments; suture material and knots; suturing techniques; haemostasis; urinary diversion; dressing.

Positioning

Hypospadias repair is a demanding operation that means the surgeon's head, neck and shoulders are leaning forward for an hour at least. Most surgeons prefer to bring the patient's waist near the edge of the operating table and the surgeon sits either on the side or at the foot of the table. Sitting has the advantages that it reduces fatigue and enables others to see the procedure clearly. Sitting alongside the operating table allows smooth movement of the operating hand; thus, precise cutting and suturing can be achieved.

Magnification

Magnification has contributed dramatically to progress and better results in hypospadias surgery. The aim is to achieve fine tissue approximation and fine cauterisation of bleeding points. The advantages of optical magnification were stated quite concisely by Dr. Norman Hodgson (Wacksman 1984):

> This concept [optical magnification] is important since magnification does more than just make the tissues larger. It develops a conscious awareness of fine vessels and their handling in ensuring the ultimate best result. With the delicate instrumentation and technology now available one can assure the successful result in the majority of patients in this early age group.

Rees et al. (1981) wrote that the use of magnification helps to avoid piercing the epithelial lining of the neourethra when it is being tubed and reduces the chance of fistula formation. Wacksman (1984) reported the use of optical magnification in hypospadias surgery (magnification 2–5 times). The use of optical magnification with fine suture material leads to a low overall complication rate. Magnification, either with loupes or an operating microscope, helps to preserve blood supply and allow the operator to perform accurate, meticulous anastomosis.

To facilitate the use of magnification, bright spot illumination of the operative field is needed and may need to be augmented by the use of a head lamp.

Traction, Retraction and Tension

The first step in the operation is to apply traction and maintain stabilisation of the penis. The is achieved by placing a traction suture in the glans penis using a fine non-absorbable material (5-0 nylon or silk on a small rounded needle). Although many surgeons prefer a longitudinal suture, I prefer a transverse one as it is less likely to cut through the tissues and may provide more stability and decrease torsion.

To minimise trauma to the tissues, I prefer to use stay sutures or skin hooks for traction rather than retractors.

Another important point is that one should avoid tension of the flaps, as this may interfere with the blood supply to the flap through the pedicle. One should also avoid tubularisation of the neourethra

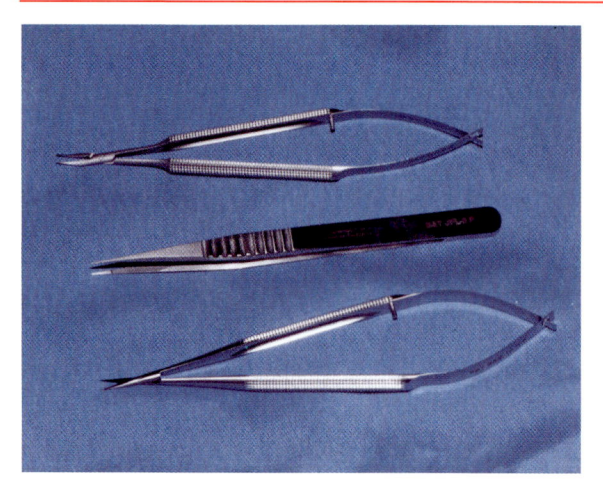

Fig. 8.1. Fine instruments used in hypospadias surgery

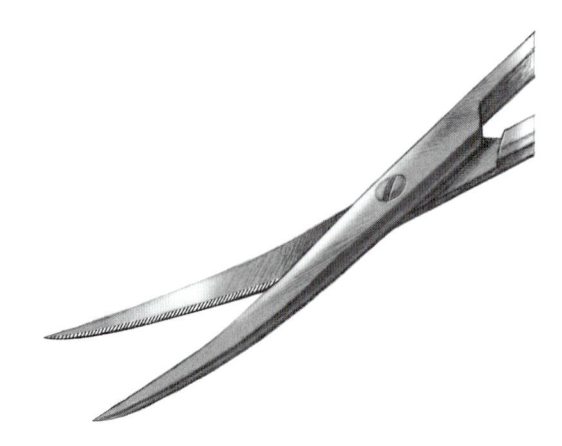

Fig. 8.2. Super Cut scissors with serrated blade, ideal for hypospadias surgery

under tension, as this will definitely interfere with the capillary circulation of the flap tissue and will lead to ischaemia and failure.

Tissue Handling and Viability

The tissues of the penis are very sensitive to trauma (like the eyelids). A simple common example is the oedema that affects the prepuce after any rough manipulation. A common finding in surgical training centres is that although residents in training may be strictly supervised and perform proper surgical techniques, unless they handle tissues delicately the results may be far from those desired. One should handle the tissues as the lioness holds her babies with her teeth, without hurting them. This is a very important point and cannot be overstressed. To achieve this one should use hooks or very fine toothed instruments to support the tissues rather than grasping the tissues.

Another important point is tissue dryness and ischaemia. One must constantly ensure adequate tissue hydration simply by continuously adding saline and avoid ischaemia by checking the tourniquet time, avoiding tight sutures, conducting delicate fine cautery of the bleeding points and avoiding haematomas.

Instruments

For hypospadias surgery, one does not need a large number of instruments. However, the instruments must be very fine and delicate, and scissors need to be very sharp. The instruments needed include fine serrated scissors, fine needle holder, fine tissue forceps, curved mosquito forceps to hold the stay sutures and a standard rounded scalpel with a number 15 blade. The diagram in Fig. 8.1 shows an example of the instruments commonly used in hypospadias surgery. Special attention may be directed to the serrated scissors. These scissors have the advantage of being very sharp, like blades, yet they remain sharp for a long time (Fig. 8.2).

Suture Material and Knots

In surgery in general, but especially in hypospadias surgery, it is very important to choose the proper suture material that will meet the needs of the wound. There are many questions to ask before choosing a specific suture (Table 8.1): For how long is the maximum tensile length needed? What is the effect of urine on the suture? What is the minimum size of suture that will hold the tissues in place? What are the knotting characteristics of the suture material? Does the knot tend to form a fistula? Is the suture to be used for skin or deeper structures? Should one use a cutting needle or a round-bodied needle (Katz and Turner 1970; Van Winkle and Hastings 1972; Holmlund 1974; Thacker et al. 1975; Case et al. 1976)?

In general, sutures may be divided into absorbable and non-absorbable. Absorbable sutures are derived from mammals or synthetic polymers. The material is capable of being absorbed but may be treated to modify its resistance to absorption. Absorbable sutures include plain and chromic catgut, coated polyglactin 910 (Vicryl), polyglycolic acid (Dexon), polydioxanone (PDS), polygluconate (Maxon), and poliglecaprone 25 (Monocryl). Non-absorbable sutures include silk, nylon, Prolene, Mersilene, Dacron and Ti-cron.

Table 8.1. Sutures commonly used in reconstructive urology

Absorbable			
Plain surgical gut	Plain gut	Ethicon	Natural fiber
Chromic surgical gut	Chromic gut	Davis & Geck	
Coated polyglactin 910	Vicryl	Ethicon	Synthetic braided
Uncoated polyglycolic acid	Dexon "S"	Davis & Geck	Synthetic braided
Coated polyglycolic acid	Dexon Plus	Davis & Geck	Synthetic braided
Polydioxanone	PDS	Ethicon	Synthetic monofilament
Polyglyconate	Maxon	Davis & Geck	Synthetic monofilament
Poliglecaprone 25	Monocryl	Ethicon	Synthetic monofilament
Non-absorbable			
Twisted silk	Virgin silk	Ethicon, Davis & Geck	Natural fibre
Monofilament nylon	Ethilon, Dermalon	Ethicon, Davis & Geck	Synthetic monofilament
Silicone-coated polyester	Ti-Cron	Davis & Geck	Synthetic braided
Polypropylene	Prolene, Surgilene	Ethicon, Davis & Geck	Synthetic monofilament

It is generally accepted that non-absorbable sutures should be excluded from contact with urine because of the potential for stone formation. Furthermore, the genitourinary tissues regain their tensile strength rapidly and the prolonged presence of a suture is not necessary.

Most hypospadias surgeons tend to use an absorbable material to minimise fistula formation. They tend to use the smallest size that will hold the tissues together on the most gentle needle available. My personal preference is to use 6-0 or 7-0 Vicryl on a cutting needle for the urethroplasty. I prefer a cutting needle because it allows one to perform proper subcuticular suturing for the neourethra without mutilation of the tissues. Nevertheless, many hypospadiologists prefer to use fine monofilament suture material because it passes through the tissues very gently. However, when monofilament sutures are used for urethral reconstruction, urinary diversion is often needed to prevent the potential adverse effects of urine on suture integrity (El-Mahrouky et al. 1987; Edlick et al. 1987; Sebeseri et al. 1975; Holbrook 1982; Stewart et al. 1990; Cohen et al. 1987).

Suturing Techniques

For urethroplasty, a subcuticular continuous suture using a fine cutting needle is highly recommended (Fig. 8.3a). The idea is to try to have both epithelial edges in contact and to avoid eversion of edges (Hadidi 1996). Eversion of the suture line increases peri-urethral reaction, which can predispose to urine leakage and potential fistula or diverticulum formation. Ulman et al. (1997) documented a statistically significant lower fistula rate (4.9% vs 16.6%) for subcuticular repair in comparison with a full-thickness (through and through) technique. Many surgeons prefer to have urine-tight anastomosis. However, one should weigh this against the more serious danger of tissue ischaemia. Spatulated anastomosis is important to prevent leakage at the original meatus, where most fistulae occur. The suture lines of tubularised neourethra can be placed posteriorly against the corpora to bury as much of the anastomosis as possible.

Interposition of multiple tissue layers between the neourethra and the skin, and avoiding the crossing of suture lines are essential to hypospadias repair (Retik et al. 1988). Attention to these points has helped to improve the results of hypospadias repair dramatically.

For skin closure, many surgeons prefer to use interrupted subcuticular rapidly absorbable material to avoid fistula formation. However, this is rather meticulous and continuous transverse mattress suturing gives very good results (Fig. 8.3c).

Haemostasis

Careful haemostasis is a very important factor in hypospadias repair. Inadequate haemostasis predisposes to haematoma formation and infection. On the other hand, excessive cauterisation causes tissue necrosis and may result in infection and failure of repair.

For distal hypospadias, intraoperative bleeding can be minimised during dissection by the intermittent use of an elastic tourniquet for periods of up to 30 min.

Redman (1986) used a rubber band tourniquet to achieve haemostasis routinely during hypospadias repairs. The tourniquet itself consists of a length of rub-

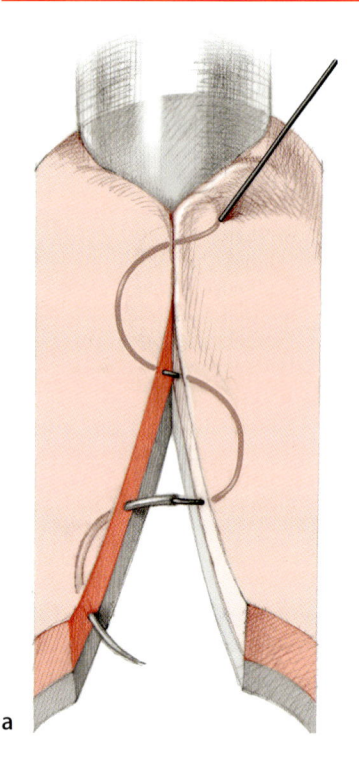

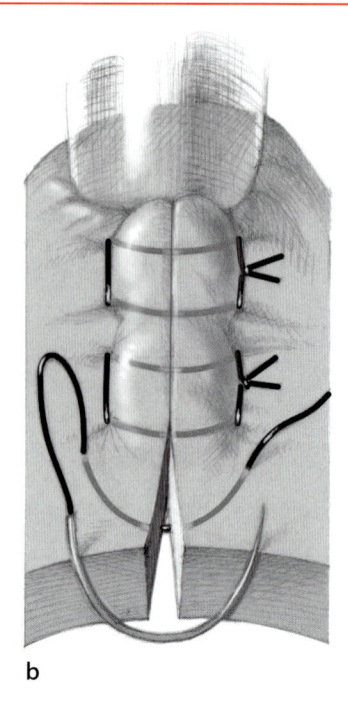

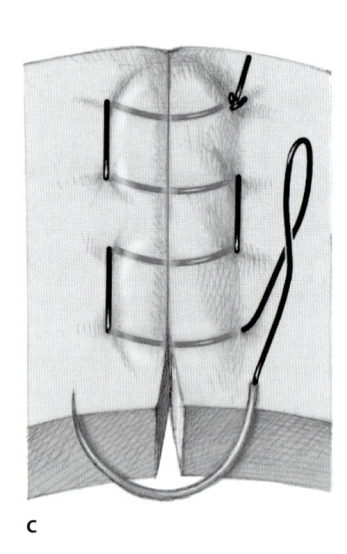

Fig. 8.3a–c. Suturing techniques. **a** A continuous subcuticular suture for urethroplasty. **b** Interrupted mattress suture for glans closure. **c** Continuous transverse suture for skin closure

ber band held in place by a haemostatic clamp after being placed proximal to the site of expected bleeding. He preferred a rubber tourniquet which is 0.1 cm thick and 1–3 cm wide.

The ischaemia time ranged from 20 to 60 min. A common fear of the use of a tourniquet in penile surgery in children is that prolonged ischaemia may result in thrombosis in the corpora. Redman stated that ischaemia under 50 min is well tolerated without complication.

Elder et al. (1987) reported the use of 1% lidocaine with epinephrine (1:100,000) to infiltrate the skin incision and the glans. They wrote that "tissue ischemia has not resulted, and it is less cumbersome than using a tourniquet".

The other alternative is to use fine bipolar diathermy to coagulate single bleeding vessels and minimise ischaemia to adjacent tissues.

Urinary Diversion

The goal of urinary diversion is to prevent urethral oedema from obstructing urine flow and to allow the neourethra to heal completely before contact with urine. Yet, the chosen device should be easy to place and remove, comfortable to wear and convenient to care for at home (Freedman 1999). Common forms of diversion include:

1. Perineal urethrostomy
2. Suprapubic cystotomy
3. Foley catheter drainage
4. Transurethral drainage (dripping stent)

Perineal Urethrostomy

The insertion of a catheter into the bladder through the bulbous urethra is known as a perineal urethrostomy. The technique varies with the type of catheter used. For example, a straight catheter can be inserted directly into the bladder and a lubricated guide then passed within the lumen of the catheter. An incision is made perineally where the guide presents as a bulge, the guide is removed, and the catheter distal to the urethrostomy is carefully pulled through the incision. The catheter should then be anchored securely to the adjacent skin, to prevent its dislodgement. If a Foley catheter is utilised, a similar procedure is carried out with the perineal incision being made over the tip of a paediatric sound.

Coran (1980) suggested a simplified technique for perineal urethrostomy using a tendon-pulling forceps. The tendon-pulling forceps is passed though the urethral meatus and pushed out on the perineum against the posterior urethra. After an incision has been made on the perineum, the forceps is pushed through and a Foley catheter is grasped. The Foley catheter is then placed into the bladder, and the balloon is inflated. As a further safety measure, the catheter is also secured to the perineal skin with a silk suture. A suprapubic cystotomy can be performed employing either a Foley or a Malecot catheter or the same forceps, by using the same principles.

Suprapubic Cystotomy

Two methods of suprapubic diversion are frequently used. The first is a standard surgical suprapubic cystotomy with a small incision and direct placement of a Malecot catheter in the bladder.

The recently introduced commercially available percutaneous trocar cystotomy sets with silicone Malecot catheter or 8-F silicone tubing has essentially replaced surgical cystotomy. Ease of replacement, diminished bladder spasm, and non-incorporation into the dressing have made this form of diversion popular for extensive hypospadias repairs requiring long periods of urinary diversion (Cromie and Bellinger 1981).

Urethral Catheterisation

The most common non-surgical form of intubated diversion is the self-retaining Foley urethral catheter. Moulded silicone catheters, 8, 10 and 12 F in size, are currently available for use in the hypospadias patient. Because of its moulded nature, the internal diameter of the catheter is maximised, providing adequate drainage. Ease of placement, plus the fact that it serves as a stent for the repair, represents a significant advantage for this form of diversion (Cromie and Bellinger 1981).

Some authors (Duckett and Baskin 1996) do not favour this type of diversion, citing potential infection from bacterial migration along the catheter or damage to the repair by inadvertent removal. Additionally, there seems to be a diversity of opinion as to whether the occurrence of bladder spasm is attributable to the Foley catheter, as the catheter balloon often rests on the trigone.

However, there appears to be a remarkable disparity of patient response to an indwelling catheter (Cromie and Bellinger 1981).

Transurethral Drainage (Dripping Stent)

If long-term diversion will be required or extensive glandular dissection is carried out in the course of the repair, a urethral form of diversion with stenting of the repair is recommended. This allows for a voiding trial at any time in the postoperative period, as well as affording protection of the glanular portion of the repair from inadvertent injury from movement of the catheter (Cromie and Bellinger 1981). Baskin et al. (1994) reported that quite good success was obtained with this technique, which allows all cases of hypospadias now to be done on an outpatient basis.

Some authors do not favour any form of urinary diversion (catheter drainage or dripping stent) in the repair of distal hypospadias. In 1987, Rabinowitz described his experience in catheterless Mathieu repair in 59 children with distal hypospadias. Rabinowitz cited that since watertight urethroplasty is performed without overlying suture lines, catheter drainage and urinary diversion may not be necessary. In 1993, Wheeler et al. supported the conclusion of Rabinowitz and stated that the urethral stent may be associated with significant morbidity without conferring any advantages in the postoperative course or the final results.

In 1996, Hakim et al. reported the results of a retrospective study to test the complication rate for Mathieu repair performed with and without a stent, and compared the results among groups. Their conclusion was that the fistula rate and overall complication rate in the stented and unstented groups were not significantly different.

In 1997, Steckler and Zaontz reported the findings of a study on stent-free Snodgrass repair. Stent-free repairs were performed in 33 children. Follow-up was obtained in 31 children. There was no postoperative urinary retention, fistulas or meatal stenosis. No unusual or prolonged discomfort distinguished these children from those who underwent a standard Snodgrass technique.

On the other hand some authors found the application of urethral stent or even suprapubic catheter mandatory: In 1994, Buson et al. stated that application of urethral stent in distal hypospadias repair is necessary to reduce the complication rate. In 1997, Demirbilek and Atayurt came to the conclusion that although urethral reconstruction without suprapubic diversion allowed early hospital discharge and outpatient treatment, the use of a suprapubic catheter for urinary diversion in hypospadias repair is to be recommended because it makes for a lower complication rate and is more comfortable for the patient during the postoperative period.

Dressings

The main purpose of a proper dressing is to provide immobilisation with prevention of haematoma and oedema. Preference for particular dressings is as varied as the other fetishes of hypospadias surgery. In fact, there may be as many different types of dressing as there are types of repair. In general, hypospadias dressings may be divided into three main categories; totally concealing, partially concealing and unconcealing. The most frequently used type is the partially concealing dressing, in its many variations. Common dressings include: cotton-ball dressing (Redman and Smith 1974), the X-shaped elastic dressing (Falkowski and Firlit 1980), silicone foam elastomer (DeSy and Oosterlink 1982), adhesive membrane dressing (Vordermark 1982), Tegaderm dressing (Patil and Alvarez 1989) sprays (Tan and Reid 1990) and Dermolite II tape dressing (Redman 1991).

The practical requirements of outpatient management after surgery dictate a simple dressing (Tegaderm or silicon foam) that does not restrict the child's mobility, or no dressing at all.

A bioocclusive membrane dressing (e.g. Tegaderm) is wrapped around the glans and shaft after the penis has been coated with an adhesive substance. It is important to keep the penis dry during application of the membrane to allow complete adhesion. In particular, the presence of dripping urine may prevent a tight seal to the glans and cause the membrane to be later dissected off by urine. The membrane is cut to a size that covers from the tip of the glans to the penoscrotal junction. The penis is then wrapped snugly with two layers. The penis can be wrapped circumferentially or with the two ends of film adhered to each other as a mesentery or "dorsal fin". It is important to include the glans in the dressing to prevent excessive glans swelling.

The major benefit of the membrane dressing is its simplicity, allowing early mobilisation and minimal home care. There are few complications, and removal is easy . The vast majority of patients with this dressing can be treated as outpatients, without hospital admission. The dressing can usually be removed easily by slipping the whole tube upward off the penis. The dressing is typically left in place for 5–7 days. The dressing not uncommonly falls off at home but rarely before the 3rd or 4th day, making its replacement unnecessary. Because the dressing is impermeable, the need for routine early dressing changes due to soiling is obviated. The transparent nature of the dressing allows observation during healing. The simplified nature of the dressing may also help to relieve parents' anxiety about taking care of the child at home.

One caution is that if the dressing begins to roll up or down the penis, it may form a tight constricting band, requiring immediate removal.

Silicone foam elastomer compound as a dressing in hypospadias surgery was first reported by DeSy and Oosterlink in 1982 and has since gained wide acceptance. The foam base and catalyst are preheated and then mixed in a syringe. The mixture is then injected into a mould (e.g. plastic coffee cup) placed around the penis, filling upward from the base. The foam sets in approximately 2 min, after which time the mould is removed. The cast can then be further anchored at the base with adhesive tape. The cast can be easily separated and removed after scoring its outer surface. The primary advantage of the foam cast is its secure immobilisation of the penis, combined with easy removal with minimal discomfort. It also provides a secure base on which to immobilise an indwelling catheter.

The role of dressings following hypospadias surgery is still controversial. In Cromie and Bellinger's interesting questionnaire (1981), 85% of the participants felt that a dressing was of importance. Van Savage et al. in 2000 and McLorie et al. in 2001 conducted a prospective study of dressing versus no dressing for hypospadias repair. They concluded that "An absent dressing simplified postoperative ambulatory parent delivered home care". They recommended that dressings should be omitted from routine use after hypospadias repair.

Hadidi et al., in 2003, having conducted a prospective randomised study to assess the role of dressing in hypospadias surgery, concluded that repair of hypospadias without dressing offers statistically significantly better results than when using dressing ($P=0.014$). The role of dressing is discussed in further detail in Chap. 27.4.

References

Baskin LS, Duckett JW, Ueoka K, et al: Changing concepts of hypospadias curvature lead to more onlay island flap procedures. J Urol. 1994;151:191.

Buson H, Smiley D, Reinberg Y, et al: Distal hypospadias repair without stents: is it better? J Urol. 1994; 151:1059–1060.

Case GD, Glenn JF, Postlethwait RW: Comparison of absorbable suture in urinary bladder. Urology. 1976; 7:165–168.

Cohen EL, Kirschenbaum A, Glenn JF: Preclinical evaluation of PDS (polydioxanone) synthetic absorbable suture vs chromic surgical gut in urologic surgery. Urology. 1987; 30:369–372.

Coran AG: A simplified technique for performing perineal urethrostomy. Surg Gynecol Obstet. 1980; 150:735.

Cromie WJ, Bellinger MF: Hypospadias dressings and diversions. Urol Clin North Am. 1981; 8:545.

Demirbilek S, Atayurt HF: One-stage hypospadias repair with stent or suprapubic diversion: which is better? J Pediatr Surg. 1997; 32:1711–1712.

De Sy WA, Oosterlink W: Silicone foam elastomer: a significant improvement in postoperative penile dressing. J Urol. 1982; 128:39.

Duckett JW, Baskin LS: Hypospadias. In: Gillenwater JY, Grayhack JT, Howards SS, Duckett JW (eds): Adult and pediatric urology, vol 3, chap 55, 3rd edn. Mosby Year Book, St Louis, pp 2549–2589; 1996.

Edlick RF, Rodeheaver GT, Thacker JG: Considerations in the choice of suture for wound closure of the genitourinary tract. J Urol. 1987; 137:373–379.

Elder JS, Duckett JW, Snyder HM: Onlay island flap in the repair mid- and distal penile hypospadias without chordee. J Urol. 1987; 138:376.

El-Mahrouky A, McElhaney J, Bartone FF et al: In vitro comparison of the properties of polydioxanone, polyglycolic acid and catgut sutures in sterile and infected urine. J Urol. 1987; 138:913–915.

Falkowski WS, Firlit CF: Hypospadias surgery: the X-shaped elastic dressing. J Urol. 1980; 123:904.

Freedman AL: Dressings, stents and tubes. In: Ehrlich RM, Alter GJ (eds): Reconstructive and plastic surgery of the external genitalia, adult and pediatric, chap 32, 1st edn. Saunders, Philadelphia, pp 159–162; 1999.

Hadidi AT: Y-V Glanuloplasty: a new modification in the surgery of hypospadias. Kasr El Aini Med J. 1996; 2:223–232.

Hadidi A, Abdaal N, Kaddah S: Hypospadias repair; is dressing important. Kasr El Aini J Surg. 2003; 4 (1): 37–44.

Hakim S, Merguerian PA, Rabinowitz R et al: Outcome analysis of the modified Mathieu hypospadias repair: comparison of stented and unstented repairs. J Urol. 1996; 156:836.

Holbrook MC: The resistance of polyglycolic acid sutures to attack by infected human urine. Br J Urol. 1982; 53:313–315.

Holmlund DEW: Knot properties of surgical suture materials. Acta Chir Scand. 1974; 140:355–362.

Katz AR, Turner RJ: Evaluation of tensile and absorption properties of polyglycolic acid suture. Surg Gynecol Obstet. 1970; 131:701–716.

McLorie G, Joyner B, Herz D, et al: A prospective randomized clinical trial to evaluate methods of postoperative care of hypospadias. J Urol. 2001; 165:1669–1672.

Patil UB, Alvarez J: Simple effective hypospadias repair dressing. Urology. 1989; 34:49.

Rabinowitz R: Outpatient catheterless modified Mathieu hypospadias repair. J Urol. 1987; 138:1074.

Redman JF: Tourniquet as hemostatic aid in repair of hypospadias. Urology. 1986; 28:241.

Redman JF: A dressing technique that facilitates outpatient hypospadias surgery. Urology. 1991; 37:248–250.

Redman JF, Smith JP: Surgical dressing for hypospadias repair. Urology. 1974; 4:739–740

Rees MJW, Sinclair SW, Hiles RW, et al: A 10-years prospective study of hypospadias repair at French Hospital. Br J Urol. 1981; 53:637.

Retik AB, Keating M, Mandel J: Complications of hypospadias repair. Urol Clin North Am. 1988; 15:223.

Schonfeld WA, Beebe GW: Normal growth and variation in the male genitalia from birth to maturity. J Urol. 1942; 48:759.

Sebeseri O, Keller U, Spreng P, et al: The physical properties of polyglycolic acid suture (dexon) in sterile and infected urine. Invest Urol. 1975; 12:490–493.

Steckler RE, Zaontz MR: Stent-free Thiersch–Duplay hypospadias repair with the Snodgrass modification. J Urol. 1997; 158:1178.

Stewart DW, Buffington PJ, Wacksman J: Suture material in bladder surgery: a comparison of polydioxanone, polyglactin, and chromic catgut. J Urol. 1990; 143:1261–1263.

Tan KK, Reid CD: A simple penile dressing following hypospadias surgery. Br J Plast Surg. 1990; 43:628–629

Thacker JG, Rodeheaver G, Moore JW, et al: Mechanical performance of surgical sutures. Am J Surg. 1975; 130:374–380.

Ulman I, Erikci V, Avanoglu A, et al: The effect of suturing techniques and material on complication rate following hypospadias repair. Eur J Pediatr Surg 1997; 7:156.

Van Savage JG, Palanca LG, Slaughenhoupt BL: A prospective randomized trial of dressings versus no dressings for hypospadias repair. J Urol. 2000; 164:981–983.

Van Winkle W, Hastings JC: Considerations in the choice of suture material for various tissues. Surg Gynecol Obstet. 1972; 135:113–126.

Vordermark JS Jr: Adhesive membrane; a new dressing for hypospadias. Urology. 1982; 20:86.

Wacksman J: Results of early hypospadias surgery using optical magnification. J Urol. 1984; 131:516.

Wheeler RA, Malone PS, Griffiths DM, et al: The Mathieu operation: is a urethral stent mandatory? Br J Urol. 1993; 71:492.

Analgesia and Pain Control

John Currie

Preparation

The birth of a child with any sort of deformity is a devastating experience for the parents. They will of course be anxious that all can be put right, with the minimum of distress, both physical and emotional, to the child and his family.

With the treatment of any child, the medical team always has more than one patient. The whole family need support and reassurance through the different stages of treatment. Hypospadias repair is seldom a single-stage process, and if any of the episodes lead to distress and distrust in any member of the family then subsequent treatments will be far more difficult to manage (Lepore and Kesler 1979; Denson and Terry 1988).

The correct approach is essential from the very first consultation. The family will have fears to express, and if these are dealt with properly then subsequent meetings will be far more a matter of the family working with the surgical team, rather than submitting to treatment (Robertson and Walker 1975). Children are very adept at picking up the attitudes and emotions of their parents. If the mother is anxious coming into hospital, and in particular going with the child to the operating theatre, then the child will be anxious too. They will become distressed, and a rapidly deteriorating situation will then develop with the parents becoming upset and the child feeling unsupported and terrified.

The initial consultation is then very important. This will usually be with the surgeon, whose main task is to assess the degree of hypospadias and decide on the best operation or course of treatment. The surgeon will have to deal with the initial anxiety as to the danger for the child of surgery and anaesthesia. If there is the opportunity for a combined consultation with the anaesthetist then this can be extremely useful, but this is a resource issue and seldom practical. There will be a degree of guilt on the part of the parents. They will wonder if they did anything wrong, or whether there is a problem with their family genetic make-up that has resulted in this deformity in their child. This anxiety can be expressed as aggression, and fathers in particular can be hostile at the consultations. The father may feel responsible for the problem. He may be thinking something like "my son can only have inherited this deformity from me". These fears will be expressed in questions such as: "What can have gone wrong?", which are of course very difficult to answer.

So an approach of "It's no-one's fault" and "We can do a lot to restore normal appearance and function" is essential. The parents will then want to discuss the operation and the anaesthesia. If you ask parents what they fear most about their child's surgery, many will say that it is the anaesthetic. The surgeon can then reassure as to how anaesthesia techniques have developed rapidly in the recent past, and how well pain control has advanced. The surgeon can also reassure them that they will have ample opportunity to discuss these matters with the anaesthetist prior to surgery.

The Preanaesthetic and Preoperative Visits

This is an opportunity to explain to the parents and the child what will happen and to answer any questions that they may have. Often the family will have thought of things to ask that slipped their minds at the surgical outpatient consultation. The anaesthetist therefore must be prepared to face questions about the surgery as well as the anaesthesia. It is of course ideal if the anaesthetist is used to working with that particular surgeon, and so will be able to add to the explanation given by the surgeon. If he or she is not so familiar with the proposed procedure then further explanation is better left until the surgeon's preoperative visit.

The anaesthetist's tasks at the preoperative visit are firstly to put the parents and child at ease. This will be helped by a show of familiarity with the operation and the treatment plan for their son that the surgeon will have outlined. Feeling that they are to be treated by a cohesive team is very reassuring for the family. The anaesthetic technique must then be explained to the parents and to the child. Depending on the age of the child, an explanation must be given to him of what is to happen and what he should expect postoperatively.

One of the great advantages in the team approach to paediatric surgery is the ability to predict or anticipate difficulties that may face other members of the team. Familiarity with the nuances of a particular surgeon's technique greatly adds to the quality of anaesthetic management and the optimum operating conditions at each stage of the procedure. Conversely the surgeon will benefit from knowledge of the anaesthetic techniques to be employed.

Premedication

Premedication is now not widely used in modern anaesthetic practice. The problems of bradycardia associated with the older anaesthetic agents no longer occur. Operations such as hypospadias repair stimulate the vagus nerve and hence may lead to intraoperative bradycardia; however, with local anaesthetic techniques this is rarely a problem. The very anxious or uncooperative child may need a sedative premedication. The most usual agents are temazepam or Vallergan (Bramwell and Manford 1981); these agents must be used with caution, however, as if the dose is inadequate hyperactivity and disinhibition may occur. This is particularly true with Vallergan. Even with adequate doses timing is crucial, and any delay to the list may lead the patient having recovered from the effects of the premedication. It must be remembered that agents such as temazepam or Vallergan are more sedative than anxiolytic in their action, and a patient who is fearful enough will overcome the effects of the drug. The response to these drugs is very variable. To give a dose high enough to be certain of the effects would lead to some patients being very deeply sedated. Some units prefer this approach, and the nurses are trained to look after deeply sedated children.

One of the major advances in paediatric anaesthesia has been the ability to make the skin analgesic using either Emla cream or Ametop. This is applied preoperatively and should result in painless venous cannulation. Distracting the child while venipucture is performed is extremely useful. Despite assurances of a pain-free jab, the very thought of a needle may distress the child.

The Parent in the Anaesthetic Room

It is now usual for one or both parents to accompany the child into the anaesthetic room prior to surgery. Our own preference is for only one parent to be present, as this aids focus and makes it easier for the parent to become part of the team (Daniels and Visram 2002). At the preanaesthetic visit the proposed method of anaesthesia will be discussed with the parent and also with the child if he is old enough. Intravenous induction is preferred, but children's veins may be difficult to cannulate and the possibility of change to inhalational induction must always be discussed with the family. It is not uncommon when the child has had multiple operations for an inhalational induction to be requested. It is useful to have the smaller child or infant sitting on the parent's knee for induction. They can be hugged by the parent and the chosen hand placed under the parents arm so that cannulation may be performed out of sight of the child with adequate time for local anaesthetic cream to work. In this way, cannulation can often be achieved without the child being aware of it. As the induction dose is then given, the parent is asked to support the child's head carefully. The child is then placed gently on the anaesthetic trolley for anaesthesia to be continued. It is essential that someone is available to escort the parent from the anaesthetic room as soon as the child loses consciousness. This will ensure smooth continuation of the anaesthetic and allow the anaesthetist and assistants to deal with any of the common minor complications associated with induction.

If cannulation cannot be achieved it is better not to persist in multiple attempts. Although the skin may be have sufficient analgesia, having his hand held soon becomes distressing for the child. With agents such as sevoflurane, inhalational induction can be achieved in about a minute, and it is a bonus if the child is cooperative for any of this period. The older child may well perform his part faultlessly and the younger child can also often be encouraged to assist in the process, particularly if blowing up balloon games are practised preoperatively. In the case of a very uncooperative child, the parent can be a major help in expediting the process.

Occasionally the parents are as anxious or more anxious than the child. In such a case, whether the mother or father should come to the anaesthetic room at all should be discussed, given how readily children pick up on their parents' body language and level of anxiety.

Anaesthesia can be achieved with any of the common induction agents. In our practice propofol is most commonly used. In smaller children with very small veins thiopentone may be a better alternative,

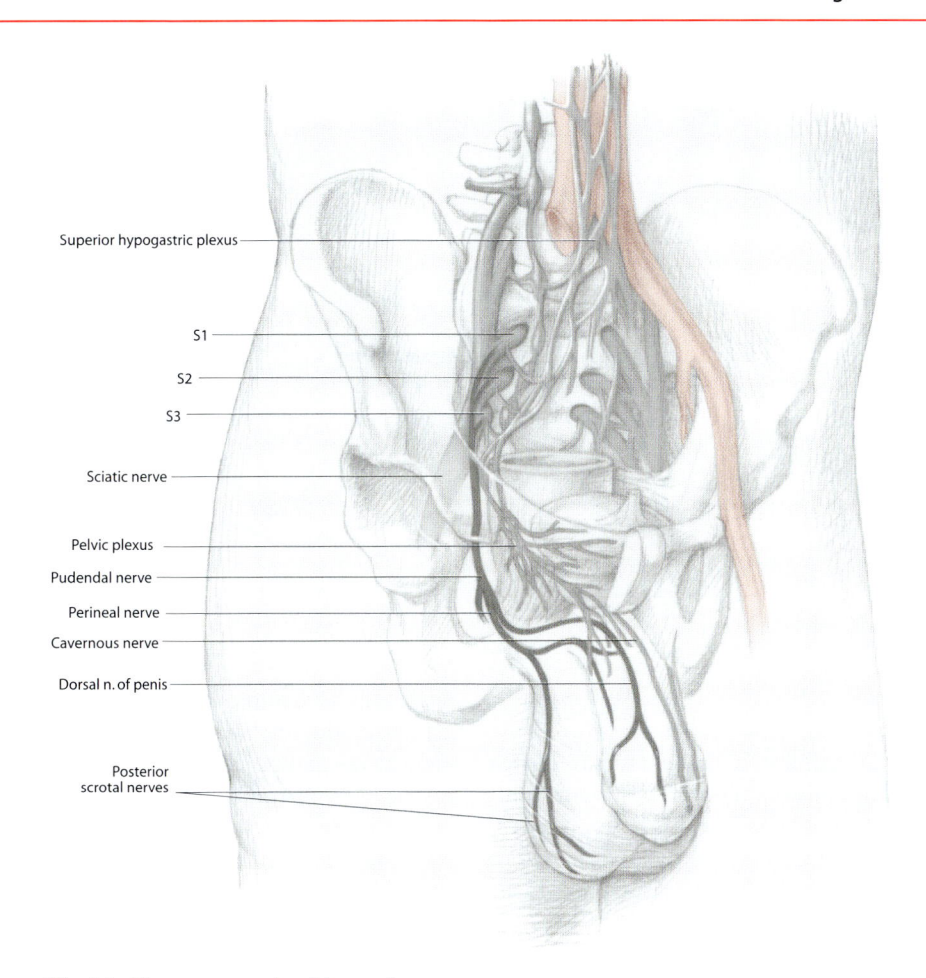

Fig. 9.1. The nerve supply of the penis

as it is less painful on injection. Anaesthesia can be maintained with any of the inhalation agents; our usual practise is to use isoflurane in nitrous oxide and oxygen. Sevoflurane is an alternative, although there are reports of excessive excitation on recovery (Murat and Constant 2000). Desflurane is a good alternative if it is preferred that the child wake up more rapidly at the end of the procedure (Hatch 1999).

The airway is maintained with a laryngeal mask airway of appropriate size if there is any worry about the child's upper airway or respiratory function intubation and ventilation is the preferred option.

Pre-emptive Analgesia

It is an old adage that it is easier to keep pain away than to take pain away. Achieving a good analgesic block prior to surgery has many real and theoretical advantages (Atallah et al. 1993; Katz 1995; McQuay 1995). There is no need to deepen the anaesthesia excessively to cover the surgical stimulus, and the stress response to surgery can be obtunded. When this technique is employed the children are much better postoperatively and require less analgesia. They also seem to be less troubled by nausea and vomiting. There is also increasing evidence that the trigger for chronic pain of the neuropathic type is more common if the painful stimulus is not controlled during surgery. It is our practice, therefore, to establish a good neurological block prior to the commencement of surgery.

Local Anaesthetic Techniques

The nerve supply of the penis is shown in ◉ Fig. 9.1.

There are two major methods of achieving nerve block for hypospadias surgery. Local infiltration or a penile block may be employed. In our experience these are insufficiently effective and do not provide adequate postoperative analgesia. Also the problem of penile erection during surgery is not always solved by these techniques. Epidural or caudal anaesthesia is much the preferred option.

Fig. 9.2. Caudal analgesia

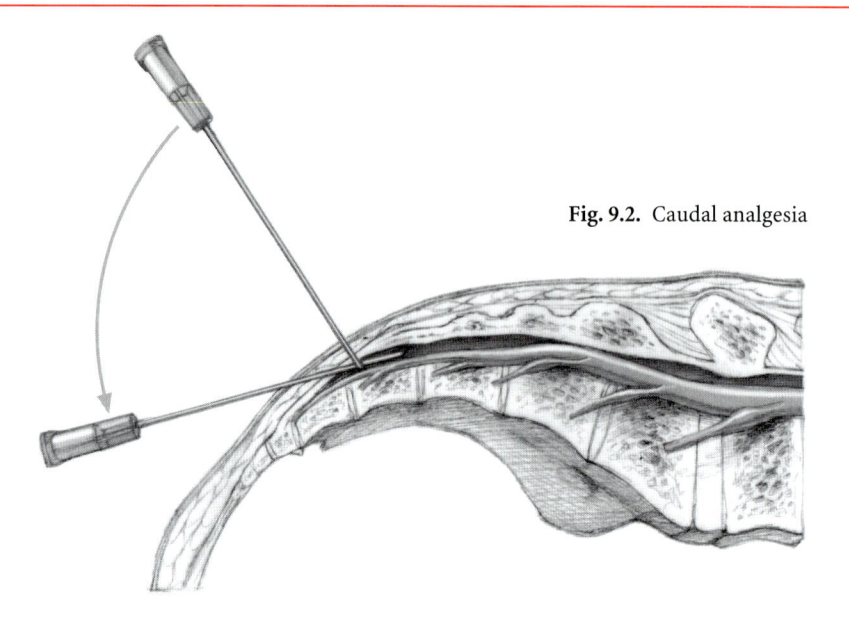

Caudal Analgesia

Instilling local anaesthetic into the caudal canal is highly effective in blocking the nerves supplying the penis (Heinen et al. 1985). The chief supply is the pudendal nerve, which has its roots at vertebrae S2 and S4. This nerve is reliably reached by local injection by the caudal root. Full precautions must be taken to ensure sterile conditions. The child is placed on his side – the left side for a right-handed anaesthetist, the right side for a left-handed anaesthetist. Generally for the age group requiring this surgery a 22-gauge needle is used. Alternatively, a cannula may be inserted into the canal. It is important that the bevel of the needle faces posteriorly so that if an epidural vein is entered this will be obvious. With the bevel facing anteriorly the vein may be compressed against the anterior wall of the canal and the fact that the needle is in the vein may not be realised (Fig. 9.2). A dose of 0.5 ml 0.25% bupivacaine per kilogram bodyweight is used. The newer agents such as ropivacaine and chirocaine are safer agents and are replacing bupivacaine in our practice. We routinely add 1 mg clonidine per kilogram, which has the effect of extending the block for as much as 24 h or even slightly longer (De Negri et al. 2001).

Epidural Analgesia

Epidural analgesia is more complicated to perform but allows for top-ups to be administered. It is technically slightly more difficult as the catheter has to be directed caudally if the lumbar route is used. The angle of the lamina will tend to direct the needle cephalad, and the Huber point of the needle gives an inadequate change in angle of insertion of the cannula (Fig. 9.3). The catheter may also be inserted via the caudal route. I personally do not use this method as I find the catheter difficult to fix in place. It is also very difficult to keep the area of insertion sterile postoperatively.

When the catheter is in place a loading dose of local anaesthetic should be injected, and here the volumes allow for 0.5% to be used. This gives a dense block which will obtund the reaction to surgery with the advantages detailed above.

The best analgesia postoperatively is achieved by an infusion of 0.125% of bupivacaine. Top-up doses may be used if nursing staff are unfamiliar with the infusion technique. This has the advantage of there being an anaesthetist present when the top-up is given to deal with any complications. The major disadvantage is that the pain will recur prior to the top-ups and a much bigger dose of local anaesthetic will be required for maintaining analgesia in the postoperative period (Morton 1999).

Penile Block

The dorsal penile nerves are blocked using an approach slightly off midline (10:30 and 1:30 positions), where the dorsal penile nerves lie on each side of the dorsal penile vein (Fig. 9.4). A small-gauge, short bevelled needle is inserted perpendicular to the skin and advanced to the symphysis pubis. Then, while withdrawing the needle, the placement is tested by

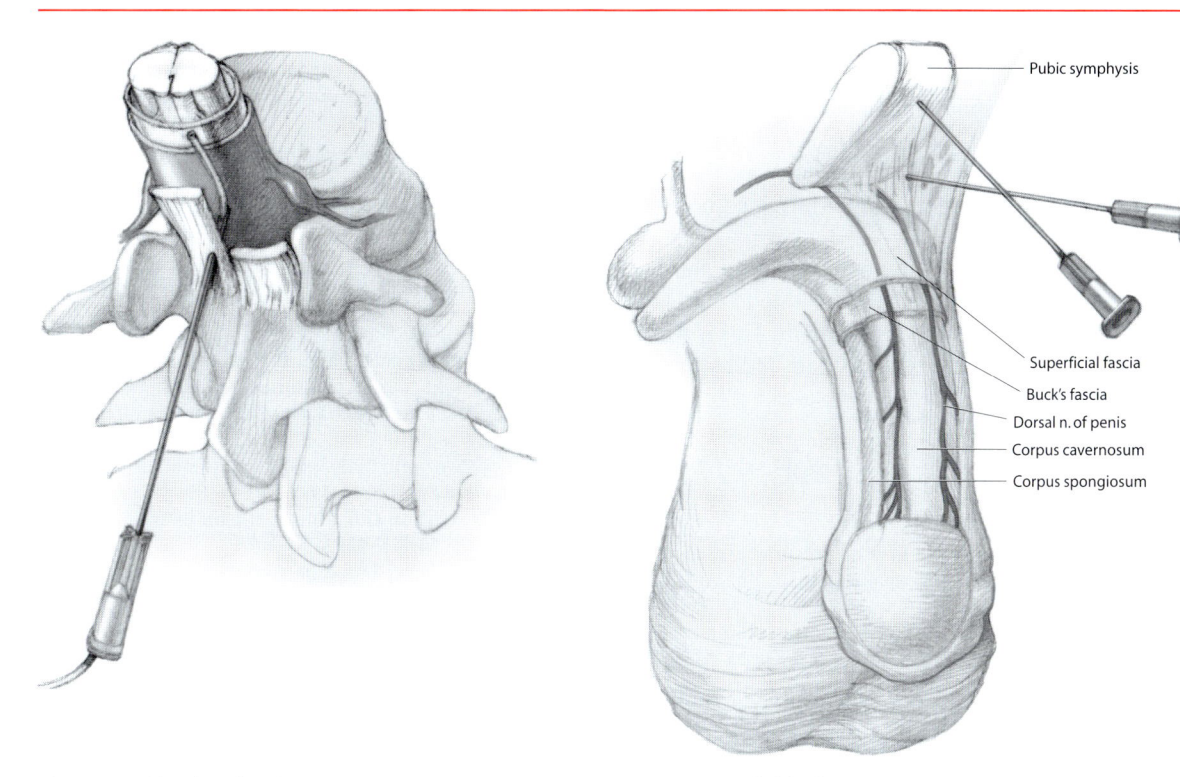

Fig. 9.3. Epidural analgesia

Fig. 9.4. Penile block

depressing the plunger of the syringe and noting when resistance is lost. This enable's one to locate Buck's fascia, where the anaesthetic solution is to be deposited. Care should be taken not to penetrate the corpora cavernosa just inferior and to avoid the dorsal penile vein. Doses for the anaesthetic range from 1 ml to 5 ml of 0.25% bupivacaine, depending on the age and weight of the patient. A potential complication is injection of the corpora with the possibility of thrombosis (Chhibber et al. 1997).

Local Application

Local application of an anaesthetic agent is useful as an adjunct to the other blocks and also postoperatively prior to any dressing change or bath. The first bath after this operation can be an unpleasant experience, and 2% lignocaine half an hour beforehand works wonders.

Summary of Agents Used

- *Local anaesthetics:* Bupivacaine, ropivacaine, chirocaine, lignocaine.
- *Adjuvants:* Clonidine, ketamine, methadone.

- *Supplementary pain management:* For dressing changes local anaesthetic gel may be employed as detailed above. Another useful technique is to use entonox, which is extremely effective in the older cooperative child (Carbajal 1999). Many other techniques have been used for sedation, including morphine and temazepam. In general, however, scheduling an anaesthetic for these events is preferable to achieving near-anaesthesia by excessive sedation. Considerable doses may be needed to achieve a dressing change, and when the stimulus is removed the child may have a level of sedation that is dangerous from the point of view of respiration and airway control.
- *Sedation agents:* Morphine, temazepam, diazepam, Vallergan, Trichlophos.

Preparation for Subsequent Surgery

As stated earlier, often several operations are required to repair hypospadias, and life is much easier if the first operation goes well. Seeing familiar faces at each admission can be very reassuring to both the child and parents, and I believe the development of surgical and anaesthetic teams that are used to working together has been a major advance (Watson et al.

2002). This is true from the point of view of the best possible surgical outcome and minimal trauma to the family. An attempt should be made to see the family when the child has fully recovered, in addition to the routine postoperative visits. The event can then be discussed and any changes or fine-tuning agreed for the next admission.

The art in all this is really attention to detail by personnel with the experience to be able to concentrate on the finer points of management. This is what makes the difference between adequate and best possible practice.

References

Atallah MM, Saied MM, Yahya R, et al: Presurgical analgesia in children subected to hypospadias repair. Br J Anaesth. 1993; 71:418–421

Bramwell RG, Manford ML: Premedication of children with trimeprazine tartrate. Br J Anaesth. 1981; 53:821–826

Carbajal R: [Analgesia using a 50/50 mixture of nitrous oxide/oxygen in children]. Arch Pediatr. 1999; 6:578–585

Chhibber AK, Perkins FM, Rabinowitz R, et al: Penile block timing for postoperative analgesia of hypospadias repair in children. J Urol. 1997;158:1156–1159

Daniels L, Visram A: Should parents be present and assist during inhalational induction of their child? A survey of the APA. Paediatr Anaesth. 2002; 12:821

De Negri P, Ivani G, Visconti C, et al: How to prolong postoperative analgesia after caudal anaesthesia with ropivacaine in children: S-ketamine versus clonidine. Paediatr Anaesth. 2001; 11:679–683

Denson CE, Terry WJ: Hypospadias repair. Preoperative preparation, intraoperative techniques, postoperative care. AORN J. 1988; 47:906–915, 918–924

Hatch DJ: New inhalational agents in paediatric anaesthesia. Br J Anaesth. 1999; 83: 42–49

Heinen M, Magna C, Corti A: [Caudal anesthesia for hypospadias operations in children]. Pediatr Med Chir. 1985; 7:879–880

Katz J: Pre-emptive analgesia: evidence, current status and future directions. Eur J Anaesthesiol Suppl. 1995; 10:8–13

Lepore AG, Kesler RW: Behavior of children undergoing hypospadias repair. J Urol. 1979; 122:68–70

McQuay HJ: Pre-emptive analgesia: a systematic review of clinical studies. Ann Med. 1995; 27:249–56

Morton NS: Prevention and control of pain in children. Br J Anaesth. 1999; 83:118–129

Murat I, Constant I: Excitation phenomena during induction and recovery using sevoflurane in paediatric patients. Acta Anaesthesiol Belg. 2000; 51:229–232

Robertson M, Walker D: Psychological factors in hypospadias repair. J Urol. 1975; 113:698–700

Watson A, Srinivas J, Daniels L, et al: An interim analysis of a cohort study on the preoperative anxiety and postoperative behavioural changes in children having repeat anaesthetics. Paediatr Anaesth. 2002; 12:824

Operative Hypospadias Surgery

Chordee (Penile Curvature)

Amir F. Azmy

Chordee With Hypospadias

Three distinct pathologic types of chordee with hypospadias were described by Horton and Devine (1973). In the first type the spongiosum is absent in the distal penis, an abnormal fibrous layer prevents the penis from being straight and the urethra is often paper thin. In the second type, the urethra is completely developed but Buck's fascia and the dartos fascia are abnormal. The third type was described as a skin chordee and is due to abnormality of the superficial dartos fascia. A fourth type was described by Kramer et al. (1982) and may be the result of disproportional growth of the dorsal portion of the corporal bodies causing downward deflection.

Chordee Without Hypospadias

Chordee without hypospadias was first described by Siever in 1926. Since then there have been a number of reports on its description and treatment (Belman 2002; Speakman and Azmy 1992). Horton and Devine (1973) described three forms of chordee without hypospadias:
1. Deficient spongiosum with thin urethra
2. Normal corpus spongiosum with abnormal Buck's fascia and dartos fascia
3. Normal urethra, corpus spongiosum and Buck's fascia with abnormal dartos fascia

Artificial Erection Test

Gittes and McLaughlin in 1974 introduced the artificial erection test to assess the degree of chordee and the point of maximum curvature and to check the results of chordee correction. Before the use of artificial erection, many cases of hypospadias were repaired without coexisting chordee being detected. As a result, residual curvature was found during follow-up.

A red rubber catheter is used as a tourniquet at the base of the penis, and normal saline is injected into a corporal body or into the glans through a 23-G butterfly needle. Both corporeal bodies are filled and show the extent of curvature (Fig. 10.1). This is repeated after excision of fibrous chordee or after dorsal plication to assess the completion of the correction of chordee before proceeding with the repair of the hypospadias.

Operative Correction of Chordee Without Hypospadias

Degloving of the penile skin is necessary to assess the degree of penile chordee and to free the shaft of the penis from its attachment to the symphysis pubis. When freeing of 1–2 cm has been achieved, the artificial erection test is carried out to identify the site of maximum curvature and clarify the anatomy of the defect. In the case of skin and dartos defects, the chordee is corrected by degloving of the penis and skin coverage using Byars flaps.

Correction of Short Urethra

Dissect and excise periurethral fibrous tissue, leaving the sulcus between the two corpora and the urethra clean. This may be enough to correct the defect. However, if curvature persists proceed to Nesbit dorsal plication (Nesbit 1965) or excise an ellipse of tunica albuginea at the maximal point of curvature with preservation of the neurovascular bundle. The length achieved by degloving the penis will compensate for the shortening created by the tunica plication. Several posterolateral Nesbit procedures may be required in persistent chordee.

Fig. 10.1. The artificial erection test

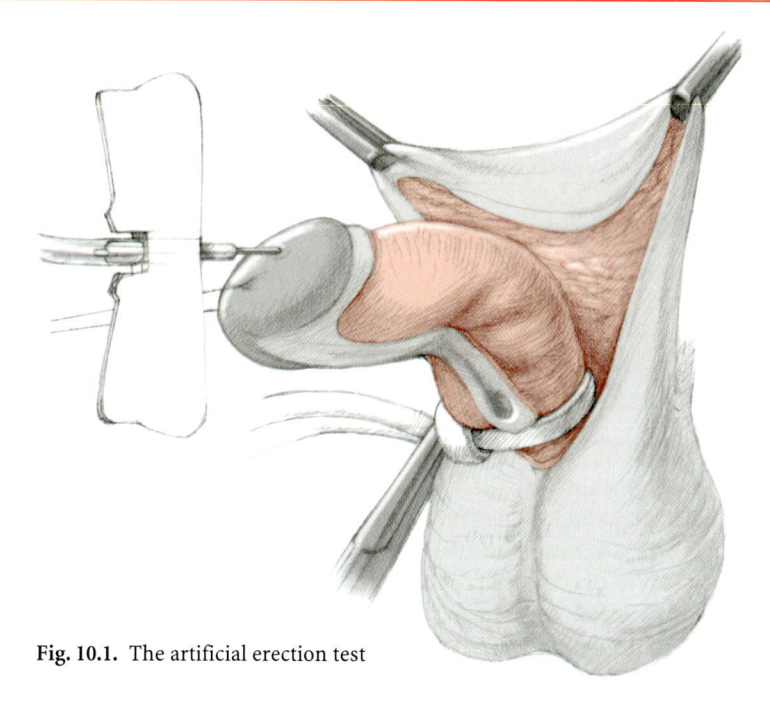

Correction of Glanular Tilt

Correction of glanular tilt is achieved by undermining the posterior subcoronal mucosa and picking up the edge of the glans and fascia by means of placing subcutaneous sutures.

Correction of the Paper-Thin Urethra

Correction of the inelastic thin urethra is achieved by dissection and excision of the fibrous bands of the periurethral tissue. Dissection under the spongiosum-covered urethra may allow some untethering.

Correction of the severe form may require resection of the abnormal urethra, correction of chordee and reconstruction of the urethra.

Correction of Chordee With Hypospadias

A survey covering current practice patterns concerning congenital chordee with hypospadias was sent to 236 members of the American Academy of Pediatrics, Section of Urology. Correction of chordee was the primary concern in hypospadias surgery for 31% of those responding, while for 54% it was not. Significant chordee is clinically defined as curvature greater than 20°. Seventy-five of the respondents would not proceed with further intervention. Placement of plicating sutures was the most common therapy chosen for 20° chordee, 50% electing this approach. Ninety-nine per cent of respondents agreed on intervening at 30° curvature; 48% used an incisional Nesbit procedure. As the degree of curvature increased, division and mobilisation of the urethral plates became the most common intervention. With 50° chordee urethral plate manipulation was used 34% of the time. It was concluded that curvature of less than 50° is best approached dorsally, while curvature of more than 50° should be approached ventrally (American Academy of Pediatrics, Section of Urology 1999).

The most popular method of correcting chordee is by dorsal plication, described by Nesbit in 1965. Nesbit excised a wedge of corporal fascia to correct the penile bend, approximating the fascial edges with buried sutures. This procedure was later modified by plication of the tunica albuginea and suturing two parallel incisions with non-absorbable stitches (Baskin and Duckett 1994). Absorbable sutures could be used, but slowly absorbed PDS (polydioxanone) is preferable.

Baskin et al., in 1998, recommended positioning the dorsal plicating sutures in the midline, as they found that the neurovascular bundle is not present at the 12 o'clock position, but rather splays out laterally from the 11 and 1 o'clock positions ventrally to the spongiosum.

Chordee correction by corporal rotation, the split and roll technique, was used as an alternative approach to correction of severe chordee. Division of the urethral plate and partial splitting of the septum between the corpora cavernosa with a ventral midline incision facilitates corporal rotation. Access is gained to the dorsal aspect of the corpora cavernosa by dissecting Buck's fascia with its encased neurovascular bundle. After artificial erection, non-absorbable sutures are placed in the area of maximal curvature. Working from the dorsal lateral aspect so that the corporal bodies are rotated toward the dorsal midline, this method does not require incision into the corporal substance, involved no use of grafts and does not cause shortening of the phallus. The neurovascular bundle is preserved and not compressed by rotational sutures (Decter 1999). Kaplan and Lamm in 1975 found that ventral penile curvature persisted in 44% of aborted fetuses through the gestational age and concluded that chordee is a normal phase of development. The degree of severity of chordee is generally proportional to the degree of hypospadias (Kaplan and Lamm 1975).

Dermal grafts harvested from non-hair-bearing inguinal skinfolds were placed in 51 patients during a 5-year period; 36 of these patients had penoscrotal or perineal hypospadias. The authors (Lindgren et al. 1998) concluded that a single dermal graft is sufficient in 57% of cases. In cases of incomplete straightening they placed an additional graft or performed dorsal plication. They believe that additional penile length achieved with dermal grafting results in a straight penis and that the cosmetic outcome is preferable to that with plication alone.

Pope et al. (1996) reported their experience with the use of dermal grafts for the correction of significant residual chordee during a 5-year period. Fifty-one patients were reviewed, of whom 41 had severe hypospadias. The dermal grafts were harvested from the hairless skin of the inguinal region and were used to fill a tunical defect created by incising the tunica at the point of maximal penile curvature. At a mean follow-up of 27 months, all patients had excellent cosmetic and functional results and the investigators concluded that in patients with significant residual chordee, a dermal graft provides a straight phallus with a minimal complication rate.

Perovic et al., in 1998, described a penile disassembly technique to avoid penile shortening in curvature repair. They used the technique in 87 patients ranging from 12 months to 47 years old (mean 4.5 years) between 1995 and 1997. The method consisted of complete disassembly of the penis: the glans cap with its neurovascular bundle dorsally; the urethra ventrally, or with coexisting hypospadias the urethral plate; and the corpora cavernosa, which may be partially separated in the midline. This disassembly technique seems to be a most effective procedure in selected cases of severe curvature of the penile shaft, marked glans tilt and a small penis. Penile disassembly combined with extensive urethral mobilisation resolves the hypospadiac meatus and there is no need to fashion a neourethra.

Correction of Penile Curvature with the Essed–Schroder Technique

A retrospective analysis carried out by Friedrich et al. (2000) used a detailed questionnaire to ascertain the long-term functional results and quality of life in patients who had undergone the Essed–Schroder procedure for correction of penile curvature.

Follow-up data were collected from completed questionnaires on 31 out of 40 patients with a median duration of follow-up of 22 months. Sexual intercourse was originally uncomfortable or impossible in 84% of cases because of penile curvature, but after surgery the cosmetic and functional results were good or sufficient in 81%; all were able to have intercourse without any problem. The investigators concluded that penile curvature correction by the Essed–Schroder technique of corporoplasty yields satisfactory results.

The technique as described begins with an incision in the penile skin, which is then retracted. A tourniquet is applied at the base of the penis and an artificial erection test is performed to define the point of maximal curvature or angulation. Then, one to three pairs of inverting non-absorbable sutures are placed in each side of the corpora cavernosa depending on the degree of curvature. The result of correction of curvature is evaluated by repeating the artificial erection test. The plication technique of tunica albuginea described by Essed and Schroder offers good correction for patients with congenital curvature of the penile shaft.

Chordee Without Hypospadias in Men

Devine et al. (1991) reported their experience over a 2 year period with 26 young men with chordee without hypospadias. Many of the patients had had straight erections as children, but ventral curvature appeared as they approached puberty. The authors performed a circumcising incision and reflection of skin to expose the shaft of the penis; the corpus spongiosum containing the urethra was mobilised by resecting the dysgenetic tissue in the dartos and Buck's fascia. This was sufficient to straighten the penis in one case. The other 25 patients required mobilisation of the neurovascular bundle and removal of one or several ellipses of tunica albuginea to equalise the length of ventral and dorsal aspects of the corpora cavernosa. The ventral curvature was resolved in 24 patients with one operation; only 2 required a second procedure.

Late-Onset Recurrent Penile Chordee After Successful Correction of Hypospadias Repair

Long-term follow-up is necessary to detect late recurrence of penile chordee.

Twenty-two patients were seen again 10 years after successful hypospadias repair (Vandersteen and Husmann 1998) because of recurrent chordee. Thirteen had had penoscrotal and 9, proximal penile hypospadias. All had originally required chordoplasty for the release of chordee, including the Nesbit procedure in 19 patients and a tunica vaginalis flap in 3. The urethra was reconstructed using a full-thickness preputial free graft in 11 cases, a bladder mucosal graft in 7 and a transverse island flap in 4.

Chordee developed again during puberty, with a median age of onset of 16 years. The median age at presentation for surgical correction was 21 years. Recurrent chordee was due to extensive fibrosis of the reconstructed urethra in seven cases, to corporal disproportion in eight and to both conditions in seven patients. Successful artificial erection at hypospadias surgery does not preclude late onset of recurrent chordee; recurrence of chordee may be secondary to the redevelopment of corporeal disproportion and/or extensive urethral fibrosis.

References

American Academy of Pediatrics, Section of Urology: Varied opinionsand treatment as documented in a survey of the American Academy of Pediatrics, Section of Urology. Urology. 1999; 53:608–612.

Baskin L, Duckett JW: Dorsal tunica albuginia plication (TAP) for hypospadias curvature. J Urol. 1994; 151:1668.

Baskin LS, Erol A, Li YW, et al: Anatomical studies of hypospadias. J Urol. 1998; 160:1108.

Belman AB: Hypospadias and chordee. In: Belman AB, King LR, Kramer SA (eds): Clinical pediatric urology, 4th edn. Dunitz, London, pp 1061–1092; 2002.

Bologna RA, Noah TA, Nasrallah PF, et al: Chordee: varied opinions and treatments as documented in a survey of the American Academy of Pediatrics, Section of Urology. Urology. 1999; 53:608–612

Decter RM: Chordee correction by corporal rotation, the split and roll technique. J Urol. 1999; 162:1152–1154.

Devine CJ, Blackly SK, Horton CE, et al: The surgical treatment of chordee without hypospadias in men. J Urol. 1991; 146:325–329.

Friedrich MG, Evans D, Noldus J, et al: The correction of penile curvature with the Essed-Schroder technique: a long-term follow-up assessing functional aspects and quality of life. BJU Int. 2000; 86:1034–1038.

Gittes R, McLaughlin AI: Injection technique to induce penile erection. Urology. 1974; 4:473.

Horton CE, Devine CJ Jr: In: Horton E (ed): One stage repair in plastic and reconstructive surgery for the genital area. Little Brown, Boston, p 278; 1973.

Kaplan W, Lamm DL: Embryogenesis of chordee. J Urol. 1975; 114:769.

Kramer SA, Aydin G, Kelalis PP: Chordee without hypospadias in children. J Urol. 1982; 128:539.

Lindgren BW, Reda EF, Levitt SB, et al: Single and multiple dorsal grafts for the management of severe penile curvature. J Urol. 1998; 160:1128–1130.

Nesbit RM: Congenital curvature of the phallus, a report of three cases with description of corrective operation. J Urol. 1965; 93:230.

Perovic SW, Vukadinovic V, Djordjevic ML, et al: The penile disassembly technique in hypospadias repair. BJU. 1998; 81:479–487.

Pope JC 4th, Kropp BP, McLaughlin KP, et al: Penile orthoplasty using dermal grafts in the outpatient setting. Urology. 1996; 48:124–127

Siever R: Anomalien auf Penis: ihre Beziehung zur Hypospadie und ihre Deutung. Z Chir. 1926; 199:286.

Speakman MH, Azmy AF: Skin chordee without hypospadias – an under-recognised entity. Br J Urol. 1992; 69:428–429.

Vandersteen DR, Husmann DA: Late onset recurrent penile chordee after successful correction of hypospadias repair. J Urol. 1998; 160:1131–1133.

Meatal Advancement and Glanuloplasty (MAGPI) Procedure

Yegappan Lakshmanan, John P. Gearhart

Introduction

Hypospadias reportedly occurs in about 1 in 125 male newborns (Sweet et al. 1974; Paulozzi et al. 1997). Recent evidence suggests that the incidence and severity of hypospadias has increased over the past 30 years (Paulozzi et al. 1997). This is thought to be a result of multiple factors, including exogenous hormone usage during gestation and environmental pollutants. About 50–70% of cases of hypospadias are classified as distal or anterior, when the meatus is located in a glanular, coronal or subcoronal location. In the past, surgical correction of these distal defects was not undertaken due to the morbidity involved with urethroplasties. It was considered that the minimal functional and cosmetic defects suffered did not warrant the potential complications of the corrective procedures. Improved surgical techniques and the increasing concern expressed by parents and older patients about appearance have changed prevailing attitudes in favor of surgical correction. Duckett, in 1981, described the meatal advancement and glanuloplasty or MAGPI procedure for the repair of distal hypospadias, renewing interest in this challenging endeavor. Since its initial description, the MAGPI operation has been performed worldwide in its original form as well as in multiple variations.

Selection of Patients

The key to a successful outcome with MAGPI is careful selection of appropriate patients. A good understanding of the nature of the defect this procedure was designed to correct is integral to the patient selection process. The MAGPI procedure is applicable to most cases of anterior hypospadias without a chordee. A glans tilt or a minor degree of chordee is not an absolute contraindication, and the insight and experience of the operator should help guide the decision-making at the time of surgery. The location and size of the meatus, the quality of the parameatal skin and the configuration of the glans are the main determinants (Duckett and Snyder 1990).

A glanular, coronal, or distal location of the meatus with a mobile distal urethra is ideal for a MAGPI operation. A more proximal hypospadias, especially with a chordee, is unsuitable. Lifting the skin below the meatus and pulling it up along with the urethra helps one to judge whether there is enough urethral mobility for the meatus to be positioned at the tip of the glans.

The size of the meatus determines the extent of lateral dissection of the glans. With a large meatus, as in the "megameatus intact prepuce" (MIP) variant, an adequate glanuloplasty may not be achieved and an alternative procedure needs to be employed.

The glans should be of adequate dimensions to allow wrapping around the advanced meatus, providing ventral support as well as a normal conical appearance. A good "ventral cushion" prevents fistulas and meatal retraction and enhances aesthetics.

A thick and pliable parameatal skin that can be dissected off the distal urethra is essential. If the skin overlying the urethra is thin and shiny, or adherent, cutting back to healthy skin would result in a more proximal defect, unsuitable for MAGPI.

Operative Technique

Meatoplasty

A polypropylene traction suture is positioned in the glans, and a combination of epinephrine (adrenaline) 1:100,000 and 1% lidocaine (lignocaine) is used for hemostasis. This can either be injected directly into the glans tissue or applied topically with a soaked sponge. The meatus, glans, and perimeatal skin are carefully inspected again to determine the most suitable repair. If the above-mentioned criteria are applicable, then MAGPI is performed. When a previous hypospadias repair has failed with a regressed meatus, we do not consider a repeat MAGPI con-

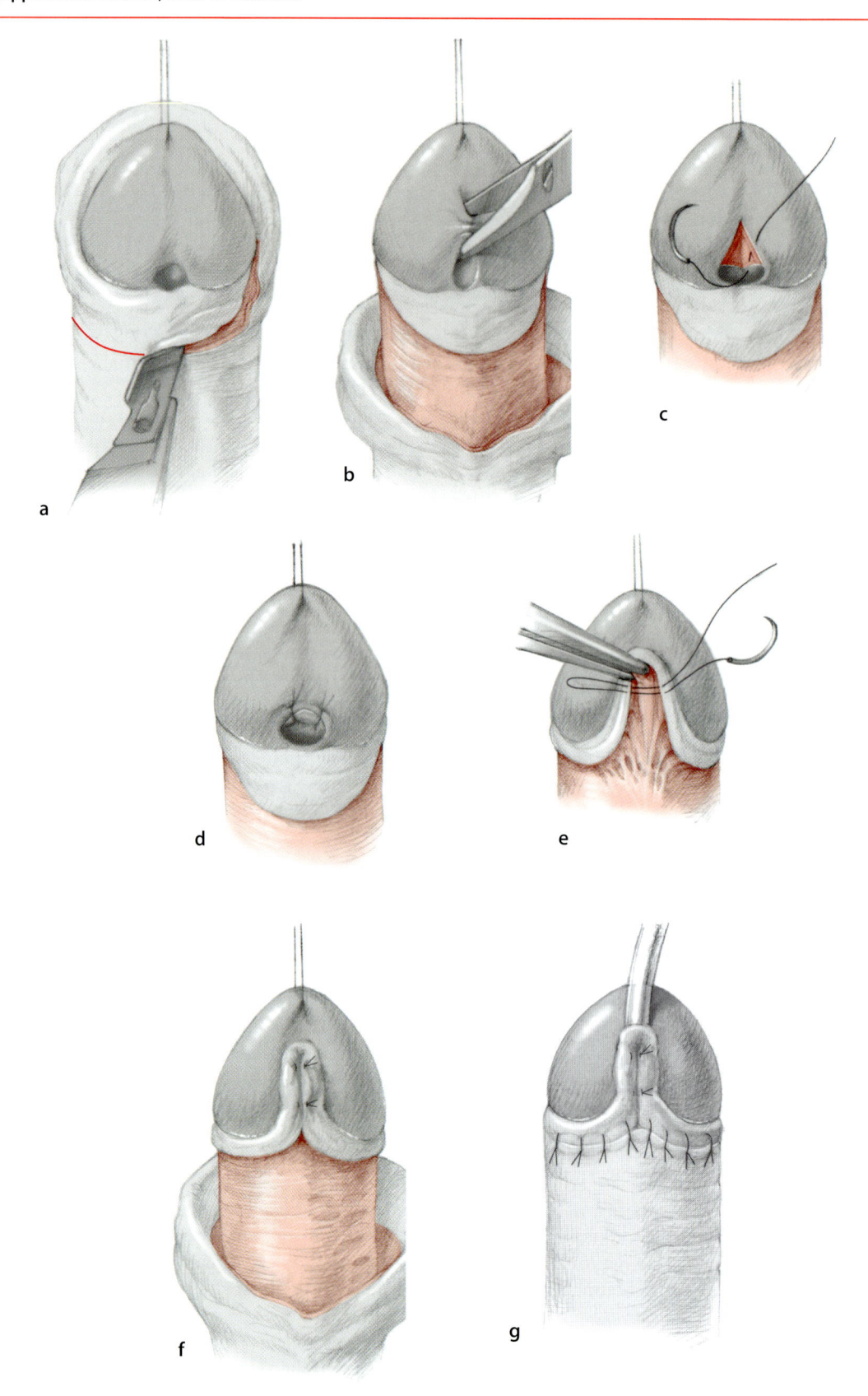

Fig. 11.1a–g. The MAGPI procedure. **a** Circumferential subcoronal incision 8 mm proximal to the meatus. **b–d** Excision of bridge of tissue between meatus and glanular groove and transverse Heineke–Mikulicz closure. **e, f** Two-layer closure of the glans edges reconfigures a conical meatus. **g** Sleeve reapproximation for skin coverage

traindicated, provided the remaining ventral skin is adequate and the meatus remains mobile enough to be advanced (Issa and Gearhart 1989).

A circumcoronal incision is made about 8 mm proximal to the urethral meatus, and the penile shaft skin degloved to the penoscrotal junction. Any fibrous tethering bands in the fascia causing chordee are released. An artificial erection may be induced to confirm that all bands have been released and to exclude any persistent curvature.

A longitudinal incision is made, starting from inside the dorsal aspect of the meatus and extending distally to the end of the glanular groove. The incision should be deepened if the glanular groove is shallow, to accommodate the urethra. Occasionally a prominent transverse "lip" of tissue in the glans, distal to the meatus, causes deflection of the urinary stream. This may be removed with a wedge excision, if not adequately flattened by the initial incision. The edges of this longitudinal incision are brought together in a horizontal Heineke–Mikulicz manner, effectively advancing the dorsal aspect of the meatus to the distal end of the glans groove. The sutures used are absorbable 6-0 Vicryl or Dexon (Fig. 11.1).

Glanuloplasty

Obtaining good glans coverage ventrally is vital for the support of the advanced meatus. To accomplish this, the ventral edge of the meatus is retracted distally toward the glans, using a stay suture or a skin hook. This brings the edges of the glans up toward the meatus in the shape of an inverted V. The skin edges of the glans wings are trimmed to expose glans tissue in order to promote good healing. This also serves to tailor the glans wings to provide a normal conical configuration. The glans tissue is approximated in the midline in two layers with interrupted absorbable sutures, completing the glanuloplasty. While a solid glans approximation prevents meatal retraction, care should be exercised to prevent compression and narrowing of the urethral lumen. Calibration of the urethra and meatus, before and after glanuloplasty, or intubation of the urethra may help avoid a tight closure.

Routine circumferential penile skin closure is performed with fine absorbable sutures. If ventral skin is deficient, skin flaps may be rotated from the dorsum. For primary repairs, catheters or stents are not required. In repeat MAGPI procedures, we leave a stent in for 3–5 days. A Tegaderm dressing is applied to provide the necessary compression and isolation.

Modifications

Many modifications of the MAGPI repair have been described. Some were meant to address known complications, while others were aimed at expanding the indications of MAGPI (Arap et al. 1984; Decter 1991).

In our experience, the MAGPI technique works well for the classically described indications. In cases where the urethral meatus and the overlying skin are mobile, and the urethral plate is of good quality, we have extended the use of MAGPI to a slightly more proximal hypospadias in a subcoronal location. The modification that allows this to succeed is the lateral mobilization of the glans wings to insure adequate glans coverage and support for the advanced urethra. As previously mentioned, we also use repeat MAGPI procedures for failed hypospadias repairs with a retracted meatus, provided the remaining ventral skin is adequate and the meatus is mobile. Similar experience has been reported by Marte et al. (2001), with good results in 18 of 21 patients using MAGPI for meatal regression after failed Duplay, Mathieu, Snodgrass, and onlay buccal mucosa graft, at a mean follow-up of 3.5 years. Use of preoperative testosterone helps to improve the vascularity and substance of local tissues in such cases.

Results

Ten years and more than 1000 patients after the original description of the MAGPI procedure (Duckett 1981), Duckett and Snyder (1990) reported an overall incidence of complications requiring a second operation in 1.2% of cases: 5 urethrocutaneous fistulas (0.45%), 7 meatal retractions (0.6%), and 1 persistent ventral curvature (0.09%). No meatal stenosis was noted. The MAGPI repair was adopted widely in the 1980s as a simple, same-day procedure for distal hypospadias. During the same period, others reported generally satisfactory results, albeit in smaller groups of patients (Hensle et al. 1983; Livne et al. 1984), while higher complication rates also became evident (Ozen and Whitaker 1987; Hastie et al. 1989). Meatal regression and stenosis were the two commonly cited problems. The proponents considered these complications related to improper selection, so that those operated on included patients with the meatus located too far proximal and with chordee. The opponents declared that lesser degrees of meatal regression were ignored by those reporting excellent results and that their follow-up was inadequate.

Several groups have stressed the importance of careful selection of the appropriate patients and not "stretching the indications" for MAGPI, to avoid such complications (Gibbons 1985; Issa and Gearhart 1989; Duckett and Snyder 1992). This is underscored by a recent report from Ghali et al. (1999), who had a 10% complication rate with 92 MAGPI repairs. The authors stated that "with increasing experience of the surgeon, avoidance of the use of MAGPI when the meatus was hypoplastic or fixed to the underlying spongiosum resulted in better cosmetic results". A recent outcome study surveyed the parents of a group of 100 children who had undergone MAGPI repairs between 1985 and 1990. These repairs were similar to the original description except in cases of hypoplasia of the distal spongiosum, where the lateral Y-shaped limbs were mobilized and approximated in the midline, or a flap of preputial subcutaneous tissue was used to cover the spongiosum. Minor complications were seen in 6% of cases and the telephone survey demonstrated a high level of parent satisfaction at a mean interval of 5.7 years after surgery (Park et al. 1995).

Complications

The reported incidence of complications after the MAGPI procedure ranges from 1.2% (Duckett and Snyder 1992) to 10% (Ghali et al. 1999). Meatal stenosis and meatal regression are the problems most commonly encountered, while other infrequent complications include urethrocutaneous fistulas and chordee.

Meatal retraction can become pronounced with growth of the penis and result in splaying of the stream, often necessitating sitting to void the bladder. Retraction may be a result of local ischemia or inflammation after surgery. Meticulous attention to tissue handling and avoidance of undue tension on the repair helps avoid this troublesome and unsightly complication. A tight glans wrap constricting the distal urethra and meatus should be avoided by mobilizing the glans wings further laterally if necessary. Such tight wraps exert tension on the glanular closure, resulting in glans separation and meatal retraction. The skin edges are trimmed to bring glans tissue together in the midline for optimal healing and ventral support of the advanced meatus. Supple perimeatal tissues and a mobile distal urethra prevent late retraction.

Strategies to avoid meatal stenosis include a meatoplasty extending into the dorsal part of the meatus, thus widening its caliber, and a deep incision of a shallow glanular groove.

Distal hypospadias is rarely associated with significant chordee. Such patients may benefit from either a meatal-based or an onlay type of flap repair after chordee correction, rather than a MAGPI repair. The risk of urethrocutaneous fistulas with MAGPI is comparatively low due to the avoidance of a sutured urethroplasty.

Conclusions

The MAGPI procedure is a dependable operation that yields good results. It has renewed interest in the surgical correction of distal hypospadias over the past two decades. While it continues to be the bulwark of surgical options for the correction of "minor hypospadias", the importance of selecting the right patient for this procedure cannot be stressed enough.

References

Arap S, Mitre AI, de Goes GM: Modified meatal advancement and glanuloplasty repair of distal hypospadias. J Urol. 1984; 131:1140–1141.

Decter RM: M inverted V glansplasty: a procedure for distal hypospadias. J Urol. 1991; 146:641–643.

Duckett JW: MAGPI (meatal advancement and glanuloplasty): a procedure for subcoronal hypospadias. Urol Clin North Am. 1981; 8:513–519.

Duckett JW, Snyder HM: The MAGPI hypospadias repair in 1111 patients. Ann Surg. 1990; 213:620–626.

Duckett JW, Snyder HM: Meatal advancement and glanuloplasty hypospadias repair after 1000 cases: avoidance of meatal stenosis and regression. J Urol. 1992; 147:665–669.

Ghali AMA, El-Malik EMA, Al-Malki T, et al: One-stage hypospadias repair. Eur Urol. 1999; 36:436–442.

Gibbons MD: Nuances of distal hypospadias. Urol Clin North Am. 1985; 12:169–174.

Hastie KJ, Deshpande SS, Moisey CU: Long-term follow-up of the MAGPI operation for distal hypospadias. Br J Urol. 1989; 63:320–322.

Hensle TW, Badillo F, Burbige KA: Experience with the MAGPI hypospadias repair. J Paediatr Surg. 1983; 18:692–694.

Issa MM, Gearhart JP: The failed MAGPI: management and prevention. Br J Urol. 1989; 64:169–171.

Livne PM, Gibbons MD, Gonzales ET: Meatal advancement and glanuloplasty: an operation for distal hypospadias. J Urol. 1984; 131:95–98.

Marte A, di Iorio G, de Pasquale M: MAGPI procedure in meatal regression after hypospadias repair. Eur J Paediatr Surg. 2001; 11:259–262.

Ozen HA, Whitaker RH: Scope and limitations of the MAGPI hypospadias repair. Br J Urol. 1987; 59:81–83.

Park JM, Faerber GJ, Bloom DA: Long-term outcome evaluation of patients undergoing the meatal advancement and glanuloplasty procedure. J Urol. 1995; 153:1655–1656.

Paulozzi LJ, Erickson D, Jackson RJ: Hypospadias trends in two US surveillance systems. Paediatrics. 1997; 100:831–834.

Sweet RA, Schrott HG, Kurland R, et al: Study of the incidence of hypospadias in Rochester, Minnesota, 1940–1970, and a case-control comparison of possible etiologic factors. Mayo Clin Proc. 1974; 49:52–58.

Urethral Advancement, Glanuloplasty and Preputioplasty in Distal Hypospadias

Dimitris Keramidas, Michael Soutis

Glanular, coronal and subcoronal hypospadias are mild forms of distal hypospadias, rarely associated with true fibrous chordee. Deviation of the urinary stream is usually the only functional problem and because of that not all the patients were treated surgically in the past. However, the abnormally situated urethral meatus and unsightly appearance of the prepuce may cause psychological stress.

Following publication of the Mathieu procedure in the year 1932, several techniques have been employed for the treatment of distal hypospadias using either the ventral penile skin (Gonzales et al. 1983) or tubularised skin flaps (Mustarde 1965; Kim and Hendren 1981; King 1981). Fistulae and meatal stenosis have been reported as postoperative complications. A new procedure for subcoronal hypospadias known as MAGPI (meatal advancement, glanuloplasty and preputioplasty incorporated) was described by Duckett in 1981. The MAGPI procedure is a simple operation, yields a cosmetically acceptable penis and has a minimal complication rate (Hensle et al. 1983; Man et al. 1984; Linve et al. 1984; Duckett and Snyder 1991). However, it is not generally applicable to all forms of distal hypospadias. Severe ventral tilt of the glans, especially in cases with preoperative ventriflexion, has been reported (Gibbon and Gonzales 1983; Mitchell 1993; Arap et al. 1984; Nasrallah and Minnot 1984; Paulus et al. 1993). As an alternative, modifications of either the Mathieu (de Jong and Boemers 1993) or the Barcat (Koff et al. 1994) techniques were used. With these techniques the prepuce is not retained, and with the Barcat procedure meatal stenosis, diverticulum or sebaceous cyst formation and urinary infection can occasionally occur. In order to overcome these problems, we have used a procedure which incorporates urethra advancement, glanuloplasty and preputioplasty (URAGPI; Keramidas and Soutis 1995). This procedure is based on the amenability of the urethra to mobilisation and advancement to the tip of the glans (Koff 1981; Hamdy et al. 1999; Caione et al. 1997).

Operative Technique

At the beginning of the operation an indwelling catheter is put into the bladder and an ischaemic tie is placed around the base of the penis. A submeatal crescent-like incision of the skin a is made few millimetres below the meatus. Two vertical incisions beginning from the lateral ends of the submeatal incision are made to converge at the tip of the glans, thus forming a triangular configuration around the meatus and the glanular groove (Fig. 12.1a). By sharp and blunt dissection, the meatus is circumscribed and the mobilisation of the distal urethra begins. There is a plane behind the urethra easily reached from the top of the triangular incision. Following this plane the dissection of the urethra from the glans and corpora cavernosa on the one hand and from the skin of the ventral surface on the other hand is generous. At this step of the operation special attention is paid to preservation of the integrity of both the urethra and the thin penile skin, thus avoiding the risk of postoperative fistula formation. The mobilisation of the urethra is completed when the urethral meatus can reach the top of the glans without tension. In order to release any remaining chordee, two lateral incisions are made along the coronal sulcus, each of them including up to one quarter of the circumference of the sulcus (Fig. 12.1b). The reconstruction starts after completion of mobilisation of the urethra. The meatus is sutured to the tip of the glans using interrupted stitches of 5-0 or 6-0 polyglucolic acid material. The two halves of the glans are sutured over the urethra, burying it without tension (Fig. 12.1c). The preputial skin is shaped to normal appearance by incising its ventral parts transversally on each side and stitching it vertically, thus circumscribing the glans (Fig. 12.1d). After completion of the operation the penis appears normal with the meatus at the tip of the glans and the preputial skin surrounding the glans (Fig. 12.2). The indwelling catheter is removed on the 6th postoperative day and the patient is discharged as soon as he has voided urine.

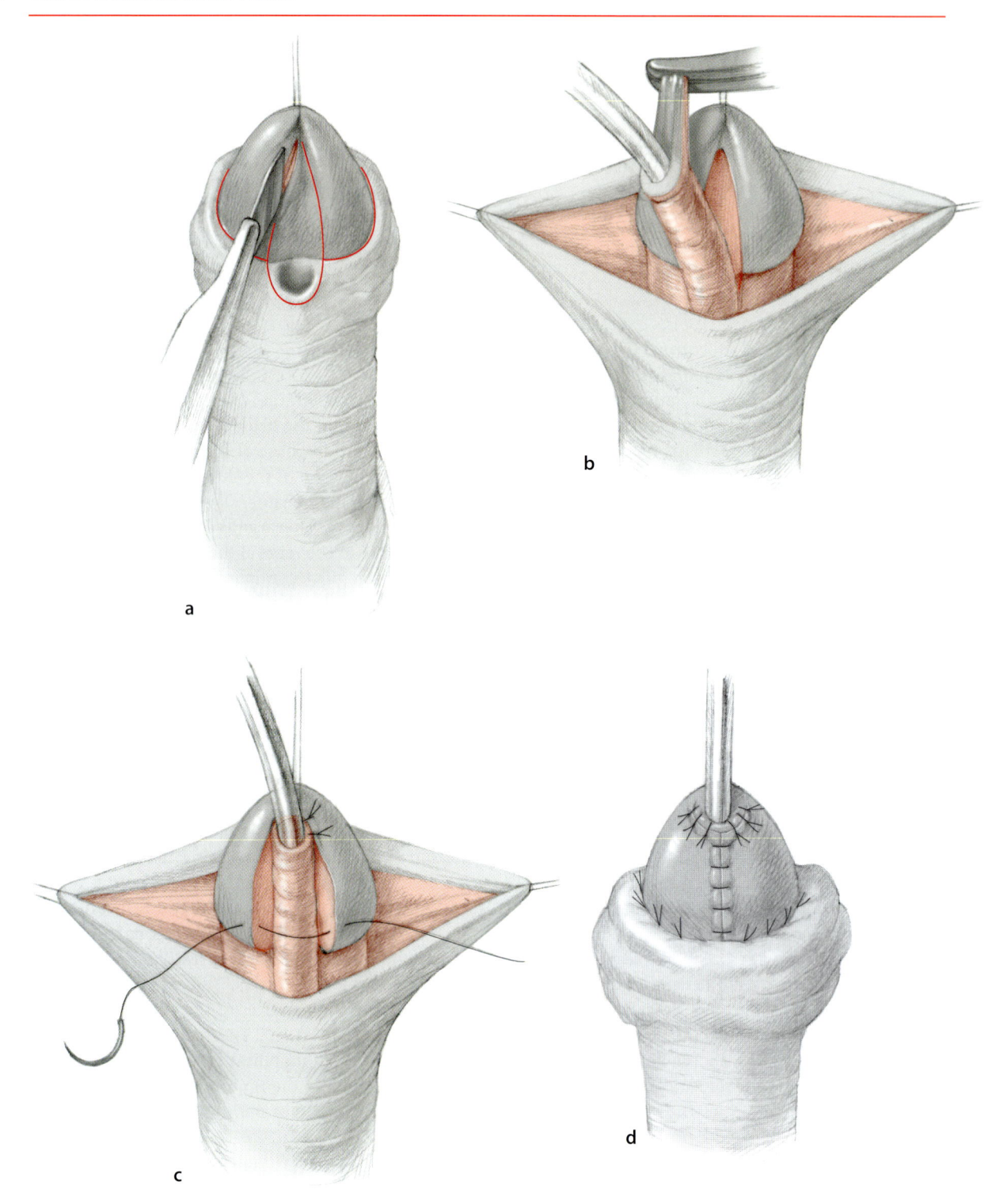

Fig. 12.1. a Triangular configuration of incisions around the meatus and the glanular groove. **b** Dissection of the urethra from the glans, corpora cavernosa and ventral skin. Lateral incisions along the coronal sulcus. **c** Fixation of the meatus to the tip of the glans and reconstruction of the glans. **d** Vertical stitching of the transversally incised ventral parts of the prepuce

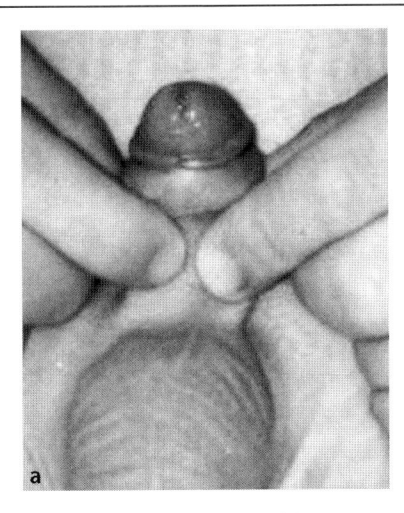

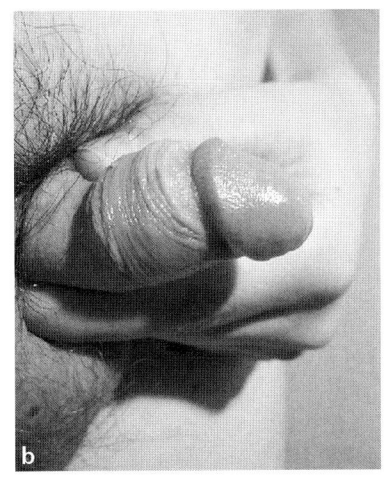

Fig. 12.2 a, b. Appearance of the penis a 6 months and b 10 years after the operation

Complications

Repair of possible complications by using preputial skin is an additional advantage of prepuce preservation. Postoperative complications are urethrocutaneous fistula (6; 12%) due to urethral damage during dissection and urethral retraction (3; 26%) due to inadequate mobilisation. They were noted early in our series of 245 patients (aged 16 months to 14 years) of whom 106 had glanular and 139 had coronal or subcoronal hypospadias. Postoperative complications were easily dealt with by reoperation using the Mathieu procedure (Keramidas and Soutis 1995).

Comments

Our experience with URAGPI and postoperative results make it necessary to emphasise the following:
1. The converging vertical incisions from the lateral ends of the submeatal incision up to the tip of the glanular groove (a) facilitate the creation of a dissection plane and mobilisation of the urethra from the glans and corpora cavernosa and (b) provide slight mobilisation of the lateral wings of the glans, so that the distal urethra can be buried in a bed between them without tension.
2. The lateral incisions along the coronal sulcus release any remaining skin chordee and straighten the penis.
3. The transverse incision of the prepuce and longitudinal suturing reconstruct the prepuce to a normal shape.

The *disadvantage* of URAGPI versus MAGPI is that both operation time and hospital stay are longer. *Advantages* of the procedure are (a) applicability to almost any type of distal hypospadias regardless of severity of glanular ventriflexion, (b) normal appearance of the penis and (c) good functional results.

References

Arap S, Mitre A, Menezes de Goes G: Modified meatal advancement and glanduloplasty repair of distal hypospadias. J Urol. 1984; 131:1140–1141.

Caione P, Capozza N, Lais A, et al: Long term results of the distal urethral advancement glanduloplasty for distal hypospadias. J Urol. 1997; 158:1168–1171.

De Jong T, Boemers TM: Improved Mathieu repair for coronal and distal hypospadias with moderate chordee. Br J Urol. 1993; 72:972–974.

Duckett JW: MAGPI (meatal advancement and glanduloplasty). A procedure for subcoronal hypospadias. Urol Clin North Am. 1981; 8:513–519.

Duckett JW, Snyder H: The MAGPI hypospadias repair in 1111 patients. Ann Surg. 1991; 213:620–626.

Gibbons MD, Gonzales ET: The subcoronal meatus. J Urol. 1983; 130:739–742.

Gonzales ET, Veeraraghavan KA, Delaune J: The management of distal hypospadias with meatal-based vascularized flaps. J Urol. 1983; 129:119–120.

Hamdy H, Awadhi MA, Rasromani KH: Urethral mobilization and meatal advancement: a surgical principle in hypospadias repair. Pediatr Surg Int. 1999; 15:240–242.

Hensle T, Badillo F, Burbige K: Experience with MAGPI hypospadias repair. J Pediatr Surg. 1983; 18:692–694.

Keramidas DC, Soutis ME: Urethral advancement, glanduloplasty and preputioplasty in distal hypospadias. Eur J Pediatr Surg. 1995; 5:348–351.

Kim SH, Hendren WH: Repair of mild hypospadias. J Pediatr Surg. 1981; 16:806–811.

King L: Cutaneous chordee and its implication in hypospadias repair. Urol Clin North Am. 1981; 8:397–402.

Koff S: Mobilization of the urethra in the surgical treatment of hypospadias. J Urol. 1981; 125:394–397.

Koff S, Brinkuian J, Ulrich J, et al: Extensive mobilization of the urethral plate and urethra for repair of hypospadias. The modified Barcat technique. J Urol. 1994; 151:466–469.

Linve P, Gibbons D, Gonzales E Jr: Meatal advancement and glanduloplasty: an operation for distal hypospadias. J Urol. 1984; 131:95–98.

Man DWK, Hamdy MH, Bisset WH: Experience with meatal advancement and glanduloplasty (MAGPI) hypospadias repair. Br J Urol. 1984; 56:70–72.

Mathieu P: Traitement en un temps de l'hypospadias balanique et juxtabalanique. J Chir. 1932; 39:481–486.

Mitchell M. In: Hensle T et al: Experience with the MAGPI hypospadias repair. J Pediatr Surg. 1993; 18:692–694.

Mustarde JC: One stage correction of distal hypospadias and other people's fistulae. Br J Plast Surg. 1965; 18:413–422.

Nasrallah PF, Minnot HB: Distal hypospadias repair. J Urol. 1984; 131:87–91

Paulus C, Dessouki T, Chelade M, et al: 220 cases of distal hypospadias. Results of MAGPI and Duplay procedures. Retrospective place of glanduloplasty and urethroplasty. Eur J Pediatr Surg. 1993; 3:87–91.

Thiersch–Duplay Principle

Moneer Hanna, Adam C. Weiser

Introduction

In 1869, Professor C. Thiersch reported that in 1857 and 1858 he had tubularized the urethral plate to form a urethral canal in a child born with epispadias. He credited the technique to August Brauser, his one-time assistant. Thiersch's classic article illustrated the design of the flaps and the asymmetric lateral incisions so that the urethral suture lines are unopposed. In 1874, Duplay described the tubularization of the urethral plate distal to the urethral orifice. His first successful hypospadias repair with this technique was achieved in five stages. In 1880, Duplay observed the capacity of the urethral plate to tubularize over a catheter. He wrote: "Although the catheter is not actually covered entirely by skin, I am convinced that this has no ill effect on the formation of the new urethra; stricture formation does not occur so long as half of the urethral wall is supplied by skin". This concept was popularized by Denis Browne in 1949, when he described the buried skin strip method for hypospadias repair.

Mettauer first reported the concept of skin chordee in 1842, and subsequently D.R. Smith reported it in 1967. In 1968 Allen and Spence utilized the technique of degloving the penile skin and performed foreskin transposition to correct coronal hypospadias with moderate to severe chordee. King (1970) incorporated the concepts of Mettauer and Thiersch–Duplay to correct midshaft hypospadias and brought the meatus to the coronal sulcus.

In early years glanular and subcoronal hypospadias were often not repaired, because the complications of repair often overshadowed the benefits of surgical correction. Duckett's (1981) meatal advancement and glanuloplasty technique (MAGPI) was designed to reduce the risks of formal urethroplasty in distal hypospadias. Time and experience demonstrated that this technique could not be universally applied to all patients with distal hypospadias. Arap et al. (1984) modified the MAGPI technique to repair a more proximal meatus. Decter (1991) described the technique of an "M inverted V" glanuloplasty and utilized the Mathieu (1932) principle. Both Arap's and Decter's methods were designed to reduce the chance of meatal retraction, which is sometimes seen after conventional MAGPI repair, and to improve the cosmetic result of the glans penis. However, neither achieved wide acceptance.

Zaontz, in 1989, applied the Thiersch–Duplay principle to the repair of distal hypospadias. He reported excellent results with the glans approximation procedure (GAP). The operation was indicated for patients with coronal or glanular hypospadias, deep glanular groove and a fish-mouth meatus. The GAP eliminated the ventral glanular tilt, meatal retraction and splaying of the urinary stream that was seen at times in meatal advancement and glanuloplasty procedures. Van Horn and Kass (1995) modified King's (1970) approach by extending the paraurethral incision to the tip of the glans penis and used a two layer ventral closure of the glans penis. They found that very few children were not candidates for this technique of glanuloplasty and in situ tubularization for the repair of distal hypospadias. They achieved better cosmetic results than with either the Mathieu or the MAGPI procedure.

In 1997 Stock and Hanna reported the largest documented series of Thiersch–Duplay repairs. Combining the principles of Heineke–Mikulicz meatoplasty to widen the meatus dorsally at 12 o'clock with Thiersch–Duplay tubularization of the urethral plate, they noted a low complication rate of 2.1% in 512 children.

While some were embracing the Thiersch–Duplay principle, others looked to the meatal-based flap technique of Mathieu, which also uses the urethral plate as the dorsal wall of the urethra. In 1969, Barcat modified the Mathieu technique, using apposing epithelial flaps based at the meatus to create a neourethra and dissecting the urethral plate from its bed. He then incised the glans penis and placed the urethral tube within the newly created sulcus. With the Barcat technique the configuration of the glans or meatus did not matter. However, the post-operative incidence of fistulae (15–20%) somewhat dampened the enthusiasm for this technique (Redman 1987). Koff et al. (1994) modified the Barcat technique and interposed a second layer of tissue over the neourethra, thus reducing the fistula rate to 2%. Koff noted that the only contraindication for this technique was in cases where a large amount of chordee was caused by factors distal to the hypospadiac meatus, whereby transection of the urethral plate was required. Barthold et al. reported their experience with 295 cases in 1996. All of these surgical modifications, including the Mathieu technique, share the inherent potential complications of raising and rotating a random skin flap.

Midline incision of the urethral plate was first reported by Reddy in 1975. He performed the incision to excise "fibrous tissue" in the midline that he believed to be the cause of the chordee. He then combined this with the Thiersch–Duplay principle and tubularized the urethral plate. Rich et al. (1989) described a technique for the creation of a normal vertical slit-like meatus by hinging the distal urethral plate longitudinally in the midline. This modification was applied to a variety of meatal-based flaps and achieved excellent cosmetic results. In 1994 Snodgrass reported on the technique of a tubularized incised plate urethroplasty (TIP) for distal hypospadias. A deep sagittal incision of the urethral plate was made from the meatus to the tip of the glans penis. This incision facilitates tubularization of the plate and results in a normal slit-shaped meatus. Furthermore, the deep incision prevents tension on the ventral suture line, thus acting as an internal relaxing incision. Hinging allows the urethral plate to be tubularized even when its width would ordinarily be inadequate to construct a neourethra of sufficient caliber.

We find the Thiersch–Duplay procedure offers several advantages. It utilizes the tissues that were embryonically destined to form a urethra; there is minimal disturbance of the blood supply of the urethral plate, which is often well vascularized, there is hardly any contracture of the tubularized plates, and stricture formation is indeed a rare complication.

Preoperative Evaluation

A routine urologic history is taken and physical examination conducted. Questions regarding maternal prenatal history and family history of hypospadias are also asked.

On physical examination one notes the position of the urinary meatus and quality of the perimeatal skin, the depth of the glanular groove, presence and degree of chordee, penile torsion, penoscrotal transposition and whether the child has been circumcised. The presence or absence and location of the testicles are recorded, and if undescended testicle is diagnosed in conjunction with any degree of hypospadias, intersex workup is requested.

In children with proximal and especially in perineoscrotal hypospadias, voiding cystography is recommended, as we encountered a significantly large prostatic utricle in approximately 25% of children. We also encountered vesicoureteral reflux in 15% of the patients we studied (unpublished data).

We currently perform surgery when the patient is 6 months old. In the child with a small phallus, 50 mg of testosterone is given intramuscularly 3–4 weeks preoperatively.

Patient Selection

We began using the Thiersch–Duplay principle in 1987 for children with a meatus at or just proximal to the coronal sulcus. When the meatus was stenotic, or a prominent shelf was encountered, we performed a Heineke–Mikulicz meatoplasty at 12 o'clock. Our experience in 512 consecutive cases was reported previously (Stock and Hanna 1997). We have subsequently extended the use of the Thiersch–Duplay technique to proximal hypospadias with chordee due to skin tethering or mild chordee (<30°), due to corporal disproportion, which was corrected by the Nesbit (1967) procedure of tunica albuginea placation (TAP) (Daskalopoulos et al. 1993). Early in our series the absence of a deep glanular groove and/or the presence of hypoplastic thin skin at the urinary meatus were considered contraindications to the Thiersch–Duplay technique. The addition of the Reddy-Rich-Snodgrass incision of the urethral plate and distally in the glans penis allowed for repair of hypospadias in children with a shallow or minimal glanular groove. Currently in our practice, the only contraindication to the Thiersch–Duplay repair is the presence of moderate or severe ventral chordee of >30°, due to corporal disproportion. In such cases we divide the urethral plate and place a dermal graft to lengthen the ventral wall of the corpora, rather than shorten the dorsal walls by the Nesbit or the TAP procedure.

Operative Management

A 5/0 silk stay suture is placed in the glans penis dorsal to where the future meatus will be. If the

Thiersch–Duplay Principle

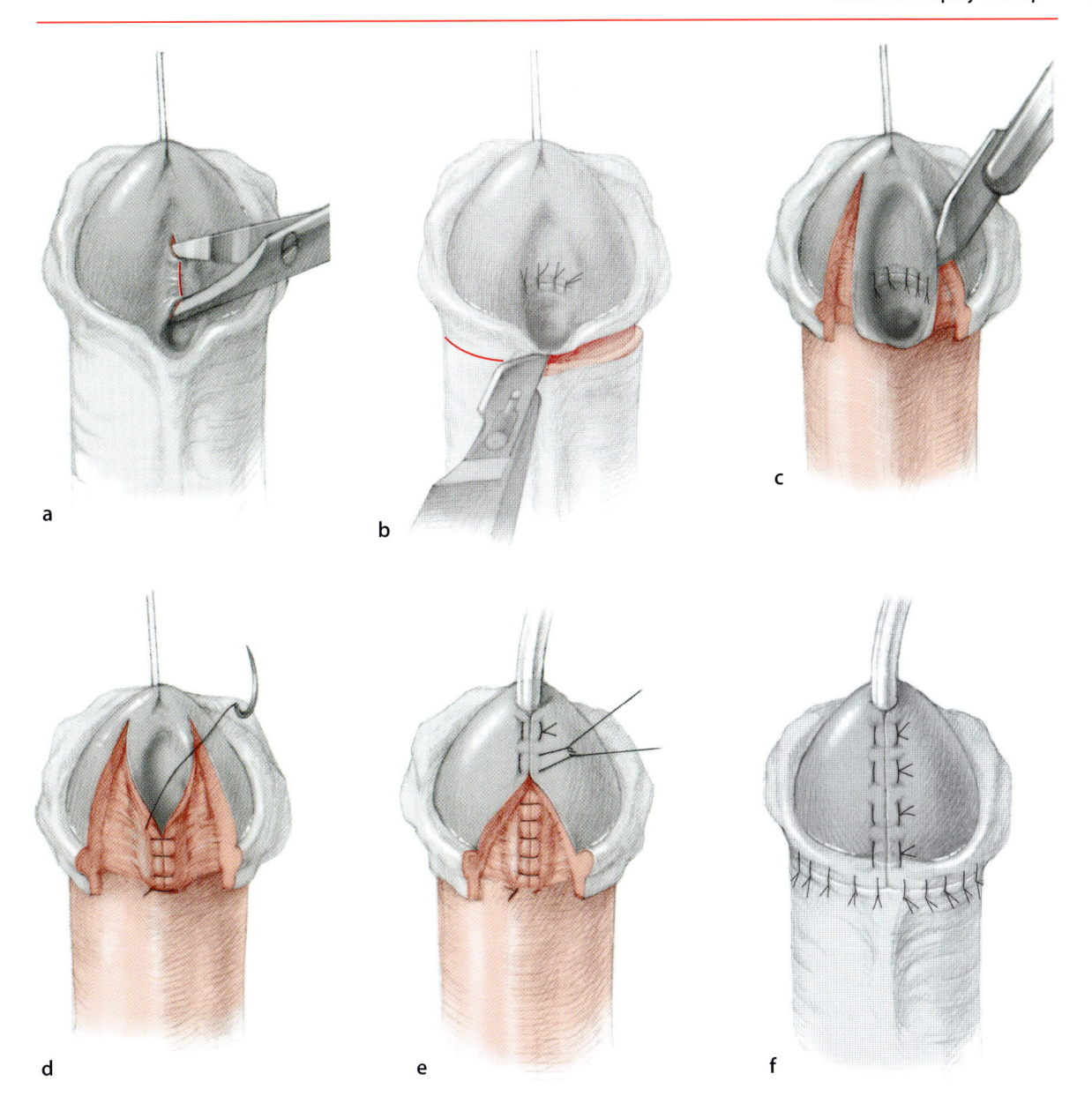

Fig. 13.1.1a–f. Diagrammatic illustration of the Thiersch–Duplay repair of distal hypospadias. **a** A longitudinal midline incision is made at 12 o'clock. This incision is closed transversely in Heineke–Mikulicz fashion. **b** A subcoronal incision is made around the glans penis. **c** An incision is made dorsally, laterally and ventrally around the meatus; the width of the urethral plate is 12 mm, leaving 2 mm of skin around the meatus. **d** The urethral plate is tubularized over the catheter using a running suture. **e** The glanular skin is approximated with horizontal mattress interrupted 7-0 polyglycolic sutures. **f** The available skin and its blood supply dictate the final closure

meatus is stenotic a longitudinal midline incision is made at 12 o'clock. This incision is closed transversely in a Heineke–Mikulicz fashion with interrupted 7-0 polyglycolic suture (Fig. 13.1.1a). An 8-F feeding tube is inserted in the urethra. If the perimeatal skin is thin and hypoplastic an incision is made ventrally until healthy skin is seen. The incised skin edges are then approximated with interrupted 7-0 polyglycolic sutures (Fig. 13.1.2). A subcoronal incision is made dorsally, laterally and ventrally around the meatus; the width of the urethral plate is 12 mm, leaving 2 mm of skin around the meatus (Fig. 13.1.1b, c). The skin and dartos fascia are dissected circumferentially proximally and the penis is degloved. In some cases deep dissection of the penoscrotal junction is necessary to completely straighten the penis. An artificial erection test is performed by placing a vessel loop as a tourniquet around the base

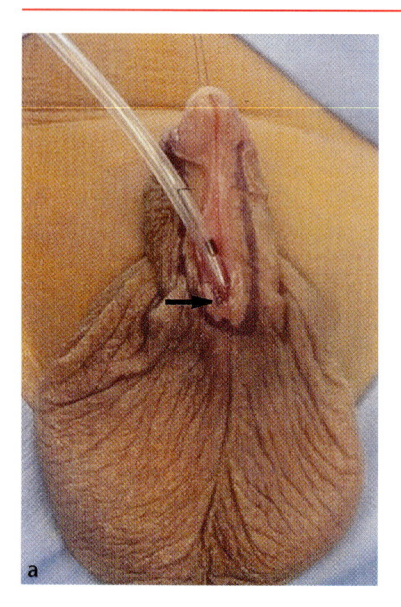

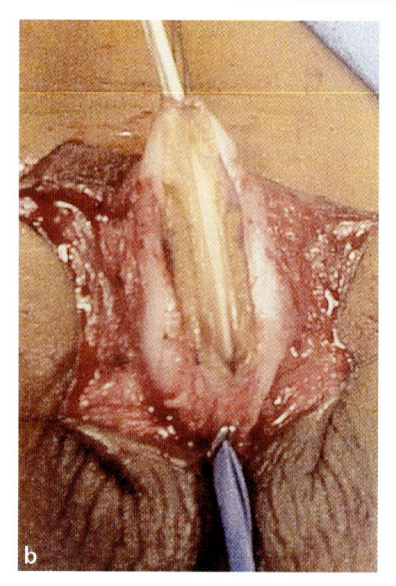

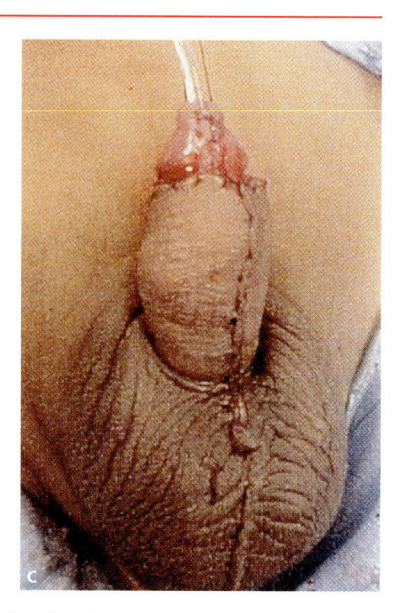

Fig. 13.1.2a–c. Thiersch–Duplay repair of proximal hypospadias. **a** Penoscrotal hypospadias and hypoplastic meatal skin: ventral meatoplasty at 6 o'clock. **b** Lateral skin incisions and denudation of glanular skin on either side of deep glanular groove. **c** Completed repair: the suture line is covered with dartos flap prior to skin closure

of the penis, then injecting the corpora with normal saline. In the case of residual mild curvature <30°, we used to use the Nesbit procedure or TAP modification. However, we have recently adopted the Baskin et al. (1998) method for chordee repair. If the glanular groove is deep, we find it unnecessary to incise the glans penis on either side and prefer to denude the skin by excising two wedges of glanular skin on either side, similar to the GAP (Fig. 13.1.3). If the glanular groove is inadequately shallow, we incise the glans penis in the midline at 12 o'clock to avoid any tension on the ventral suture line. The feeding tube is then removed and either a Silastic urethral catheter or a silicone splint of appropriate size is placed and secured. The urethral plate is then tubularized over the catheter using a running subcuticular 7-0 polydioxanone suture (PDS) (Fig. 13.1.1d). A dartos flap is raised, mobilized from the dorsal penile skin, then rotated and sutured to cover the urethral suture line. The glanular skin is approximated with horizontal mattress interrupted 7-0 polyglycolic sutures (Fig. 13.1.1e). For resurfacing the penis we often adopt Byars flaps (1955), which create a midline ventral raphe. However, the available skin and its blood supply dictate the final closure (Fig. 13.1.1f). Duoderm dressing is applied around the penis and secured with Op.site transparent adhesive. The catheter drains into a double diaper and the child is discharged the same day. In distal hypospadias repair a catheter is seldom used, but for proximal repairs the catheter and dressing are necessary and are removed 3–5 days postoperatively. Prolonged urinary drainage is frequently associated with catheter obstruction and bladder spasm, which only serve to complicate matters.

Results

The Thiersch–Duplay principle with or without hinging of the urethral plate is now widely accepted and practiced by many surgeons.

The main complications in the reported series are urethrocutaneous fistula and stricture formation. Table 13.1.1 summarizes the surgical morbidity in the largest reported series of cases using the Thiersch–Duplay principle. It is inevitable that there are subtle variations of the surgical technique, and these are hard to quantify. However, in our experience the major factors that determine success and complications are primary vs reoperative repair, and distal vs proximal hypospadias. In comparing our early series (1987–1994), which included 512 children with distal hypospadias (coronal or juxtacoronal meatus), with our second series of 265 children with proximal hypospadias (penile, midshaft and penoscrotal meatus), it became apparent that surgical complications were more often encountered (8.6%) in proximal than in distal repairs (2.9%).

The interposition of a healthy de-epithelialized skin flap, as described by Durham Smith (1973), reduces the incidence of urethrocutaneous fistula. We

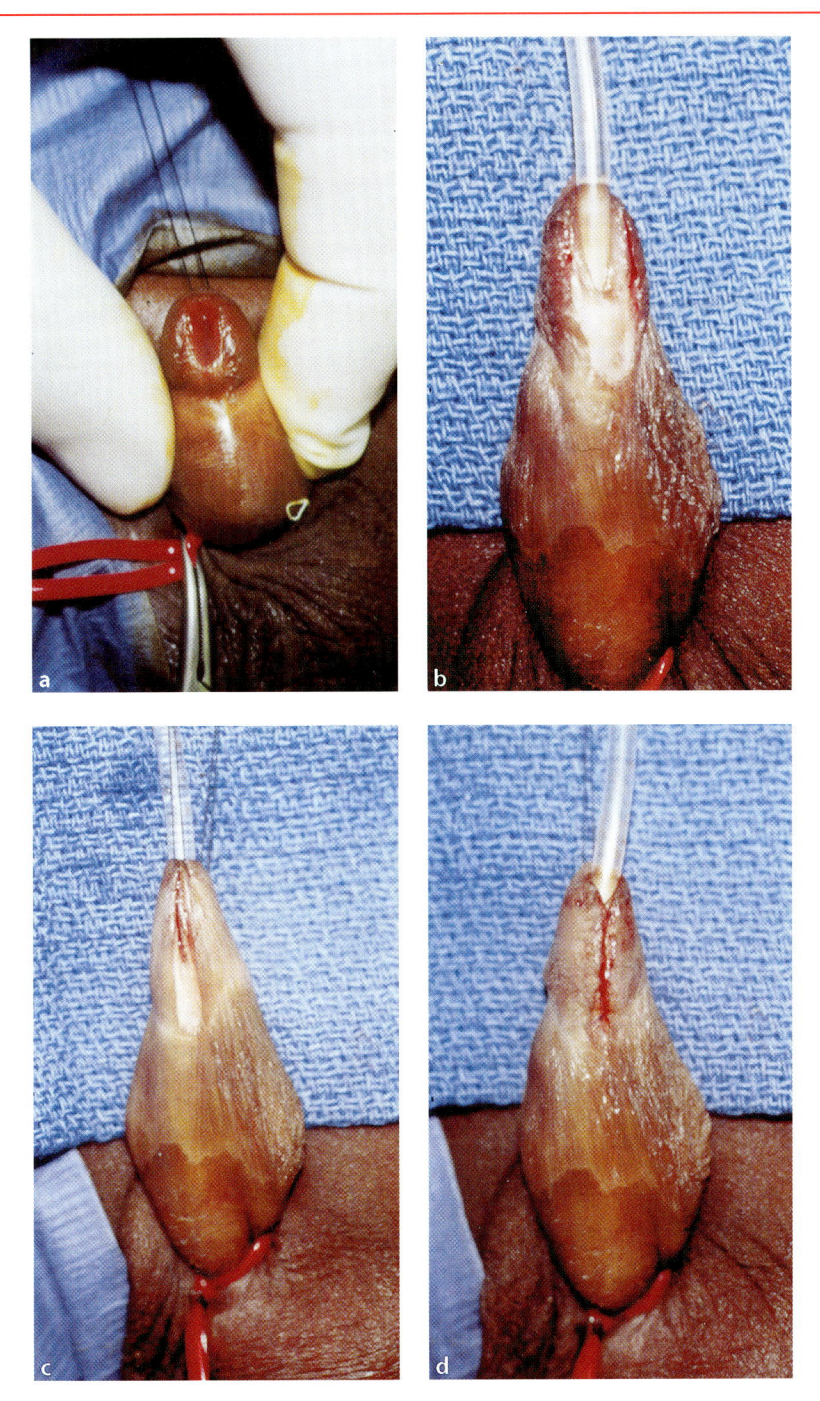

Fig. 13.1.3a–d. GAP procedure. **a** Megameatus with deep groove. **b** Glanular skin is excised on either side. **c** The urethral plate is tubularized using continuous subcuticular sutures. Note placement of ventral stay sutures aligns the tissues. **d** Skin closure using horizontal mattress sutures

Table 13.1.1. Surgical morbidity in the major reported series of patients operated on using the Thiersch–Duplay principle

Reference	Number of patients	Primary vs secondary repair	Location	Complications – Meatal stenosis	Complications – Fistula
Zaontz 1989: GAP	24	Primary	Coronal 11, proximal 13	0	1
Kass 2000: glanuloplasty (no hinging)	308	Primary	Coronal/glans 84%, midshaft 9%, prox./penoscrotal 7%	Diverticulum 2 (0.6%)	28 (9.1%): distal 6.2%, mid. 17.9%, proximal 42.9%
Snodgrass et al. 1996	148	Primary	Distal	3	Fistula 5, glans dehiscence 3
Ross and Kay (1997)	18	Primary 15, secondary 3	Distal or midshaft	0	0
Stock and Hanna (1997)	512	Primary	Distal	2	Initial 5 (4 small fistulae diagnosed after toilet training)
Steckler and Zaontz (1997)	33	Primary	Distal 31, midshaft or proximal 2	0	0
Snodgrass et al. (1998)	27	Primary	Midshaft, penoscrotal	1	Fistula 1, glans dehiscence 1
Stock and Hanna (1997)	265	Primary	Midshaft to proximal, penoscrotal	Stricture 3, diverticulum 2	Fistula 16, dehiscence 2
Decter and Franzoni (1998)	197 (156 hinged)	Primary	Glans 52, coronal 101, proximal 44	Meatal retraction 4	Fistula 5
Dayanc et al. (2000)	25	Primary 23, secondary 2	Distal 20, midshaft 11	Mid-penile 1 (primary), distal 1 (primary)	Distal 1 (secondary)
Hayashi et al. (2001)	13	Secondary	Distal 5	0	Distal 1 (secondary)
Shanberg et al. (2001)	13	Secondary	Distal	1	Fistula + glans dehiscence 1
Smith (2001)	64	Primary	Distal 53, midshaft 11	0	0
Yang et al. (2001)	25	Secondary	Distal 10, midshaft 9, proximal 4, penoscrotal 2	13 (3 in patients with unaltered urethral plate and no preoperative fistula)	7 (0 in patients with unaltered urethral plate and no preoperative fistula)

often raise a dartos flap from the dorsal penile skin and rotate it to cover the ventral urethral suture line (Fig. 13.1.4).

Conclusions

Hypospadias surgery provides ample opportunity for modification by any surgeon who wishes to establish his individuality. Some authors claim originality of idea, but it behooves us all to credit those who pioneered current surgical concepts and principles,

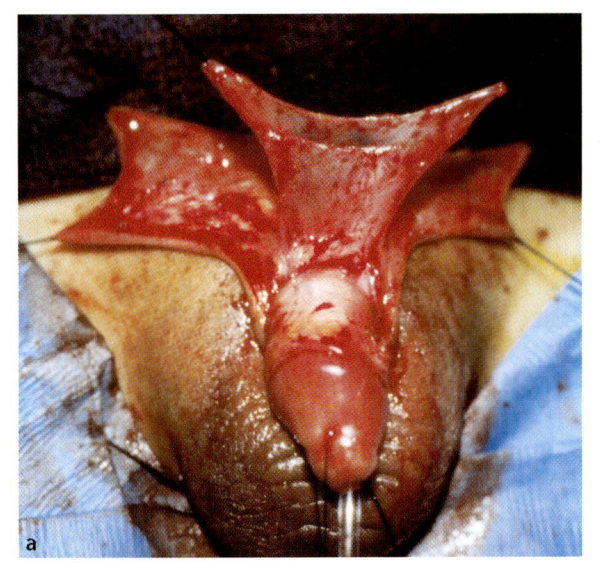

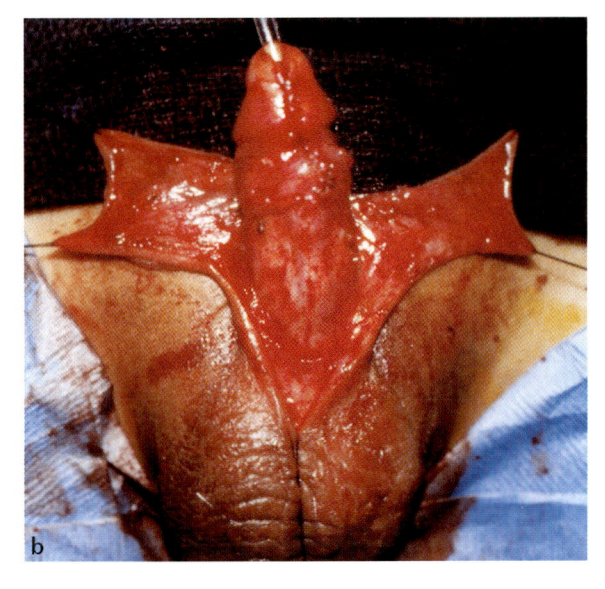

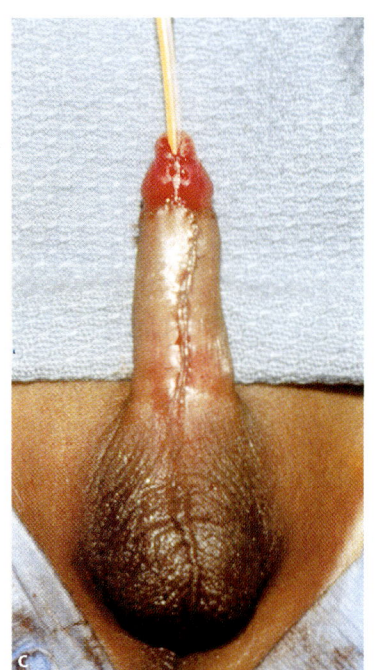

Fig. 13.1.4a–c. Dartos flap and penile resurfacing. **a** Dartos flap is raised from dorsal prepuce and is dissected proximally to avoid rotational deformity. **b** Flap is rotated and covers ventral suture line. **c** Completed repair

thus preserving our surgical heritage. We submit that the Thiersch–Duplay principle represents the basic foundation for all the surgical methods that utilize the urethral plate to construct a urethral tube.

References

Allen TD, Spence HM: The surgical treatment of coronal hypospadias and related problems. J Urol. 1968; 100: 504.

Arap S. Mitre AI, de Goes GM: Modified meatal advancement and glanuloplasty repair of distal hypospadias. J Urol. 1984; 131:1140.

Barcat J: L'hypospadias. III. Les urethroplasties, les resultats – les complications. Ann Chir Infant. 1969; 10:310.

Barthold JS, Tell TL, Rodman JF: Modified Barcat balanic groove technique for hypospadias repair: experience with 295 cases. J Urol. 1996; 155:1735.

Baskin LS, Erol A, Li YW, et al: Anatomical studies of hypospadias. J Urol. 1998; 160:1108.

Browne D: An operation for hypospadias. Proc. R Soc. Med. 1949; 41:466.

Byars LT: A technique for consistently satisfactory repair of hypospadias. Surg Gynecol Obstet. 1955; 100:184.

Daskalopoulos BI, Baskin L, Duckett JW, et al: Congenital penile curvature (chordee without hypospadias). Urology. 1993; 42:708.

Dayanc M, Tan MO, GoKalp A, et al: Tubularized incised plate urethroplasty for distal and mid penile hypospadias. Eur Urol. 2000; 37:102–125.

Decter RM: M inverted V glansplasty: a procedure for distal hypospadias J Urol. 1991; 146:641.

Decter RM, Franzoni DF: Distal hypospadias repair by the modified Thiersch–Duplay technique with or without hinging the urethral plate: A near ideal way to correct distal hypospadias. J Urol. 1998; 162:1156.

Duckett JW: MAGPI (meatal advancement and glanuloplasty): a procedure for subcoronal hypospadias. Urol Clin North Am. 1981; 8:513.

Duplay S: De l'hypospadias perineo-scrotal et de son traitement chirugical. Arch Gen Med. 1874; 1:613:657.

Duplay S: Sur le traitement chirugical de l'hypospadias et de l'epispadias. Arch Gen Med. 1880; 5:257.

Hayashi Y, Kojima Y, Mizuno K, et al: Tubularized incised-plate urethroplasty for secondary hypospadias surgery. Int J Urol. 2001; 8:444–448.

Kass EJ, Chung AK: Glanuloplasty and in situ tubularization of the urethral plate: Long-term follow up. J Urol. 2000; 164: 991.

King LR: Hypospadias – a one stage repair without skin graft based on a new principle: chordee is sometimes produced by skin alone. J Urol. 1970; 103:660.

Koff SA, Brinkman J, Ulrich J, et al: Extensive mobilization of the urethral plate and urethra for repair of hypospadias: the modified Barcat technique. J Urol. 1994; 151: 466.

Mathieu P: Traitment en un temps de l'hypospadias balanique et juxta-balanique. J Chir (Paris). 1932; 39:481.

Mettauer JP: Practical observations on those malformations of the male urethra and penis, termed hypospadias and epispadias with an anomalous case. Am J Med Sci. 1842; 4:43.

Nesbit RM: Operation for correction of distal penile ventral curvature with or without hypospadias. J Urol. 1967; 97: 470.

Reddy LN: One stage repair of hypospadias. Urology. 1975; 5:475.

Redman JF: The Barcat balanic groove technique for the repair of distal hypospadias. J Urol. 1987; 137:83.

Rich MA, Keating MA, Snyder HM III, et al: Hinging the urethral plate in hypospadias meatoplasty. J Urol. 1989; 142:1551.

Ross JH, Kay R: Use of de-epithelialized local skin flap in hypspadias repairs accomplished by tubularization of the incised urethral plate. Urology. 1997; 50:110.

Shanberg AM, Sanderson K, Duel B: Re-operative hypospadias repair using the Snodgrass incised plate urethroplasty. BJU Int. 2001; 87:544–547

Smith DR: Repair of hypospadias in the pre-school child. A report of 150 cases. J Urol. 1967; 97:723.

Smith ED: A de-epithelised overlap flap technique in the repair of hypospadias. Br J Plast Surg. 1973; 26:106.

Smith DP: A comprehensive analysis of a tubularized incised plate hypospadias repair. Urology. 2001; 57:778.

Snodgrass W: Tubularized, incised plate urethroplasty for distal hypospadias. J Urol. 1994; 151:464.

Snodgrass W, Koyle M, Manzoni G, et al: Tubularized incised plate hypospadias repair: results of a multicenter experience. J Urol. 1996; 156:839.

Snodgrass W, Keys M, Manzoni G, et al: Tubularized incised plate hypospadias repair for proximal hypospadias. J Urol. 1998; 159:2129.

Steckler RN, Zaontz MR: Stent free Thiersch–Duplay hypospadias repair with the Snodgrass modification. J Urol. 1997; 158:1178.

Stock JA, Hanna MK: Distal urethroplasty and glanuloplasty procedures: Results of 512 repairs. Urology. 1997; 49:449.

Thiersch C: Über die Entstehungweise und operative Behandlung des Epispadie. Arch Heilkd. 1869; 10:20.

Van Horn AC, Kass FJ: Glanuloplasty and in situ tubularization of the urethral plate: simple reliable technique for the majority of boys with hypospadias. J Urol. 1995; 154:1505.

Zaontz MR: The GAP (glans approximation procedure) for glanular/coronal hypospadias. J Urol. 1989; 141:359.

Megameatus Intact Prepuce Variant

Amir F. Azmy

The prominent or deep glanular groove variety of distal hypospadias associated with megameatus is often hidden by an intact prepuce; a large number of children have been circumcised due to the apparently normal appearance of the prepuce and surgical options may then be limited due to the circumcision. The megameatus and intact prepuce variant of anterior hypospadias was described by Duckett and Keating in 1989 and is characterised as a subcoronal wide-mouth meatus with deep glanular groove associated with normal prepuce and no chordee. It was thought possibly to be due to maldevelopment of the glanular epithelial infolding and misdirected correcting of the glans proceeding down the already fused distal urethra, creating a megaurethra and keeping the foreskin intact (Duckett and Keating 1989).

Nonomura et al., in 1998, postulated that the megameatus intact prepuce (MIP) deformity might occur after completion of penis formation and be due to external compression of the penis in utero. The urethral plate in MIP is always wide and elastic and there is no chordee.

Duckett and Keating, in 1989, described the pyramid procedure for the MIP repair by creating lateral incisions along the glanular plate and a horseshoe-shaped incision over the meatus, with wide mobilisation of the megameatus from the penile skin. The meatus is tailored (if necessary) and the glanular plate is tubularised into a neourethra. Skin cover is completed with approximation of the glanular flap.

In the Duckett and Keating procedure (Fig. 13.2.1) a tennis-racket incision is made beside the glanular groove and around the edges of the megameatus; this section is carried out approximately below the corona, mobilising the urethra to the apex of the pyramid and deepening the edges of the glanular groove to develop glanular wings from the urethral plate. The distal urethral plate is left wide and intact dorsally. The widened distal urethra is tailored in continuity with the urethral plate by removing a small wedge of ventral tissue. The urethra and the glans strips are tubularised to form the new urethra and the glanular repair is performed. Dressings are applied and removed after 48 h by the parents, and the stent is removed after 5–7 days.

Hill et al., in 1993, described their experience with pyramid hypospadias repair in 37 patients with distal or subcoronal hypospadias. The pyramid repair was used as a primary procedure in 35 patients; the other two had had a previous Thiersch–Duplay repair with resultant malposition of the neourethra on the shaft. A large proportion of the patients had been circumcised due to an apparently normal prepuce, limiting the surgical options. Hill and colleagues included a de-epithelialised perimeatal tissue flap to cover the ventral suture line. This technique was originally described by Smith in the context of a two-stage repair and resulted in a low complication rate (one fistula in 51 repairs) (Smith 1973). The use of a de-epithelialised flap has been described by Retik et al (1988) and Belman (1988).

The pyramid modification included de-epithelialisation of the Mathieu flap, leaving only a proximal horseshoe-shaped skin margin around the meatus. The de-epithelialised Mathieu flap is brought over the ventral suture line, effecting a two-layer closure.

It is important that the glanular plate is adequate to allow tubularisation with compliant glans to cover the neourethra without compression. The presence of a silicone stent may exert tension on the suture line and result in fistula formation. Successful operation without a stent reduces complications; a second layer of viable tissue is very important to prevent fistula (Fig. 13.2.2, p. 137).

Nonomura et al. (1998) used a parameatal-based foreskin flap for urethroplasty, harvested from either a ventral (Mathieu) or a unilateral site. The glans is split along the cleft glanular groove to create glans wings. The flap is laid on the urethral plate to form the neourethra and glanuloplasty is completed by approximation of the glanular wings. Byars flaps are then used to cover the ventral surface of the penile shaft. This is shown in Fig. 13.2.3, p. 138.

Attalla (1991) proposed a surgical repair which combines reconstruction of the glanular urethra and

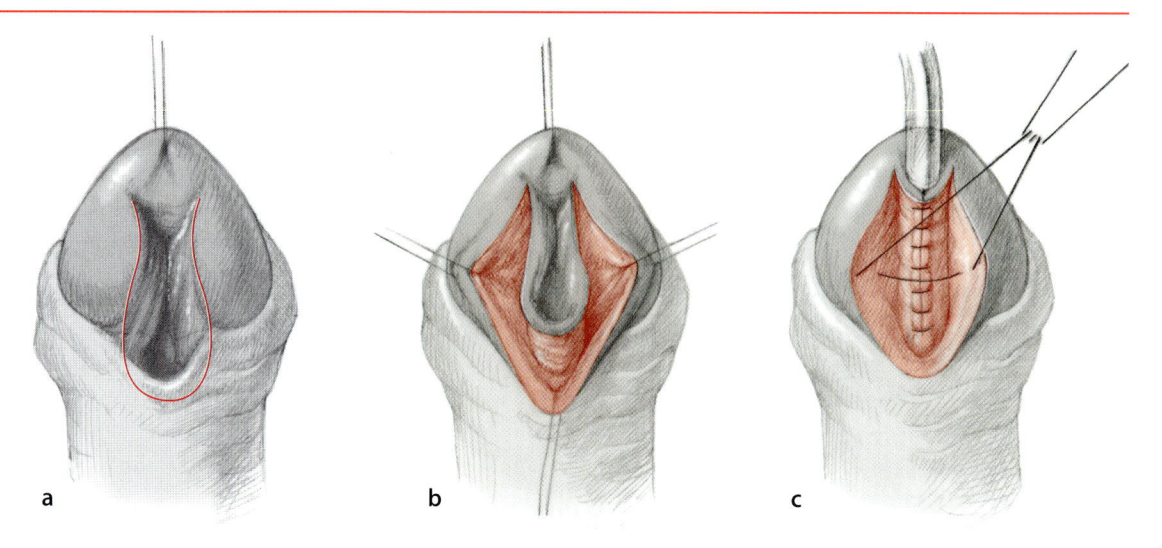

Fig. 13.2.1. Steps of the pyramid proceduce. **a** Tennis-racket incision. **b** Mobilisation of the distal urethra. **c** Urethroplasty and glanuloplasty

fashioning of the neomeatus with circumcision. In this procedure, the prepuce is divided in the dorsal midline from its free edge to 5 mm from the coronal sulcus. An approximately rectangular flap is created from the ventral external preputial skin and lining. The preputial flap is raised. A vertical glanular incision is made on each of the two navicular ridges and deepened enough to create thick urethral and glanular lips. The lateral edges of the preputial flaps are sutured to the glanular incisions in two layers; circumcision is then completed. Follow-up showed no fistula, breakdown or recession of the meatus with satisfactory cosmetic and functional results.

Docimo, in 2001, described a technique employing a subcutaneous frenulum flap for iatrogenic or primary megameatus and reoperative hypospadias repair. Using an inferiorly based island flap of the frenulum, the skin is de-epithelialised and advanced over the urethral repair, yielding in a satisfactory cosmetic result and providing added elasticity in these relatively unusual cases in which a dorsal or meatal-based flap is not feasible.

Although a meatal advancement and glanuloplasty procedure may correct the deformity, the presence of a wide meatus represents a major disadvantage as the advancement of such a meatus will result in an unacceptably patulous neomeatus and sprayed urine stream.

References

Attalla ML: Subcoronal hypospadias with complete prepuce: a distinct entity and new procedure for repair. Br J Plast Surg. 1991; 44:122–125.
Belman AB: Deepithelialized skin flap coverage in hypospadias repair. J Urol. 1988; 140:1273
Docimo SG: Subcutaneous frenulum flap (SCFP) for iatrogenic or primary megameatus and re-operative hypospadias repair. Urology. 2001; 58:261–273
Duckett JW, Keating MA: Technical challenge of the megameatus intact prepuce hypospadias variant. The pyramid procedure. J Urol. 1989; 141:1407–1409
Hill GA, Wacksmann J, Lewis AG, et al: The modified pyramid hypospadias procedure: Repair of megameatus and deep glandular groove variants. J Urol. 1993; 150:1208–1211.
Nonomura K, Kakizakia H, Shomoda N, et al: Surgical repair of anterior hypospadias with fish-mouth megameatus and intact prepuce based on an anatomical characteristics. Eur Urol. 1998; 34:368-371.
Retik AB, Keating M, Mandell J: Complications of hypospadias repair. Urol Clin N Am. 1988; 15:223
Smith D: A deepithelialized overflap flap technique in the repair of hypospadias. Br J Plast Surg. 1973; 26:106

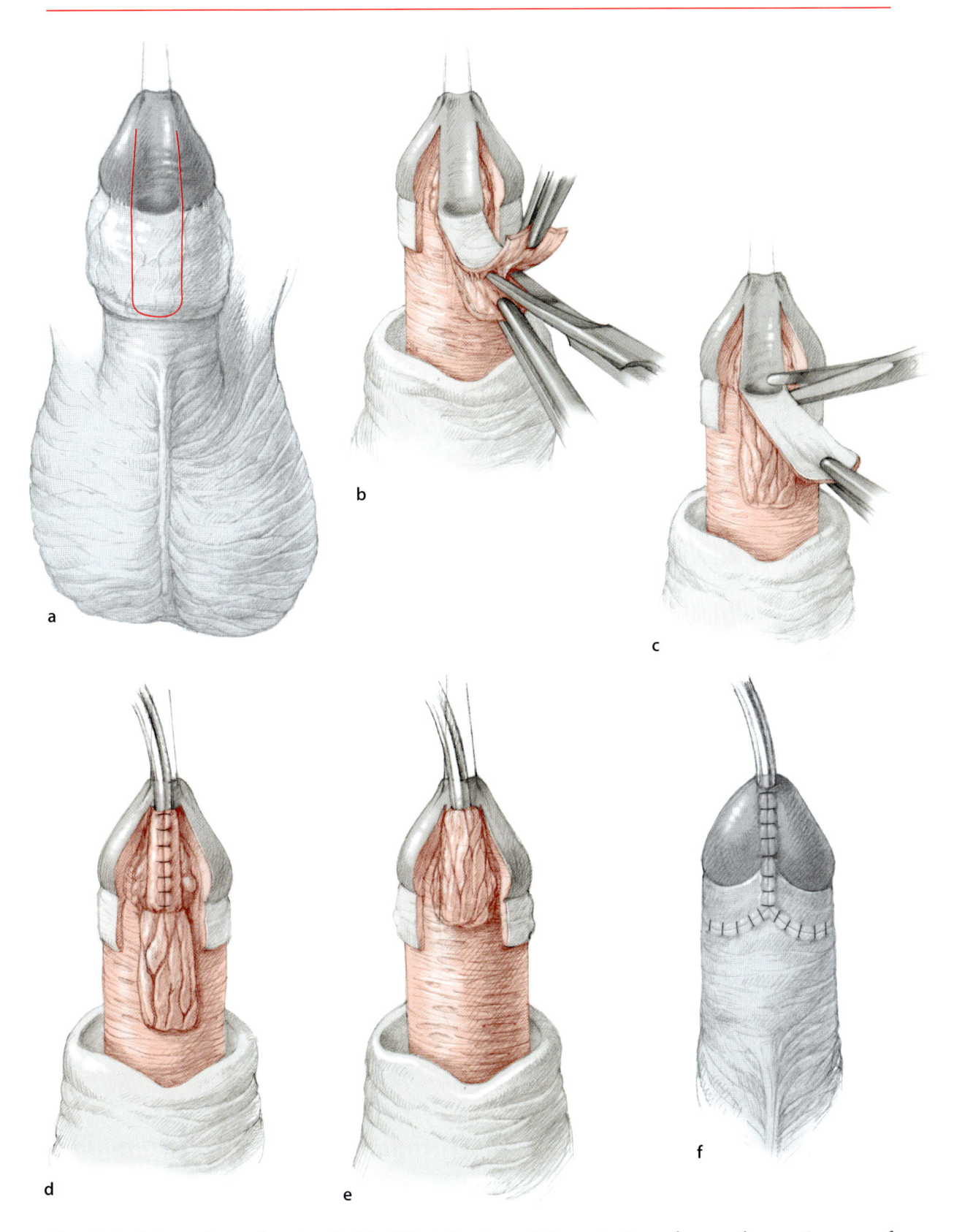

Fig. 13.2.2a–f. Steps of procedure described by Hill et al. (1993). **a** Creation of meatal-based flap. **b** Penile skin is mobilised: glans flaps and perimeter-based flap and development. **c** Skin flap is excised, leaving its vascularised mesentery. **d** Reconstruction of neourethra. **e** Coverage of neourethra suture line by the vascularised mesentery. **f** Appearance after approximation of glanular wings

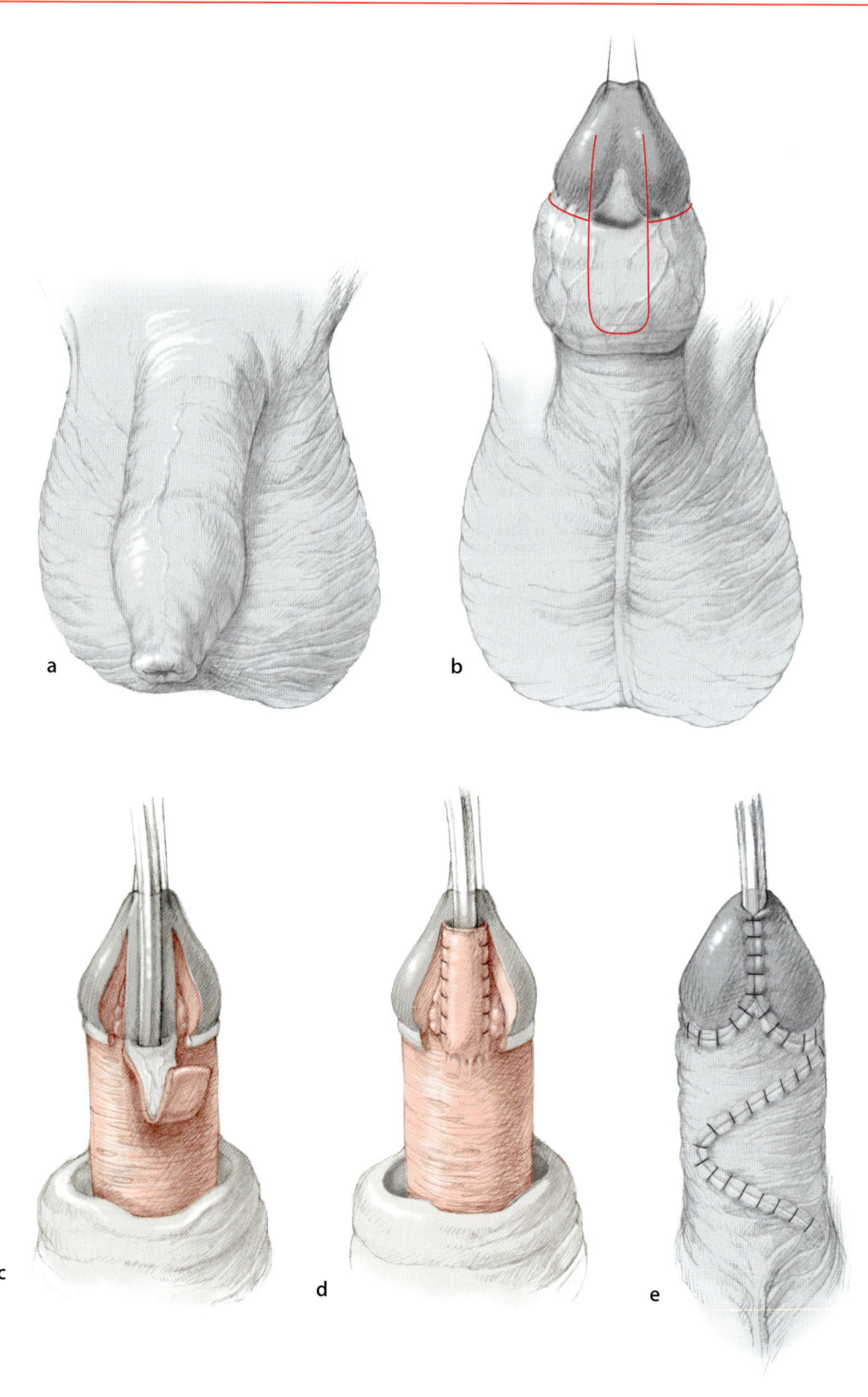

Fig. 13.2.3a–e. Surgical repair of anterior hypospadias with fish-mouth meatus and intact prepuce as described by Nonomura et al. (1998). **a** Appearance of intact prepuce. **b** Subcoronal wide-mouth meatus with deep glanular groove. **c** Creation of Mathieu parameatal flap and glans wings. **d** Parameatal flap onlaid to the urethral plate. **e** Final appearance after completion of meatoglanuloplasty

The Meatal-based Flap "Mathieu" Technique

Cenk Büyükünal

Introduction

Bouisson (1861) may have been be the first to use a rotated pedicled scrotal flap for creation of the ventral surface of the neourethra. In 1875 Wood presented the "meatal-based flap" technique which was a prototype of Mathieu's procedure (cited in Mayo 1875). Bevan, in 1917, designed a rectangular-shaped meatal-based flap technique, and this procedure can be considered the father of the Horton–Devine flip-flap technique. We think Mathieu's technique is also based on the proximal skin flap repair introduced by Ombredanné (1925). In the 21st century, the single-stage flip-flap procedure of Horton and Devine and the meatal-based flap technique of Mathieu seem to be the most popular 'local-flap techniques' for distal types of hypospadias without chordee or with minimal chordee.

The Mustardé Procedure

Mustardé's technique was described in 1965 (Mustardé 1965). A wider meatal-based flap is created and the whole flap is designed for tubularization of the new urethra. A triangular glanular flap is prepared for the construction of the glanular part of the urethra (Fig. 14.1.1) The most important problems were: (a) a higher incidence of meatal stenosis and (b) technical problems related to the coverage of the large ventral skin defect (Belman 1982, 1992; Duckett 1998; Mustardé 1965; Roth 1999; Smith 1990; Wacksman 1981).

The Horton–Devine Flip-Flap Procedure

In 1973 Horton and Devine presented a meatal-based flap technique, a modification of Bevan's and Mustardé's operation. This single-stage procedure allowed release of chordee in the distal shaft and helped to form a glanular meatus (Baran and Çenetoğlu 1993, unpublished data; Belman 1986, 1992; Devine and Horton 1977). The indications for the Horton–Devine technique are: (a) distal hypospadias without chordee or with moderate chordee; (b) a meatus that is still localised on the distal third of the penile shaft after the chordee release; (c) well-vascularised and reasonably thick skin proximal to the hypospadiac meatus. In this flip-flap procedure, the length of the penile flap should be equal to the distance between the hypospadiac urethral meatus and the tip of the penis (Fig. 14.1.2). After the precise measurement of this distance, a triangular meatal-based flap is prepared from the penile skin proximal to the meatus (Fig. 14.1.2a). A triangular glanular flap is prepared from the middle third of the glans (Fig. 14.1.2b). To prevent meatal stenosis a small dorsal meatotomy incision is performed in the penile skin-flap (Fig. 14.1.2b, c). Lateral glanular flaps are prepared with deep dissection in the plane of the corpus cavernosum (Fig. 14.1.2c). The penis is degloved and meticulous chordee release between the meatus and glans is performed. An erection test is done to make sure that there is no residual chordee or glanular tilt. Anastomosis between the triangular glanular flap and ventral flap is completed (Fig. 14.1.2d). Lateral glanular wings are reapproximated and coverage of the penile shaft is completed by ventrally rotated Byars flaps (Fig. 14.1.2e, f). A silicone Foley catheter is routinely used for urinary diversion (Baran and Çenetoğlu 1993, unpublished data; Belman 1986; Bocchiotti et al. 1982; Brodsky 1980; Devine and Horton 1977; Duckett 1998; Smith 1990; Woodard and Cleveland 1982).

The major advantages of the Horton–Devine technique can be stated as follows: (a) the risk of meatal stenosis is decreased by the aid of a triangular glanular flap; (b) this was a single-stage operation with a reasonable complication rate. The disadvantages of the technique were: (a) the characteristic snub-nosed appearance of the glans and (b) an ugly-looking meatus.

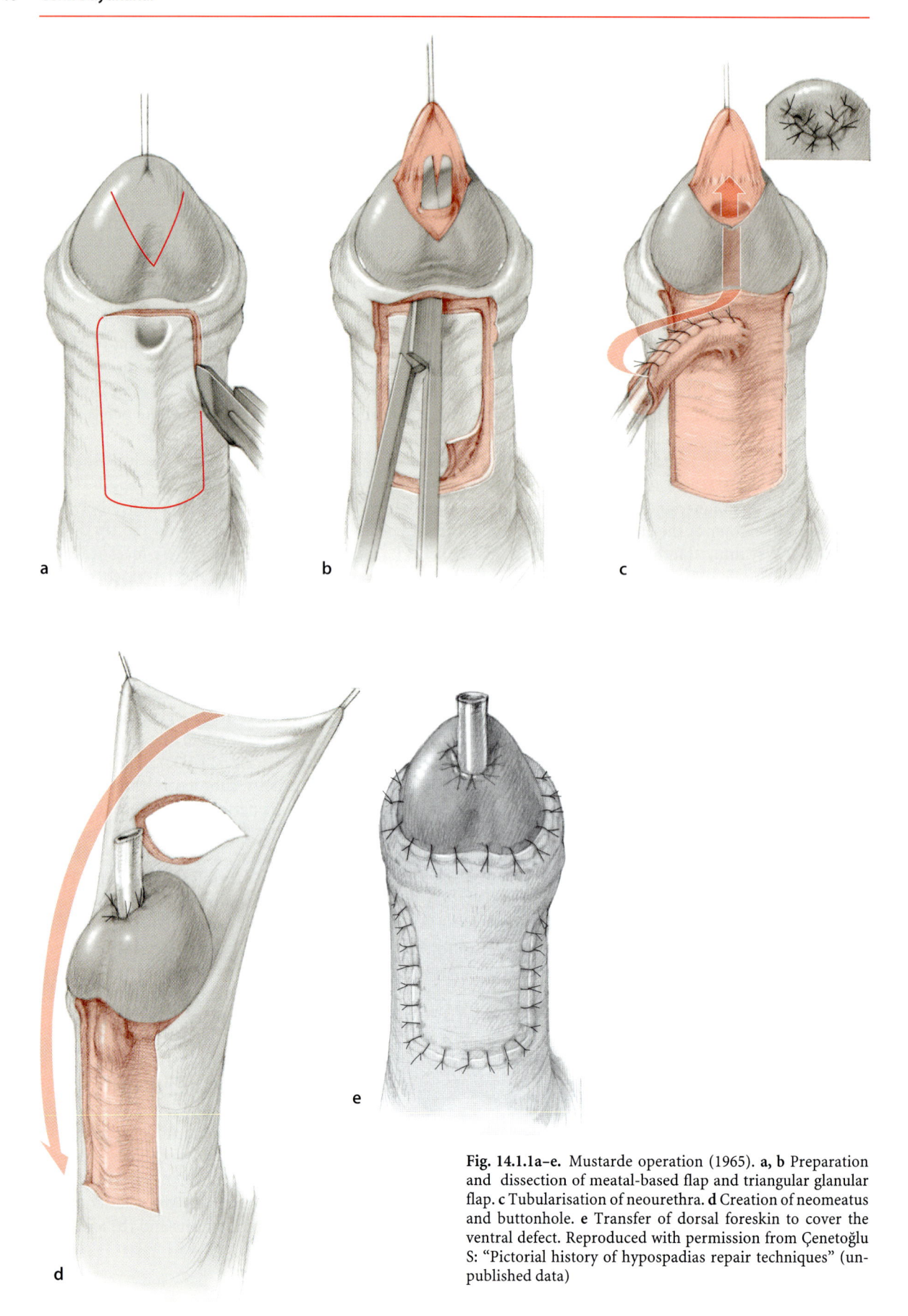

Fig. 14.1.1a–e. Mustarde operation (1965). **a, b** Preparation and dissection of meatal-based flap and triangular glanular flap. **c** Tubularisation of neourethra. **d** Creation of neomeatus and buttonhole. **e** Transfer of dorsal foreskin to cover the ventral defect. Reproduced with permission from Çenetoğlu S: "Pictorial history of hypospadias repair techniques" (unpublished data)

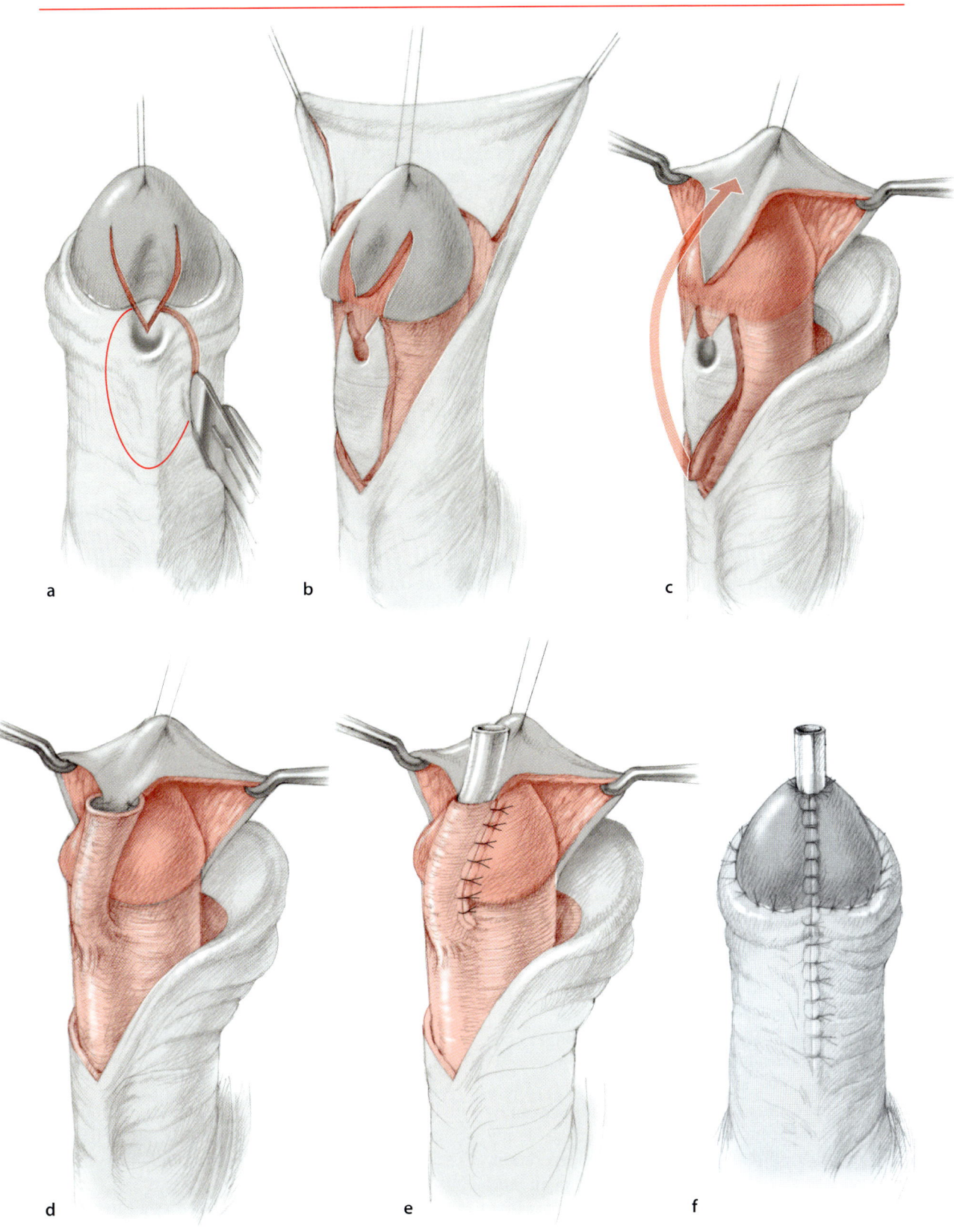

Fig. 14.1.2a–f. Horton–Devine operation (1973). **a** Preparation of triangular meatal-based flap. **b, c** Small dorsal meatotomy to prevent meatal stenosis; creation of triangular glanular flap. **d, e** Anastomosis between the glanular and the ventral flap; preparation of Byars flaps. **f** Coverage of ventral defect. Reproduced with permission from Çenetoğlu S: "Pictorial history of hypospadias repair techniques"

The Mathieu Procedure

In 1928 Mathieu described a single-stage, meatal-based flap technique to repair the distal forms of hypospadias. The detail of this operation with its preliminary results was reported in 1931 (Mathieu 1932; Rabinowitz 1987). Since then, due to the successful results achieved, the technique has been popularised by Gonzales et al. (1983), Rabinowitz (1987), Rabinowitz and Hulbert (1999), Kim and Hendren (1981) and Belman (1986, 1988, 1992). Wacksman, in 1981 presented this technique as a modification of the Mustardé and Horton–Devine procedures; however, his technique was almost the same as Mathieu's procedure. However, his technique was almost the same as Mathieu's procedure.

Preoperative Evaluation and Patient Selection

This procedure is ideal for distal shaft, coronal or subcoronal hypospadias. The ideal candidate for Mathieu's operation should have a straight penis. However, a glanular tilt and/or limited distal chordee can be easily corrected by the techniques of Nesbit's or Baskin's dorsal plication methods. A wide glanular groove is very important in order to perform a successful Mathieu repair. Problems related to the width of the glanular plate can easily be resolved by the aid of "hinging or incising the urethral plate" (Rich and Keating 1999).

Contraindications of the Mathieu Procedure

- Midshaft or proximal-shaft types, severe chordee.
- Cone-shaped glans with a shallow groove.
- A very small amount of unhealthy skin over the distal urethra (this may be the most important factor).

Stenotic hypospadiac meatus can be easily treated by a dilatation or a meatotomy. It is no longer considered as a contraindication to Mathieu repair.

A preoperative testosterone injection is not a routine pretreatment method for all Mathieu candidates. If there is an indication, testosterone, 25 mg i.m, monthly, three times before the operation, enlarges the size and vascularity of the penis and foreskin, thus enhancing the success of the operative procedure.

Operative Technique

The author uses a penile block: injecting 0.5% bupivacaine solution is very effective for analgesia in Mathieu patients. Most of these patients can be sent home the same day or the day after the operation. An oral analgesic has to be given before the termination of the effects of the bupivacaine block. A single dose of prophylactic antibiotic is given to each patient. An epinephrine solution is not used in the Mathieu operation. A tourniquet, however, consisting of a rubber vascular band, is used during the preparation of the glanular incision and the mobilisation of the glanular wing.

The Steps of Mathieu's Procedure

a) An erection test for the chordee is performed.
b) A 5-0 monofilament suture material with a round needle is inserted into the glans (just by the dorsal edge of the "neomeatus") and traction is established.
c) The distance between the hypospadiac meatus and the tip of the penis is measured. An equal distance from the meatus is measured on the skin of the proximal penile shaft and marked with a marking pen. A width of 7.5–8 mm is measured for the proximal flap. The width is tapered to 5.5–6 mm at the glanular groove (Borer 1999; Brueziere 1987; Duckett 1998; Hinmann 1994; King 1998). Longitudinal lines defining the urethral plate are then drawn as the lines of incision on either side of the glanular groove and proximal urethral flap (Fig. 14.1.3a). The width of the proximal flap has to be larger (2. 5–3 mm) than the width of the glanular flap.
d) Incise along the marks on the penile shaft (Fig. 14.1.3b). Two 6-0 traction sutures are put in the proximal edges of the proximal flap subcutaneously. The aim of these sutures is "gentle traction without any harm". A fine pair of scissors is used to get the maximum amount of vascularised subcutaneous tissue, which is attached to our proximal flap. This is one of the important tricks of this procedure!
e) The prepuce is incised 10–12 mm away from the glans. The penile skin is degloved, and all fibrotic tissues which are responsible for any minor chordee are excised.
f) A vascular rubber band is placed as a tourniquet. An incision is made along the marks in the glanular groove and the lateral glanular wings are mobilised and undermined adequately (Fig. 14.1.3b). In order to make a bloodless dissection and to obtain

The Meatal-based Flap "Mathieu" Technique   143

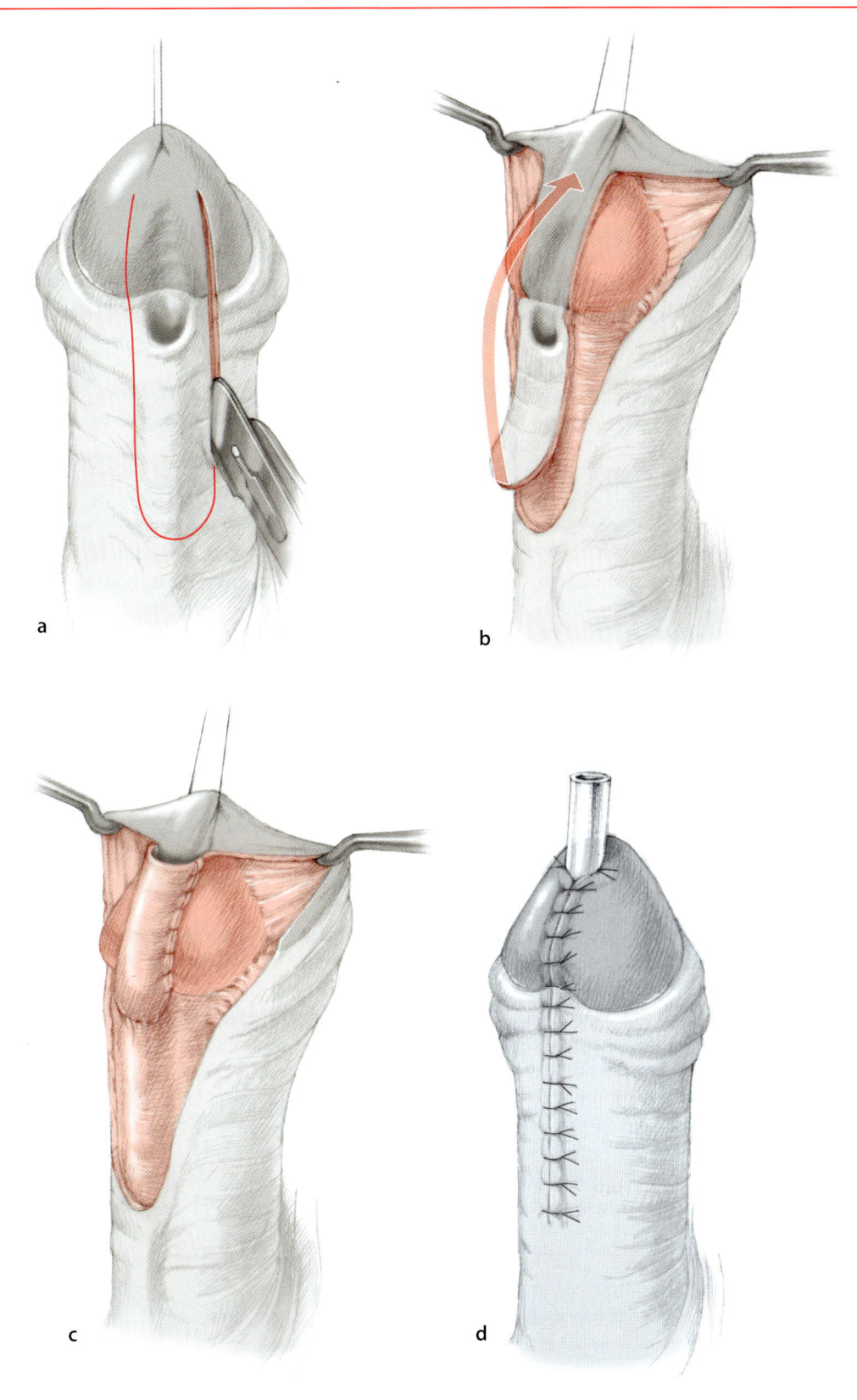

Fig. 14.1.3a–d. Mathieu technique (1932). **a** Lines defining the urethral plate are drawn. **b** Incision along the marks; preparation and mobilization of glanular wings. **c** Creation of the neourethra by means of subcuticular running sutures. **d** Prepared Byars flaps are sutured in the midline Reproduced with permission from Çenetoğlu S: "Pictorial history of hypospadias repair techniques"

vascularised and mobilised glanular wings, this dissection should be done at the tissue plane of the corpus spongiosum.

g) An 8-F silicone catheter is passed through the meatus. The proximal flap is brought over the catheter and glanular groove by gently pulling the traction sutures which are attached to the flap and lastly the glanular wings are brought over the catheter and the flap in order to test the efficacy of the mobilisation of the glanular wings. This is an important manoeuvre to prevent tension and late stricture. If tension is not present, the chordee test is repeated. In the case of tilting or the presence of minimal chordee, the dorsal plication method (Nesbit or Baskin) is performed.

h) The proximal flap is then rotated and flipped distally (thus "flip-flap") to the glanular flap so that the original proximal end becomes the neomeatus. Each lateral border is anastomosed with 7-0 Vicryl or PDS subcuticular running sutures (Fig. 14.1.3c), which has the advantage of inverting the edges, thus reducing the risk of fistula formation (Aktuğ et al. 1992; Rabinowitz and Hulbert 1999). At this point, it is advised to add a protective layer to prevent fistula formation. If there is enough vascularised subcutaneous tissue attached to the proximal flap, this should be used to provide additional coverage over the closure. The tissue is wrapped around the anastomosis and the edges are attached to the penile shaft with a couple of 7-0 sutures, thereby decreasing the occurrence of fistulae. In some cases the subcuticular tissue may be weak. In this case, it is better to use the dorsal dartos subcutaneous flap to wrap the neourethra (Belman 1988; Churchill et al. 1996; Ravasse et al. 2000; Wheeler et al. 1993). Some authors prefer to use "tunica vaginalis blanket wrap" (Snow et al. 1995) if there is any problem with dorsal preputial excessive skin.

i) Another technical modification has to be considered after the completion of anastomosis: a "V" excision or the so-called MAVIS technique which was mentioned recently by Boddy and Samuel (2000). A V-shaped piece of tissue from the anterior face of the tip of the neourethra is excised. This is an important manoeuvre to get a "slit-like-meatus" and prevent stricture formations. After the MAVIS procedure, the 8-F catheter is taken out and a 6-F silicone catheter is inserted into the bladder.

j) The glanular wings and mucosal collar of the glans are reapproximated and sutured with 6-0 Vicryl or PDS. One medial suture (to the tip of the V excision) and four lateral sutures (two in each side) are used for the anastomosis between the neomeatus and the tip of the neourethra. The hooded foreskin is spilt in the midline and rotated ventrally as Byars flaps. The flaps are sutured in the midline (Fig. 14.1.3d). Silicone foam or Tegaderm dressing are the dressing materials of our choice. The author prefers to fix silicone foam to the skin around the penile base with three sutures (at the 3, 7 and 11 o'clock positions) We prefer to keep the catheter and foam dressing for 5 days. In some cases the foam can be taken off after the 2nd postoperative day.

The Mathieu Technique and Relevant Modifications and Controversies

Stenting

A modification of the Mathieu repair eliminating stenting or catheterisation, described by Rabinowitz (1987), makes the technique more convenient for outpatient surgery. Since then Aktuğ et al. (1992), Buson et al. (1994) and Retik et al. (1994), Borer (1999); Wheeler et al. 1993) have described a modification of the Mathieu repair using a subcuticular suture for urethroplasty. No catheter, stent or suprapubic drainage is used in these patients. A relatively high complication or reoperation rate (as much as 18–20%) is reported (Aktuğ et al. 1992; Buson et al. 1994). However, there was no incidence of urethrocutaneous fistula in the series of Retik et al. where a dorsal subcutaneous dartos wrap was used to cover the neourethra (Ravasse et al. 2000).

Wheeler et al. (1993) suggested the Mathieu operation without a catheter. Although the patients could be discharged the same day, the complication rate was around 15%. Gough et al. in 1995 presented a prospective randomised trial of the Mathieu operation. Their complication rate with 2–5 days' urinary diversion and Silastic foam dressing was less than 5%. They do not recommend a catheterless technique due to the higher incidence of immediate dysuria and an apparent increase in late complications.

In 1996 Hakim et al. presented the results of four different centres ($n=300$ patients). They reported an extremely low complication rate, with no statistically significant difference between catheterised and non-catheterised patients. In the author's experience, 3–5 days' catheterisation is the policy of choice, at least for the prevention of immediate dysuria syndrome. We think Silastic foam dressing plus a double-diaper–free-dripping Silastic catheter method does not create much trouble for the family and for children who are not toilet-trained.

Reinforcement of the Neourethra Using Local Tissues

Belman, in 1988, presented his "deepithelialised skin flap coverage" procedure in 84 hypospadias patients whose treatment included Mathieu urethroplasty. He applied a flap of de-epithelialised preputial skin over the neourethra and reported a 3.5% rate of fistula formation. In 1994 Retik et al. reported the results of a "dorsal dartos subcutaneous flap" to wrap the neourethra after a Mathieu repair. There was no evidence of urethrocutaneous fistula among 204 patients. Churchill et al. (1996) presented excellent results with a dartos flap in reoperations. Ravasse et al. (2000) used a foreskin subcutaneous connective tissue pedicled flap to reduce the rate of fistula formation, which for them was 6%. Snow et al. (1995) reported a 0% complication rate in their patients, who were treated with microscopic magnification plus a "tunica vaginalis blanket wrap" technique. Today, many paediatric urologist and paediatric surgeons prefer to use subcutaneous tissue which is attached to the flip-flap to cover the neourethra in the Mathieu technique (Belman 1986, 1988; DeJong and Boemers 1993; Oswald et al. 2000; Ravasse et al. 2000). If there is no enough tissue attached to the flap, wrapping the neourethra with the vascularised dartos tissue from the inner surface of the preputial foreskin can prevent fistula formation.

How To Improve the Appearance of the Meatus in Mathieu Cases

In 2000 Boddy and Samuel reported the "V"-incision sutured MAVIS technique to provide a cosmetically acceptable natural slit-like meatus in Mathieu cases. We have been using the MAVIS technique since 1999 (Tekand et al. 2000) as one of the important steps in the Mathieu operation. Since then we have encountered neither meatal stenosis nor the horizontal buckethandle meatus problem. All patients have a slit-like meatus with the proper calibre (Fig. 14.1.4).

Chordee

Some surgeons prefer to use dorsal plication techniques (Nesbit or Baskin type) for glanular tilt and moderate chordee (DeJong and Boemers 1993; Hinmann 1994). De Grazia et al. (1997) mentioned a 12.5% incidence of distal curvature and advised the mobilisation of the urethral plate and extensive removal of ventral chordee elements beneath the

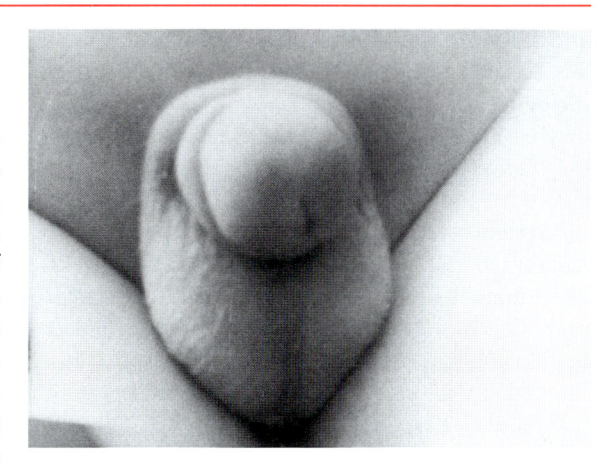

Fig.14.1.4. Slit-like meatus after Mathieu operation and MAVIS modification

plate. We consider that fibrotic elements should be dissected and the dorsal plication procedure should be applied to a selected group of Mathieu cases.

Hinging of Urethral Plate

Rich and Keating (1999) advised "hinging of the urethral plate" to lower the glanular groove and create a vertical urethral meatus. This modification enhances the enlargement of a narrow glanular groove and thus may change the spectrum of indications for the Mathieu procedure.

Mathieu as a Rescue Operation

Hayashi et al. (2001), Ravasse et al. (2000) and Simmons et al. (1999) reported their experience with the Mathieu operation in secondary cases. Their data suggest a success rate exceeding 85%. The author has performed 24 of his 143 Mathieu operations in secondary, complicated cases. Mathieu has been used as a rescue operation after the complications of MAGPI and distal problems in transverse island flap techniques.

Results and Complications

Fistula formation, meatal stenosis, stricture, meatal retraction and the dehiscence of glans sutures are the most frequent complications of the Mathieu operation (Elder et al. 1987; Gough et al. 1995; Mollard et al. 1987; Smith 1990). During the past decade, the improvements seen in suture materials, magnification and suture techniques and the application of vascularised flaps around the neourethra have reduced the incidence of these complications. A hair-bearing urethra may be the most distressing complication of the Mathieu operation. Longer flaps are not only at risk for devascularisation with complications of distal stenosis and stricture but also may incorporate hair-bearing skin (Belman 1986, 1992). The risk of development of a urethral beard in adolescence is very high in these patients. 'Half-moon' or 'bucket-handle' meatus is not a real complication but an important and distressing aesthetic problem (Boddy and Samuel 2000; Mouriquand and Mure 2001). We believe that the MAVIS "V excision" modification is a better alternative.

Murphy (2000) reviewed the literature in 1999 and investigated the complication rates in a series of 792 Mathieu operations. There were only 16 complications (9 fistulae and 7 meatal stenoses – a 2% incidence. We have collected a group of Mathieu series involving 1,060 cases. The incidence of complications varied between 1.5% and 11.2% (Bevan 1917; Boddy and Samuel 2000; Dolatzas et al. 1994; Elder et al. 1987; Gonzales et al. 1983; Gough et al. 1995; Minevich et al. 1999; Ravasse et al. 2000) (Table 14.1.1).

Our Experience

Since 1980 more than 500 patients with various types of hypospadias have been treated in the Paediatric Surgical Department of the Cerrahpaş Medical Faculty of the University of Istanbul. Of these, 143 with distal hypospadias were treated by Mathieu's operation. In 24 of the 143, the Mathieu technique was used as a secondary operation to treat complicated cases.

The author has personal experience of Mathieu operations in 68 patients. Of these, 32 were treated without using the dorsal dartos flap modification or the MAVIS procedure. There have been five complications in this group (two apparent, three pinpoint fistulae). Since 1999, 36 of these 68 patients have been treated with the dorsal dartos flap wrapping modification and the MAVIS technique. Neither fistula formation nor stricture stenosis occurred in this group (Tekand et al. 2000). All of these patients had a slit-like meatus with sufficient calibre. A silicone foam dressing and 3–5 days' free dripping catheterisation (average 4.2 days) with a double-diaper application was used. The average duration of hospitalisation was 1.5 days.

In conclusion, we think Mathieu's urethroplasty technique is an effective procedure for distal hypospadias cases with moderate chordee and as a salvage operation for secondary complicated cases.

Table 14.1.1. The complication rate in the Mathieu operation

Reference	Number of patients ($n=1060$)	Complication rate
Boddy and Samuel (2000)	64	3%
DeJong and Boemers (1993)	116	3.4%
Dolatzas et al. (1994)	180	11.2%
Elder et al. (1987)	56	1.8%
Gonzales et al. (1983)	63	8%
Gough et al. (1995)	95	4.7%
Minevich et al. (1999)	202	1.5%
Oswald et al. (2000)	30	10%
Ravasse et al. (2000)	50	6%
Retik et al. (1994)	204	0%

References

Aktuğ T, Akgür FM, Olguner M, et al: Outpatient catheterless Mathieu repair: how to cover ventral penile skin defect. Eur J Pediatr Surg. 1992; 2:99–101.

Belman AB: The modified Mustardé hypospadias repair. J Urol. 1982; 127:88–90.

Belman AB: Hypospadias. In: Welch KJ, Randolph JG, Ravitch MM, O'Neill JA Jr, Rowe MI (eds) Pediatric surgery, 4th edn, vol 2. Year Book, Chicago, pp 1286–1302; 1986.

Belman AB: De-epithelialized skin flap coverage in hypospadias repair. J Urol. 1988; 140:1273–1276.

Belman AB: Hypospadias and other urethral abnormalities. In: Kelalis PP, King LR, Belman AB (eds) Clinical pediatric urology, vol 1, 3rd edn. Saunders, Philadelphia, pp 619–663; 1992.

Bevan A: A new operation for hypospadias. JAMA. 1917; 68:1032–1034.

Bocchiotti G, Bruschi S, Bosetti P, et al: Technical considerations using the Horton-Devine technique in distal hypospadias. Ann Plast Surg. 1982; 9:164–166.

Boddy SA, Samuel M: A natural glanular meatus after "Mathieu and V incision sutured" MAVIS. BJU Int. 2000; 86:394–397.

Borer JG, Retik AB: Current trends in hypospadias repair. Urol Clin North Am. 1999; 26:15–37.

Bouisson MF: De l'hypospadias et de son traitment chirurgical. Trib Chir. 1861; 2:484.

Brodsky MA: Reconstruction of the urethra in hypospadias according to Horton-Devine. Ann Chir Gynaecol. 1980; 69:23–31.

Brueziere J: How I perform the Mathieu technique in the treatment of anterior penile hypospadias. Ann Urol. 1987; 21:277–280.

Buson H, Smiley D, Reinberg Y, et al: Distal hypospadias repair without stents: is it better? J Urol. 1994; 151:1059–1060.

Churchill BM, van Savage JG, Khoury AE, et al: The dartos flaps as an adjuant in preventing urethrocutaneous

fistulas in repeat hypospadias surgery. J Urol. 1996; 156: 2047–2049.
De Grazia E, Cigna RM, Cimador M: Modified Mathieu's technique: a variation of the classical procedure for hypospadias repair. Eur J Pediatr Surg. 1997; 8:98–99.
DeJong TP, Boemers TM: Improved Mathieu repair for coronal and distal shaft hypospadias with moderate chordee. Br J Urol. 1993; 72:972–974.
Devine CJ Jr, Horton CE: Hypospadias repair. J Urol. 1977; 118:188–193.
Dolatzas T, Chiotopoulos D, Antipas S, et al.: Hypospadias repair in children: review of 250 cases. Pediatr Surg Int. 1994; 9:383–386.
Duckett JW: Hypospadias. In: Walsh PC, Retik AB, Vaughan ED Jr, Wein AJ (eds) Campbell's urology, 7th edn, vol 2. Saunders, Philadelphia, pp 2103–2119; 1998.
Elder JS, Duckett JW, Snyder HM: Onlay island flap in the repair of mid and distal penile hypospadias without chordee. J Urol. 1987; 138:376–379.
Gonzales ET Jr, Veerarghaven KA, Delaune J: The management of distal hypospadias with meatal-based vascularized flaps. J Urol. 1983; 129:119–122.
Gough DCS, Dickson A, Tsung T: Mathieu hypospadias repair: postoperative care. In: Thüroff JW, Hohenfellner M (eds) Reconstructive surgery of the lower urinary tract in children. ISIS Medical Media, Oxford, pp 55–58; 1995.
Hakim S, Merguerian PA, Rabinowitz R, et al: Outcome analysis of the modified Mathieu hypospadias repair: comparison of stented and unstented repairs. J Urol. 1996; 156:836–838.
Hayashi Y, Sasaki S, Kojima Y, et al.: Primary and salvage urethroplasty using Mathieu meatal-based flip-flap technique for distal hypospadias. Int J Urol. 2001; 8:10–16.
Hinmann F Jr: Atlas of pediatric urologic surgery. Saunders, Philadelphia, pp 581–582; 1994.
Kim SH, Hendren WH: Repair of mild hypospadias. J Pediatr Surg. 1981; 16:806–811.
King LR: Hypospadias. In: King LR (ed): Urologic surgery in infants and children. Saunders, Philadelphia, pp 194–208; 1998.
Mathieu P: Traitement en un temps de l'hypospadias balanique et juxta balanique. J Chir. 1932; 39:481–484.
Minevich E, Pecha BR, Wacksman J, et al.: Mathieu hypospadias repair:An experience in 202 patients. J Urol. 1999; 162:2141–2143.
Mollard P, Mouriquand PDE, Basset T: Le traitement de l'hypospade. Chir Pediatr. 1987; 28:197–203.
Mouriquand PDE, Mure PY: Hypospadias. In: Gearhardt JP, Rink RC, Mouriquand PDE (eds) Pediatric urology. Saunders, Philadelphia, pp 713–728; 2001.
Murphy JP: Hypospadias. In: Ashcraft KW, Murphy JP, Sharp RJ, Sigalet DL, Snyder CL (eds) Pediatric surgery, 3rd edn. Saunders, Philadelphia, pp 763–782; 2000.

Mustardé JC: One-stage correction of distal hypospadias and other people's fistulae. Br J Plast Surg. 1965; 18:413–422.
Ombrédanne L: Précis clinique et opératoire de chirurgie infantile. Collection de Précis Médicaeux Masson et Éditeurs, Paris, 1925.
Oswald J, Körner I, Riccabona M: Comparison of the perimeatal-based flap (Mathieu) and the tubularized incised-plate urethroplasty (Snodgrass) in primary distal hypospadias. BJU Int. 2000; 85:725–727.
Rabinowitz R: Outpatient catheterless modified Mathieu hypospadias repair. J Urol. 1987; 138:1074–1076.
Rabinowitz R, Hulbert WC: Meatal-based flap Mathieu procedure. In: Ehrlich RM, Alter GJ (eds) Reconstructive and plastic surgery of the external genitalia. Adult and pediatric. Saunders, Philadelphia, pp 39–43; 1999.
Ravasse P, Petit T, Delmas P: Anterior hypospadias: Duplay or Mathieu? Prog Urol. 2000; 10:653–656.
Ravasse P, Petit T: Mathieu's urethroplasty in surgery for hypospadias: postoperative complications. Ann Urol. 2000; 34:271–273.
Retik AB, Mandell J, Bauer SB, et al.: Meatal based hypospadias repair with the use of dorsal subcutaneous flap to prevent urethrocutaneous fistula. J Urol. 1994; 152: 1229–1231.
Rich MA, Keating MA: Hinging the urethral plate. In: Ehrlich RM, Alter GJ (eds): Reconstructive and plastic surgery of the external genitalia. Adult and pediatric. Saunders, Philadelphia, pp 63–65; 1999.
Roth DR: Hypospadias. In: Gonzales ET, Bauer SB (eds): Pediatric urology practice. Lippincott Williams and Wilkins, Philadelphia, pp 487–497; 1999.
Simmons GR, Cain MP, Casale AJ, et al: Repair of hypospadias complications using the previously utilized urethral plate. Urology. 1999; 54:724–726.
Smith ED: Hypospadias. In: Ashcraft KW (ed): Pediatric urology. Saunders, Philadelphia, pp 353–395; 1990.
Snow BW, Cartwright PC, Unger K: Tunica vaginalis blanket wrap to prevent urethrocutaneous fistulas. A 8-year-experience. J Urol. 1995; 153:472–473.
Tekand G, Beşik C, Emir H, et al.: Is it possible to create slit-like meatus without incising urethrael plate? IIIrd congress of Mediterranean Association of Pediatric Surgeons, Corfu, Greece, 12–15 Oct, abstracts, 2000, p 67.
Wacksman J: Modification of one-stage flip-flap procedure to repair distal penile hypospadias. Urol Clin North Am. 1981; 8:527–530.
Wheeler RA, Malone PS, Griffiths DM, et al: The Mathieu operation. Is urethral stent mandatory? Br J Urol. 1993; 71:492–495.
Wood J (1875): Cited by Mayo CH: JAMA. 1901; 36:1157.
Woodard JR, Cleveland R: Application of Horton-Devine principles to the repair of hypospadias. J Urol. 1982; 127:1155–1158.

The Y-V Glanuloplasty Modified "Mathieu" Technique

14.2

Ahmed T. Hadidi

Introduction

In Chap. 14.1, Prof. Büyükünal presents an excellent, up-to-date detailed account of the Mathieu technique, describing the historical background, evolution and most of the current modifications.

The major drawback of the original Mathieu technique (Mathieu 1932) is the final appearance of the meatus (a smiling meatus that is not very terminal). Two recent important modifications correct this drawback. The first is the Y-V glanuloplasty described by Hadidi in 1996. This technique helps to use the Mathieu operation in all forms of hypospadiac glans in distal hypospadias and results in a terminal, slit-like meatus.

The other modification is the MAVIS technique described by Boddy and Samuel in 2000. In this technique a triangle is excised from the apex of the parameatal flap, facilitating a slit-like meatus.

This section deals with the Y-V modification of the Mathieu procedure. I believe that Y-V glanuloplasty avoids the drawbacks of the original Mathieu technique and helps to make it an excellent option for the treatment of distal hypospadias.

Patient Selection

The Y-V glanuloplasty modified Mathieu technique may be applied to most forms of distal hypospadias. By distal we mean all types of hypospadias where the meatus is just distal to the midpoint of the shaft. The reason is to avoid hair-bearing skin. This will include about 70–80% of patients with hypospadias. The only contraindication is the presence of severe chordee distal to the hypospadiac meatus, (a flat-looking glans is not a contraindication). In the majority of cases of distal hypospadias, chordee, if present, is usually a cutaneous form that is almost always released by simply freeing the proximal skin adequately.

The Y-V technique has been used successfully in recurrent cases of distal penile hypospadias, provided there is a good quality of skin proximal to the meatus for flap reconstruction (i.e. the potential flap skin should not be scarred or fibrosed). The details of the technique are described in the following section.

Operative Technique

The author prefers to use caudal block to avoid any change in tissue planes. The patient may be brought close to the edge of the table and the surgeon sits; alternatively, the patient lies in the traditional middle-of-table position if the surgeon prefers to stand.

Step 1: A 5-0 nylon traction suture is placed on the glans. It should be central, transversely applied and just dorsal to the site of the "neomeatus".

Step 2: A tourniquet is placed at the root of the penis after compressing the penis.

Step 3: The erection test is applied and any chordee present is evaluated.

Steps 4, 5, 6: Y-V Glanuloplasty

Step 4: A Y-shaped incision is outlined on the glans. The centre of the Y is exactly at the tip of the glans and where the tip of the neomeatus will be located. Each limb of the Y is 0.5 cm long, and the angle between the upper two limbs of the Y is 60° (👁 Fig. 14.2.1a). The Y-shaped incision is made deep and results in three flaps, one upper(median) and two lateral (👁 Fig. 14.2.1b).

Step 5: The three flaps are elevated and a core of soft tissue is excised from the bed of each flap to create a space for the neourethra.

Step 6: The Y shape is sutured as a V using continuous through-and-through 6-0 Vicryl or similar suture (👁 Fig. 14.2.1c). This means that the upper flap is sutured to the lateral limbs, making sure to keep the "dog-ears" at the upper ends of the V suture lines. These dog-ears are important because, when opened,

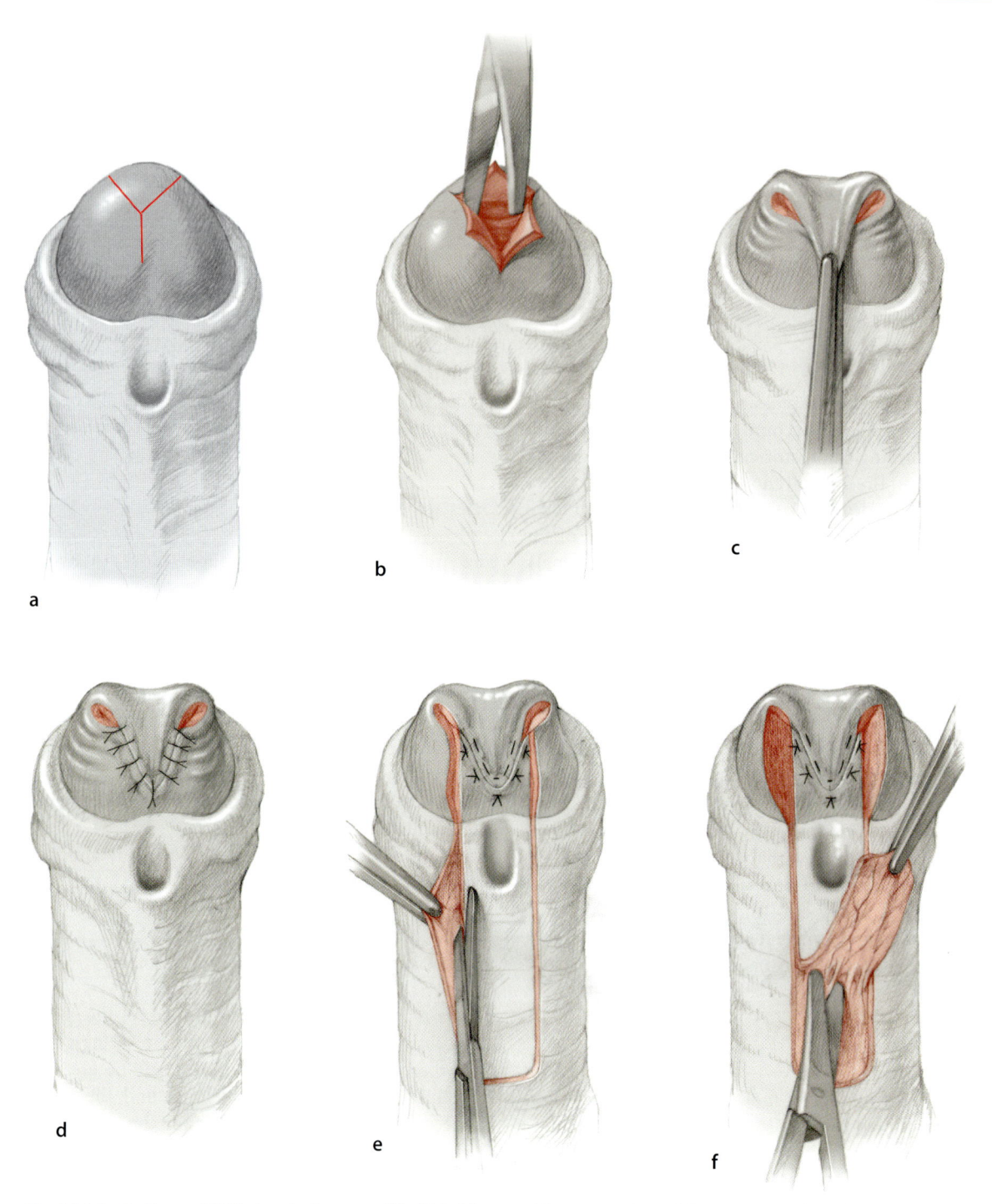

Fig. 14.2.1a–j. Steps of Y-V glanuloplasty modified Mathieu technique. **a** Y incision. **b** Elevation of the three flaps and coring to make a space for the neourethra. **c, d** Y sutured as V with preservation of dog-ears. **e** U-shaped flap. **f** The flap is elevated, taking care to preserve its fascia. **g–j** see p. 151

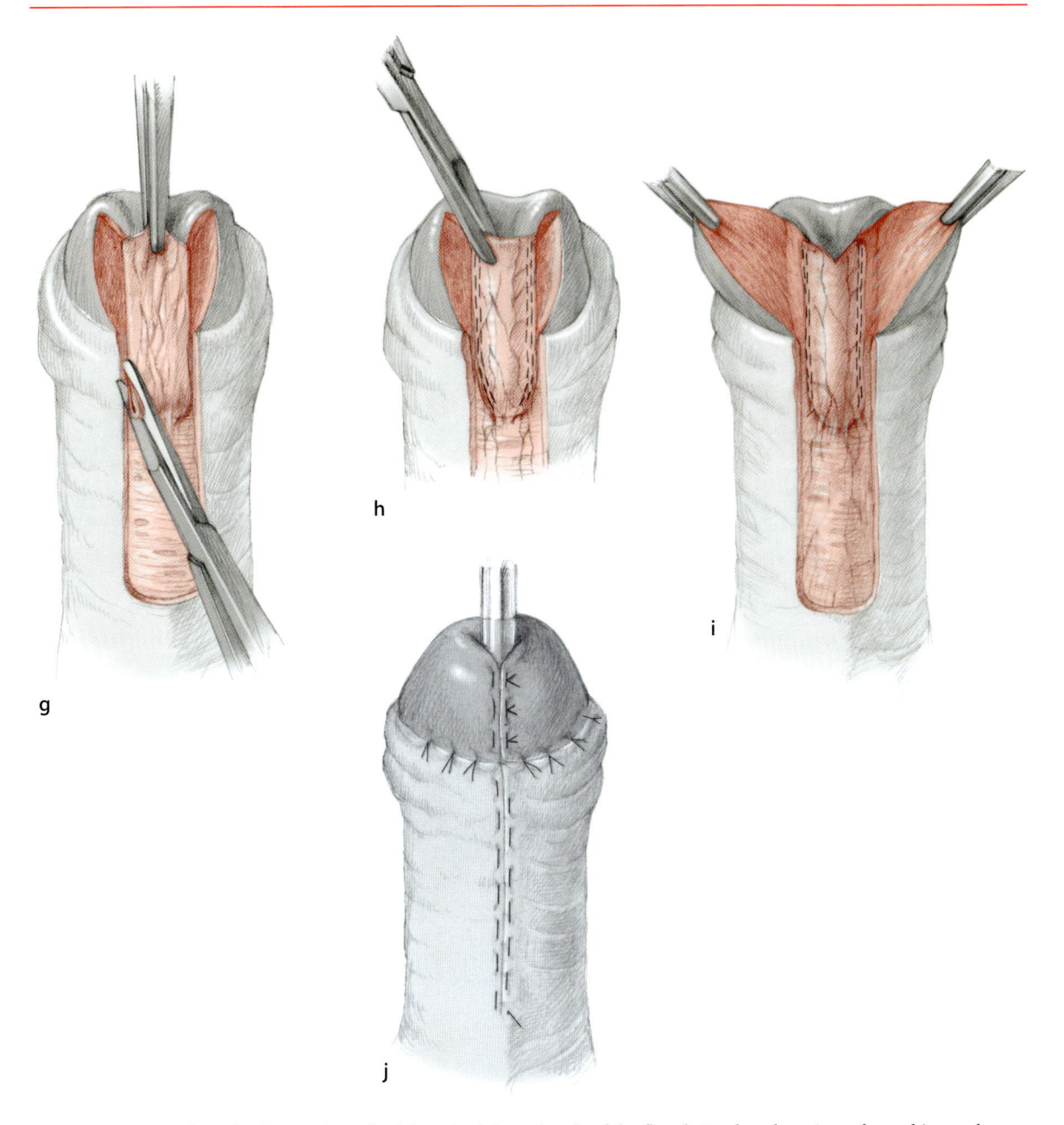

Fig. 14.2 (*continued*). **g** The dog-ear is excised from both lateral ends of the flap. **h** Urethroplasty is performed in two layers. **i** A V is excised from the tip of the flap. **j** Meatoplasty and glanuloplasty

they will enlarge the circumference of the tip of the glanular wings by 1 cm at least (Fig. 14.2.1d).

Step 7: The hypospadiac meatus is evaluated. If the meatus is narrow, it should be dilated to accommodate a size 10 F catheter. If the skin proximal to the meatus is thin, transparent, it should be excised until we reach a normal healthy skin. A size 10 F catheter is inserted into the meatus down to the root of the penis.

Parameatal Flap Design

Step 8: The U-shaped incision is made taking the following points into consideration: (a) The length of the flap is slightly longer than the distance between the meatus and the designed tip of the neomeatus. (b) When designing the two longitudinal incisions, they have to diverge away from the hypospadiac meatus to allow for adequate blood supply to the flap. (c) When the U-shaped incision reaches the tip of the glans, it will open the dog-ears wide as one opens a book. (d)

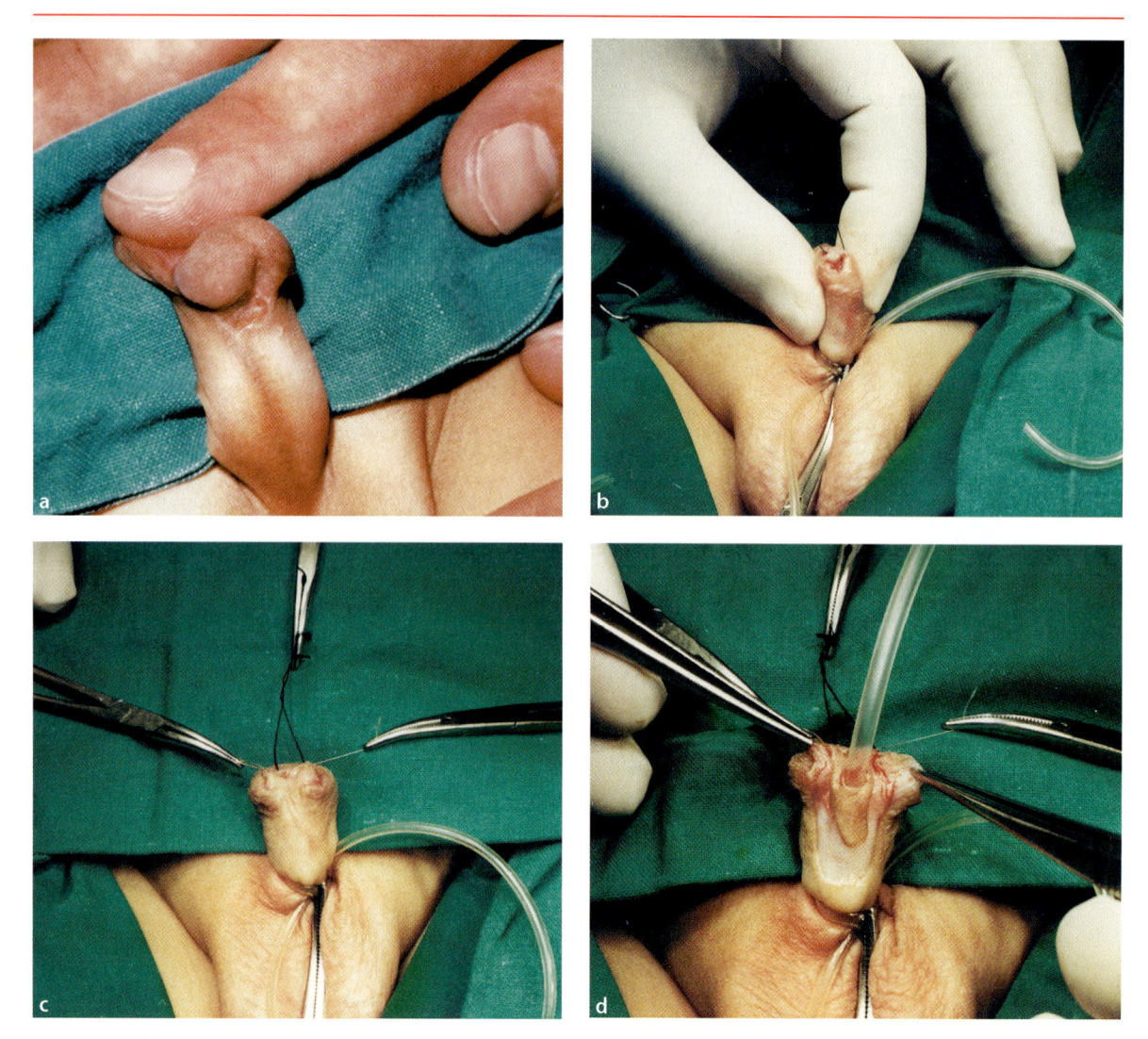

Fig. 14.2.2a–h. Y-V glanuloplasty modified Mathieu technique. **a** Preoperative view; **b** Y incision; **c** V closure with preservation of dog-ears; **d, e** U-shaped incision; **f, g** urethroplasty; **h** final postoperative result. **e–h** see p. 153

When mobilising the flap, one should be holding the opposite skin edge and not the flap skin edge. This has two advantages, minimising flap tissue injury and increasing the amount of subcutaneous tissue and fascia for a multilayer closure. (e) When the flap is elevated, there will be two small dog-ears on either end of the original meatus. This is better excised as it is a common site for fistula formation (Fig. 14.2.1e, f).

Neourethra Reconstruction

Step 9: I prefer to use a continuous subcuticular running Vicryl 6-0 suture on a *cutting* or *taper needle*. I start a few millimetres proximal to the original meatus. This helps to have the knot away from the neourethra. The subcuticular suture is continued until I reach the tip of the glans, then I go back with the same stitch doing a running stitch approximating the flap fascia to the depth of the glans and the shaft of the penis *(double breasting)*. Thus, one will have only one knot for the whole two layers (Fig. 14.2.1g).

Meatoplasty and Glanuloplasty

Step 10: A small V is excised from the apex of the parameatal flap and the meatus is reconstructed with fine simple Vicryl 6-0 sutures (Fig. 14.2.1h). This helps to achieve a slit-like meatus. The glanular wings are

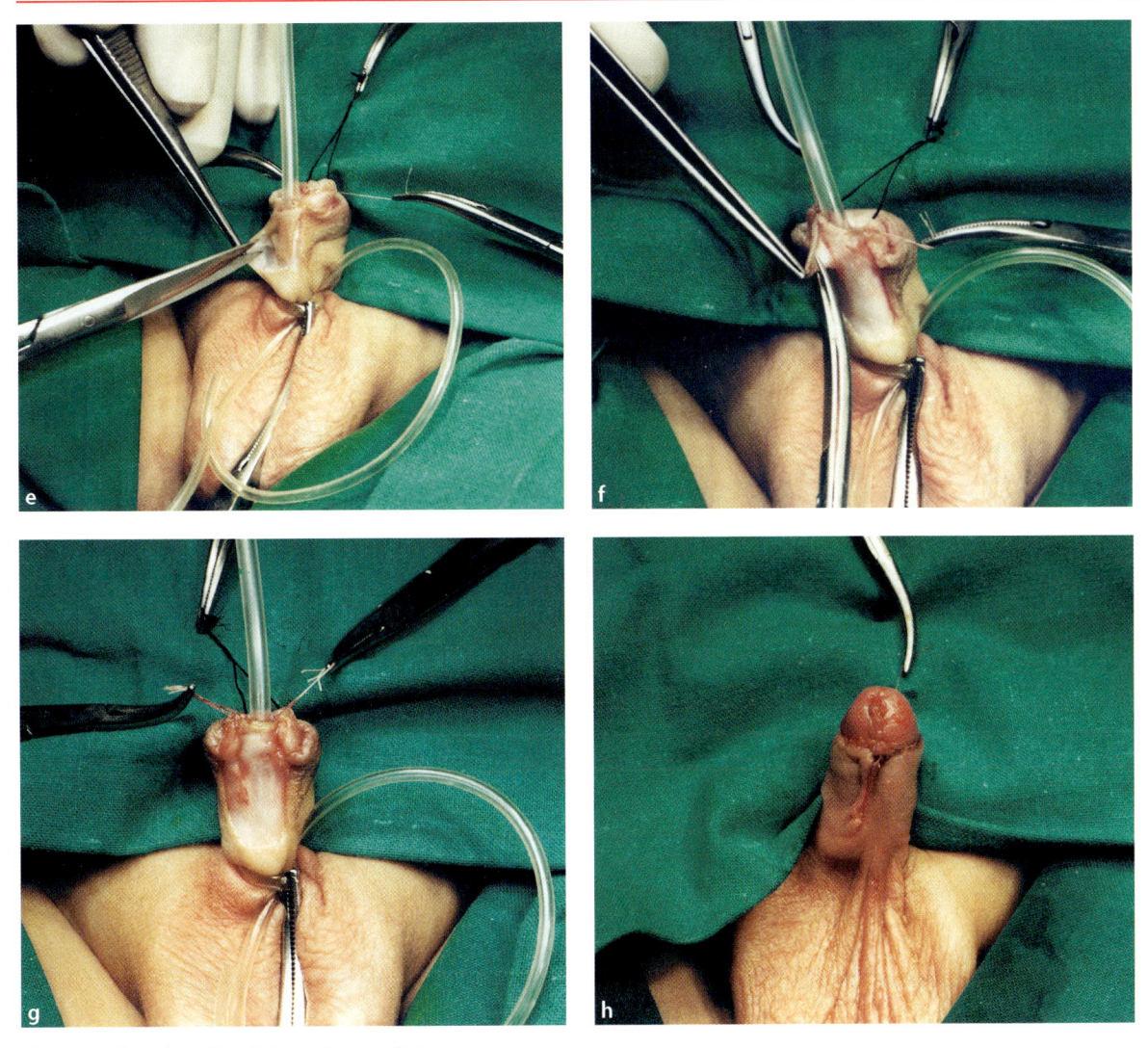

Fig. 14.2.2 (*continued*). e–h Legend see p. 152

closed using Vicryl 6-0 *transverse mattress interrupted sutures*. The remaining wound is closed using continuous mattress or interrupted subcuticular Vicryl stitches (👁 Fig. 14.2.1i, j).

Urinary Diversion

Step 11: I have stopped putting a catheter or a stent inside the urethra as a routine since 1992. It is my belief that it causes more irritation and complications (just like wearing a shirt for 7 days, it will most likely result in skin maceration and infection).

Dressing

Step 12: A local gentamycin ointment is applied. A compression dressing is applied for 6 h for haemostasis, then removed. The operation is performed as an outpatient procedure and the patient is discharged home on the same day on local gentamycin ointment and oral sulphamethoxazole-trimethoprim.

Results and Conclusion

Between January 1992 and July 2002, 384 Y-V glanuloplasty modified Mathieu procedures were performed 👁 (Fig. 14.2.2). Early in the study, three patients developed meatal stenosis that responded to dilatation. There were five fistulas, one wound disruption for severe infection, and one patient came back 5 days later with secondary bleeding due to infection (complication rate 2%). There was no need to leave a catheter inside the urethra and no need for calibration or dilatation. The Mathieu procedure combined with Y-V glanuloplasty is an excellent technique for distal hypospadias that has stood the test of time.

References

Boddy SA, Samuel M: A natural glanular meatus after "Mathieu and V incision sutured" MAVIS. BJU Int. 2000; 86:394-397.

Hadidi AT: Y-V Glanuloplasty: a new modification in the surgery of hypospadias. Kasr El Aini Med J. 1996; 2:223–233.

Mathieu P: Traitment en un temps de l'hypospadias balanique et juxta balanique. J Chir. 1932; 39:481–484.

Tubularized Incised Plate Urethroplasty

Warren Snodgrass

Introduction

Midline incision into the urethral plate widens it sufficiently for urethroplasty and heals without stricture. These observations form the basis for the tubularized incised plate (TIP) hypospadias repair, first described in 1994 (Snodgrass 1994). Following that report, clinical experience from many institutions has shown that the technique is applicable to essentially all cases of distal hypospadias, without concern for the specific meatal configurations that determine the applicability of other procedures discussed in this textbook. Furthermore, TIP may be preferable to many alternative options since it is versatile, easily performed, has few complications, and always results in a vertically oriented meatus.

Several recent reports (Snodgrass et al. 1998; Chen et al. 2000; Borer et al. 2001; Snodgrass and Lorenzo 2002b) also indicate that TIP is being increasingly used to repair proximal hypospadias. From these publications it appears that contraindications for the procedure include ventral curvature that requires transection of the urethral plate with substitution urethroplasty and the occasional finding that the incised plate is unsatisfactory for tubularizing. Furthermore, the operation has been used successfully for selected reoperations when the urethral plate is intact and appears supple (Shanberg et al. 2001; Borer et al. 2001; Snodgrass and Lorenzo 2002a).

Preoperative Evaluation

In my experience, incision of the glanular aspect of the urethral plate always widens it sufficiently for tubularization without supplemental skin flaps. Accordingly, I routinely perform TIP for distal hypospadias regardless of the specific location or appearance of the meatus. The authors of first multicenter study of the procedure for distal repairs (Snodgrass et al. 1996) found this simplification of decision-making an appealing aspect over other choices for urethroplasty.

It is generally not possible to assess whether or not TIP can be used for a boy with proximal hypospadias based upon any preoperative consideration. Even what appears to be severe ventral penile curvature sometimes will be found intraoperatively to be correctable without transecting the urethral plate. Similarly, before surgery the plate may appear to be only a very narrow strip of epithelium, yet with incision open into a broad sheet of tissue that is satisfactory for urethroplasty. Therefore, when the penis obviously is curved I inform the family of the possibility that the repair will be done in stages, but always begin the operation preserving the urethral plate while degloving the penis.

For reoperations, preoperative assessment simply involves confirming that the urethral plate is intact and not grossly scarred. The final decision regarding urethroplasty is deferred until the plate is incised to determine whether it seems sufficiently "supple" for tubularization.

The underlying principle of this evaluation is that the decision for urethroplasty is no longer made before surgery. Consequently, all operations begin with the presumption that TIP repair will be done, which means the urethral plate is initially preserved, the penis is straightened as required, and the plate is incised before the means of urethroplasty is determined.

Another consideration regards use of testosterone, especially for proximal hypospadias and reoperations. It is my impression that the size of the phallus often is underestimated in boys with proximal defects and ventral curvature. Therefore, I use testosterone sparingly before surgery, primarily when the glans is small. I have not used hormone stimulation routinely for reoperations since I do not create skin flap urethroplasties.

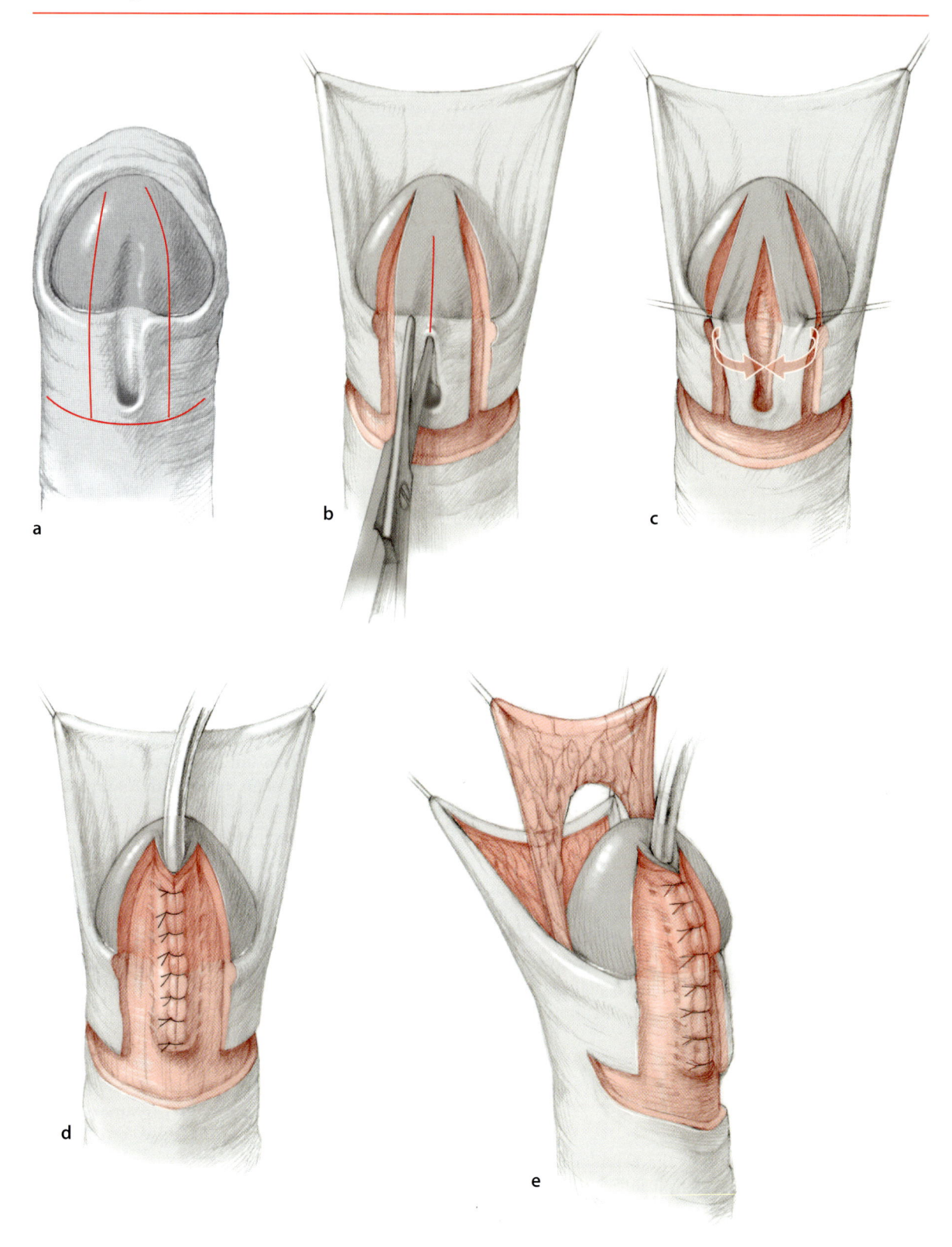

Fig. 15.1a–g. TIP for distal hypospadias repair. **a** *Horizontal line* indicates circumscribing incision to deglove the penis. *Vertical lines* indicate incisions along the lateral margins of the urethral plate. **b** Glans wings have been mobilized. **c** Relaxing incision widens the urethral plate. **d** Urethral plate is tubularized with a two-layer running subepithelial absorbable suture, beginning at approximately the midglans level. Note the large, oval neomeatus. **e** A dartos pedicle flap obtained from the dorsal prepuce and the shaft skin is buttonholed and transposed ventrally to cover the entire neourethra. **f, g** see p. 157

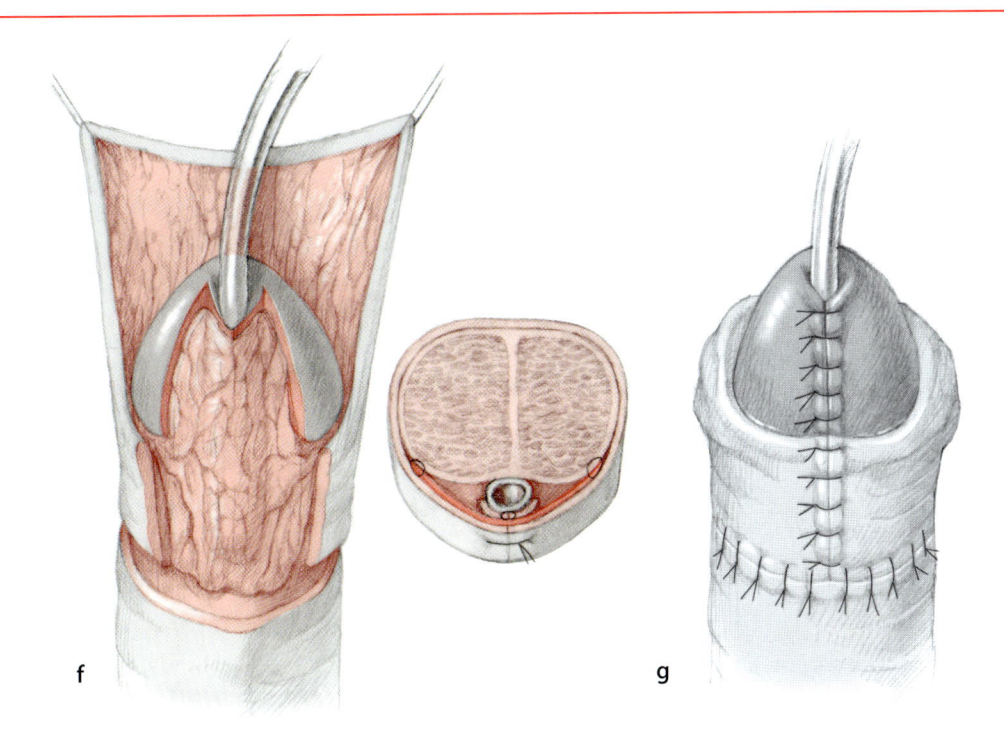

Fig. 15.1 (*continued*). **f** Glanuloplasty begins with approximation of the glans wings at the corona. The mucosal collar is also closed in the midline with subepithelial stitches. **g** The meatus is sewn to the glans at 5 and 7 o'clock. Skin closure is completed using subepithelial stitches

Operative Technique

Distal Hypospadias Repair

The technique of distal hypospadias repair is shown in Fig. 15.1.

Degloving the Penis

A 5-0 polypropylene traction suture is placed in the glans just beyond the anticipated dorsal lip of the neomeatus. Then a sound is passed to assess the urethra and overlying skin. Because the normal corpus spongiosum investment over the urethra often terminates proximal to the hypospadiac meatus, and dartos tissues are frequently deficient on the ventrum of the penis, the quality of the distal portion of the urethra varies and it may be quite thin and adherent to the skin. Most often, a circumscribing skin incision is made 1–2 mm proximal to the meatus and the shaft skin is degloved to the penoscrotal junction. If a portion of the native urethra is excessively thin, however, a U-shaped incision is made extending to more healthy tissues.

Penile curvature occurs in approximately 15% of cases of distal hypospadias, so artificial erection should be performed routinely. When bending is encountered in these cases, it is usually mild and readily corrected by dorsal plication. I recently adopted Baskin's recommendation and place a single plicating stitch of 6-0 polypropylene at the 12 o'clock position–opposite the point of maximum curvature (Baskin et al. 1998).

Urethroplasty

The urethral plate is next separated from the glans wings by parallel longitudinal incisions along their visual junction. Previously, I first injected this plane with dilute epinephrine, but subsequently have found that placement of a tourniquet at the base of the penis provides better visualization of the operative field. The glans wings are mobilized laterally, taking care to avoid damage to the margins of the urethral plate.

In most cases the urethral plate is not sufficiently wide at this point to tubularize it into a functional neourethra. Therefore, a relaxing incision is made in the midline from within the meatus to the end of the plate (Fig. 15.2). I have emphasized that this incision should be limited to the urethral plate and not carried into the rim of the glans at the distal margin of the plate. The depth of the relaxing incision varies

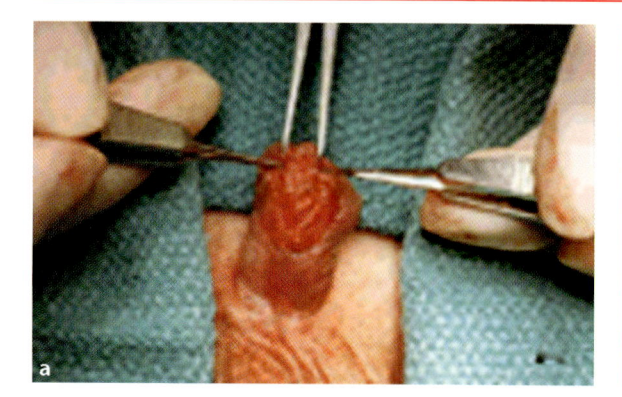

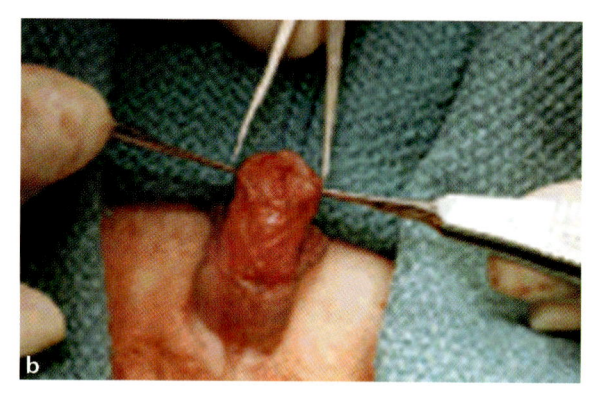

Fig. 15.2a, b. Midline relaxing incision of the urethral plate. **a** Before incision this plate was 6 mm wide. **b** Midline incision increased plate width to >12 mm

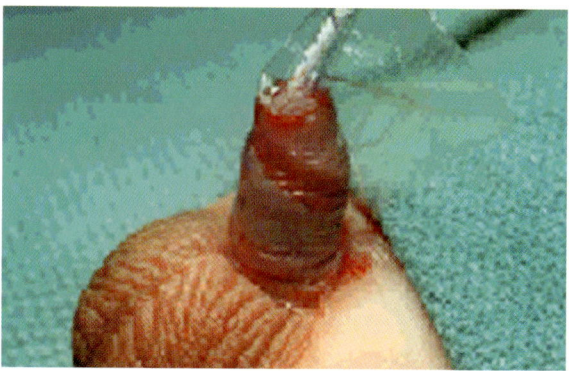

Fig. 15.3. Postoperative dressing

depending upon whether the plate is flat or grooved, but always extends through the epithelium to near the underlying corpora cavernosa. I prefer to use tenotomy scissors for this step, and have found the plate is reliably widened to create a neourethra greater than 10–12 F in children.

A 6-F stent is passed into the bladder and secured with the glans traction suture. I have used a variety of suture materials and techniques to tubularize the urethra. Currently, 7-0 polyglactin is preferred, with the first stitch placed at approximately the midglans level. Occasionally, an additional stitch is taken distal to this reference point, but the neomeatus should be generously sized with an oval, not rounded, configuration. Tubularization is completed with a two-layer running subepithelial closure.

Any adjacent dartos tissues are used to cover the neourethra and then a dartos pedicle is developed from the dorsal shaft skin, buttonholed, and transposed to the ventrum to additionally cover the repair.

Glanuloplasty

Reconstruction of the glans is a key determinant of the final cosmetic result. While tubularization of the urethral plate creates a vertically oriented meatus, a solid bridge of glans between the neomeatus and corona is needed to properly position the meatus. In the past, I closed the glans wings with vertical mattress chromic sutures, but subsequently noted cases of partial or complete dehiscence. Today, I first approximate the coronal margin with subepithelial 6-0 polyglactin and have found that this provides a more secure closure. Then the skin edges of the glans are sutured, and the meatus is matured at the 5 and 7 o'clock positions with 7-0 ophthalmic chromic catgut.

Skin Closure

The mucosal collar is approximated with subepithelial absorbable sutures. Then Byars flaps are created from the preputial hood to allow ventral midline skin closure to mimic the median raphe. Subepithelial stitches are used throughout to avoid suture tracks. A Tegaderm dressing is applied (Fig. 15.3) which almost always falls off within a few days. The stent is removed approximately 1 week later.

Proximal Hypospadias Repair

Degloving the Penis

For proximal hypospadias repair, the initial incision always extends along the lateral margins of the urethral plate and around the meatus. I believe it may be important to avoid the temptation of making this initial degloving incision wider than the plate, as hair follicles might be incorporated into the neourethra.

Ventral curvature occurs in more than 50% of these cases, and some other repairs begin with routine transection of the urethral plate, anticipating urethral reconstruction with skin flaps. However, the degree of bending often cannot be accurately determined until the shaft skin is released, so I always preserve the plate during the initial dissection. Mild curvature is straightened with dorsal midline plication as previously described. When there is more significant bending, I still attempt correction while maintaining the urethral plate. Consequently, in cases with moderate curvature the corpus spongiosum on either side of the plate is elevated from the corpora cavernosa, and, on occasion, this dissection extends completely under the plate as described by Mollard and Castagnola (1994). These maneuvers may resolve the curvature or diminish it sufficiently that dorsal plication may also be done. In rare cases, all these steps are inadequate and it appears best to transect the plate near the meatus and perform ventral dermal grafting to lengthen the corpora cavernosa.

Urethroplasty

Assuming the plate has been preserved during penile straightening, the midline relaxing incision is next made along its proximal aspect leaving the glanular portion intact. Most often, the urethral plate will increase in width and have a gross appearance similar to that seen in distal repairs. However, I have encountered two patients whose incised plates seemed to have deficient subepithelial tissues based upon an obviously different appearance, and TIP repair in these cases resulted in complications (Snodgrass and Lorenzo 2002b). After ensuring that the proximal plate is satisfactory, the glans wings are mobilized and the midline relaxing incision in the plate is carried to its distal extent. If the incised plate appears "unhealthy," it is excised and either a tubularized preputial flap or, in my hands, a staged repair is performed.

Tubularization of the urethral plate is accomplished in two layers using 7-0 polyglactin. The first layer consists of interrupted subepithelial stitches, followed by a running subepithelial second layer. Because fistulas have been a more bothersome problem for me in proximal repairs, I have adopted the "Y to I" closure of the corpus spongiosum over the neourethra (Yerkes et al. 2000) before the dorsal dartos pedicle is added, to provide an additional barrier layer.

Reoperations

Urethroplasty

The basic steps for TIP hypospadias reoperations are the same as described above. The key point in decision-making in these cases regards the suitability of the plate for incision and tubularization. For example, with a failed flip-flap or onlay preputial flap the urethral plate usually has been minimally traumatized, whereas after MAGPI or TIP, the midline of the plate has already been incised. I have been impressed that the plate often has a "healthy" appearance not significantly different than in primary cases, even following prior incision. Accordingly, I have performed TIP urethroplasty after a variety of failed procedures with acceptable outcomes (Snodgrass and Lorenzo 2002a), although a previous resection of the plate, or obvious gross scarring of it, are contraindications to this approach. While I have even performed TIP repair after two prior MAGPI procedures in one patient, a relative contraindication would also be multiple prior midline plate incisions.

Results

TIP repair creates a vertically oriented, slit neomeatus that closely resembles the normal urethral meatus (Fig. 15.4). This outcome does not depend upon the preoperative anatomy of the hypospadiac meatus or upon its location from the glans to the perineum. No other procedure consistently gives this result, which accounts for the rapid, worldwide acceptance of TIP urethroplasty. Furthermore, no other techni-

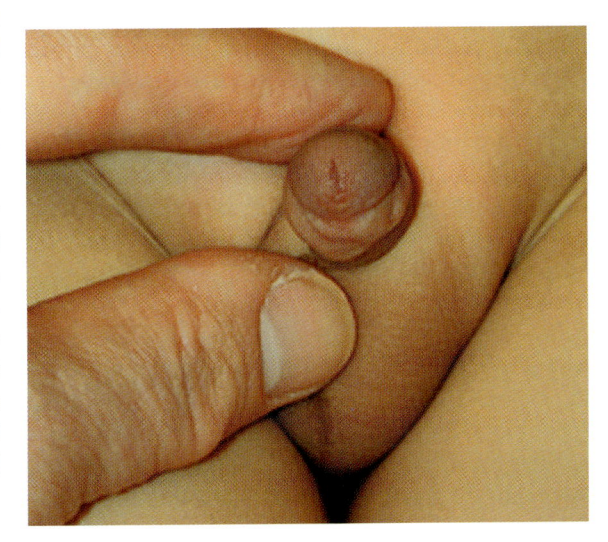

Fig. 15.4. Postoperative outcome

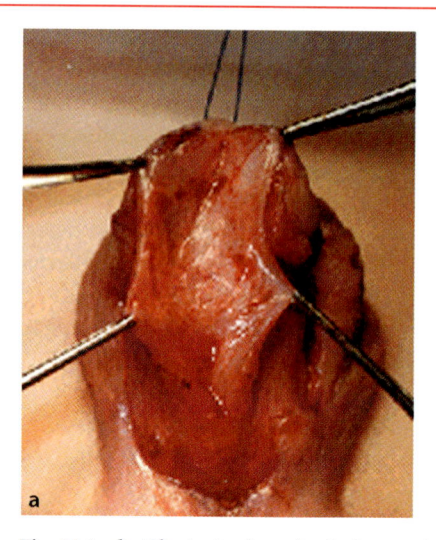

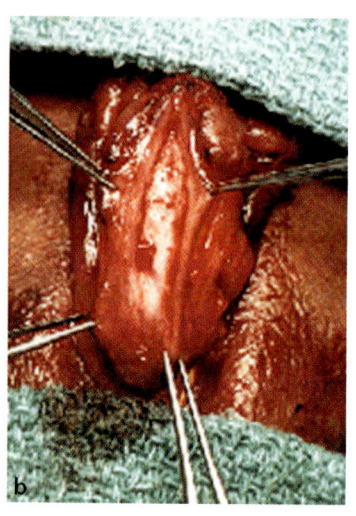

Fig. 15.5a, b. The incised urethral plate. a A supple plate. b A patient with dehiscence

que offers the versatility of TIP repair for distal, proximal, and reoperative hypospadias.

I have found TIP urethroplasty applicable to essentially all cases of distal hypospadias, and in a recent series of 150 consecutive patients did not resort to any other technique for distal shaft, subcoronal, or glanular repair (Snodgrass, unpublished data). Use of the technique in proximal hypospadias depends first upon whether curvature can be corrected without transecting the plate. In a consecutive series of 47 boys, this extent of penile curvature was encountered in 4 (8%) (Snodgrass, unpublished data). I have also observed an occasional incised plate to have an "unhealthy" appearance during proximal surgery (Fig. 15.5), and recommend it not be tubularized in this situation. Initial experience with TIP reoperations indicates that the urethral plate usually remains supple despite prior surgery, even in some cases after TIP and MAGPI in which the plate was incised (Shanberg et al. 2001; Borer et al. 2001; Snodgrass and Lorenzo 2002a).

TIP urethroplasty results in a functional urethra. Calibration of the neourethra consistently shows it to be at least 10–12 F, regardless of urethral plate width before incision. Urethroscopy has been performed in all patients requiring reoperation for complications or cosmetic improvements, such as correction of penoscrotal transposition. A neourethral stricture was encountered in one boy operated on for midshaft hypospadias at the original site of the meatus. In all other cases, following both distal and proximal hypospadias repair the urethra had a smooth and normal appearance without gross scarring where the dorsal incision was made (Lorenzo and Snodgrass 2002).

Complications

A compilation of published outcomes for TIP urethroplasty between 1994 and 1999 found an overall complication rate of 5.5% in series primarily comprised of distal repairs (Snodgrass 1999a). As in all other hypospadias reconstructions, the most common problem is fistulas. Their incidence is minimized by in-turning all epithelium when tubularizing the neourethra, and then covering the repair with a dorsal dartos pedicle. While these precautions reduce the likelihood of this complication to less than 2% in my experience with distal repairs, similar steps during proximal hypospadias surgery are still associated with a significantly higher fistula rate (Snodgrass and Lorenzo 2002b). This suggests that the glans wings, which cover essentially all the neourethra in distal repairs, provide superior protection to that afforded by dartos. Accordingly, I now routinely mobilize the corpus spongiosum alongside the urethral plate and close it over the neourethra during proximal hypospadias surgery to provide a similar, vascularized barrier between the urethral suture line and overlying skin closure.

The second most frequent complication is meatal stenosis. This was reported to occur in 1.5% of the 328 patients in the combined series mentioned above. I have had only two patients with meatal stenosis, of whom one appeared to have developed balanitis xerotica obliterans 6 years postoperatively. Most cases of stenosis probably reflect technical error, notably overzealous closure of the neourethra distally. As emphasized above, the neomeatus should be oval, not circular, to avoid this problem. Obviously, it is also necessary to deeply incise the urethral plate before tubularization to gain maximal width and ensure an adequate neourethral diameter. Initially, I routinely calibrated the neourethra postoperatively every 3 months for 1 year, but never detected meatal stenosis (Snodgrass 1999b). Today I only calibrate the repair once at 6 months and then dismiss healthy patients from further follow-up (Lorenzo and Snodgrass 2002).

Both stricture and diverticulum formation in the neourethra have been rare complications after TIP repair. Partial glans dehiscence has been noted occasionally, and prompted a change in suture material. Initially, I closed the glans wings using ophthalmic chromic suture, which may have dissolved too quickly. Today, I approximate the wings at the corona with subepithelial 6-0 polyglactin for a more secure closure.

Reported outcomes of TIP reoperations are encouraging, with complications noted in 15–24% of patients (Shanberg et al. 2001; Borer et al. 2001; Snodgrass and Lorenzo 2002a). The most common problem has been fistulas, especially when barrier layers were not used between the neourethra and skin (Borer et al. 2001). Despite prior surgery, including previous incision into the urethral plate, urethral healing has occurred without stricture.

Conclusions

TIP repair is still a new procedure lacking long-term follow-up. Preliminary experience using the operation across the spectrum of hypospadias is favorable, with complication rates the same, or less than, those of other modern techniques currently in use. Furthermore, the cosmetic outcome of the neomeatus and glans closely resembles normal anatomy. Given its versatility and these results, the operation has rapidly become a preferred means worldwide for hypospadias urethroplasty.

References

Baskin LS, Erol A, Li Y, et al: Anatomic studies of hypospadias. J Urol. 1998; 160:1108.

Borer JG, Bauer SB, Peters CA, et al: Tubularized incised plate urethroplasty: Expanded use in primary and repeat surgery for hypospadias. J Urol. 2001; 165:581.

Chen SC, Yang SS, Hsieh CH, et al: Tubularized incised plate urethroplasty for proximal hypospadias. BJU Int. 2000; 86:1050.

Lorenzo AJ, Snodgrass WT: Regular dilatation is not unnecessary after tubularized incised plate hypospadias repair. BJU Int. 2002; 89:94.

Mollard P, Castagnola C: Hypospadias: The release of chordee without dividing the urethral plate and onlay island flap (92 cases). J Urol. 1994; 152:1238.

Shanberg AM, Sanderson K, Duel BP: Reoperative hypospadias repair using the Snodgrass incised plate urethroplasty. BJU Int. 2001; 87:544.

Snodgrass WT: Tubularized incised plate urethroplasty for distal hypospadias. J Urol. 1994; 151:464.

Snodgrass WT: Tubularized incised plate hypospadias repair: Indications, technique and complications. Urology. 1999a; 54:6.

Snodgrass WT: Does the tubularized incised plate hypospadias repair create neourethral strictures? J Urol. 1999b; 162:1159.

Snodgrass WT, Lorenzo A: Tubularized incised plate urethroplasty for hypospadias reoperation. BJU Int. 2002a; 89:98.

Snodgrass WT, Lorenzo A: Tubularized incised plate urethroplasty for proximal hypospadias. BJU Int. 2002b; 89:90.

Snodgrass WT, Koyle M, Manzoni G, et al: Tubularized incised plate hypospadias repair: Results of a multicenter experience. J Urol. 1996; 156:839.

Snodgrass WT, Koyle M, Manzoni G, et al: Tubularized incised plate hypospadias repair for proximal hypospadias. J Urol. 1998; 159:2129.

Yerkes E, Adams M, Miller DA, et al: Y to I wrap: use of distal spongiosum for hypospadias repair. J Urol. 2000; 163:1536.

The Island Onlay Hypospadias Repair

Howard Snyder

Introduction

In patients with hypospadias sufficiently severe to require a substitution urethroplasty, for many years the most commonly utilized technique at the Children's Hospital of Philadelphia has been the island onlay one-stage hypospadias repair (Elder et al. 1987). Even for the most severe hypospadias, it has been this author's practice to carry out one-stage repairs.

The concept of a vascularized preputial island flap was introduced by Hook in 1896 (Horton et al. 1973). It was, however, Asopa and colleagues in Agra, India who developed the first very effective use of inner preputial skin for a substitution urethroplasty in hypospadias (Asopa et al. 1971). Duckett developed this by describing a transverse island tube repair in 1980. This was an era when it was presumed that if there was a need for a substitution urethroplasty, the urethral plate would be abnormal and require division. In the routine division of the urethral plate, since the plate was of elastic tissue, it would retract, supporting the then held view that the division was required. Gradually, it became recognized as the 1980s wore on that most chordee in hypospadias is due to simply the skin asymmetry and subcutaneous tissue. Controversy grew about the significance of the spongiosum, with some prominent surgeons continuing to recommend excision. Histologic work by Avellán and Knuttsson in 1980, Baskin et al. in 1998 and then in 2000 by Snodgrass et al., who carried out histologic examination of the spongiosum, indicated that the spongiosum really was not dysplastic at all and indeed was a vascularized healthy layer that could be incorporated into a hypospadias repair to provide healthy vascularized tissue for the anastomosis of a neourethra. With experience, we recognized that only a minority of hypospadias cases require division of the urethral plate – on the order of about 10% of major hypospadias cases at the Children's Hospital of Philadelphia today (Hollowell et al. 1990). It also was recognized that a minor bend of less than 30° after penile degloving can be adequately treated by dorsal midline plication without disturbing the neurovascular supply of the penis. It is, however, possible that this treatment is not essential, since in the era prior to the artificial erection we would never have identified this minor residual bend when we carried out a first-stage hypospadias repair. It is interesting to see that hypospadias patients are infrequently seen in adult sexual dysfunction clinics, suggesting that we have not undertreated chordee in the past, in an era when minor residual bend was probably undetected.

Operative Technique

Timing

Surgery for hypospadias is generally carried out between 6 and 12 months of age. This is after children reach the age where they will have the same anesthetic risks that they will have throughout childhood and yet well below the age of genital awareness which occurs at about 18 months. This timing follows the recommendations of the Urologic Section of the American Academy of Pediatrics.

Design of Glanuloplasty

The determination of the apex of the glanuloplasty ventrally is the single most important initial decision that must be made (Fig. 16.1.1a). This point is where the flat ventral surface of the glans begins to curve around the meatus. If holding stitches are placed in the abortive foreskin, in the majority of cases, the insertion of the foreskin into the glans will show where the flat surface can be traced up to where it begins to curve around the meatus. If the apex is held with forceps on each side, then the amount of epithelium that will be within the meatus can be determined. It will be readily appreciated that if the apex point is picked too high, it will compromise the size of the meatus. Conversely, placement of the apex

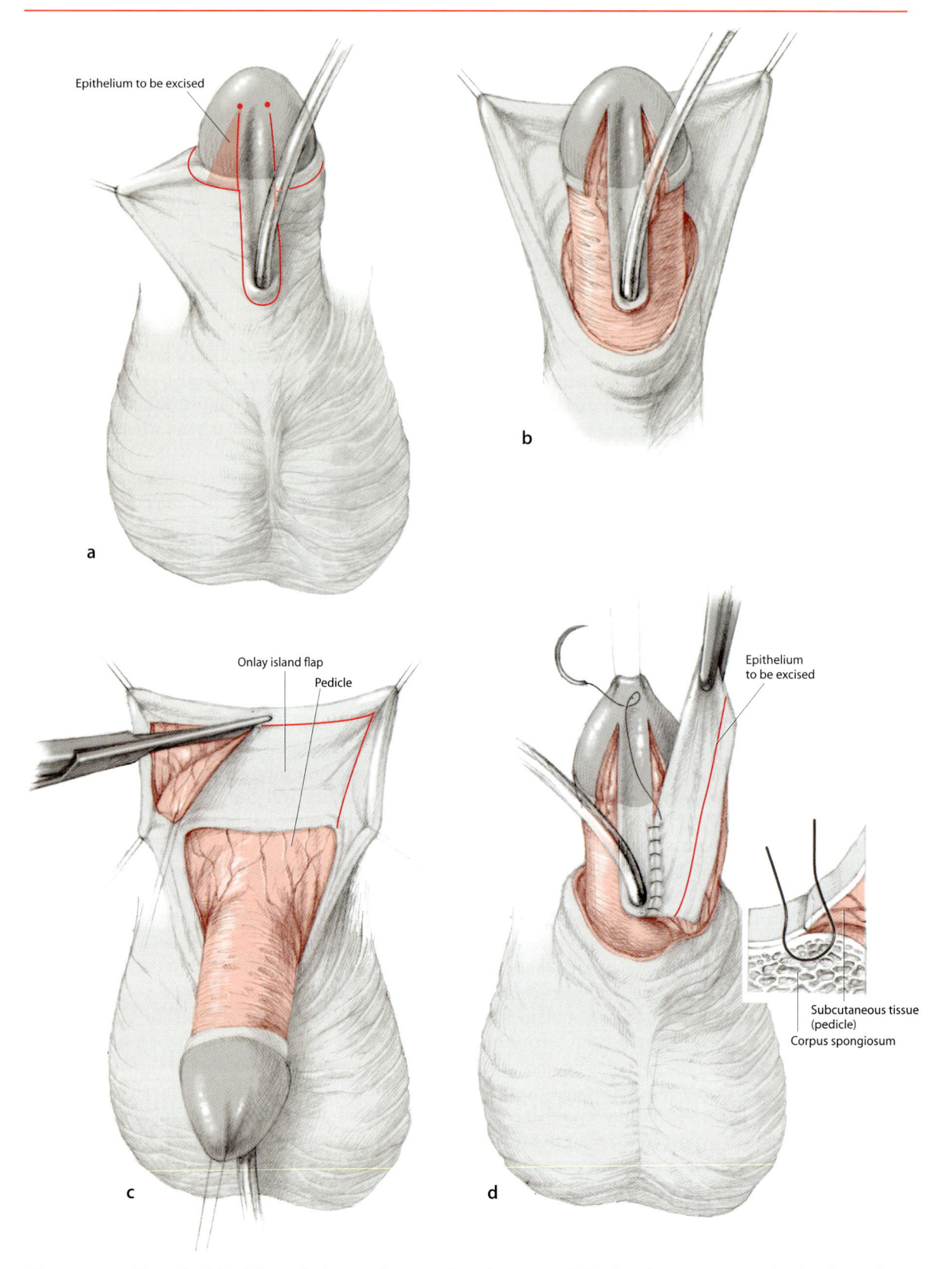

Fig. 16.1.1a–e. The onlay island flap technique. **a** The apex of glanuloplasty is identified (marked by *dots*). The *shaded triangle* shows the epithelium to be excised. A subcoronal incision encircles the glans and continues around the urethral plate. **b** The penile skin is dropped back and the glanular wings are mobilised. **c** The inner preputial onlay flap with its pedicle is developed and separated from the dorsal penile skin. **d** Suturing the onlay flap to the urethral plate incorporates generous bites of the spongiosum. **e** see p. 165

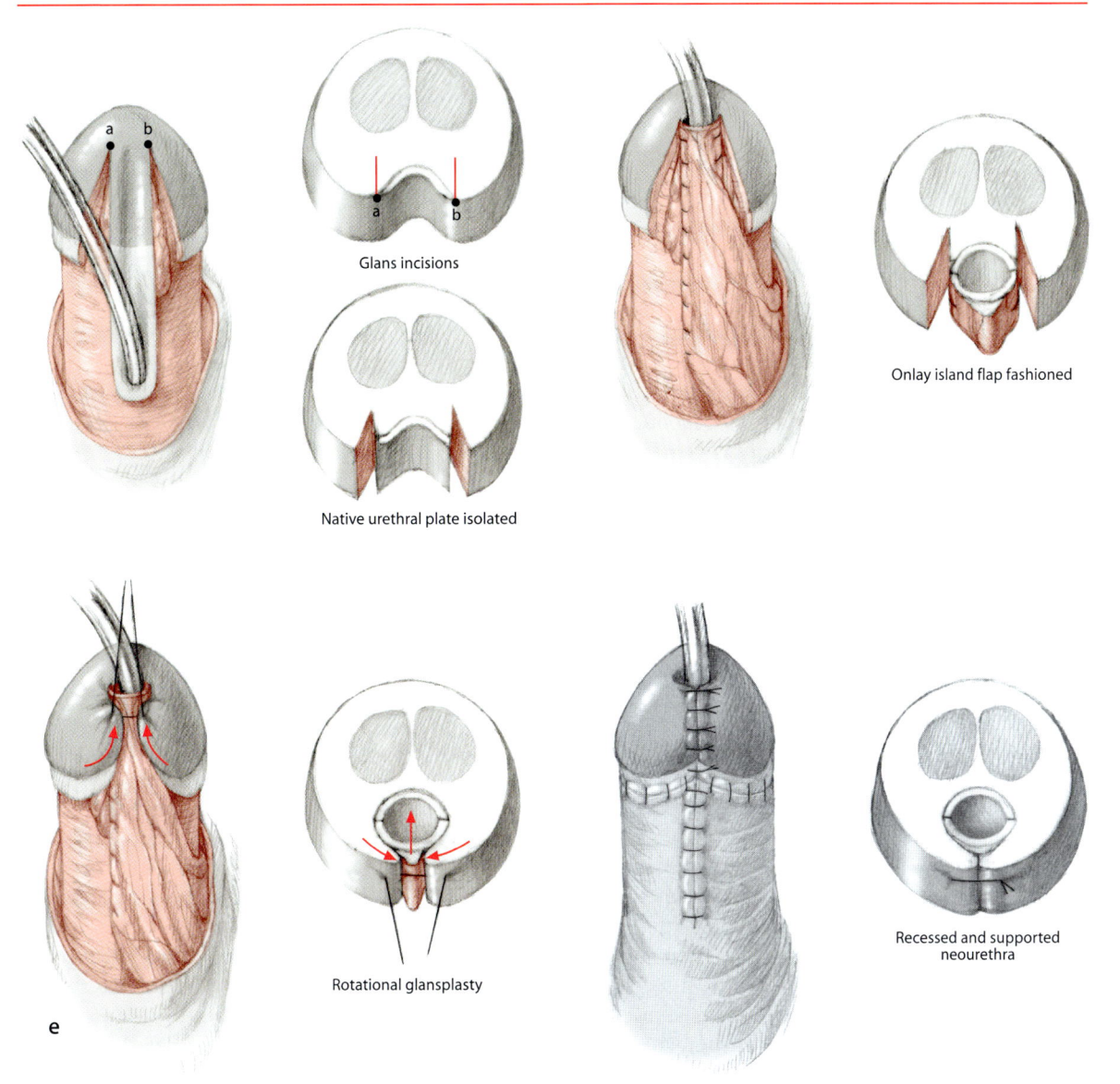

Fig. 16.1.1 (*continued*). **e** The glanuloplasty is the completion of the medial rotation of the glanular wings that has failed during development

too low leaves unsightly bumps on either side of the meatus after the glanuloplasty is completed. If the width and depth of the glanular groove is inadequate, then steps to deepen and widen the groove are appropriate. In infant boys a groove 12–14 mm is appropriate and in a teenager, 25 mm. A dorsal vertical incision is made until the width of the glanular groove is adequate for the meatus (Rich et al. 1989). While in the past we closed this in a Heineke–Mikulicz transverse fashion to create an epithelial-to epithelial-anastomosis, today it is our practice to follow Snodgrass' suggestion and leave the vertical incision open without closure (Snodgrass 1994). Secondary epithelialization occurs very rapidly and satisfactorily and gives a more normal slit-like configuration to the meatus.

Incisions

It is our practice to outline the incisions for a penile hypospadias repair at a subcoronal level, incorporating ventrally skirt flaps as described by Firlit in 1987. The incisions on either side of the urethral plate are right at the junction with the normal ventral skin. The incisions ventrally are kept very superficial, just going through the skin in order to avoid injury to the underlying spongiosum. The incisions continue up on either side of the glanular groove to the apex of the glanuloplasty. By use of xylocaine with epinephrine and careful following of dissection planes away from the vascular supply (described below), a tourniquet is not required.

Penile Skin Dropped Back

a) *Ventrally*. The skin drop-back is maintained just below the intrinsic blood supply of the ventral skin, carefully keeping the scissors' tip parallel to the skin so as not to injure the intrinsic blood supply of the skin (Fig. 16.1.1b). It is important to remember that the spongiosum inserts into both the overlying skin and the corporal bodies. Accordingly, a plane of dissection just below the intrinsic blood supply must be established laterally and then sharp dissection used to separate the skin from the underlying spongiosum. Meticulous attention to the plane of dissection avoids trauma to the delicate spongiosum and does not disturb the spongiosum's insertion into the glans. Starting the dissection distally and working proximally up the shaft has been easiest in my experience.
b) *Dorsally*. The plane of dissection is kept deep to the four small arteries that constitute the pedicle to the preputial flap. These four vessels are the distal end of the pudendal artery system and reliably provide excellent blood flow for the preputial flap.
c) *Laterally*. The dissection progresses to join the deep plane of dissection dorsally with the superficial plane ventrally lateral to the dorsal preputial pedicle and lateral to the spongiosum with an incision running parallel to the spongiosum and just outside its border.
d) *The Pedicle*. The pedicle is then separated from the outer preputial skin in a plane just below the intrinsic blood supply of the outer prepuce. Holding stitches are placed on the prepuce, flattening it (Fig. 16.1.1c).

Elevation of Glans Wings

The elevation of the glans wings will permit them to be rotated around the urethroplasty. The plane of dissection is established laterally just outside the corporal bodies and then carried medially, preserving an adequate amount of spongiosum with the urethral plate for a healthy reconstructed urethra. Care is taken not to divide the spongiosum insertion into the glans. Glans wing elevation usually continues until approximately the mid coronal plane of the glans. The blood supply to the glans in hypospadias is via the dorsal vascularity and no glans jeopardy is created by this mobilization.

Artificial Erection

An artificial erection is now routinely carried out unless the family reports perfectly straight erections. Normal saline for injection and a 23-scalp vein needle is utilized with a tourniquet at the base of the penis usually from a rubber band. It is important not to overfill the corporeal bodies.

Design of Island Onlay Flap

In general, the urethral plate after the skin drop-back measures 5 to 6 mm in width in small infants. Accordingly, a maximum of only a 1-cm wide onlay flap is required. At each end of the flap it should taper, as there is no need to introduce new epithelium. Distally, the amount of epithelium within the urethral meatus will be determined by the dorsal tissue rearrangement opposite the apex of the ventral glanuloplasty. Leaving too much neourethra distally can lead to distention and kinking to create the physiology of an anterior urethral valve which will eventually then lead to the formation of a sizable urethral diverticulum. Having designed the onlay flap, it is sutured into place beginning with the suture line underneath the pedicle utilizing running 7–0 polydiaxanone suture. The monofilament nature of this suture helps to avoid the frustrating drag through the tissues that is seen with braided sutures. Generally the stitches are placed from inside the native urethra outward in order facilitate gathering up a good bite of the supporting spongiosum (Fig. 16.1.1d). As the second suture line is completed distally opposite the pedicle, the glans should be drawn together setting up the first stitch of the glanuloplasty ventrally at its apex. Before the glanuloplasty is begun, redundant tissue from the pedicle is tacked over the suture lines with interrupted 7-0 polydiaxanone suture. This creates further vertical displacement of suture lines and contributes to avoidance of fistulas.

Glanuloplasty

Rotation medially of the mobilized glans wings is carried out with interrupted 6–0 polydiaxanone sutures. The stitches are placed parallel to the surface of the glans and 2 to 3 mm from the cut edge of the flat glans surface. This completes the rotation of the glans into a conical configuration that was aborted embryologically. A second just immediately subcuticular 7–0 Maxon layer ensures a smooth approximation of the glans edge and should result in an almost imperceptible eventual scar (Fig. 16.1.1e).

As the glanuloplasty is completed, it will bring to the midline the Firlit skirt flaps that were designed with the initial incisions. The skirt flaps are sutured into position with subcuticular stitches. The soft tissues associated with the skirt flaps may further contribute to separation of suture lines and avoidance of fistulas. The rotated broad surface of the glans brought together in the glanuloplasty achieves the same goal.

Skin Closure

The dorsal preputial skin is split in the midline and then there is a slide-around step to move it ventrally for a midline closure. In the careful dropping back of the ventral skin in the plane just below its intrinsic blood supply, one has abundant protected blood supply to the ventral skin to permit it to be closed in the midline. This creates the illusion of a normal penile ventral midline raphe. Having anchored the outer skin carefully, ventrally and dorsally, care is taken to be certain, by precise measurement, that the same amount of epithelium is left on all sides of the penis. Asymmetry in residual skin on the shaft will give a lopsided appearance and yield an unsatisfactory eventual cosmetic result. Having trimmed the excess skin, the closure is completed with subcuticular 7–0 polydiaxanone suture. Usually the designing of the closure proceeds most smoothly if the ventral midline closure is completed first before trimming the excess skin on either side. A subcuticular closure reliably avoids dermal suture sinuses later.

Urethral Stenting

A 15-cm length of 6-F medical grade silicone tubing obtained from the manufacturer who fashions this same material into ventriculoperitoneal shunts is used for urinary diversion. Extra holes are placed on the bladder end of the tube and it is threaded into place protruding about 2 cm outside the urethral meatus. If there is any difficulty threading the stent into place, this may indicate the presence of a utricle, as is fairly commonly seen in significant hypospadias. Either utilizing a small probe to anteriorly direct the stent, or utilizing the slightly stiffer 6-French Kendal catheter made of polyurethane, which tends to pop over the entrance to the utricle, will deal satisfactorily with the placement of a catheter into the bladder. The diverting stent is secured by a 5-0 Prolene suture placed on the inner aspect of the urethral meatus in order to avoid any suture marks on the surface of the glans postoperatively.

Dressing

We continue to utilize Duckett's "sandwich" dressing. This consists of pieces of telfa and gauze on either side of the penis which is then compressed against the lower abdominal wall aimed at the umbilicus and held down by a piece of Tegaderm.

Aftercare

The child is sent home on the day of the surgical procedure in all cases. The family is instructed to use for pain medication acetaminophen with codeine in a dose of 0.5–1 mg/kg every 4 h. Bladder spasms are minimal with the soft Silastic plastic stent but are dealt with by routine oxybutynin 0.2 mg per kilo every 8 h for the first 48 h. After that, most parents find they can reduce the dosage to just one dose given before the child is put to sleep. We utilize antibiotic prophylaxis with Trimethoprim-Sulfamethazole at $1/2$ to 1 teaspoon per day until the urethral stent has been removed.

Thirty-six hours after the procedure, the family teases the Tegaderm off the skin and then soaks off the remainder of the dressing in a tub. Subsequent care comprises merely soaking the child in a comfortable tepid tub twice a day for 15–20 min. As long as there is just clean water in the tub, there does not seem to be any adverse effect from having the urethral stent go below the surface of the water. Families are instructed to avoid straddle-type activities for the child until the urethral stent is removed. They are encouraged to give the child extra fluid to drink as it is very rare to see these small stents become obstructed unless the child develops significant dehydration and amorphous phosphate crystals plug the tube. The child returns at 10–14 days after surgery for division of the Prolene suture holding the stent in place and its removal. Generally, children void without any discomfort because epithelialization will have been complete by the time the silastic stent is removed.

Outcome

In a personal series reported by Cooper, a two-year experience between February 1997 and 1999 was summarized (Cooper et al. 2001). Thirty-six island onlay hypospadias repairs were carried out in sequence without one fistula. However, no hypospadias surgeon is immune from that complication, and patients of mine have had fistulas subsequent to that series. In this series of 36 consecutive patients, it is of importance to realize that only four needed a midline plicating stitch for minor residual bending of the penis. Three in the series, however, did come to redo surgery for the development of a urethral diverticulum. As none had meatal stenosis, the cause was almost certainly excess epithelium incorporated into the repair distally.

Conclusion

With our current understanding of hypospadias surgery, the meticulous design of the surgery from the beginning, paying particular attention to the fine points of the glanuloplasty, will permit an operation to start out on the right foot. If errors in design are made initially, it is very difficult to rescue the situation later. An understanding of the vascular anatomy of hypospadias, avoiding entry into the dorsal pedicle or the spongiosum ventrally, will make for a hemostatic procedure with minimal blood loss. With meticulous attention to dissection, there can be consistent preservation of the spongiosum, which can then be incorporated into the repair. Leaving the spongiosum maximally inserted into the tunica albuginea avoids injury to this delicate vascular structure. The spongiosal support contributes to a lower complication rate, particularly the fistula rate, which from our institution had previously been reported at 6%. For these reasons, if a substitution urethroplasty is required, the island onlay operation continues to be this reconstructive surgeon's operation of choice.

References

Asopa HS, Elhence IP, Atri SP, et al: One stage correction of penile hypospadias using a foreskin tube. Int Surg. 1971; 55:435

Avellán L, Knuttson F: Microscopic studies of curvature-causing structures in hypospadias. Scand J Plast Reconstr Surg. 1980; 14:249–258.

Baskin LS, Duckett JW, Ueoka K, et al: Changing concepts of hypospadias curvature lead to more only island flap procedures. J Urol. 1994; 151:191–196.

Baskin LS, Erol A, Li YW, et al: Anatomic studies of hypospadias. J Urol. 1998; 150:1108.

Cooper CS, Noh PH, Snyder HM: Preservation of urethral plate spongiosum technique to reduce hypospadias fistulas. Urology. 2001; 57:351–354

Duckett JW: Transverse preputial island flap technique for repair of severe hypospadias. Urol Clin North Am. 1980; 7:423.

Duckett JW: Hypospadias. Contemp Urol. April; 1992

Elder JS, Duckett JW, Snyder HM: Onlay island flap in the repair of mid and distal penile hypospadias without chordee. J Urol. 1987; 138:376–379.

Firlit CF: The mucosal collar in hypospadias surgery. J Urol. 1987; 127:80–82.

Hollowell JG, Keating MA, Snyder HM III, et al: Preservation of the urethral plate in hypospadias repair: extended applications and further experience with the onlay island flap urethroplasty. J Urol. 1990; 143:98–100.

Horton CE, Devine CJ Jr, Barcat N: Pictorial history of hypospadias repair techniques. In: Horton CE (ed): Plastic and reconstructive surgery of the genital area. Little Brown, Boston, pp 237–248; 1973.

Rich MA, Keating MA, Snyder HM, et al: "Hinging" the urethral plate in hypospadias meatoplasty. J Urol. 1989; 142:1551.

Snodgrass WT: Tubularized incised plate urethroplasty for distal hypospadias. J Urol. 1994; 151:464.

Snodgrass WT, Patterson K, Plaire JG, et al: Histology of the urethral plate: implications for hypospadias repair. J Urol. 2000; 164:988.

Tubularised Preputial Island Flap

16.2

Ahmed T. Hadidi, Amir F. Azmy

Dr. Howard Snyder has written an excellent description of the modified onlay procedure that grants the patient a near-normal looking penis at the end of the day (Chap. 16.1).

However, many surgeons (including the authors) have a different view concerning the nature of chordee and whether it should be excised. Snodgrass et al. (2002) suggested that if the chordee is causing 30% curvature of the penis or less they would prefer to perform dorsal plication. In our hands, 80% of patients with proximal types of hypospadias have severe chordee that needs careful dissection and excision. It is true that when the surgeon applies the artificial erection test after chordee excision, the penis may have some degree of curvature. This is similar to the situation when a person has his elbow in plaster of Paris for a month. One should not expect him to be able to extend his elbow completely immediately after plaster removal. The penis has been in "plaster" (chordee) for several months before birth and a few months, at least, after birth. One should expect some residual curvature to remain temporarily after chordee excision.

Surgeons who prefer to excise the deep fibrous chordee associated with proximal hypospadias may prefer to use the transverse preputial island flap popularised by Duckett (1980) or one of its modifications. Duckett used a glans channel when he described the technique. This is no longer recommended as meatal stenosis is liable to occur. We prefer to make a deep Y-shaped incision of the glans and mobilise freely the two lateral glanular wings.

Operative Steps

A deep Y-shaped incision is made on the glans. The centre of the Y is where the tip of the neomeatus will be located. The upper two short limbs of the Y are each 0.5 cm long. The long vertical limb of the Y extends down the whole length of the glans penis to the coronary sulcus (Fig. 16.2.1a).

The resultant three flaps are elevated and a core of soft tissue is excised to create a space for the neourethra. A subcoronal circumferential incision is made 3 mm below the coronal sulcus and an artificial erection is performed. Meticulous excision of any chordee or fibrous bands is carried out. This fibrous tissue is particularly heavy in the midline but may extend well laterally (Fig. 16.2.1b). Some surgeons correct residual penile curvature by dorsal plication; we prefer not to do so, as the curvature disappears spontaneously in most patients. The urethral meatus is circumcised to free the urethra from the overlying skin. The distal urethra and meatus are trimmed back to good spongiosum, and the cutaneous edges are removed. The proximal spatulated meatus and urethra are fixed to the corpora in a splayed-out fashion to receive the proximal end of the obliqued neourethra.

The penile and preputial skin is dissected free off the shaft from distal to proximal close to Buck's fascia, preserving the arteries that constitute the pedicle to the preputial flap. A 1.5-cm-wide rectangular flap is prepared. The length must suffice to bridge the gap between the meatus and the tip of the glans (Fig. 16.2.1c). Extra length can be obtained by going down into the penile skin in a horseshoe fashion on either side.

The flap is tubularised around a 12-F (according to patient's age) catheter and sutured into the meatus. The calibre of the new urethra should be 12 F when completed. Polyglactin 7–0 continuous subcuticular sutures are used with a cutting needle. Interrupted sutures are used on the ends so that excess length may be excised (Fig. 16.2.1d).

Then, the pedicle is separated from the outer preputial skin in a plane just below the intrinsic blood supply of the outer prepuce down to the root of the penis. The flap is usually rotated so that the right side of the flap is attached to the proximal urethral meatus. An oblique anastomosis is made, freshening up the proximal urethra so that good tissue along with spongiosum is sutured to the tube. The suture line of the neourethra lies against the corporal groove. The

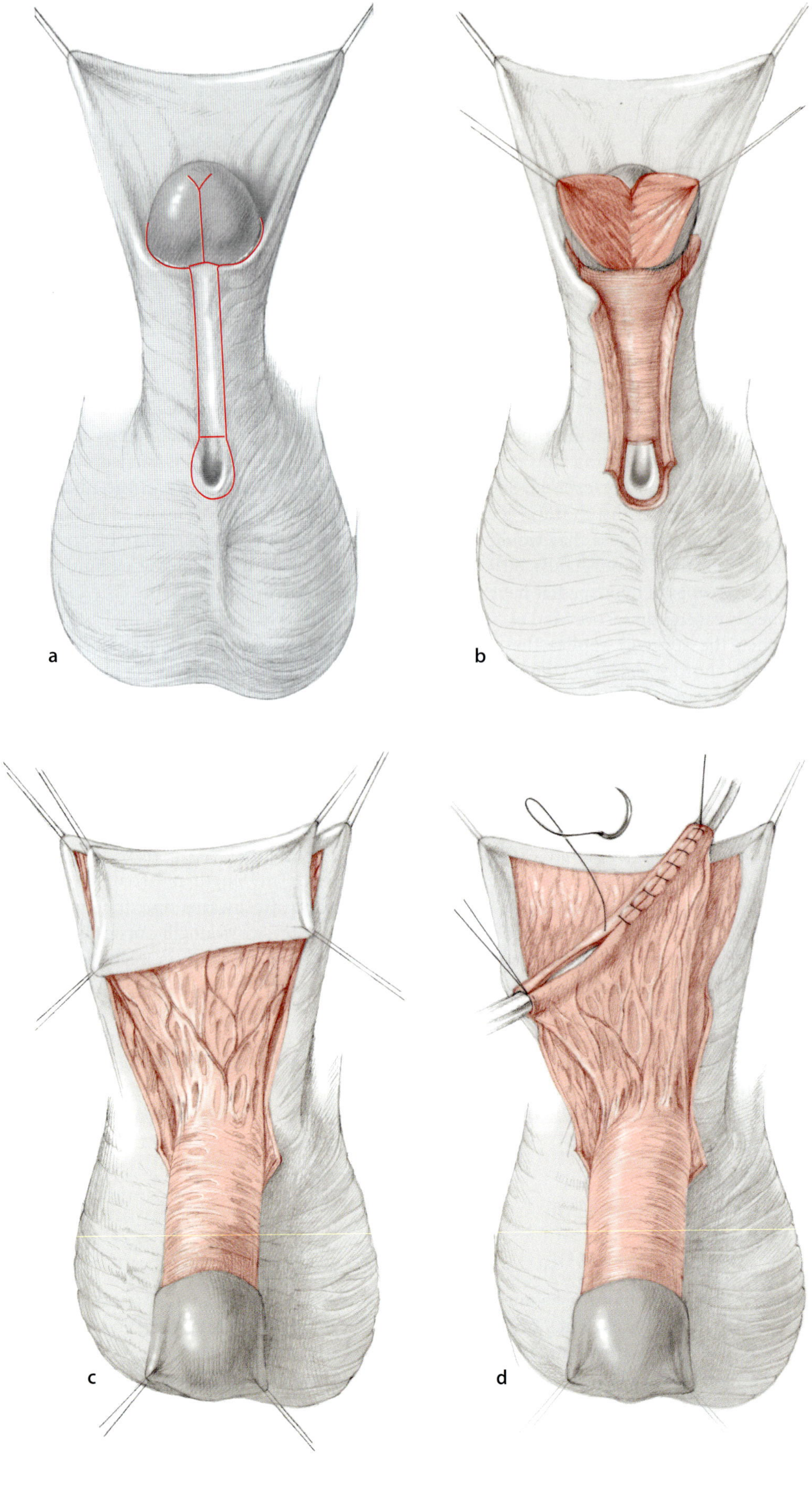
a
b
c
d

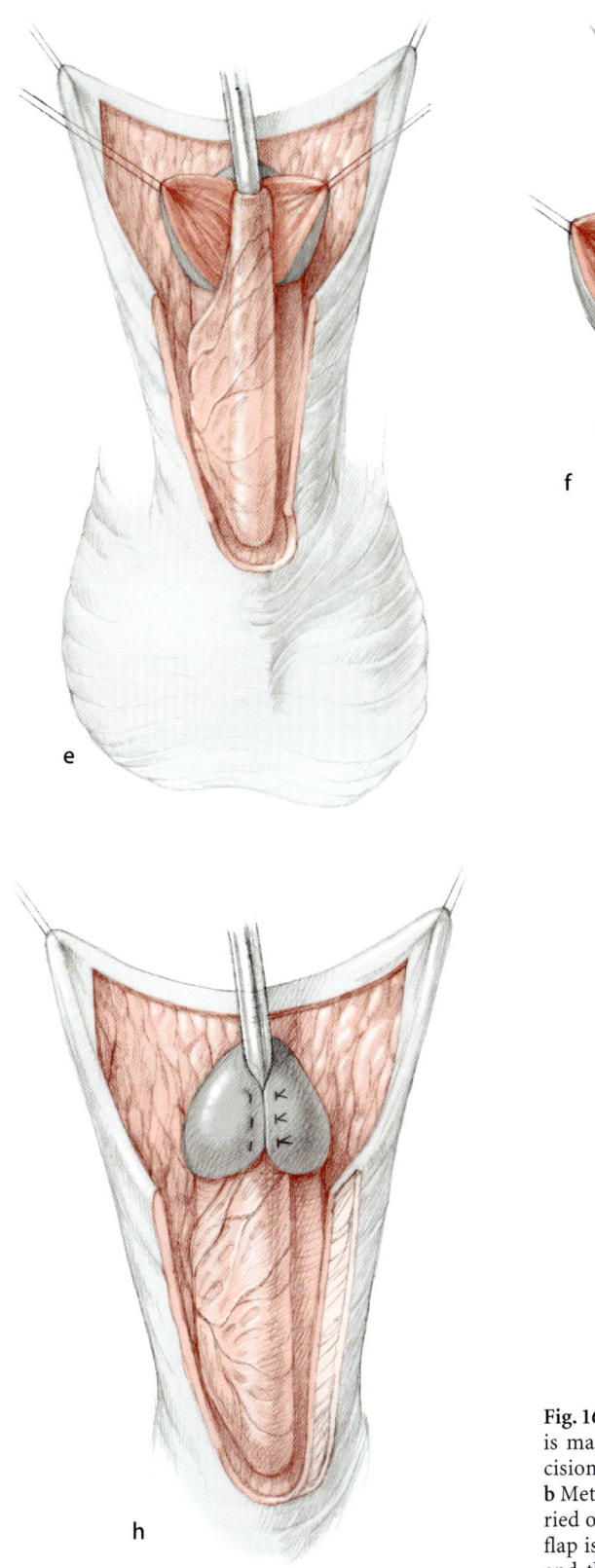

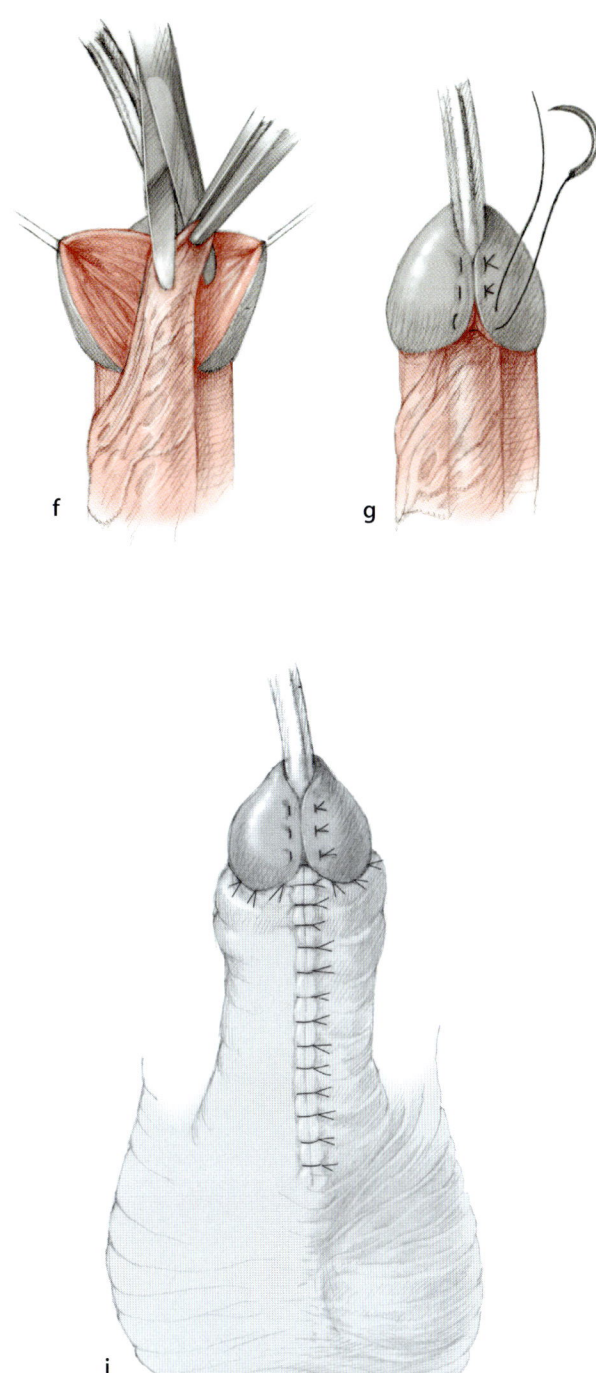

Fig. 16.2.1a–i. Transverse preputial island flap. **a** A Y incision is made on the glans and a subcoronal circumferential incision is made, and an artificial erection is performed. **b** Meticulous excision of any chordee or fibrous bands is carried out. **c** A 1.5-cm-wide rectangular flap is prepared. **d** The flap is tubularised. **e** The lower end is sutured to the meatus and the upper median flap is sutured to the upper end of the tube. **f** A small V is excised from the tip of the tube. **g** The mobilised glans wings are rotated medially and three transverse mattress sutures maintain firm approximation of the glanular wings in the midline. **h, i** De-epithelialisation of skin to protect the neourethra

proximal anastomosis is fixed to the tunica albuginea of the corpora. The neourethra is gently pulled distally toward the glans to avoid redundancy of the tube and kinking of the proximal anastomosis. Any excess length of the tube is excised. The upper small median flap resulting from the Y incision is sutured to the upper dorsal end of the tube (👁 Fig. 16.2.1e).

A small V is excised from the tip of the neourethra to obtain a slit-like meatus (👁 Fig. 16.2.1f). The mobilised glanular wings are rotated medially around the neourethra. Three transverse mattress sutures maintain firm approximation of the glanular wings in the midline (👁 Fig. 16.2.1g).

The remaining part of the prepuce is divided in the midline and wrapped around the penis. We prefer to use Smith's de-epithelialisation technique to have a protective intermediate layer (Smith 1973; Telfer et al. 1998) (👁 Fig. 16.2.1h, i).

References

Duckett JW: Transverse preputial island flap technique for repair of severe hypospadias. Urol Clin North Am. 1980; 7:423

Duckett JW, Baskin LS: Hypospadias. In: Gillenwater JY, Grayhack JT, Howards SS, Duckett JW (eds): Adult and pediatric urology, 3rd edn. Mosby-Year Book, St. Louis, pp 2549–2589; 1996.

Smith D: A de-epithelialized overlap flap technique in the repair of hypospadias. Br J Plast Surg. 1973; 26:106–114.

Snodgrass WT, Baskin LS, Mitchell ME: Hypospadias. In: Gillenwater JY, Grayhack JT, Howards SS, Mitchell ME (eds): Adult and pediatric urology, 4th edn. Lippincott Williams and Wilkins, Philadelphia, pp 2509–2532; 2002.

Telfer JRC, Quaba AA, Kwai B, et al: An investigation into the role of waterproofing in a two-stage hypospadias repair. Br J Plast Surg. 1998; 51:542-546.

Single-Stage Procedure for Severe Hypospadias: Onlay-Tube-Onlay Modification of the Transverse Island Preputial Flap

Jyoti Upadhyay, Anthony Khoury

Recent advances in hypospadias repair enable excellent functional and cosmetic results for treatment of severe hypospadias. We have utilised flaps rather than grafts in almost all cases. In this chapter, we illustrate our current approach to single-stage repair of severe penoscrotal/perineal hypospadias. In most of these cases, division of the urethral plate, which is often necessary, is performed in the midportion to allow a "combination flap" for the urethroplasty. Here we describe our technique with special emphasis on the correction of severe chordee utilising ventral lengthening procedures rather than dorsal plication in addition to a combined onlay-tube-onlay preputial flap for the urethroplasty.

Introduction

Irrespective of the classification utilised for major or severe or proximal hypospadias, increased cosmetic expectations along with a better understanding of the pathophysiology of this deformity have resulted in an array of new surgical techniques and modifications. Two major components of all repairs are reconstruction of the urethra with a normally positioned meatus (urethroplasty) and correction of the curvature (orthoplasty).

Urethral reconstruction may incorporate adjacent skin flaps, free skin grafts, and mobilised vascularised flaps. It was not until the 1970s that the procedures for severe hypospadias dramatically changed with the work of Asopa, Duckett, Snyder, Mollard and their coworkers (Asopa et al. 1971; Duckett 1981; Elder et al. 1987; Mollard et al. 1991). Regardless of the technique used, vascularised flaps have been reported to be generally superior to free skin grafts (Borer and Retik 1999). There has also been a change with regard to the management of the urethral plate for repair of curvature (Baskin et al. 1994; Borer and Retik 1999). In the past, the urethral plate was often excised because it was thought to be responsible for the severe curvature associated with more proximal cases of hypospadias (Baskin et al. 1994; Duckett 1980)

Recognition that excision/division of the urethral plate was not routinely necessary for correction of the curvature increased the number of onlay flaps for hypospadias repair (Baskin et al. 1994; Elder et al. 1987; Gearhart and Borland 1992; Hollowell et al. 1990). In the past few years, several modifications of the onlay flap for hypospadias repair have been reported (Gonzalez et al. 1996; Rushton and Belman 1998). The modern approach to repair of severe hypospadias attempts to preserve the urethral plate if possible. Nevertheless, in cases of severe chordee associated with an atretic or underdeveloped urethral plate, resection of the fibrovascular tethering tissue may be necessary as a component of orthoplasty. In this scenario, the transverse preputial island tube flap as reported by Asopa and Duckett (Asopa et al. 1971; Duckett 1981) is the most commonly performed repair.

Historically, management of severe proximal hypospadias with chordee was by utilising a two-stage repair in an attempt to avoid higher complication rates including urethral fistula and strictures. Using various techniques, chordee was repaired during the first stage and subsequently an urethroplasty was performed (Horton 1973). With the introduction of techniques for artificial penile erection during hypospadias repair, chordee correction was amenable to complete repair during the initial surgery (Gittes and McLaughlin 1974). This innovation, along with other technical advances utilising various vascularised flaps (such as preputial island flaps), free grafts, bladder and buccal mucosa, brought the conceptual change from a two-stage to a one-stage repair (Devine and Horton 1977; Duckett 1981; Elder et al. 1987; Frey and Bianchi 1989; Hollowell et al. 1990; Mollard et al. 1991; Rober et al. 1990; Sauvage et al. 1993; Wacksman 1986). Early experiences with various one-stage techniques have demonstrated that in the hands of experienced surgeons comparable complication rates and cosmetic results can be achieved using a one-

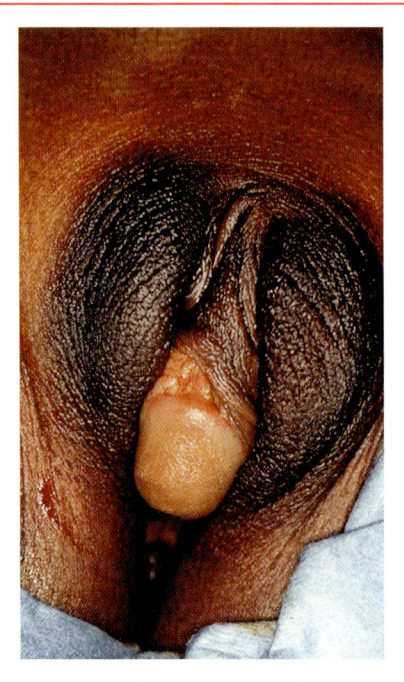

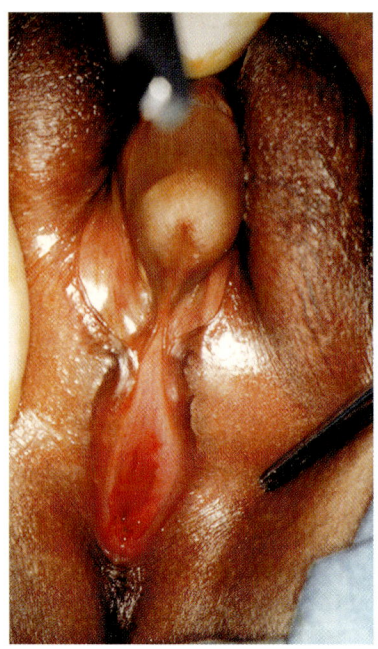

Fig. 17.1. A case of severe perineal hypospadias with a poorly developed atretic urethral plate, severe chordee, and penoscrotal transposition

stage approach (Kelalis et al. 1977). Since the late 1970s, the one-stage approach has gained popularity. Although some controversy exists in using a two-stage approach (Greenfield et al. 1994; Retik et al. 1994), and some still prefer a two-stage approach (Bracka 1995), currently a one-stage repair for both the orthoplasty and urethroplasty in proximal hypospadias repair is the approach preferred by most experienced paediatric urologists in large centres.

The tubularised incised plate (TIP) technique described by Snodgrass was originally described for repair of distal hypospadias with a 7% complication rate (Snodgrass 1994, 1999). Recently, it has been advocated for more proximal hypospadias repair, with a reported complication rate of 11% (Snodgrass et al. 1998). We do not advocate the TIP technique for severe proximal hypospadias. The long-term outcome, and whether the neourethra will be adequate in calibre 10–15 years later, is not known.

We utilise a preputial transverse island onlay or tube flap or a combination of the two, an onlay-tube-onlay flap, for repair of the majority cases of of severe proximal hypospadias at our institution. In the following, we will review current concepts for management of severe proximal hypospadias with emphasis on our preferences for a single stage procedure for the urethral reconstruction using an onlay-tube-onlay modification of the transverse island preputial flap in addition to a tunica vaginalis-augmented pericardial patch ventral lengthening procedure for chordee correction.

Surgical Treatment

A two-stage repair for patients with proximal hypospadias commits 100% of the patients to more surgery. We believe a planned one-stage repair can offer comparable results and may spare the patients further surgical interventions. Even if there is a higher chance of secondary procedures (20–30%), approximately two thirds of the cases of hypospadias will be corrected with one intervention. Furthermore, a well-performed single-stage repair does not compromise availability of vascular tissue for subsequent procedures. Furthermore, in our analysis, a single-stage repair does not compromise functional or cosmetic outcome for the patients.

Patients with severe penoscrotal or perineal hypospadias and a short atretic urethral plate with significant chordee are candidates for this procedure. Severe curvature after degloving the penis is a common finding in these patients and needs to be corrected simultaneously. An atretic urethral plate requiring transection is another common finding in this selected group of patients (Fig. 17.1).

A prerequisite for a one-stage repair is the presence of appropriate dorsal hood foreskin for a preputial-based island flap. Adequate penile length (girth/length >10th percentile for age) is another precondition for a successful outcome. All hypospadiac patients with one undescended testicle and all patients with bilateral undescended testes undergo preoperative karyotyping. Vesicourethrography to evaluate for a müllerian remnant is only performed if the child has severe hypospadias and a history of urinary tract infections. Müllerian remnants are usually asymptomatic and we do not believe that they require routine surgical resection.

Choice of Repair

A primary determinant in successful repair of severe hypospadias is the decision regarding the type of the repair. This decision is based on the quality and length of the urethral plate, the amount of foreskin available and the degree of persistent curvature after penile degloving. We believe the decision on which repair to use can only be taken intraoperatively. Although the choice of repair can be individualised based on the surgeon's experience/preference, some general principles apply and are agreed upon. If there is a poorly developed urethral plate requiring transection, a transverse island tube flap has been recommended as the repair of choice. If, however, the urethral plate is well developed and has a good calibre without associated severe chordee, which is seldom the case in severe hypospadias, an onlay flap or a Duplay-type repair has been advocated (Elder et al. 1987; Snodgrass et al. 1998)

In cases with a short-tethering, poorly developed urethral plate and severe chordee, we prefer to divide the urethral plate in the middle which provides an opportunity to incorporate the vascularised urethral plate at the proximal and distal ends into the repair. We prefer a preputial transverse onlay flap proximally and distally combined with a central tubularised modification of the flap, which we refer to as the onlay-tube-onlay modification. Also, we find the double-face split preputial flap modification extremely helpful in situations in which there is severe deficiency in ventral skin coverage (Rushton and Belman 1998).

General Principles

For these select cases of severe penoscrotal/perineal hypospadias, we recommend adherence to certain guidelines or principles to assure optimal results:
1. Attempt not to use a free graft.
2. Lengthening the penis is better than shortening it.
3. Use a single-stage repair, making sure to preserve the blood supply so one can subsequently repair any small fistulas that may develop.
4. Use a double-faced preputial flap if ventral skin coverage is compromised so as to avoid a central suture line covering the urethroplasty.
5 Repair penoscrotal transposition during the same procedure.

A 5-0 Prolene suture is placed in the glans penis as a holding stitch. A 10-F urethral Silastic catheter is passed into the hypospadiac meatus to assess the ventral urethral lumen proximally after degloving the penis. An atretic distal opening with underdeveloped ventral urethral tissue can be identified by using the "white line test" of the Silastic catheter. The penile skin is degloved dorsally and followed around ventrally approximately 2–3 mm lateral to the urethral plate and the meatal opening proximally. The skin dissection is performed in order to create a 6- to 8-mm Firlit mucosal collar (Firlit 1987). As one proceeds ventrally, care must be taken when dissecting the skin off the spongiosum, where it is usually adherent. It is vital to approach this part of the dissection from lateral to medial and to stay closer to the skin then one thinks is necessary to avoid bleeding from the underlying splayed spongiosal tissue (👁 Fig. 17.2). If excessive spongiosal tissue bleeding is encountered, then the dissection is being carried out in the wrong plane. Proximally, care is taken to separate the underlying urethra, albeit an often atretic one, from the ventral skin to prevent injury to the urethra. Often the urethra is tethered down between the bifid scrotum, requiring wider mobilisation to free the proximal urethral opening from the adjacent tissues. This can create excessive bleeding if the dissection is performed too deep or compromise the blood supply to the urethra if performed too superficially. After degloving is complete, a tourniquet is applied to the base of the penis and an artificial erection is created utilising lactated Ringer solution and a 25-gauge butterfly needle (Gittes and McLaughlin 1974).

Atraumatic minimal tissue handling is crucial for a successful repair. We utilise a tourniquet only during evaluation of chordee and occasionally during glanuloplasty for adequate visualisation. The key to bloodless hypospadias surgery is knowledge of the anatomy of the defect and being in the correct planes. Epinephrine or other vasocontrictive agents have been advocated for improved operative visualisation (Duckett 1996). We have not found this necessary and have not utilised this approach. In fact, constriction of vessels with vasoactive agents may result in more delayed bleeding.

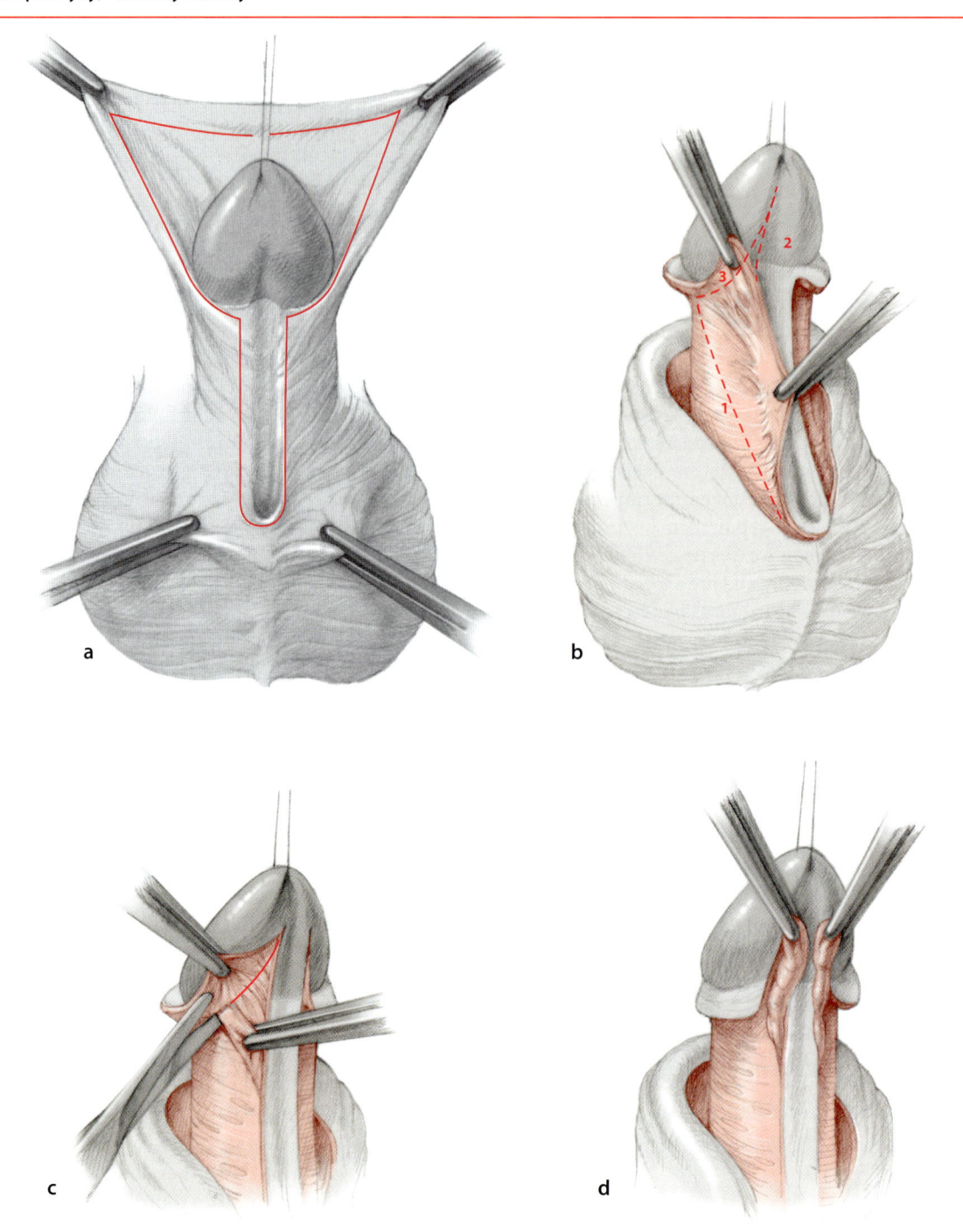

Fig. 17.2a–d. Spongioplasty. **a** Dotted outline of the penile degloving incision. **b** The spongiosal dissection provides the road map for creation of the glans wings. First, the spongiosum is dissected off the tunica albuginea laterally and followed to its point of insertion under the glans (*1*). Next, superficial incisions parallel to the urethral plate are performed and deepened (*2*). A third incision (*3*) medially following the spongiosal tissue to the tips of the corporal bodies within the glans tissue towards incision 2 provides a road map for the proper location, depth and angle for the creation of the glans wings. **c** Spongiosal dissection is performed sharply in an avascular plane underneath Buck's fascia in a lateral to medial direction. Note the spongiosum inserts under the glans. The spongiosal tissue is dissected from underneath the glans. The spongiosal tissue is then free and the glans wings are mobilised. **d** The spongiosal tissue can be approximated medially and serve as a second-layer closure after the urethroplasty is performed

Spongioplasty/Glanuloplasty

Embryologically, the corpus spongiosum surrounds the urethra circumferentially. However, the ventral spongiosum is severely deficient in severe hypospadias and remains splayed laterally adjacent to the urethral plate, inserting at the 4 and 8 o'clock positions (ventrolaterally) under the glans. Rather than excising the spongiosum, we routinely dissect this tissue and if enough tissue is present incorporate it into a non-constricting second-layer coverage of the urethral repair.

The spongious tissue is separated from the underlying tunica albuginea and used to cover the suture line of the urethroplasty. The steps utilised in performing the spongioplasty/glanuloplasty are shown in diagram form in Fig. 17.2a–d. The dissection of the spongious tissue is performed in an avascular plane deep to Buck's fascia, which is followed distally to its insertion under the glans (step 1). Next, separate superficial incisions parallel to and at the edge of the urethral plate are made and slightly deepened (step 2). A third incision following the spongious tissue to the tip of the corporal body in the glans is made, curved towards the urethral plate and connected to the incisions made parallel to the urethral plate (step 3). Hence, the spongious dissection provides a road map for the proper location, depth and angle for the creation of the glans wings (Fig. 17.2b).

Repair of Chordee

Penile curvature in severe hypospadias is secondary to a combination of deficiency of skin, dartos fascia, urethral plate, spongiosal tissue and corpora cavernosa disproportion. Some curvature improves after degloving the penis (King 1981). If curvature persists after these manoeuvres, which it usually does in severe cases, orthoplasty prior to urethroplasty is necessary. Persistent curvature is related to deficient growth of the corpora cavernosa on the ventral aspect. The principle of repair, therefore, can be divided into procedures aimed at shortening the corpora dorsally and those that lengthen the corpora ventrally.

Historically dorsal plication has been performed in mild to moderate curvatures using the Nesbit technique or various modifications (Baskin and Duckett 1994; Nesbit 1967). Recent anatomical studies demonstrate that the course of the dorsal neurovascular bundles is lateral and not at 12 o'clock on the corpora cavernosa as presumed previously (Baskin et al. 2000). Therefore, our current technique for dorsal plication utilises a midline vertical incision at the point of maximum curvature and subsequent transverse closure using interrupted 4-0 Prolene sutures with inverted knots. We believe that dorsal plication invariably results in shortening of the penile shaft, especially in more severe cases of proximal hypospadias. We do a dorsal plication in minor cases of hypospadias with a residual glans tilt after skin degloving or in cases with adequate penile length and only mild to moderate chordee.

Our belief is that the penis will be as long as its shortest aspect. Therefore, correction of more severe penile curvatures may require additional techniques to increase the length of the ventral aspect of the corpora cavernosa. This has been achieved using dermal grafts, allogenic and synthetic materials (Borer and Retik 1999; Devine and Horton 1975; Hendren and Keating 1988). We have performed ventral lengthening procedures using all three types of materials.

Our preferred choice of correction of moderate to severe curvature is a cadaveric pericardial graft with an additional tunica vaginalis flap for coverage of the repair. A schematic illustration of our approach to correction of chordee is given in Fig. 17.3. The urethral plate is completely mobilised and lifted away from the underlying corpora cavernosa. A transverse incision is made at the point of greatest curvature through the tunica albuginea (Fig. 17.3a). The tunica albuginea is lifted from the underlying corpora cavernosa. The linear incision becomes an ellipsoid defect, and the curvature is corrected by unhinging the corpora bodies from the overlying tunica (Fig. 17.3b). The created defect is closed with a cadaveric pericardial patch that is at least 20% larger than the defect itself to prevent contracture-induced recurrent curvature (Fig. 17.3c). The patch is then covered with an onlay flap of tunica vaginalis which serves as a second layer and separates the free pericardial graft from the urethral plate (Fig. 17.3d).

We use the technique described by Khoury et al. (1989) and Hafez et al. (2001) for raising the tunica vaginalis flap. Briefly, the skin and dartos of the hemiscrotum are incised and the testis within its tunica vaginalis covering is delivered into the surgical field. The tunica vaginalis is incised longitudinally anteromedially so as to preserve the posteriorly based blood supply that originates from the cremasteric artery. The flap is then trimmed and the superficial mesothelial layer is anastomosed to the tunica albuginea in order to cover the underlying pericardial patch.

a b c d

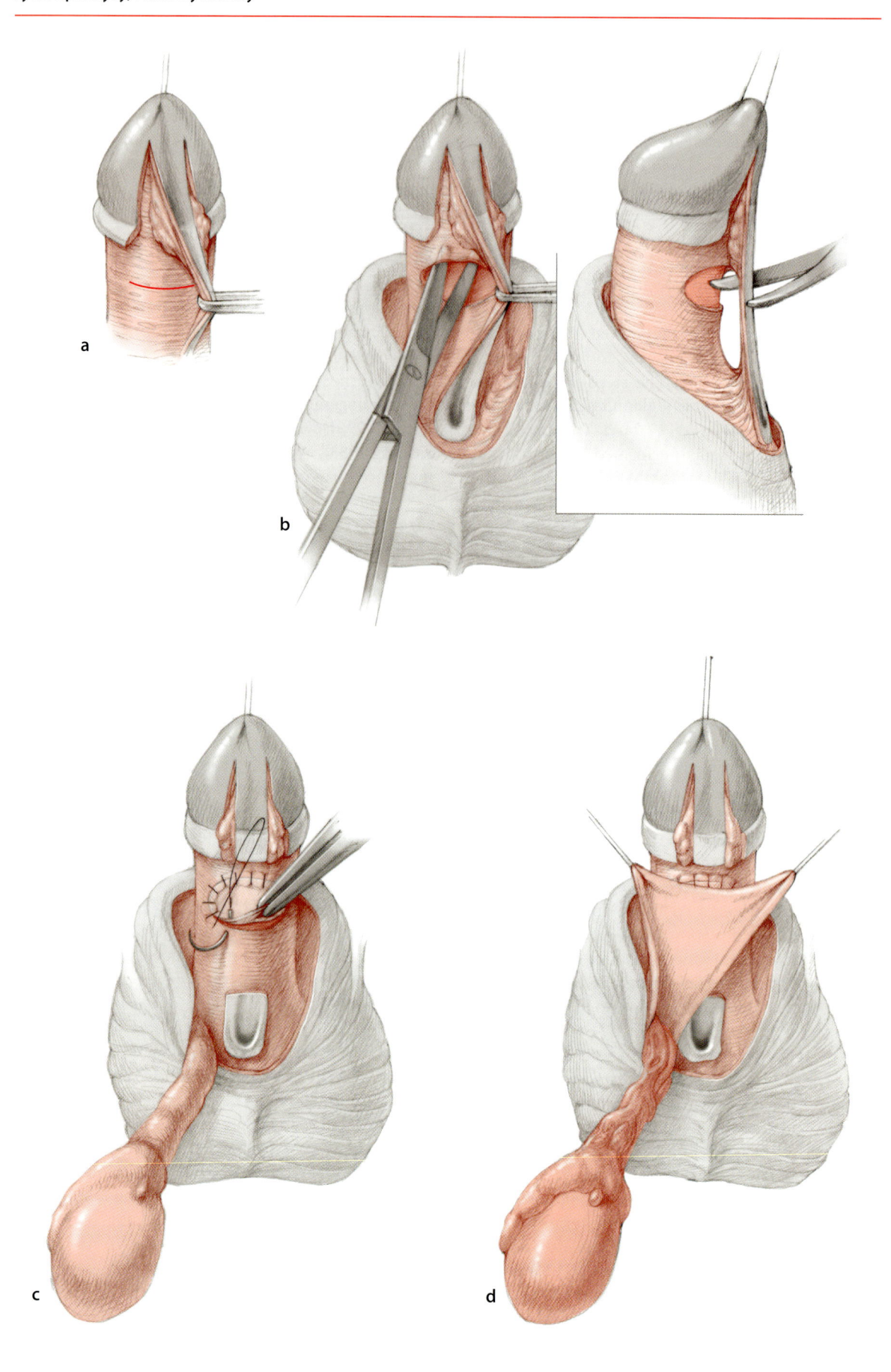

◀ **Fig. 17.3a–d.** Chordee correction using a ventral lengthening procedure (cadaveric pericardial graft covered with a tunica vaginalis flap). **a** Diagram of erection test showing site of incision ventrally at point of maximum curvature after the urethral plate is mobilised off the underlying corpora cavernosa. The dotted outline of the axis of the penis anticipated after ventral lengthening procedure is complete. **b** Ellipsoid defect created after an incision is made and the underlying corpora cavernosa is mobilised using sharp dissection. *Inset:* Lateral view of large ventral defect with resultant straightening of penile axis and division of the urethral plate in the midportion. **c** Cadaveric pericardial patch utilised to cover the ventral defect with a running suture. **d** An onlay flap of tunica vaginalis is used to separate the free pericardial graft from the urethral plate

Urethroplasty

Clearly, the type of urethroplasty depends on whether the plate has to be divided or not. The manner in which we have dealt with the urethral plate in this select group of patients with the most severe forms of proximal hypospadias has changed over time. In the past, the plate was completely excised with creation of the neourethra using a preputial tubular flap. Later, we divided the urethral plate distally, excised the atretic middle portion of the plate and then performed an onlay proximally with a tubularisation of the flap distally. Our technique has continued to evolve, and now we divide the plate in the middle, in the most atretic area, so as to maximise the available healthy tissue for the urethroplasty at the most proximal and distal ends.

Today our techniques for urethroplasty for severe proximal hypospadias include an onlay flap with an additional transverse island preputial tubular flap component of the preputial skin. We preferably perform an onlay flap in cases with a well developed urethral plate with good blood supply requiring no division. If the urethral plate is deficient or has to be transected, a transverse island tubular flap with a proximal and distal spatulated onlay of the same preputial skin (onlay-tube-onlay modification) is our procedure of choice.

Preputial Transverse Island Combined Onlay-Tube-Onlay Flap

This repair is our primary choice in penoscrotal/perineal hypospadias with a short deficient urethral plate in cases of severe proximal hypospadias (👁 Fig. 17.4). We believe that a spatulated onlay of the tubular flap minimises the risk of ischaemia and resultant stricturing at the anastomotic sites. The cosmetic result is more pleasing with a decreased rate of meatal stenosis and meatal regression noted distally at the neomeatus. We believe the spatulated anastomosis of the tubular flap in an onlay fashion maximises the blood supply of the flap at the most caudal and cranial locations and ultimately results in less stricturing and obstruction of urinary flow, hence less chance of fistula formation, than utilising just a tubular flap.

After degloving of the penile shaft, the chordee is repaired as indicated previously. Traction sutures are placed on the dorsal preputial edges after performing the degloving circumcision incision and correction of chordee (👁 Fig. 17.4a).

The stretched length of the urethral defect is then measured and the preputial flap is harvested. While harvesting the preputial skin flap, we loosely apply a compressive dressing around the shaft of the penis if any minor oozing is present. This flap is based on the vascular supply of the inner prepuce originating from the external pudendal artery. The blood supply to the flap is centrally positioned and proximally lies from the 11 to 1 o'clock location; distally, it fans out more laterally to the 2 to 10 o'clock position. To harvest the flap the dissection is first carried out parallel to the pedicle on the shaft skin side. If the dissection is in the right plane and superficial, no bleeding is encountered. A transversely oriented rectangle from the inner prepuce is allocated for the urethroplasty to cover the distance between the urethral opening and the tip of the glans. The width of the flap utilised is 15–20 mm, depending on the age of the child. The lateral edges of the flap are tapered proximally and distally prior to the anastomosis (👁 Fig. 17.4b). The middle portion of the inner prepuce is ultimately tubularised over a 10-F Silastic catheter using a 7-0 Vicryl subcuticular stitch after a spatulated anastomosis of the most proximal end of the preputial flap to the native urethra. The tubularised neourethra is created after completion of the anastomosis of the flap to the proximal end of the native urethra in an onlay fashion with interrupted 6-0 Vicryl (👁 Fig. 17.4c). The key here is to cut back the underdeveloped ventral urethral tissue of the native urethra to the point where one has an opening, albeit more proximal in location, that has a healthy wide urethral plate with well-formed urethral and spongiosal tissue circumferentially. In a similar fashion the most distal aspect of the tubularised flap remains spatulated and is sutured in an onlay fashion to create a neomeatus (👁 Fig. 17.4d). An interrupted 6-0 Vicryl suture is used to create a neomeatus in the glans. The neomeatus is placed at a position on the glans where the normal urethral landmarks are present. In some

180   Jyoti Upadhyay, Anthony Khoury

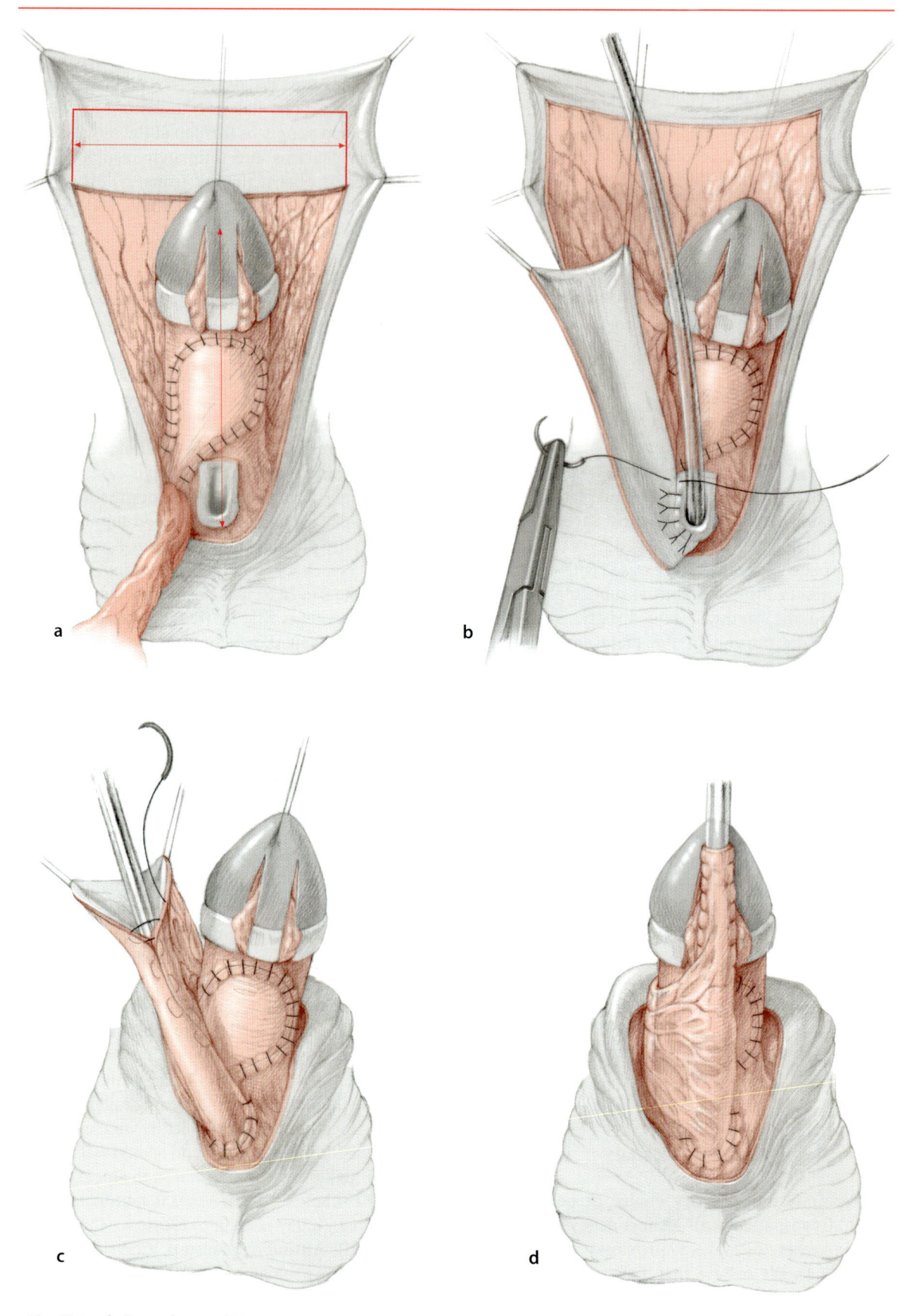

a

b

c

d

Fig. 17.4a–d. Legend see p. 181

superficially. We have stopped using deep reapproximating sutures, as we have not found them necessary to maintain glans approximation and configuration. We have found that a deep stitch at times serves as an iatrogenic point of narrowing. We believe the key factor in achieving a normal looking glans without obstruction is to have good dissection and mobilisation of the glans wings.

Often, cases of severe penoscrotal/perineal hypospadias are associated with a small, underdeveloped glans penis. This may make the placement of the neourethra in the anatomical position in the glans difficult. In such cases, a neourethra located at the coronal/subcoronal level may be the best result possible. If any further revision of the neourethra is needed it can be carried out with ease in the future. Often, these are the cases that may benefit from postoperative testosterone injections to improve the girth and vascularity of the penis and glans.

Skin Coverage

In cases of severe hypospadias, skin coverage can be challenging at times. Skin closure is performed using a 5-0 chromic suture. In cases with severely deficient ventral skin, we perform a modification of the double-onlay flap (Gonzalez et al. 1996; Rushton and Belman 1998). The prepuce is split into two adjacent portions horizontally leaving the common blood supply intact. The distal prepuce is utilised for creation of the neourethra while the proximal portion provides ventral skin coverage. The split preputial flap has the advantage of providing a skin island flap that covers the suture line of the urethroplasty (Fig. 17.5). The key technical point is superficial dissection of the prepuce to allow separate use of two portions without compromising the common blood supply.

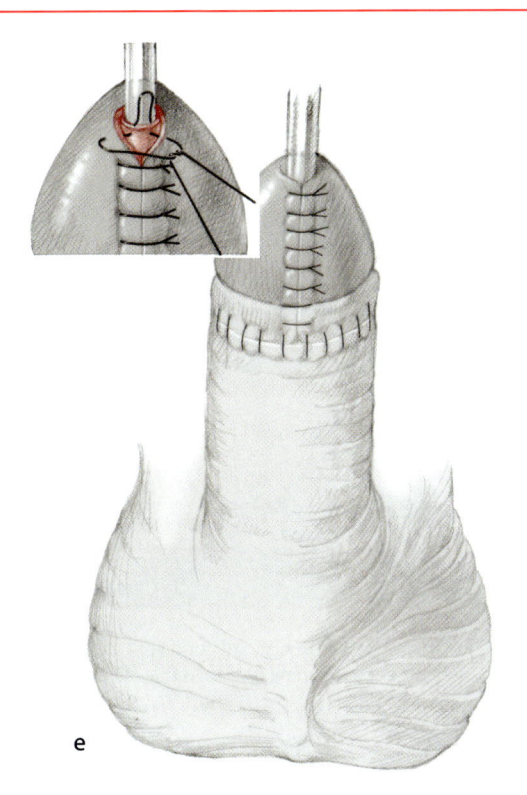

◀ **Fig. 17.4a–e.** Onlay-tube-onlay modification of the transverse island flap urethroplasty. **a** Outline of the dorsal preputial skin utilised to create the neourethra. Note the urethral defect with the proximal and distal segments of the urethral plate preserved. **b** Onlay repair of the refashioned preputial skin at the most proximal end to the native urethral opening. The lateral edges of the flap are tapered proximally and distally prior to the anastomosis. **c** Tubularisation of the middle portion of the inner prepuce over a 10-F Silastic catheter using a 7-0 Vicryl subcuticular stitch. **d** The most distal aspect of the tubularised flap remains spatulated and is sutured in an onlay fashion to create the neomeatus in the glans. **e** Superficial skin reapproximation of the glans completes the repair after using a second layer of spongiosal tissue over the urethroplasty if available. *Inset:* A 4-point stitch from the glans skin through the neourethra at the 6:00 o'clock position creating a slit-like opening of the meatus

cases, meatal advancement is performed. A dorsal vertical cut in the glans is performed to create a deep groove into which the neourethra can be positioned. This is not necessary in all cases and is referred to as a technique for dorsal advancement of the meatus. The neomeatus should have a circumference size of 10 F. Tissue provided by the spongioplasty is often available as a second layer of closure over the primary suture line. The glans is then reapproximated using 6-0 Vicryl sutures for superficial skin closure. ⊙ Figure 17.4e shows the four-point stitch from the glans skin through the neourethra at the 6 o'clock position, which creates a slit-like opening of the meatus. The glans wings are only reapproximated

Stents/Dressings

During the urethroplasty, the watertightness and calibre of the urethra can be evaluated by manual expression of urine from the bladder. If a reduced stream with spraying is noted, this manoeuvre provides an opportunity to remove any visually obstructive sutures. Also, it provides an opportunity to reinforce any areas of urinary leakage. If the urethral plate was not transected and an onlay flap has been performed for the urethroplasty, a urethral stent alone is placed for approximately 5 days. For an extensive onlay-tube-onlay repair with division of the plate, we routinely insert a suprapubic catheter to divert the

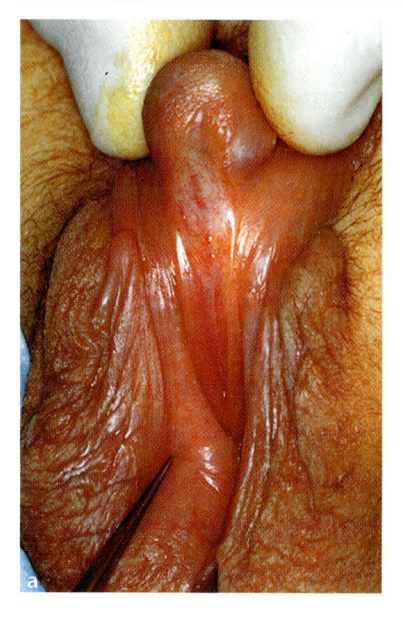

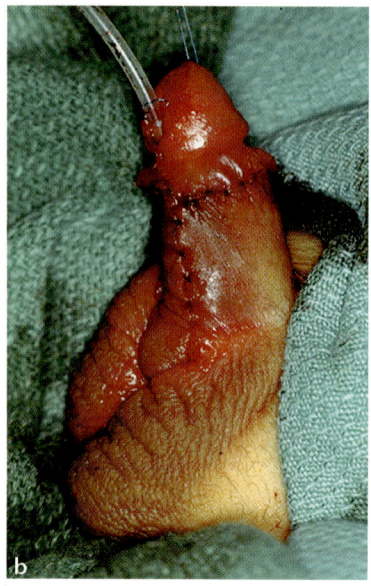

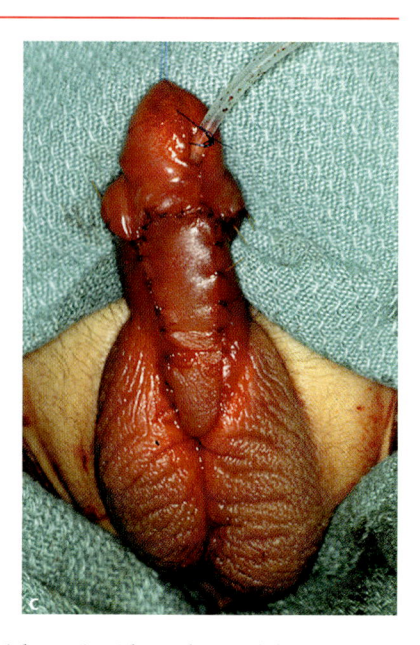

Fig. 17.5a–c. Double-faced split preputial onlay-tube-onlay repair. **a** Preoperative photo showing severe perineal hypospadias with chordee. **b** Postoperative lateral view of the repair showing a straight penis with good ventral skin coverage. **c** Postoperative frontal view of the double-faced flap

urine for 7–10 days in addition to placement of a Silastic urethral stent. The stent is removed 48 h before the suprapubic tube. We use an 8-F Silastic urethral stent with multiple side holes for all transverse island tube flap repairs. We utilise a double-diaper technique when a stent is used. The stent is left long enough to be placed outside the first diaper and placed into a second diaper to divert the urine while keeping the child's perineal skin dry. We place copious amounts of polysporin ointment over the entire perineal wound and utilise loosely placed compressive dressing circumferentially around the shaft of the penis at the completion of the operation.

Follow-up

The dressing, if used, is soaked off 24–48 h postoperatively by the parents. The dressing is soaked in mineral oil to dissolve any clots. We have found this loosens any adherent areas, and after several hours the bandage easily soaks off in the bath. The urethral stent is removed 7 days postoperatively, after which the suprapubic tube is clamped periodically for 1–2 days and removed once complete emptying is confirmed (usually in 10–12 days postoperatively). Sitz baths four times daily are utilised in the first week postoperatively. Polysporin topical ointment is applied judiciously for the next 2 weeks during the healing process. The child is seen in the outpatient clinic at 1 week to have the stent removed and then 6–8 weeks later urinary flow and postvoiding residual urine are assessed if the child is toilet trained. Follow-up is conducted six-monthly for the first year and annually thereafter, including evaluation of urinary flow as indicated. Poor flow in conjunction with symptoms such as straining to void, intermittency and a high postvoid residual are indicative of a urethral or meatal stricture. In these situations, voiding cystourethrography and/or retrograde urethrography may be employed and urethral dilation or cystoscopic examination may be required for precise anatomical evaluation prior to any repair.

Results

Various procedures have been reported for severe proximal hypospadias repair. Generally, pedicle flaps or free grafts have been utilised as onlays or tubes. Onlay urethroplasties have been associated with lower complication rates than tubularised repairs (Baskin et al. 1994; Hollowell et al. 1990). Excellent results using onlay urethroplasties have been reported in large series (Baskin et al. 1994; Elder et al. 1987; Gearhart and Borland 1992; Hollowell et al. 1990). In general, onlay procedures are believed to be associated with lower rates of long-term complications such as urethrocutaneous fistula and diverticulum formation than tubularised pedicle flaps and grafts

(Baskin et al. 1994; Gearhart and Borland 1992; Powell et al. 2000). Onlay repairs require less tissue dissection and are easier to perform. The preservation of the urethral plate is advantageous with improved vascularity of the repair. Baskin et al. (1994) reported on 65 out of 374 onlay repairs performed for proximal hypospadias. At a mean follow-up of over 2 years, the complication rate was 8.6% with an urethrocutaneous fistula rate of 6%.

Between 1995 and 2001, a total of 286 patients underwent a transverse island flap repair, of which 57 (20%) had ventral lengthening procedures for chordee correction and 23 (8%) had an onlay-tube-onlay modification for their urethroplasty. International patients with follow-up elsewhere and more recent cases without a minimum of 4 months' follow-up (altogether seven patients) were excluded from further analysis. Of the 16 preputial onlay-tube-onlay transverse island flap urethroplasties performed, 3 were performed using a split preputial double-faced modification for severely deficient ventral skin. The mean age at surgery was 25.4 months (range 11–52) and the mean follow-up was 24 months (range 6–69).

Associated genitourinary anomalies were found in 8 patients (50%) and included unilateral undescended testicle (3), bilateral undescended testicle (2), vesicoureteral reflux (1), Noonan's syndrome (45XO/46XY) with gonadal dysgenesis (1), and penoscrotal transposition (3). Karyotyping was performed in 70% of the patients, of whom 10 were 46XY (91%) and one was 45XO/46XY. Five patients with a penile size below the 10th percentile for age received preoperative testosterone injections.

Among these 16 patients, ventral lengthening procedures were performed in 11 (73%) and dorsal plication of the tunica albuginea in 4. In one patient, skin degloving, the spongioplasty and division of the urethral plate resulted in correction of the associated curvature. Postoperatively, a straight penis with maximal length of the corporal bodies was achieved in 15 of the 16 patients. One patient with residual curvature (ventral scarred tissue with skin tethering) had breakdown of the original repair and a meatus in midshaft location (Fig. 17.6).

We have satisfactory cosmetic results with the onlay-tube-onlay urethroplasty. A normal-looking penis has been achieved in 70% of cases after single-stage repair of both the chordee and urethral defect. A slit-like meatus in the glans has been achieved in 50% of cases and a coronal and subcoronal location in 4 and 3 patients, respectively.

Our complications include fistula formation in 2 cases (12.5%), urethral diverticulum in 1 (6%) and a urethral stricture in 1 (6%). Meatal stenosis occurred

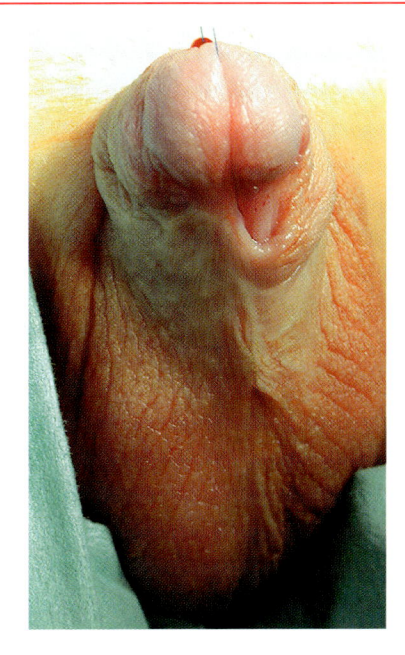

Fig. 17.6. Breakdown of the onlay-tube-onlay repair with residual chordee secondary to ventral skin tethering/scarring and a midshaft urethral opening

in no cases, while meatal regression occurred in one case secondary to distal breakdown of the repair. Redundant foreskin occurred postoperatively in one case, giving a "buried penis" which improved after postoperative utilisation of testosterone injections to promote erections and avoid skin adherence to the coronal sulcus.

Utilising the above single-stage approach, our overall secondary procedure rate was 31% (5/16). Fistula repair was performed in 2 cases utilising a local tubularisation of the vascular skin flap. Distal tubularisation of the flap was required in one case for postoperative breakdown of the urethroplasty with a resultant midshaft meatus (Fig. 17.7). Presently, this child has a well-formed coronal meatus. Cystoscopy with direct internal urethrotomy was performed in one patient for a distal urethral stricture. One patient suffered from ventral skin scarring secondary to devascularised ventral tissue, which required a revision of the transverse island flap. The defect in this child was greater than 5 cm and a double-faced flap was not used.

Acknowledgements ▶ Illustrations by Jason Sharpe, 296 Orioli Parkway, Toronto, Ontario, Canada M5P 2H5.

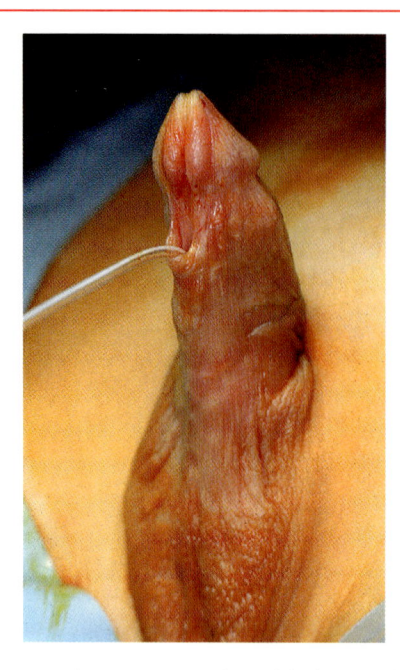

Fig. 17.7. Meatal regression with midshaft meatal opening after breakdown of distal repair. Photo depicts healthy adjacent tissue that can be used in the second operation

References

Asopa HS, Elhence IP, Atri SP, et al: One stage correction of penile hypospadias using a foreskin tube. A preliminary report. Int Surg. 1971; 55:435–440.
Baskin LS, Duckett JW: Dorsal tunica albuginea plication for hypospadias curvature. J Urol. 1994; 151:1668–1671.
Baskin LS, Duckett JW, Ueoka K, et al: Changing concepts of hypospadias curvature lead to more onlay island flap procedures. J Urol. 1994; 151:191–196.
Baskin LS, Erol A, Li YW, et al: Anatomy of the neurovascular bundle: is safe mobilization possible? J Urol. 2000; 164: 977–980.
Borer JG, Retik AB: Current trends in hypospadias repair. Urol Clin North Am. 1999; 26:15–37, vii.
Bracka A: Hypospadias repair: the two-stage alternative (see comments). Br J Urol. 1995; 76 [Suppl 3]:31–41.
Devine CJ Jr, Horton CE: Use of dermal graft to correct chordee. J Urol. 1975; 113:56–58.
Devine CJ Jr, Horton CE: Hypospadias repair. J Urol. 1977; 118:188–193.
Duckett JW, Baskin LS: Hypospadias. In: Gillenwater JY, Grayhack JT, Howards SS, Duckett JW (eds): Adult and pediatric urology, vol 3, 3rd edn.. Mosby, St Louis, pp 2549–2589; 1996.
Duckett JW Jr: Transverse preputial island flap technique for repair of severe hypospadias. Urol Clin North Am. 1980; 7:423–430.
Duckett JW: The island flap technique for hypospadias repair. Urol Clin North Am. 1981; 8:503–511.
Elder JS, Duckett JW, Snyder HM: Onlay island flap in the repair of mid and distal penile hypospadias without chordee. J Urol. 1987; 138:376–379.
Firlit CF: The mucosal collar in hypospadias surgery. J Urol. 1987; 137:80–82.
Frey P, Bianchi A: One-stage preputial pedicle flap repair for hypospadias: experience with 100 patients. Prog Pediatr Surg. 1989; 23:181–191.
Gearhart JP, Borland RN: Onlay island flap urethroplasty: variation on a theme. J Uro. 1992; 148:1507–1509.
Gittes RF, McLaughlin AP III: Injection technique to induce penile erection. Urology. 1974; 4:473–474.
Gonzalez R, Smith C, Denes ED: Double onlay preputial flap for proximal hypospadias repair. J Urol. 1996; 156: 832–834; discussion 834–835.
Greenfield SP, Sadler BT, Wan J: Two-stage repair for severe hypospadias. J Urol. 1994; 152:498–501.
Hafez AT, Smith CR, McLorie GA, et al: Tunica vaginalis for correcting penile chordee in a rabbit model: is there a difference in flap versus graft? J Urol. 2001; 166:1429–1432.
Hendren WH, Keating MA: Use of dermal graft and free urethral graft in penile reconstruction. J Urol. 1988; 140: 1265–1269
Hollowell JG, Keating MA, Snyder HM, et al: Preservation of the urethral plate in hypospadias repair: extended applications and further experience with the onlay island flap urethroplasty. J Urol. 1990; 143:98–100; discussion 100–101.
Horton CE, Devine CJ Jr, Barcat N: Pictorial history of hypospadias repair techniques. In: Horton CE (ed): Plastic and reconstructive surgery of the genital area. Little Brown, Boston, pp 237–248; 1973.
Kelalis PP, Benson RC Jr, Culp OS: Complications of single and multistage operations for hypospadias: a comparative review. J Urol. 1977; 118:657–658.
Khoury AE, Olson ME, McLorie GA, et al: Urethral replacement with tunica vaginalis: a pilot study. J Urol. 1989; 142:628–630; discussion 631.
King LR: Cutaneous chordee and its implications in hypospadias repair. Urol Clin North Am. 1981; 8:397–402.
Mollard P, Mouriquand P, Felfela T: Application of the onlay island flap urethroplasty to penile hypospadias with severe chordee. Br J Urol. 1991; 68:317–319.
Nesbit RM: Operation for correction of distal penile ventral curvature with or without hypospadias. J Urol. 1967; 97: 720–722.
Powell CR, McAleer I, Alagiri M, et al: Comparison of flaps versus grafts in proximal hypospadias surgery. J Urol. 2000; 163:1286–1288; discussion 1288–1289.
Retik AB, Bauer SB, Mandell J, et al: Management of severe hypospadias with a 2-stage repair. J Urol. 1994; 152:749–751.
Rober PE, Perlmutter AD, Reitelman C: Experience with 81, 1-stage hypospadias/chordee repairs with free graft urethroplasties. J Urol. 1990; 144:526–529; discussion 530.
Rushton HG, Belman AB: The split prepuce in situ onlay hypospadias repair. J Urol. 1998; 160:1134–1136; discussion 1137.
Sauvage P, Becmeur F, Geiss S, et al: Transverse mucosal preputial flap for repair of severe hypospadias and isolated chordee without hypospadias: a 350-case experience. J Pediatr Surg. 1993; 28:435–438.
Snodgrass W: Tubularized incised plate urethroplasty for distal hypospadias. J Urol. 1994; 151:464–465.
Snodgrass W, Koyle M, Manzoni G, et al: Tubularized incised plate hypospadias repair for proximal hypospadias (see comments). J Urol. 1998; 159:2129–2131.

Snodgrass WT: Tubularized incised plate hypospadias repair: indications, technique, and complications. Urology. 1999; 54:6–11.

Wacksman J: Use of the Hodgson XX (modified Asopa) procedure to correct hypospadias with chordee: surgical technique and results. J Urol. 1986; 136:1264–1265.

18

The Modified Asopa (Hodgson XX) Procedure to Repair Hypospadias with Chordee

Jeffrey Wacksman

Introduction

Midpenile and proximal penile hypospadias is usually associated with chordee that causes a ventral deflection of the penile shaft. The chordee may be superficial (skin and/or dartos tissue) or deep (dysplastic urethral remnants and corpus spongiosum). With cases of superficial chordee, this is usually corrected by dividing the skin and dartos tissue. In many cases, the urethral plate can be tubularized via the TIP procedure and/or onlay graft placed to repair this defect. When the chordee is more extreme, then the urethra itself will need to be constructed utilizing some type of skin, usually from the prepuce. In 1971, Asopa et al. reported on a transverse pedicle flap utilizing the underneath surface of the prepuce to replace the urethra. The major problem with this technique was penile torsion due to the transference of the entire preputial skin with the attached skin tube. Subsequent to this, Hodgson modified this approach by incising the preputial skin on a bias, leaving the newly constructed skin tube attached to the larger surface area of the incised preputial skin (👁 Fig. 18.1). This modification, termed the Hodgson XX technique, was related to me by the late Norm Hodgson as a personal communication. The technique usually has a lower fistula rate than the Duckett procedure (Duckett 1981) because the neourethra is left attached to the underneath surface of the preputial skin (Wacksman 1986). Torsion is not a problem as long as the preputial skin is totally dissected back to the penopubic angle. Because of this modification, I have been able to employ this procedure in over 250 patients with midpenile to penoscrotal hypospadias.

Operative Technique

After routine general anesthesia, the patient is moved to the foot of the operating room table and placed in a frog position. We employ the operating room microscope and usually sit to the side of the patient. A traction suture of 5-0 silk is placed through the glans, and a vessel loop is placed at the base of the penis to act as a tourniquet. An incision is made in either transverse or vertical fashion in the dysplastic urethral plate. The dysplastic tissue is resected (👁 Fig. 18.1a, b) and an artificial erection is accomplished (👁 Fig. 18.1c). If the penis is straight, then no further chordee resection is necessary. If all of the chordee tissue has been resected, but there still exists some remaining chordee, then the dissection is continued onto the dorsum of the penis. The preputial skin is dissected back to the penopubic angle. The broad-based dorsal neurovascular bundle is dissected free, and a modified Nesbit procedure is accomplished to completely straighten the phallus. I prefer two vertical incisions in Buck's fascia closed transversely with either 5-0 or 6-0 Maxon suture. There are other procedures available, but I do feel one has to incise Buck's fascia to the corporal tissue as opposed to just plicating the tunica albuginea.

Having straightened out the penis, the underneath surface of the foreskin is tented out with traction suture of 6-0 chromic. For the neourethra, we usually construct this over an 8-F Silastic stent. The underneath surface of the foreskin is cut and rolled loosely over this urethral stent. I usually mark out the suture line with several interrupted 6-0 chromic sutures followed by a running interlocking 7-0 Maxon suture. At either end of the neourethra, interrupted sutures should be placed to allow for trimming of the suture line when the neourethra is completed (👁 Fig. 18.1d). Next, I usually dissect the neourethra for a short distance from the preputial skin but leave the neourethra well attached to this underneath surface of the foreskin. Therefore, the skin and neourethra will share a common blood supply, which is totally different from the Duckett island pedicle flap procedure. Next, the preputial skin is cut on a bias. Usually, the preputial skin on the right side is large and contains the neourethra (👁 Fig. 18.1e). This is then rotated to the ventral aspect of the penis. The proximal end of the neourethra is sutured to the distal end of the proximal urethra with 7–0 Maxon over an 8-F Silastic stent. I

188 Jeffrey Wacksman

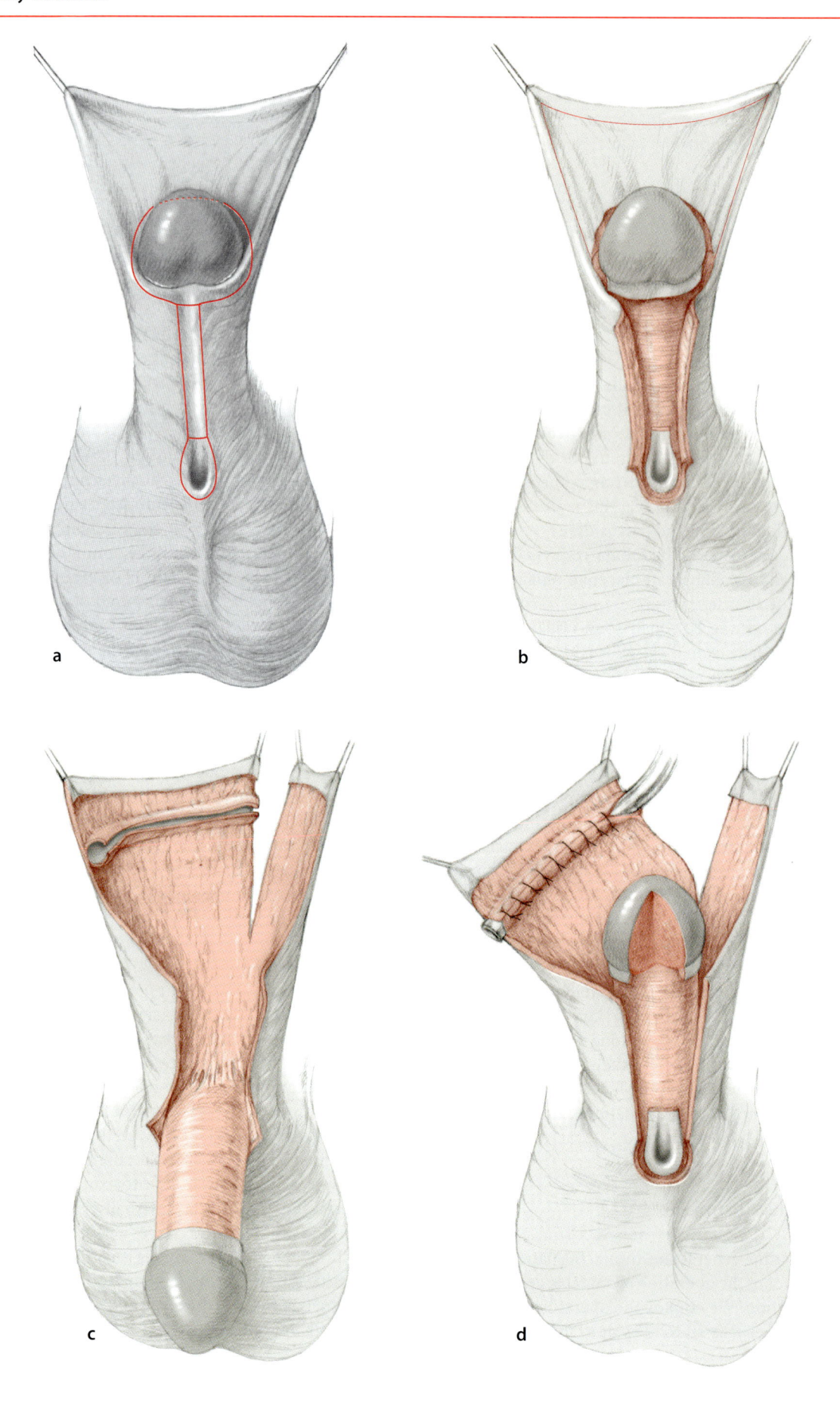

a

b

c

d

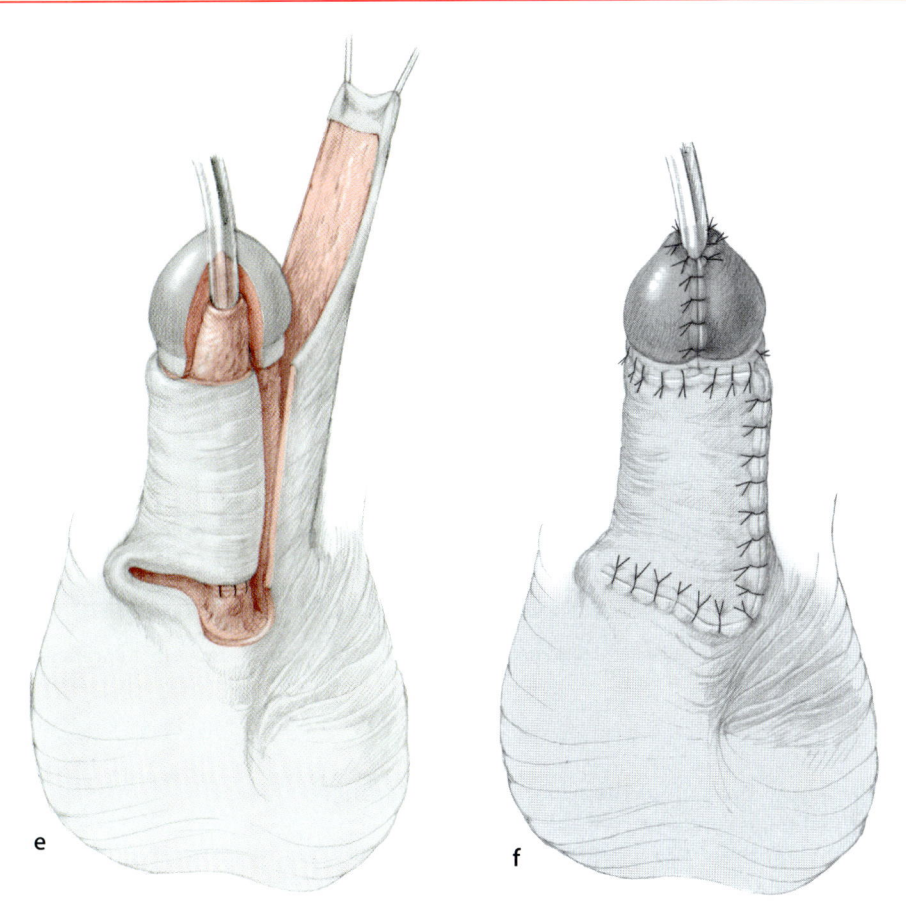

Fig. 18.1. a–c Diagram outlining chordee release and outline of neourethra from underneath surface of foreskin. **d–f** Neourethra created and rotated onto ventral surface covered with foreskin

usually spatulate the proximal urethra to assure a wide-open anastomosis. I will also remove any devascularized skin of the proximal urethra before completing the anastomosis (Fig. 18.1f).

After completing the anastomosis, we direct our attention to the glans. The glans is split in the midline and two large flaps are created. The neourethra is laid in the glanular bed, and the glans flaps are brought around the neourethra and sutured in place with two layers: an inner layer of 6-0 or 7-0 Maxon and an outer layer of 6-0 chromic. The neourethra is sutured to the glans with interrupted 6-0 chromic. The proximal anastomosis is inspected, and a second layer of tissue is brought over the urethral anastomosis. The ventral surface is covered with preputial skin, but the left side, which is the thinner side, is brought around and sutured in the midline on the ventral aspect of the penis. This will prevent any penile torsion. The ventral skin flaps are closed with a running 6-0 chromic catgut suture (Fig. 18.2a). For dressing we usually employ a single layer of Tegaderm, which will stay in place from 1 to 5 days. The urethral stent is left indwelling in the bladder to drain for 10–14 days. The patient is placed on full-strength trimethoprim sulfamethoxazole antibiotics while the stent is in place.

Conclusion

My results in over 250 cases over the past 15 years show a fairly low complication rate (Fig. 18.2b). We have had a fistula rate of around 8%, but not all patients have had follow-up for a long enough time. Occasionally, a patient may return 10 years after surgery with a small pinpoint fistula. No patient has developed a urethral stricture at the site of the anastomosis, but one patient did develop balanitis xerotica obliterans 10 years after a successful repair. Meatal stenosis has not been a problem, but we have repaired three significant urethral diverticula. Although penile swelling may initially be a concern 6 months to 1 year after surgery, this problem has usually resolved. Penile torsion has not been a problem as long as the steps described above are followed. One late complication has been either an occasional urinary infection or urinary dribbling. It appears that urinary infection

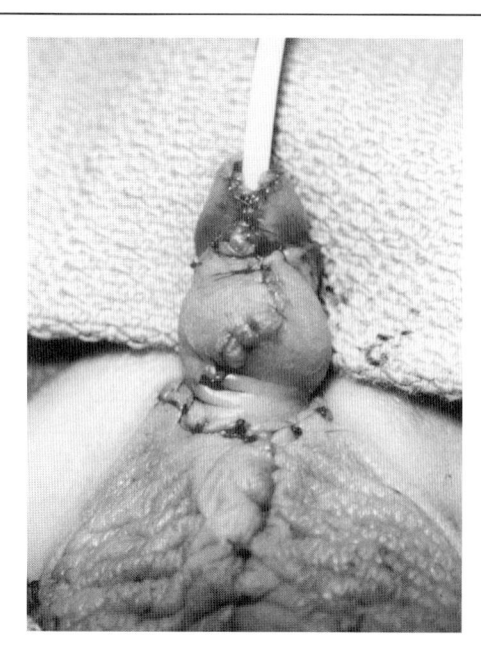

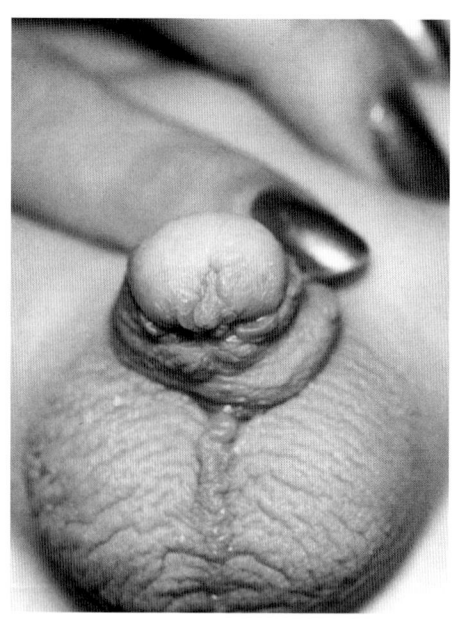

Fig. 18.2. a Completed repair with penoscrotal transposition repaired as a single stage. **b** Appearance 6 months after operation

is due to colonization of the skin of the neourethra while the urinary dribbling is related to urine collection in the neourethra. For this, I have recommended that patients concentrate on stripping the urethra following voiding. This usually solves the problem. Overall, the vast majority of patients have done quite well, and I still employ this procedure in the properly selected patient.

References

Asopa HS, Elhence EP, Atria SP, et al: One-stage correction of penile hypospadias using a foreskin tube. Int Surg. 1971; 55:435.

Duckett JW: The island flap technique for hypospadias repair. Urol Clin North Am. 1981; 8:503.

Wacksman J: Use of the Hodgson XX (modified Asopa) procedure to correct hypospadias with chordee: surgical technique and results. J Urol. 1986; 136:1264.

Koyanagi–Nonomura One-Stage Repair for Severe Perineal Hypospadias

Tomohiko Koyanagi, Katsuya Nonomura, Hidehiro Kakizaki, Masashi Murakumo, Takashi Shibata

Introduction

Considerable difficulties of various kinds accompany the surgical management of severe perineal hypospadias. Whether the case is hypospadias of the severest form or phenotypic expression of a more complicated underlying intersexuality must be verified diagnostically. To name a few characteristic features, hypospadias is exemplified by intrinsically deficient skin, a long neourethra must be constructed from the perineum to the glans, and it is associated with propenile scrotal transposition. Subsequently very few have dared to perform repair in one stage, although sporadic reports of the use of a free flap (Devine) or vascularized pedicled island skin flap (Duckett) technique are available (Ehrlich and Scardino 1982). Early in the 1980s some experts considered staged repair preferable in this group of children (Hodgson 1984; King 1984). Later Woodard and Parrott (1991) developed a one-stage repair combining the vagaries of urethroplasty. From their experience they concluded that although these patients are amenable to a one-stage procedure at an early age with a high degree of success, over one third will require a secondary procedure for complete correction of the anomaly, rendering one-stage repair a challenging issue in this particular group. Over the past several years we have addressed the issue first by reporting the technique (Koyanagi et al. 1984), then by refining and expanding our experience (Koyanagi et al. 1988, 1993), as well as by confirming the viability of a parameatal-based foreskin flap (Nonomura et al. 1992), which has been consistently used in our one-stage repair regardless of its severity (Koyanagi et al. 1994). The following is a detailed description of our technique, which has been bestowed with the eponym Koyanagi–Nonomura one stage repair (Glassberg et al. 1998).

Operative Technique

Step 1: Outlining the Skin Incision and Dartos Mobilization

A traction suture is placed on the glans and on each side of the dorsal foreskin. The meatus is dilated with the tip of a fine curved mosquito clamp, or ventral meatotomy is done in the usual fashion, wide enough to accommodate a 6-F urethral silicone catheter (Cliny Create Medic, Japan). Using gentian violet the skin is marked before incision. The incision encircles proximal to the meatus, runs laterally on both sides along the medial edge of the scrotal raphe, which by virtue of the bifid state is adherent to the lateral aspect of the penile shaft, and dorsally along the sulcus coronalis over the foreskin until it meets with its counterpart at 12 o'clock on the dorsum of the penis. Lateral parameatal skin marking should be wide, as this is to form a base for the parameatal foreskin flap, but must stay medial to the scrotal raphe so that the scrotal skin is not included or incorporated in the flap. Similarly, circumcoronal outlining of the dorsal foreskin should be away from the sulcus so that enough preputial foreskin is included, as this is where the parameatal-based pedicle foreskin flap is harvested in an extended form for eventual urethroplasty (Figs. 19.1a, 19.2a).

With fine curved iris scissors a sharp incision is made along the full circumference of the previously defined skin marking. While the glans and shaft are held under a fine dressing gauze, countertraction is applied to the dorsal foreskin by holding the traction stitches, and the skin proximal to the incision is mobilized by cutting sharply in the plane between the dartos and Buck's fascia. This dartos mobilization of the skin should be extensive enough in both the dorsal and ventral aspects of the penis so that when it is completed the penile shaft is completely degloved, being freed from the penile foreskin and lateroventrally adherent bivalved scrotum. During the mobilization of the bivalved scrotum one can often appre-

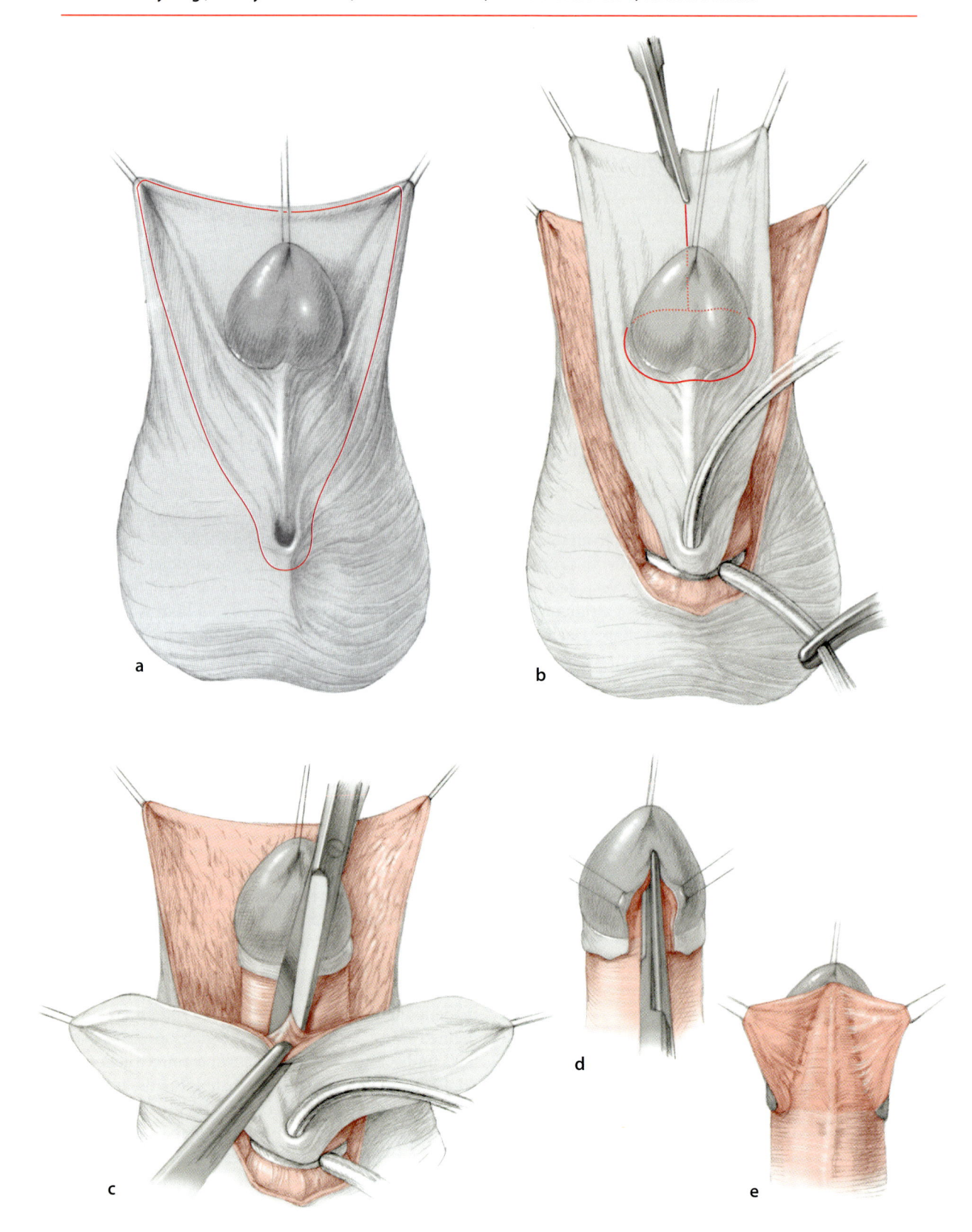

Fig. 19.1a–k. Schematic drawings of the operative technique. The *solid lines* outline the incisions (**a, d, e**). For explanation please refer to the text. **f–k** see p. 193

f g h

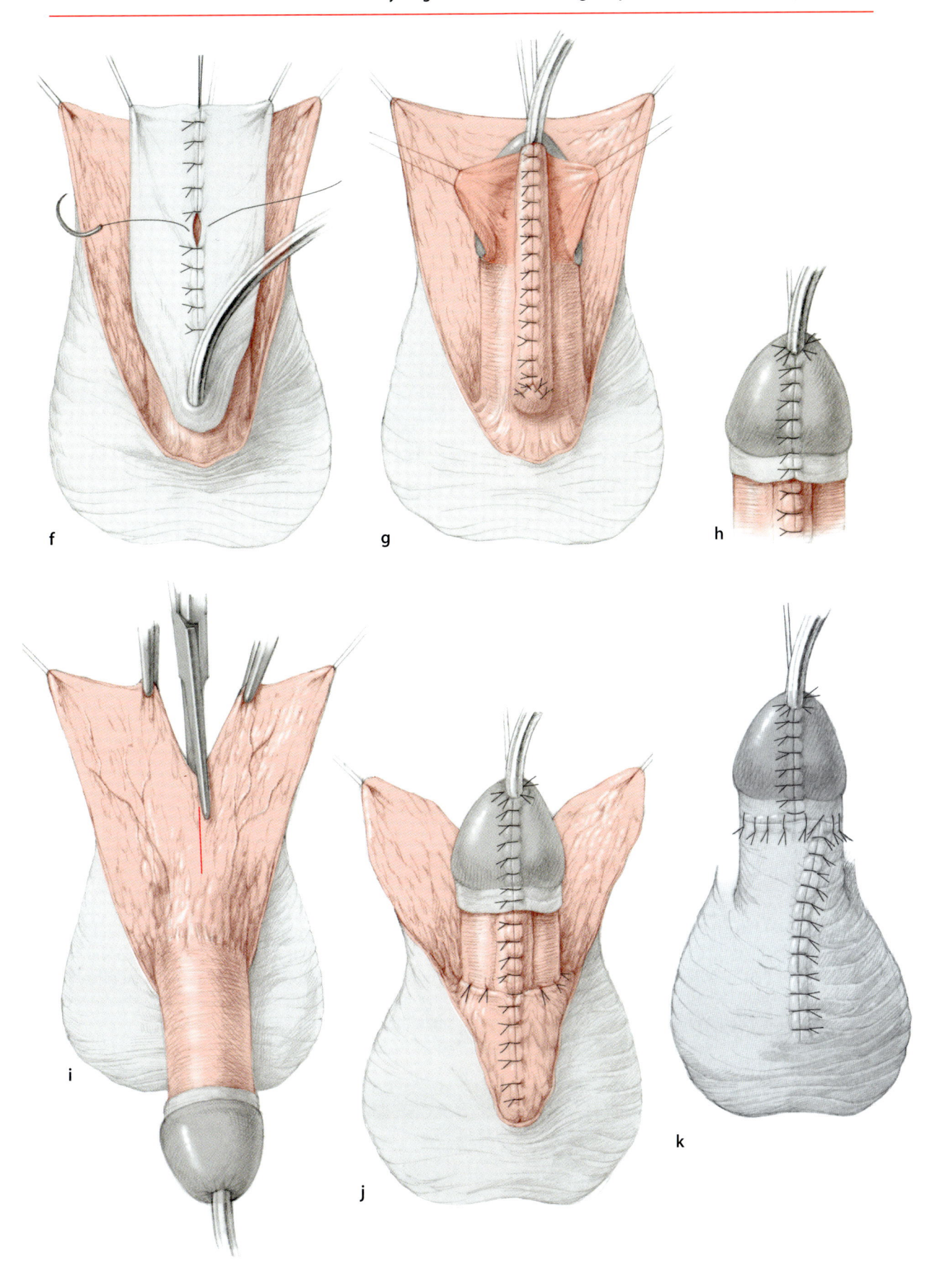

i j k

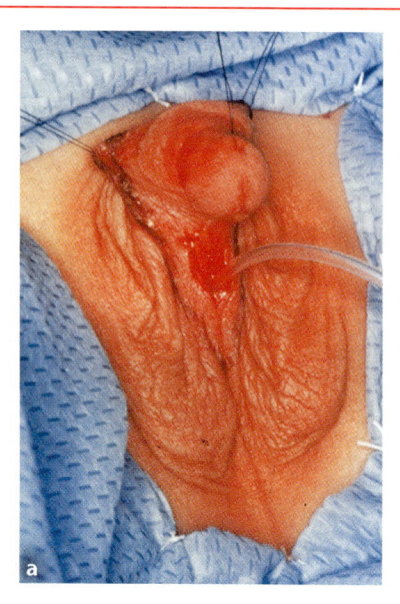

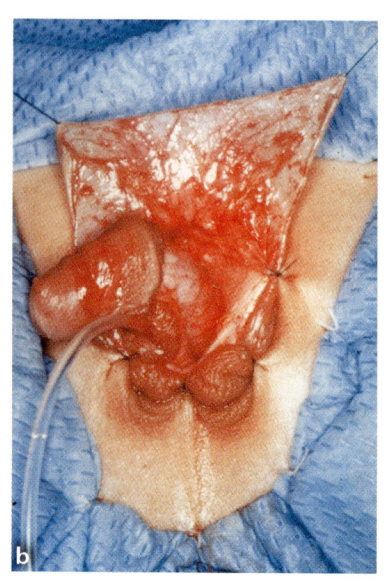

Fig. 19.2. a Outline of the skin incision. **b** Penile shaft with parameatal foreskin is degloved of phallic foreskin and bivalved scrotum after dartos mobilization

ciate that the perineal bulbocavernous muscle is also splayed out laterally in this severe hypospadias. Although the procedure is extensive, in the right plane bleeding is minimal as all the blood vessels in the skin run axially. Thus, when brisk bleeding is encountered the dissection is too deep in either the skin or the corporal body itself and must be corrected in due course. At the end of this extensive dartos mobilization the penile shaft, which was buried ventrally behind the dorsally displaced scrotum, is now fully exposed and degloved of the skin except for the distally attached foreskin. The mobilized skin is gently protected under moistened gauze until needed later (Figs. 19.1b, 19.2b).

Step 2: Chordectomy and Creation of Parameatal Foreskin Flap

Unlike distal hypospadias, dartos mobilization alone is not sufficient to restore ventriflexion of the penis, which is easily confirmed by artificial erection (Figs. 19.1c, 19.3a). In proximal hypospadias, a hypospadiac urethra distal to the meatus is literally atretic and fibrotic, adhering tightly to the ventral aspect of the penile corpora, resulting in its ventriflexion or chordee deformity (Koyanagi et al. 1983). The atretic urethra must be sharply excised, freed, and mobilized proximally enough to encounter a dorsum of intact spongy urethra. Before proceeding to this classic chordectomy by excising buried tissue (Hodgson 1984), however, another marking for the flaps for urethroplasty is made on the distal foreskin which was intentionally left attached to the distal shaft during dartos mobilization. This starts from the dorsal midline at 12 o'clock, securing enough width, and then runs circumcoronally along the sulcus on both sides of the glans until it meets in the ventral midline at 6 o'clock subfrenulum by crossing the atretic urethral plate.

Again using fine iris scissors, a flap is harvested on both sides by cutting along the proposed skin marking (Fig. 19.3b), transecting the urethral plate (Fig. 19.3c), then mobilizing the urethra while the flaps are gently protected under the moistened gauze (Fig. 19.3d). This essentially combines the classic chordee release with harvesting of parameatal-based foreskin flaps. When the urethra is mobilized sufficiently chordee is usually eliminated, which can be confirmed by another artificial erection (Fig. 19.3e). Occasionally a fibrous tissue in the intercorporal septum must be excised, and very rarely dorsal plication over the neurovascular bundle is necessary to complete the chordectomy (Nesbit 1965).

Step 3: Bisecting the Glans and Creation of Glanular Wings

The glans is bisected in the midline over the meatal pit (Barcat 1973) (Figs. 19.1d, 19.4a) and the glanular cap is lateralized on both sides by freeing it from the corporal shaft (Fig. 19.4b). By virtue of the embryologically separate origin of the corporal body, ure-

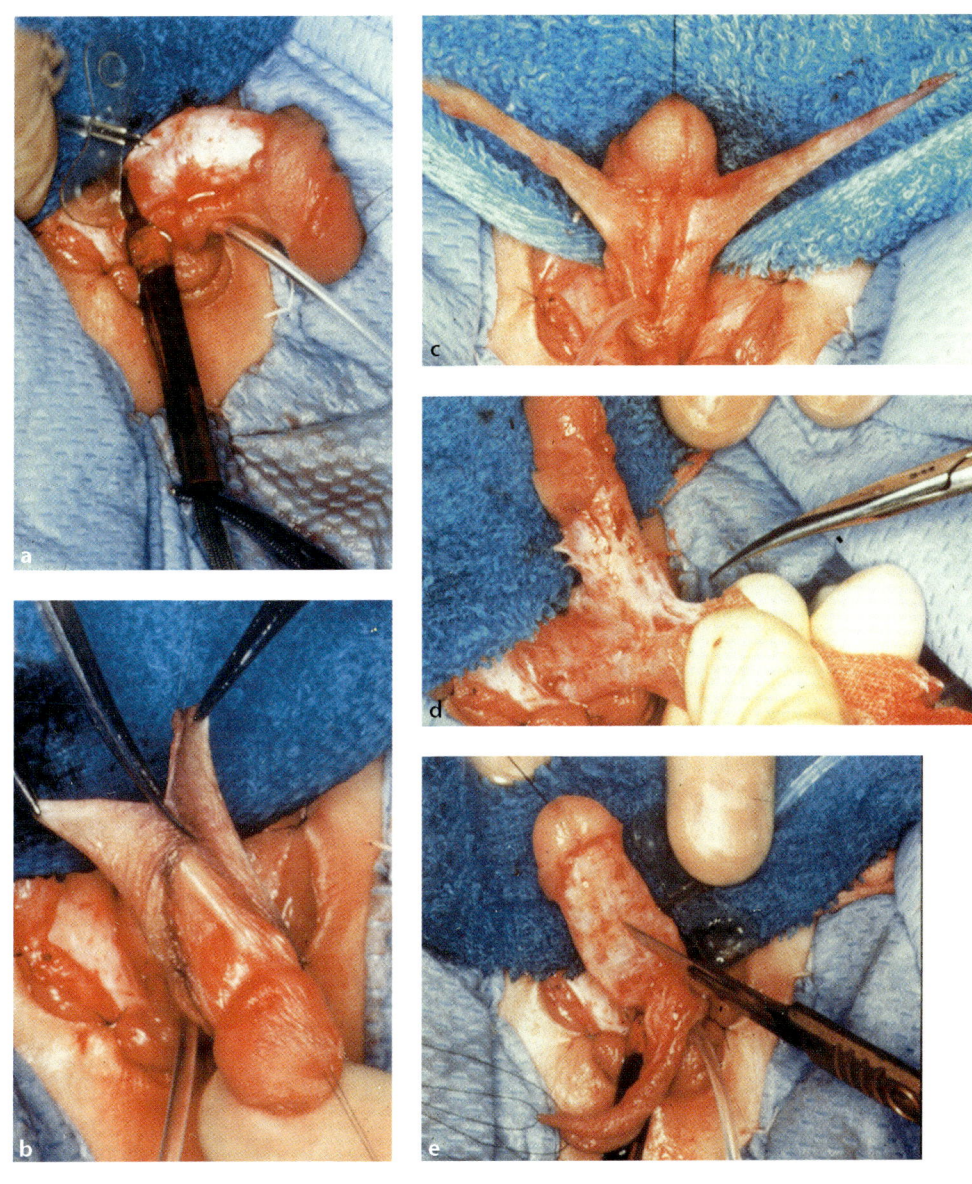

Fig. 19.3. a On artificial erection, ventriflexion of the phallus (chordee deformity) still remains. **b** Parameatal foreskin flap is harvested, by first cutting in the midline at 12 o'clock. **c** Then the incision is continued circumcoronally down to the frenulum where the hypospadiac urethra is transected. **d** The urethra with the parameatal foreskin flap is sharply detached from the ventral aspect of the of corpora as in classic chordectomy. **e** Remnant chordee tissue in the ventral septum is incised while the shaft is held in artificial erection

thral plate and glanular cap (Altemus and Hatchins 1991), this creation of glanular wings, if done in the right plane, is usually accomplished bloodlessly without the aid of a tourniquet (Redman 1987) or epinephrine injection. Lateralization of the glanular wings should be wide enough to accommodate and enroll the neourethra snugly (Figs. 19.1e, 19.4c).

Step 4: One-Stage Urethroplasty with Parameatal Foreskin Flaps (Koyanagi et al. 1987, 1994)

Parameatal based foreskin flaps are brought to the ventral aspect of the penile shaft (Fig. 19.5a) and fashioned into the neourethra, by approximating first the medial edges (Figs. 19.1f, 19.5b) and then the lateral edges (Figs. 19.1g, 19.5c) over the inlying urethral catheter. The stitches are all interrupted sutures with 7-0 polydioxanone). Free movement of the urethral catheter must be assured by occasionally

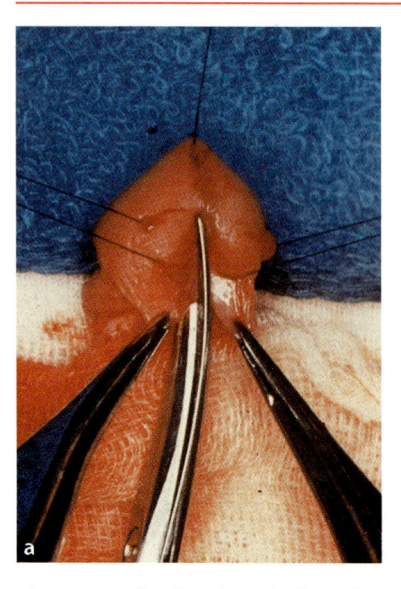

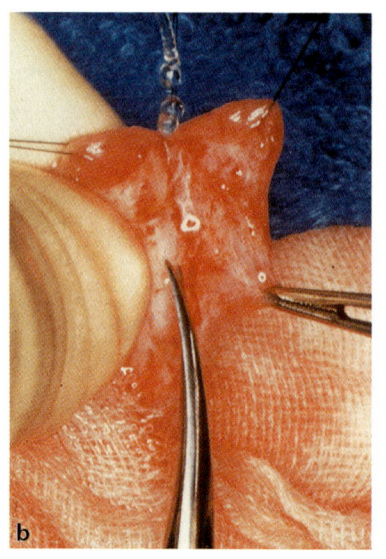

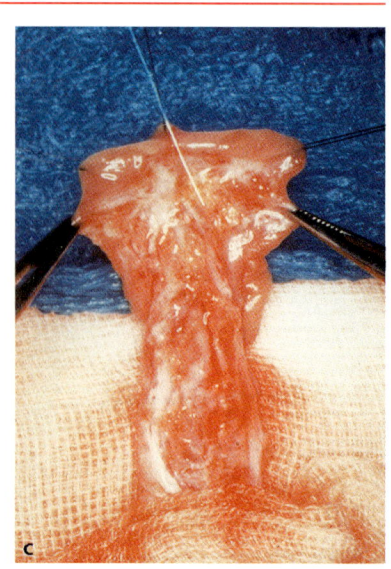

Fig. 19.4. a The glans is cut in the midline along the meatal pit all the way to the most distal edge of the glans. **b** A left glanular wing is created. Saline irrigation of the wound facilitates dissection by identifying the correct plane between the corpora and the glanular substance. **c** The glanular wings are lateralized on both sides wide enough to accommodate the formation of the neourethra

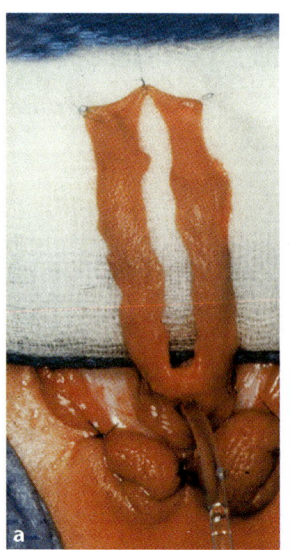

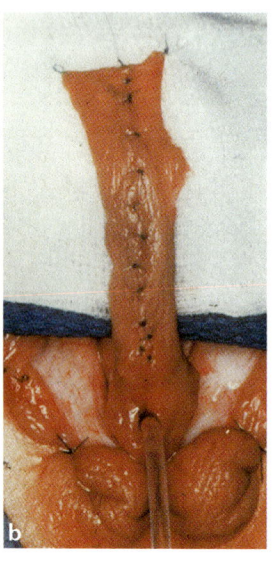

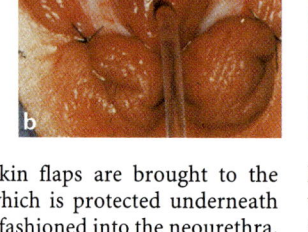

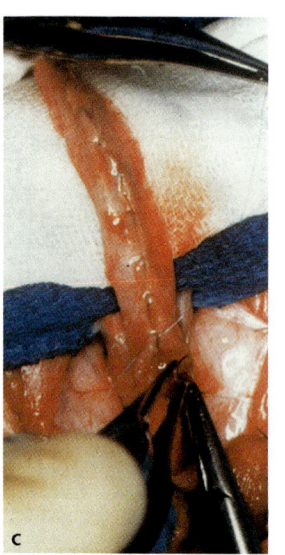

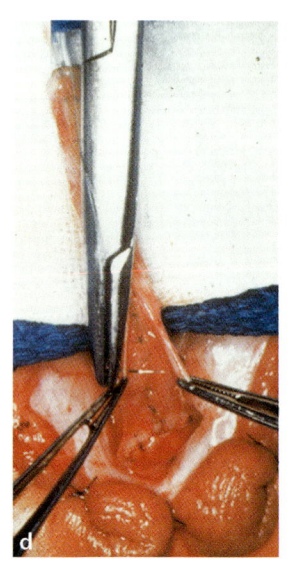

Fig. 19.5. a Parameatal foreskin flaps are brought to the ventral aspect of the shaft (which is protected underneath moistened gauze), ready to be fashioned into the neourethra. **b** The medial edges of the flaps are approximated. **c** The lateral edges over the inlying urethral catheter, all stitched with interrupted 7-0 polydioxanone, are sutured to complete the first row of the urethroplasty. **d** The neourethra is reinforced with second-layer closure

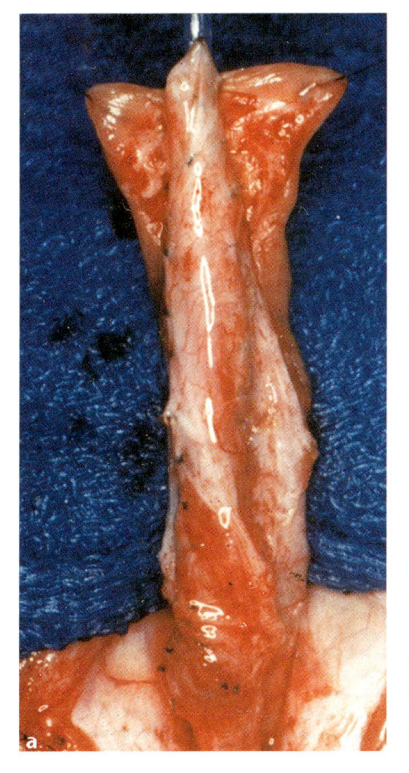

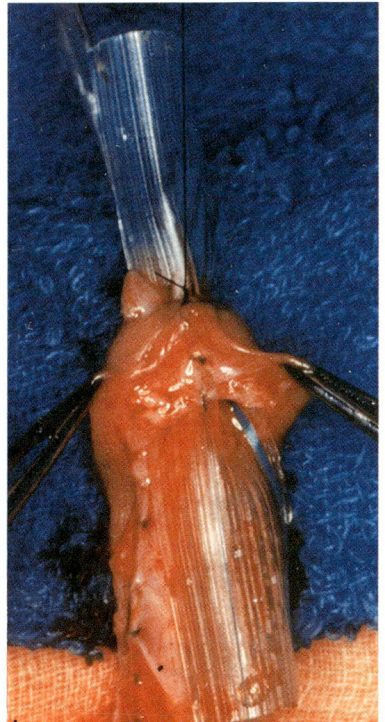

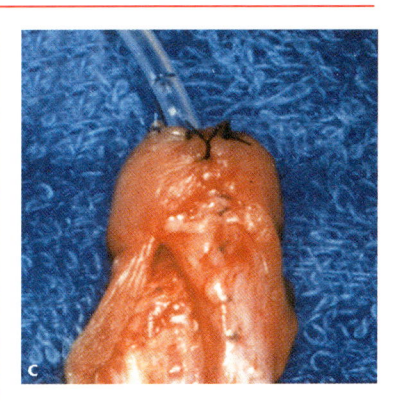

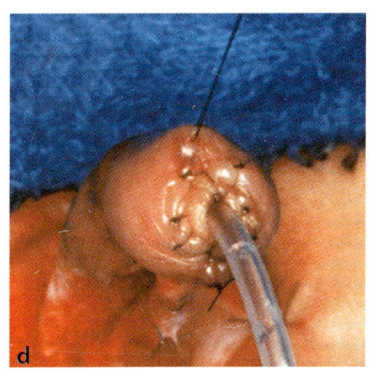

Fig. 19.6. a The neourethra is anchored to the tip of the bivalved glans. **b** The glans wings are approximated midline over the neourethra, which is temporarily protected underneath the Penrose tube. Note that subcutaneous glanular substance is approximated at the frenulum to secure two-layer closure of this portion. **c** Appearance of the glans at the end of glanulomeatoplasty. **d** Note the semicuffed appearance of the neomeatus

sliding it up and down during the fashioning of the urethra. Two-layer closure by approximating loose subcutaneous tissue of the flaps (Fig. 19.5d) secures its watertightness, which should be confirmed by saline flushing of the neourethra. While closing the proximal portion of the neourethra, the laterally splayed out bulbocavernous muscle is also brought to midline, which restores normal perineal muscular anatomy as well as reinforcing the two-layered urethral closure. Inadvertent "bite" of axially running blood vessels in the flaps should be avoided. Several reinforcing stitches may be added as needed.

Step 5: Glanulomeatoplasty

The distal end of the neourethra is anchored to the tip of the bisected glans (Figs. 19.1h, 19.6a), and then the glanular wings are approximated in the midline over the neourethra while it is held somewhat taut at 6 o'clock with a traction stitch. Temporary placement of a small Penrose drainage tube over the neourethra facilitates glans approximation without undue bite of the urethra (Fig. 19.6b). As a consequence of adequate lateralization of the glanular wings this glanuloplasty is done without any tension, which is confirmed by free movement of the Penrose tube. Usually two rows of vertical mattress sutures of 6-0 PDS are all that is necessary for glanuloplasty.

After enrollment of the neourethra with glanuloplasty and removal of the Penrose tube, the somewhat protruding ventral edge of the neourethra is flipped down so that it can be stitched to the glanular edge in a semicuffed fashion, thus completing the meatoplasty (Fig. 19.6c, d). Again, free movement of the inlying urethral catheter is to be confirmed.

Step 6: Byarsization of the Dorsal Foreskin and Its Subcutaneous Tissue for Skin Closure

The moistened gauze dressing protecting the dorsal penile foreskin is removed. Before byarsization of this flap for wound closure, another mark is added with gentian violet. On the dorsal cutaneous side, an ordinary distal half-length of the flap is satisfactory (Figs. 19.1i, 19.7a). The subcutaneous portion of the flap, however, should extend proximally deep

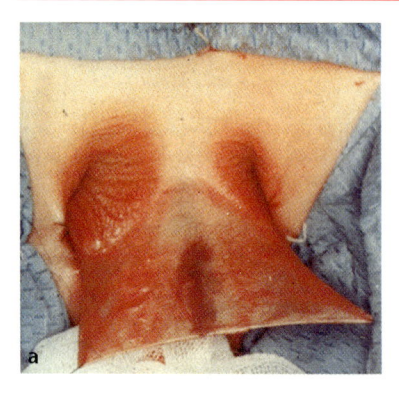

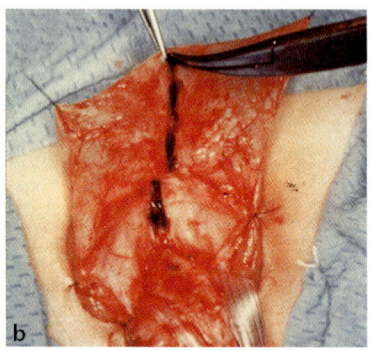

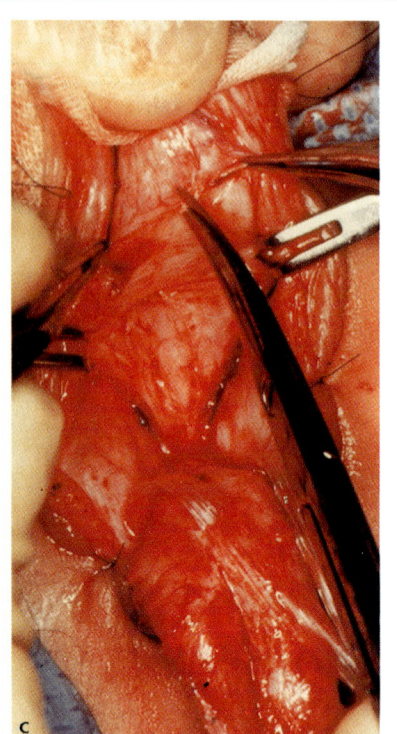

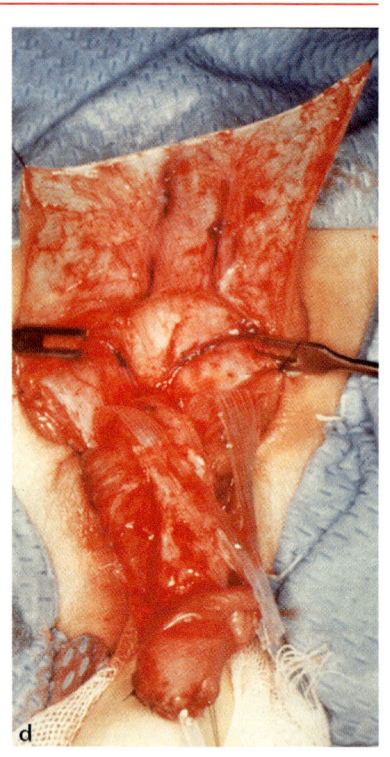

Fig. 19.7. a Dorsum of the foreskin before byarsization along the marked line. The dorsally displaced appearance of the scrotum is better appreciated. b Marking of the dorsal subcutaneous layer for byarsization. c The subcutaneous tissue is incised deep and lateralized wide to ensure snug rolling of the shaft at the ventral midline. d Note the relevance for byarsization of not only the subcutaneous tissue of the foreskin but also the dorsally displaced scrotal septum

enough to include the subcutaneous layer of the dorsally displaced scrotal tissue (Fig. 19.7b). By cutting along the proposed outline, the foreskin flap is bivalved and the proximal subcutaneous layer is lateralized judiciously so that the subcutaneous trough thus created is wide enough to enroll the penile shaft with no tension at later skin closure (Fig. 19.7c,d). Needless to say, care should be taken not to injure the axially running branches of the superficial dorsal arterial system during this byarsization.

Step 7: Skin Closure

A Penrose tube is left in the subcutaneous space as a drain and brought out through a separate incision in the perineum. The wound is closed in multiple layers. With the penis held in dorsiflexion, the subcutaneous tissue is approximated ventrally over the penile shaft proximally to distally. The most proximal part of the subcutaneous layer is not the penile foreskin but rather the dorsally displaced scrotal skin (Figs. 19.1j, 19.8a). Thanks to adequate dartos mobilization of the scrotal skin (step 1) and judicious byarsization, this subcutaneous closure is done without any tension. In so doing, the dorsally displaced scrotum is now replaced to a more natural ventriposition. Closure should be symmetrical and avoid inadvertent bite of the shaft so that it will not cause any torsion of the shaft or restrict its free movement on erection (Fig. 19.8b).

The coverage of the distal shaft is done similarly, proximally to distally in multiple layers (usually three to four) with byarsized foreskin flaps (Fig. 19.8c). The ventrally repositioned subcutaneous layer of the distal foreskin is then stitched to the subcutaneous tissue of the glans underneath the frenulum, thus securing the coverage of this portion of the urethra, which is potentially the most likely site of fistula formation (Fig. 19.8d). Once multilayered subcutaneous closure is completed, the skin edges are approximated loosely to avoid edema of the foreskin, thus concluding skin closure (Figs. 19.1k, 19.8e).

The traction suture on the tip of the glans is tied around the inlying urethral catheter, thus securing its position during the postoperative period. A fluffy compression dressing is applied to the wound, and the penis is held in dorsiflexion under the compression coverage. An antibacterial ointment is applied

Fig. 19.8. a The subcutaneous tissue of the dorsally displaced scrotal septum is repositioned ventrally while the proximal half of the wound is being closed. **b** Several layers of reinforcing subcutaneous sutures closing the scrotum are added. **c** Similar multilayer closure of the subcutaneous tissue of the foreskin flap is carried out. **d** The distal edge of the foreskin flap is stitched to the subcutaneous tissue of the glanular substance. **e** One-stage urethroplasty with simultaneous correction of a bifid scrotum is completed

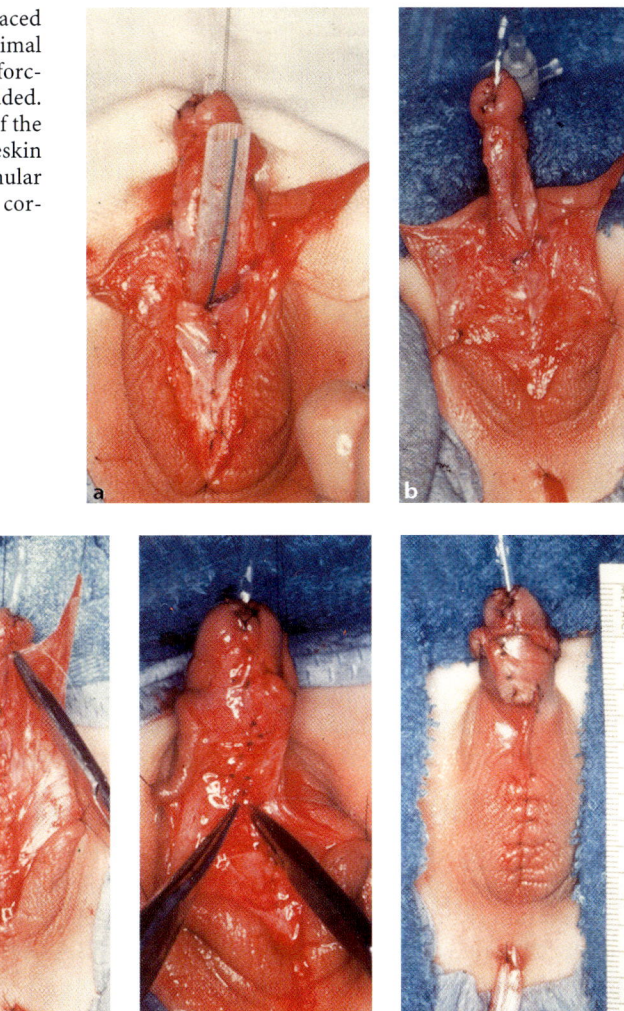

over the glans and around the meatus to prevent surface drying before the child is woken.

Postoperative Care

The Penrose drain is removed on the 1st or 2nd postoperative day. The compression coverage is released on the 4th or 5th postoperative day, and the child takes a warm sitz bath two or three times a day during hospitalization. Similarly, meatal flushing with a jet stream of normal saline should be continued to prevent crust formation around the meatus (Redman 1983; Parsons and Abercrombie 1982). The inlying urethral catheter, which should be checked daily for patency, is to be removed on the 10th to 14th postoperative day. No attempt should be made to manipulate the urethra with a catheter or a sound once the inlying catheter has been taken out.

Results

In 1995 we reported 10 years' experience based on 70 patients subjected to this technique (Koyanagi et al. 1995). Their ages ranged from 2 to 12 years (mean of 3.7 years). Primary success was obtained in 53% (37/70). Complications requiring secondary repair occurred in 33 cases: these comprised meatal stricture requiring meatal recession or glanular dehiscence with meatal recession in 12, urethrocutaneous fistula in 15 and urethral stricture in 6 cases. The patients concerned were subjected to secondary procedures such as extension urethroplasty or fistula closure, with a satisfactory result in over 90% of cases. Thus the overall success rate with this technique was 87% (61/70). This general trend has been the same over the subsequent years. The final outcome was satisfactory both cosmetically and functionally (Fig. 19.9).

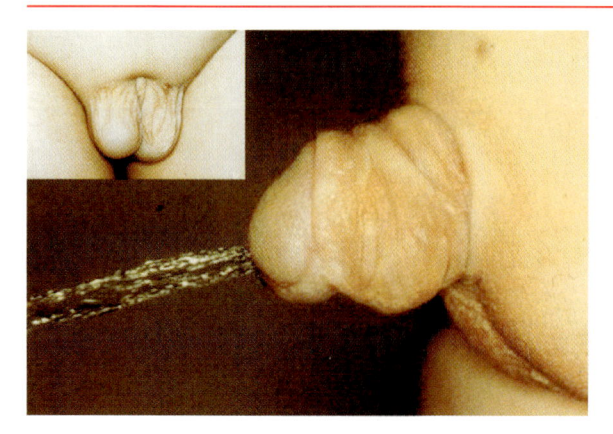

Fig. 19.9. An example of the postoperative result. *Inset:* preoperative appearance showing the distinct propenile scrotal transposition often associated with this severe perineal hypospadias

Comments

One-stage repair, which is currently considered standard in the majority of cases of distal hypospadias with or without chordee, is still a challenging issue in more severe perineal hypospadias with various degrees of scrotal transposition. We have been performing one-stage repair ever since we first reported a prototype method for this severe hypospadias with bifid scrotum (Koyanagi et al. 1984). Our method of one-stage repair, which has similarities with Russell's method (Russell 1900), has evolved since then. The refined form reported here is distinct in several aspects. First, dartos mobilization of the penile foreskin and scrotum is extensive for eventual simultaneous correction of scrotal transposition with skin closure. Second, by virtue of the natural continuity with spongy urethra, the parameatal foreskin flap maintains satisfactory microcirculatory parameters (Nonomura et al. 1992). When blood flow measured on laser Doppler was compared at the tip of the parameatal flap before and after harvesting, there was only an 18% reduction with a parameatal-based and fully extended circumferential foreskin flap. Viability of this flap is further acknowledged with its response to papaverine load. This, along with the lack of necessity of performing end-to-end anastomosis to the old urethra, is beneficial in our method. Furthermore, excision of the urethral plate while harvesting the parameatal flap militates against the recurrence of chordee (Demirbilek et al. 2001). Third, approximation of splayed out bulbocavernous musculature with formation of neourethra is expected to lessen postmicturition dribbling. Fourth, to bring the neomeatus to the most distal tip of the glans, it is bisected (Barcat 1973) rather than channeled by removing the core of glanular substance. We believe this is more anatomical in dissection (Altemus and Hatchins 1991) and corrects the rather flattened globular deformity of the glans to a more natural cone-shaped one when it enrolls the neourethra (Turner-Warwick 1979). Lastly, meatoplasty in a semicuffed fashion adds a few extra millimeters to the urethral length and prevents meatal stricture. Our complication rate of 40% is certainly higher than that of distal hypospadias, where less than 5% required a secondary procedure (Redman 1983), but not as high as our own complication rate with multistage repair for severe hypospadias (Adachi et al. 1987), and others are more candid by reporting an even higher chance (50%) of requiring a secondary or more operations in their experience with pedicle tube urethroplasty (Dewan et al. 1991). By its sheer severity, one-stage repair for this group of children is demanding. Some of our patients ($n=14$) required topical application of testosterone ointment for several weeks to months preceding the operation (Sakakibara et al. 1991) (Fig. 19.10a,b). Operation time is longer than in the distal type of hypospadias. The urethral catheter has to remain in place longer for the wound to heal. All these perioperative obstacles and difficulties notwithstanding, we still believe one-stage repair is worthy of recommendation in all children with severe proximal hypospadias, as final outcomes are satisfactory, both cosmetically and functionally, and in the long term as well (Fig. 19.10c). It is pleasing to witness satisfactory results from others who advocated our principles (Glassberg et al. 1998; Emir et al. 2000; Sugita et al. 2001).

Editorial Comment

Emir et al. (2000) described a modification of the procedure of Koyanagi et al. designed to reduce the complication rate and the need for reoperation. The meatal-based yoke is outlined and the incision is made first to allow mobilization of the urethral plate sufficiently to excise all chordee. The artificial erection test is then performed to check for residual chordee, which, if present, should be corrected at this stage. Only then is the other incision made. To preserve the vascular supply to skin flaps, the flaps are joined together to form the neourethra after being tubularized and the tip is placed on the glans after dissection or by tunneling. The repair is completed by multilayer closure and skin coverage. The focus of this modification is to preserve the lateral blood supply to the neourethral flaps.

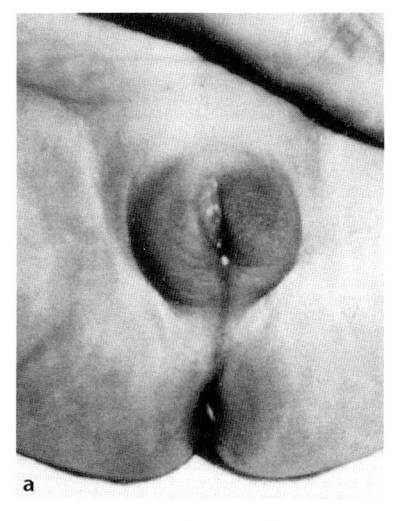

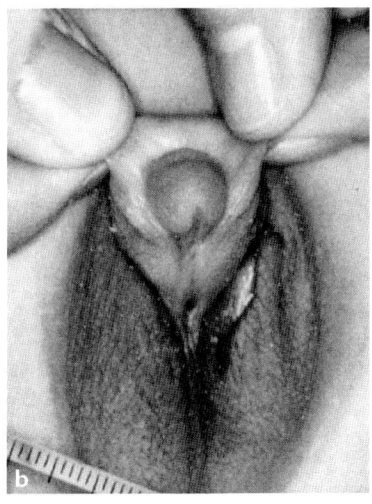

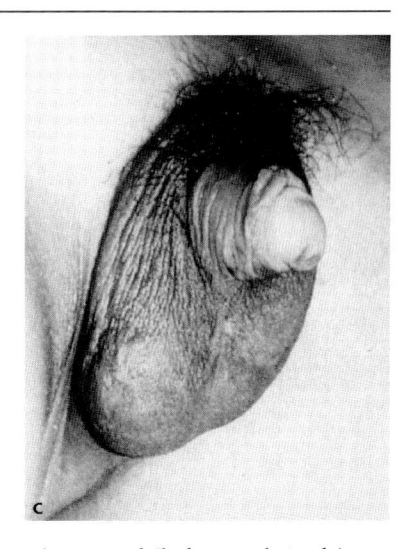

Fig. 19.10a–c. A boy with severe perineal hypospadias. a Genital appearance at the age of 11 days. b Appearance at age 3 years after nine cycles of topical application of testosterone ointment (0.2–0.4 g daily for 3 weeks/cycle) preceding urethroplasty. c Long-term outcome: appearance at age 13 years with the onset of spontaneous puberty

References

Adachi Y, Nonomura K, Togashi M, et al: Comparison of one stage and two stage urethroplasty for hypospadias. Jpn J Urol. 1987; 78:667–673.

Altemus AR, Hatchins GM: Development of human anterior urethra. J Urol. 1991; 146:1085–1093.

Barcat J: Current concepts of treatment. In: Horton CE (ed): Plastic and reconstructive surgery of the genital area. Little Brown, Boston, pp 249–263; 1973.

Demirbilek S, Kanmaz T, Aydin G, et al: Outcomes of one-stage techniques for proximal hypospadias repair. Urology. 2001; 58:267–270.

Dewan PA, Dinneen MD, Winkle D, et al: Hypospadias: Duckett pedicle tube urethroplasty. Eur Urol. 1991; 20:39–42.

Ehrlich RM, Scardino PT: Surgical correction of scrotal transposition and perineal hypospadias. J Pediatr Surg. 1982; 17:175–177.

Emir H, Jayanthi VR, Nitahara K, et al: Modification of the Koyanagi technique for the single stage repair of proximal hypospadias. J Urol. 2000; 164:973–976.

Glassberg KI, Hansbrough F, Horowitz M: The Koyanagi-Nonomura 1-stage bucket repair of severe hypospadias with and without penoscrotal transposition. J Urol. 1998; 160:1104–1107; discussion 1137.

Hodgson NB: Commentary: review of hypospadias repair. In: Whitehead ED, Leiter E (eds): The current operative urology, 2nd edn. Harper and Row, New York, pp 1233–1242; 1984.

King LR: Overview: Hypospadias repair. In: Whitehead ED, Leiter E (eds) The current operative urology, 2nd edn. Harper and Row, New York, pp 1265–1271; 1984.

Koyanagi T, Matsuno TZ, Nonomura K, et al: Complete repair of severe penoscrotal hypospadias in 1 stage: experience with urethral mobilization, wing-flap-flipping urethroplasty and 'glanulomeatoplasty'. J Urol. 1983; 130:1150–1154.

Koyanagi T, Nonomura K, Gotoh T, et al: One-stage repair of perineal hypospadias and scrotal transposition. Eur Urol. 1984; 10:364–367.

Koyanagi T, et al: One-stage urethroplasty with parameatal foreskin-flap (OUPF) for severe proximal hypospadias associated with bifid scrotum (abstract). J Urol. 1987; 137:152A.

Koyanagi T, Imanaka K, Nonomura K, et al: Further experience with one-stage repair of severe hypospadias and scrotal transposition. Modifications in the technique and its result in eight cases. Int Urol Nephrol. 1988; 20:167–177.

Koyanagi T, Nonomura K, Kakizaki H, et al: Experience with stage repair of severe proximal hypospadias: operative technique results. Eur Urol. 1993; 24:106–110.

Koyanagi T, Nonomura K, Yamashita T, et al: One-stage repair of hypospadias: is there no simple method universally applicable to all types of hypospadias? J Urol. 1994; 152:1232–1237.

Koyanagi T, Nonomura H, Kakizaki H, et al: Hypospadias repair. In: Thüroff JW, Hohenfellner M (eds) Reconstructive surgery of the lower urinary tract in children. ISIS Medical Media, Oxford, pp 1–21; 1995.

Nesbit RM: Congenital curvature of the phallus: report of three cases with description of corrective operation. J Urol. 1965; 93:230–234.

Nonomura K, Koyanagi T, Imamaka K, et al: Measurement of blood flow in the parameatal foreskin flap for urethroplasty in hypospadias repair. Eur Urol. 1992; 21:155–159.

Parsons KF, Abercrombie GF: Transverse preputial island flap neo-urethroplasty. Br J Urol. 1982; 54:745–747.

Redman JF: Experience with 60 consecutive hypospadias repairs using the Horton-Devine techniques. J Urol. 1983; 129:115–118.

Redman JF: Tourniquet as hemostatic aid in repair of hypospadias. Urology. 1987; 28:241–245.

Russell RH: Operation for severe hypospadias. Br Med J. 1900; 2:1432–1435.

Sakakibara N, Nonomura K, Koyanagi T, et al: Use of testosterone ointment before hypospadias repair. Urol Int. 1991; 47:40–43

Sugita Y, Tanikaze S, Yoshino K, et al: Severe hypospadias repair with meatal based paracoronal skin flap: the modified Koyanagi repair. J Urol. 2001; 166:1051–1053.

Turner-Warwick R: Observation upon techniques for reconstruction of the urethral meatus, the hypospadiac glans deformity and the penile urethra. Urol Clin North Am. 1979; 6:643–655.

Woodard JR, Parrott TS: Management of severe perineal hypospadias with bifid scrotum (abstract). J Urol. 1991; 145:245A.

Recommended Reading

Koyanagi T, Nonomura K: Hypospadias repair: one-stage urethroplasty with parameatal foreskin flap for all types of hypospadias. In: Ehrlich RM, Alter GJ (eds): Reconstructive and plastic surgery of the external genitalia, 1st edn. chap 19. Saunders, Philadelphia, pp 92–100; 1999.

The Yoke Hypospadias Repair

Brent W. Snow

Repair of severe hypospadias has been and continues to be a significant challenge to surgeons in the field. In the past, surgical repair has relied on staging the procedure or combinations of procedures. Often, the combination of procedures may add the complication rate of one procedure to that of another. Procedures were often designed for a specific length of hypospadias repair, and extending the indications may compromise the integrity of the original procedure design (Snodgrass et al. 2002). In order to create a repair that maintains blood supply to the neourethra for severe hypospadias patients, the yoke procedure was created (Snow and Cartwright 1994). Recognizing that most common hypospadias procedures are based on ventral perimeatal blood supply (Mathieu 1932; Mustarde 1965) or on dorsal island pedicle flap (Duckett 1980) blood supply, the repair was developed to maintain both dorsal and ventral supplies and allow a single-stage repair of complex hypospadias. This repair would avoid combining repairs and obviate the anastomotic difficulties that may occur.

Technique

The incisions are initially indicated by marking a circumcising incision. Ventrally at the location of the hypospadiac meatus, there is a gentle downward "V" of the incision towards the meatus. A second incision is marked which begins proximal to the hypospadiac meatus and then runs parallel along the urethral plate. The width of this incision is chosen remembering that the circumference of the neourethra in French measurements equals the millimeters of circumference. Thus, the parallel incisions are made as many millimeters wide as the new urethra will become in French size plus 1–2 mm that will be taken up by suturing. As the incisions approach the coronal margin, the incision is then carried around the dorsum of the penis. The measurement, then, is one-half the desired French size in millimeters plus 1–2 mm, since these two sides are going to be sutured together, both anteriorly and posteriorly (Fig. 20.1). As the incision is marked, the observer will note that the name "yoke" is derived from the resemblance of the marked incisions to the apparatus draped around the neck of working animals to which implements are attached. Once the incisions are marked, the initial incision made is the circumcising incision. The skin of the penis is degloved along Buck's fascia and the urethral plate is separated from the corpora cavernosa. Chordee correction can be undertaken according to the surgeon's preference. Once chordee has been corrected, the second incision is made taking care to incise only dermis and epidermis, not the underlying vascular pedicle. The shaft skin is then separated from the vascular pedicle for a distance of 1–2 centimeters away from the neourethra (Fig. 20.1b). It is not necessary to separate the vascular pedicle as far as one would during an island flap urethroplasty (Fig. 20.1c). Once the outer skin has been separated and the vascular pedicle developed, a buttonhole is made near where the shaft skin attaches to the vascular pedicle (Fig. 20.1d). The glans penis is drawn through this buttonhole in the vascular pedicle (Fig. 20.1e), transposing the entire urethra and vascular pedicle to the ventral aspect of the penis. A glans channel is made dissecting over the corpora cavernosa to the tip of the glans and making an adequate channel of 18–22 F in size. The neourethra that has been transferred to the ventral aspect of the penis with the buttonhole technique now has a tennis racquet appearance (Fig. 20.1f). The distal portion where the glans was has a gap which is sutured together beginning with a 7-0 absorbable suture layer, followed by a second running subcuticular 8-0 absorbable suture layer to complete the neourethra's posterior suture line. Then, a urethral catheter is placed in the urethra and the ventral suture line of the neourethra is begun by using an 8-0 absorbable suture subcuticular stitch. The distal 1 cm of the neourethra is sutured in an interrupted fashion so the length can be trimmed without

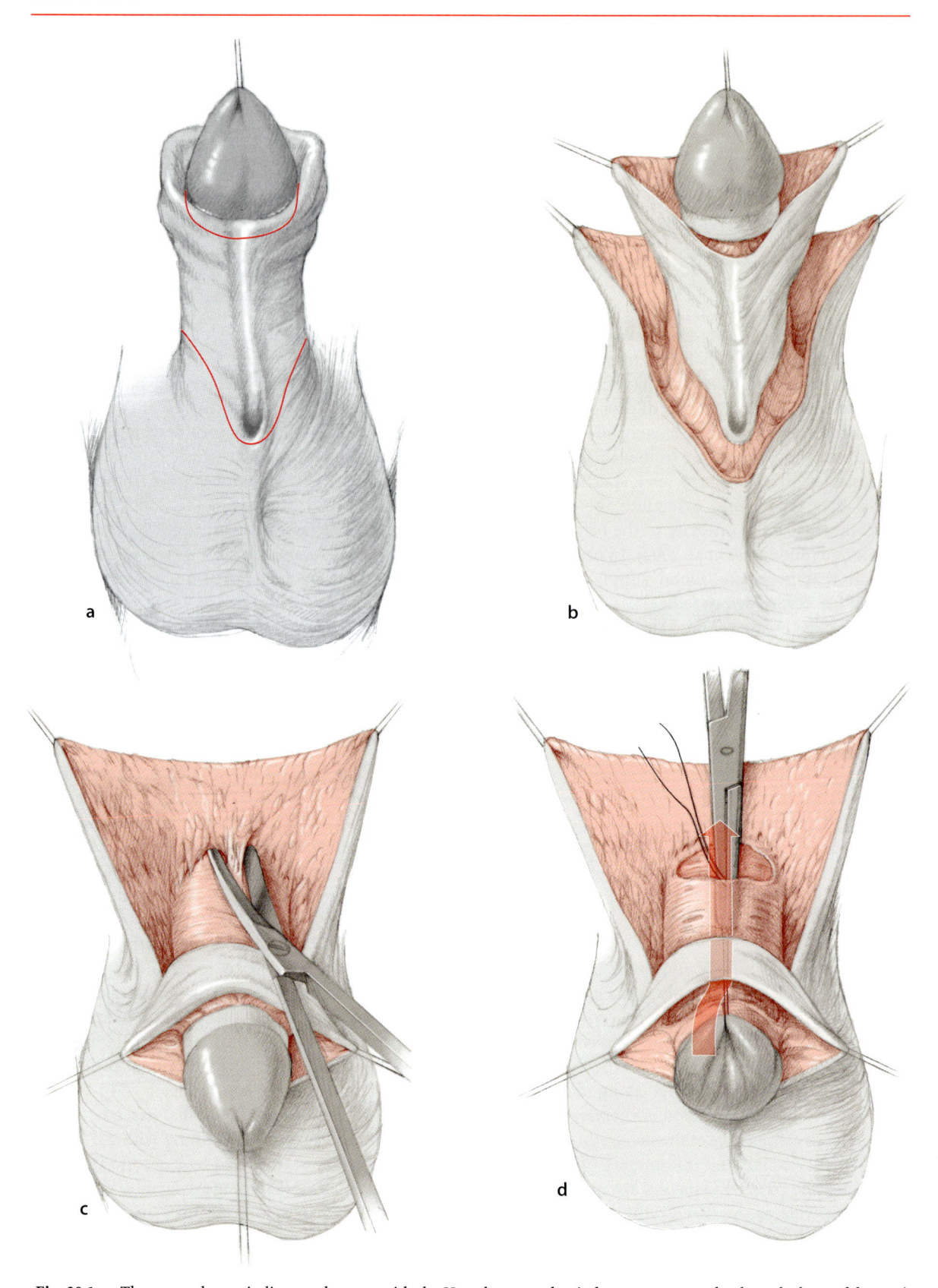

Fig. 20.1. a The coronal margin line can be seen with the V-shaped ventral incision. The parallel incision is the urethral plate. Then go around to the dorsum parallel to the coronal margin incision **b** The penis already degloved ventrally with the coronal margin incision made and the parallel urethral plate incisions and incision around the dorsal aspect of the coronal margin. **c** The vascular pedicle is developed dorsally, but note that it does not go completely to the base of the penis because in this procedure that is not necessary. **d** A dorsal view of the penis with the buttonhole having been made and a hemostat used to pull the traction suture and the glans penis through the buttonhole, transferring the neourethra to the ventral aspect of the penis. **e–i** see pp. 205, 206

The Yoke Hypospadias Repair 205

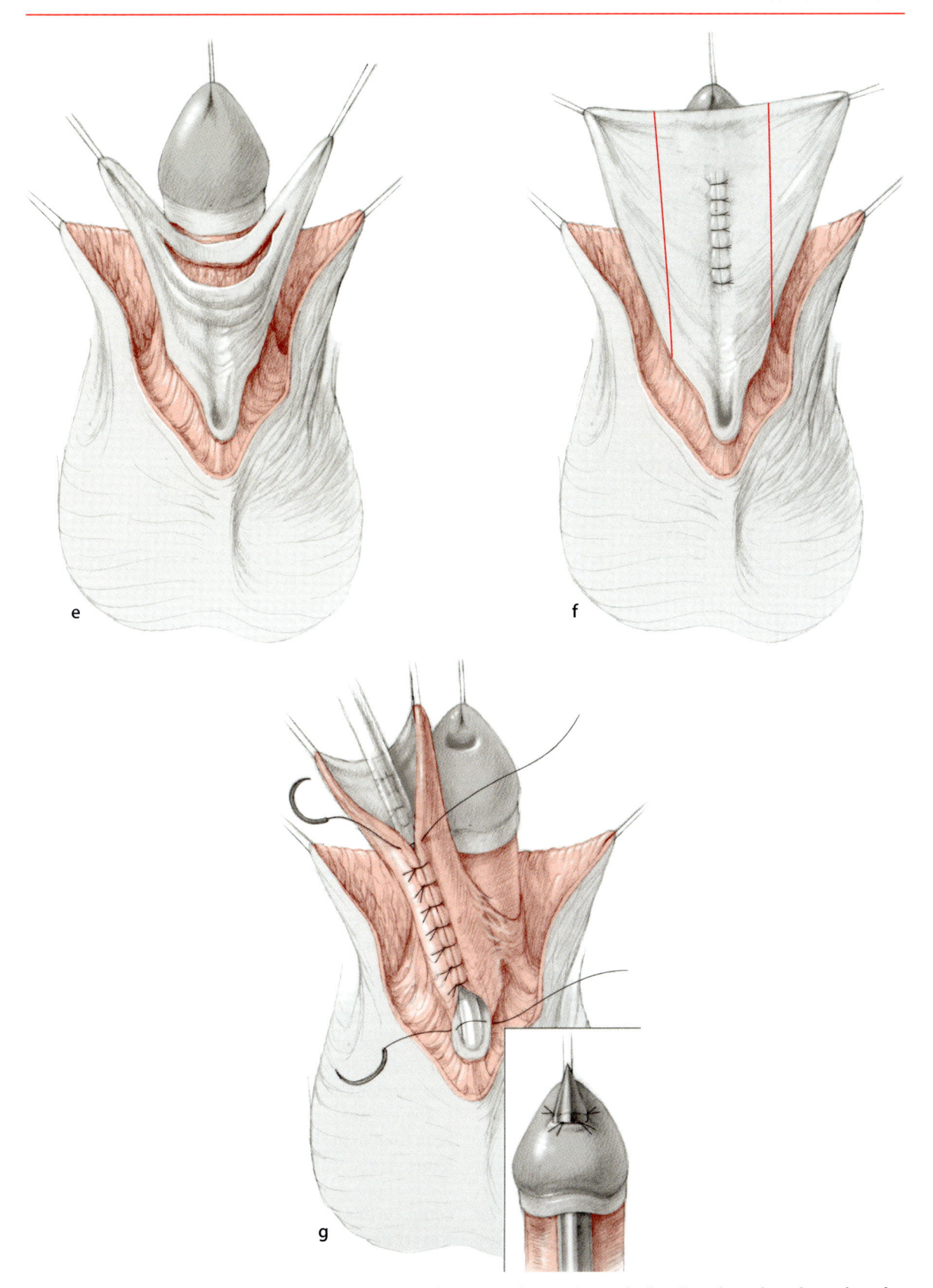

Fig. 20.1 (*continued*). **e** A ventral view at the same stage of the repair: the buttonhole remains as a gap in the neourethral plate. **f, g** The gap in the neourethral plate has been closed and the neourethra is being sutured closed to near the tip. The second view shows the hooding that takes place when the neourethra has been completed and has been passed through the glans channel. The *inset* shows this being excised. **h, i** see p. 206

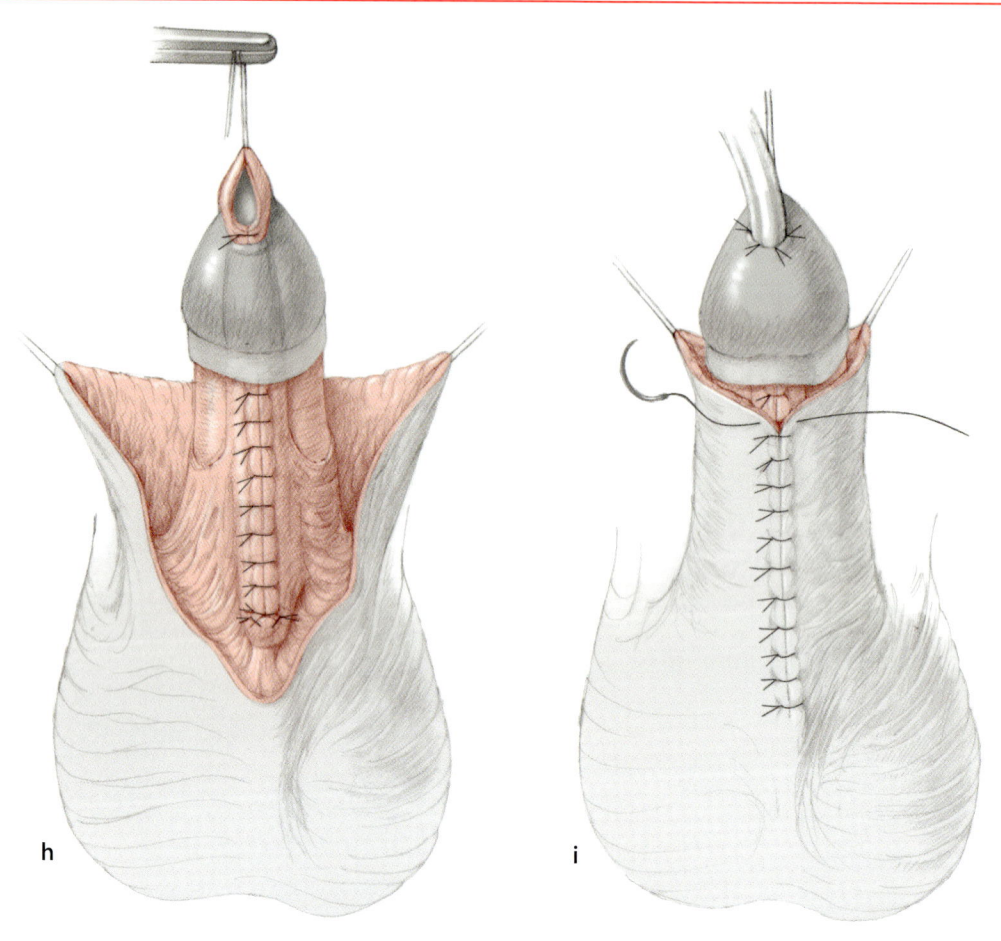

Fig. 20.1 (*continued*). **h, i** Skin coverage of the yoke procedure can easily be accomplished by suturing the circumcision site back together and performing a median raphe closure, as shown

ruining a running suture line. A second layer of 7-0 absorbable suture is completed over this, with the last centimeter again being sutured in interrupted manner (Fig. 20.1f, g). The urethral catheter is removed before the urethra is passed through the glans channel. The surgeon will note that the distal portion of the neourethra is hooded, which allows for generous pedicle blood supply. The hooded part of the neourethra is excised by removing dermis and epidermis, leaving the vascular pedicle (Fig. 20.1f, g). This hood is similar to the Turnbull modification of ileoconduit that maintains good blood supply to the meatus and minimizes stomal complications (Turnbull and Fazio 1975). The meatus is made by suturing interrupted 7-0 absorbable sutures around the tip. The shaft skin of the penis is next sutured to the coronal margin with absorbable suture, and the closure can be made in the ventral midline to mimic the median raphe (Fig. 20.1h, i). The surgical scars, when completed, go around where a circumcision scar would be and in the ventral midline along the median raphe, giving a wonderful cosmetic result (Fig. 20.2). Often, a scrotoplasty is necessary to complete the operation. A urethral catheter is left in place for 7–10 days and the surgeon's choice of dressing is applied.

The operation is based on careful dissection and maintenance of periurethral blood supply and vascular pedicle. These principles and technique are familiar to hypospadias surgeons. Those who perform surgery to correct hypospadias recognize that it is often tedious and technically demanding.

Experience with this repair is limited since it has been used in the most sever forms of hypospadias patients. Some authors have expressed concern that there would be inadequate shaft skin and foreskin to complete this operation; however, 9 cm of neourethra was created in one patient, and in no patient has there been inadequate skin to perform this operation in its entirety.

The limited experience has shown that urethrocutaneous fistula is more common than desired, and

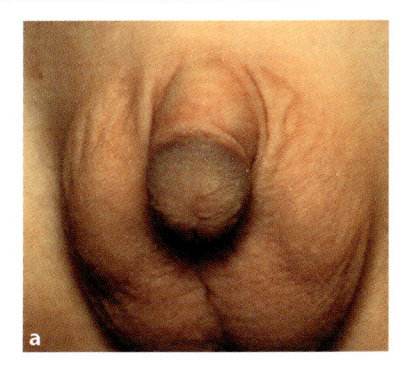

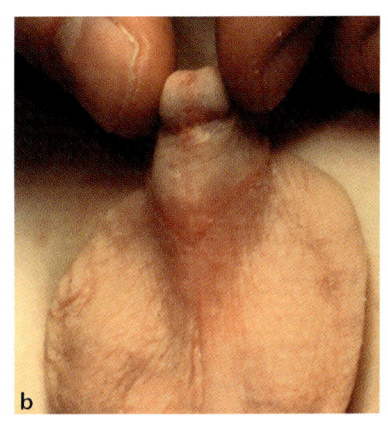

Fig. 20.2a, b. Postoperative view showing the excellent cosmetic results after a midscrotal hypospadias repair using the yoke technique

this seems always to happen near the proximal anastomosis or the penoscrotal junction. It would be recommended at this point to consider a second buttonhole to bring a dartos flap or a tunica vaginalis flap through the neourethra's vascular pedicle to cover the neourethra from the original meatus to the glans channel, which would minimize the chance of fistula formation.

Other authors in the past have had similar creative suggestions, but none with the dedication to preserving blood supply as the yoke procedure does. Russell reported parallel circumferential incisions that he called a stole procedure. His operation, published in 1900, was a two-stage procedure where the part of the urethra that was taken from the dorsum was divided and the blood supply was not preserved (Russell 1900). Koyanagi et al. developed similar incisions but divided the dorsal neourethra. Long parameatal-based flaps were created in a procedure called "wing flap-flipping urethroplasty" (Koyanagi et al. 1984). These are exceedingly long and narrow perimeatal-based flaps that did not maintain pedicle blood supply.

The yoke operation does not cause the torsion that is associated with long-pedicle urethroplasties. Since the urethra is brought ventrally through with a buttonhole technique, no bulk is added to one side of the shaft of the penis with the vascular pedicle, nor are there any twisting rotational effects. The pedicle dissection is minimized compared with traditional pedicle flap urethroplasties, and this minimizes the damage to the pedicle blood supply. The cosmetic results of the yoke hypospadias repair are excellent. The major fault of the repair is the frequency of urethrocutaneous fistulas near the proximal meatus. It is the author's recommendation that additional tissue be transposed to this area through a buttonhole to prevent this complication and accomplish repair of severe hypospadias in a single procedure.

References

Duckett JW: Transverse preputial island flap technique for repair of severe hypospadias. Urol Clin North Am. 1980; 7:423–431.
Koyanagi T, Nonomura K, Gotoh T, et al: One-stage repair of perineal hypospadias and scrotal transposition. Eur Urol. 1984; 10:364–367.
Mathieu P: Traitement en un temps de l'hypospadias balanique' et juxta-balanique. J Chir. 1932; 39:481.
Mustarde JC: One-stage correction of distal hypospadias and other people's fistulae. Br J Plast Surg. 1965; 18:413.
Russell RH: Operation for severe hypospadias. Br Med J. 1900; ii:1432–1435.
Snodgrass W, Baskin LS, Mitchell ME: Hypospadias, In: Gillenwater JY, Grayhack JT, Howards SS, Mitchell ME (eds): Adult and pediatric urology, 4th edn. Lippincot Williams and Wilkins, Philadelphia, 2002; pp 2509–2532.
Snow BW, Cartwright PC: The yoke hypospadias repair. J Pediatr Surg. 1994; 29:557–560.
Turnbull RB Jr, Fazio V: Advances in the surgical technique and ulcerative colitis surgery. In: Nybus L (ed): Surgery annual. Appleton Century-Crofts, California, USA, p 315; 1975.

Lateral-based Flap With Dual Blood Supply: A Single-Stage Repair for Proximal Hypospadias

Ahmed T. Hadidi

Introduction

Repair of severe hypospadias in one stage is among the most difficult challenges a reconstructive surgeon may face. Most procedures in the past relied on several stages, each of which had its own complication risks. More recent attempts have relied on multiple stages or combinations of other well-described repairs. However, repairs each designed for a specific purpose may not necessarily be easily combined. The combination of different techniques also often introduces another anastomosis to heal and another potential location for complications to occur.

In the attempt to solve this dilemma for patients with severe hypospadias, a repair with dual blood supply would offer many advantages. Two of the most common categories of hypospadias repairs are parameatal-based flaps and transverse preputial island pedicle flaps. Each flap has a rich blood supply from the dorsal or ventral aspect of the root of the penis. Therefore, these two types of procedure seem to represent an ideal combination of repairs to correct severe hypospadias. With these concepts in mind, the lateral-based (LB) flap repair was conceived. This procedure combines meatal-based flap and pedicle flap techniques into one procedure without the need for an intervening anastomosis. It also allows for extensive excision of ventral chordee and the urethral plate (if necessary) without damaging the flap.

Surgical Technique

The technique follows steps 1–10, illustrated in 👁 Fig. 21.1.

Step 1: Stay Suture, Erection Test and Meatal Dilatation or Incision

A traction suture of 4-0 nylon is placed through the tip of the glans. An artificial erection test is performed. The native urethral meatus is dilated with a fine curved mosquito forceps or incised proximally (if very thin) to create a wide spatulated junction.

Step 2: Y-shaped Deep Incision of the Glans

A Y-shaped incision is outlined on the glans. The centre of the Y is just below the tip of the glans and where the tip of the neomeatus will be located. The upper two short limbs of the Y are 0.5 cm long and the angle between them is 60 deg. The long vertical limb of the Y extends down the whole length of the glans penis to the coronary sulcus (similar to urethral plate incision or hinging). The Y-shaped incision is made deep and results in three flaps, one small upper (median) flap and two large lateral flaps.

The three flaps are elevated and a core of soft tissue is excised from the bed of each flap to create a space for the neourethra (👁 Fig. 21.1a, b).

Step 3: Chordectomy

Meticulous excision of any chordee or fibrous bands is carried out. This fibrous tissue is particularly heavy in the midline but may extend well laterally (👁 Fig. 21.1c).

Step 4: Outlining Skin Incision and Flap Mobilisation

Two stay sutures are placed through the outer surface of the tip of the prepuce at least 1.5 cm apart. A rectangular skin strip is outlined extending proximally from the urethral meatus staying in the midline in the scrotum to avoid potentially hair-bearing skin. The skin strip is extended distally and laterally by curving it towards the prepuce, where stay sutures are taken. This allows for formation of a very long tube that can easily reach the tip of the

210 Ahmed T. Hadidi

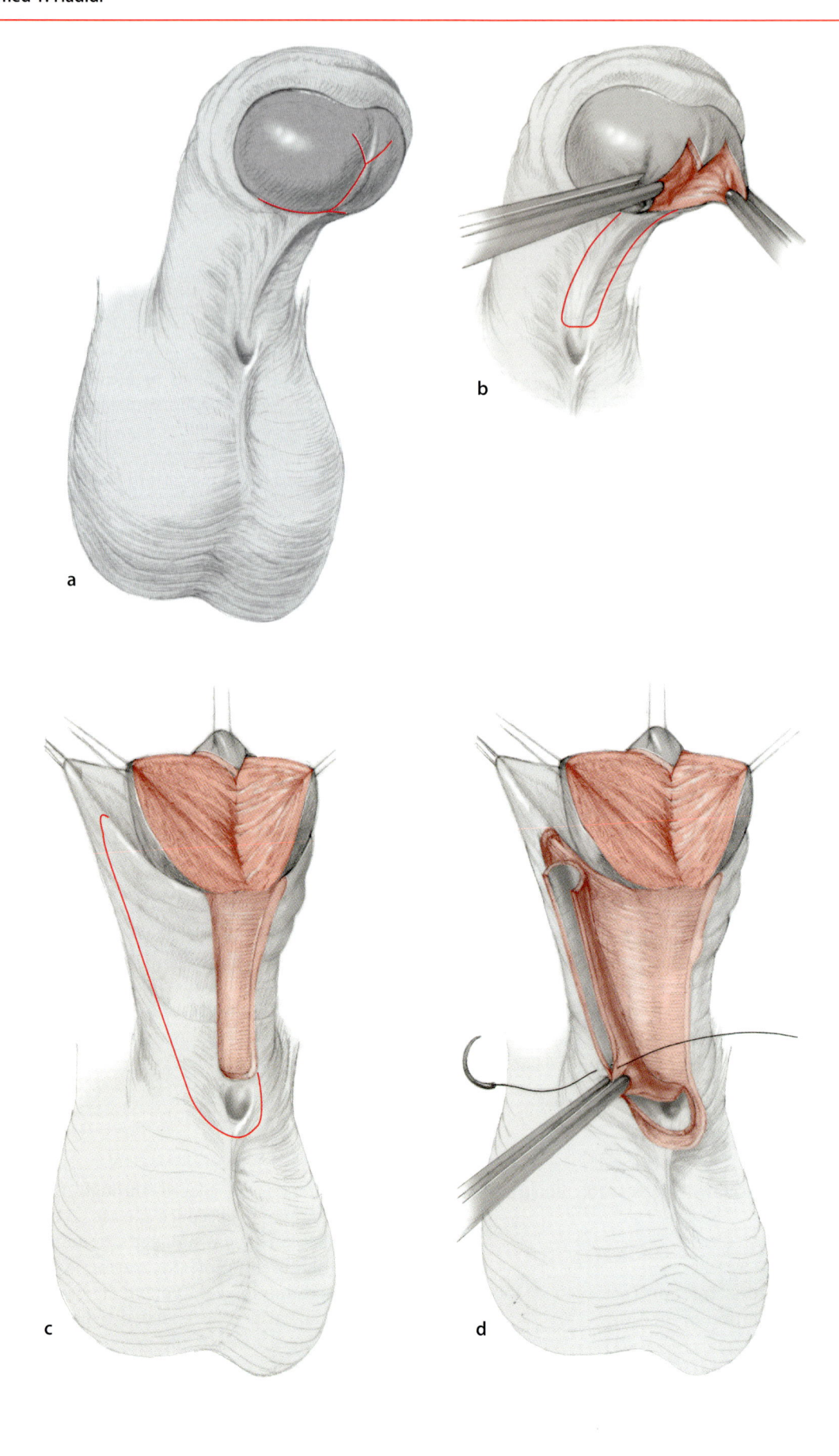

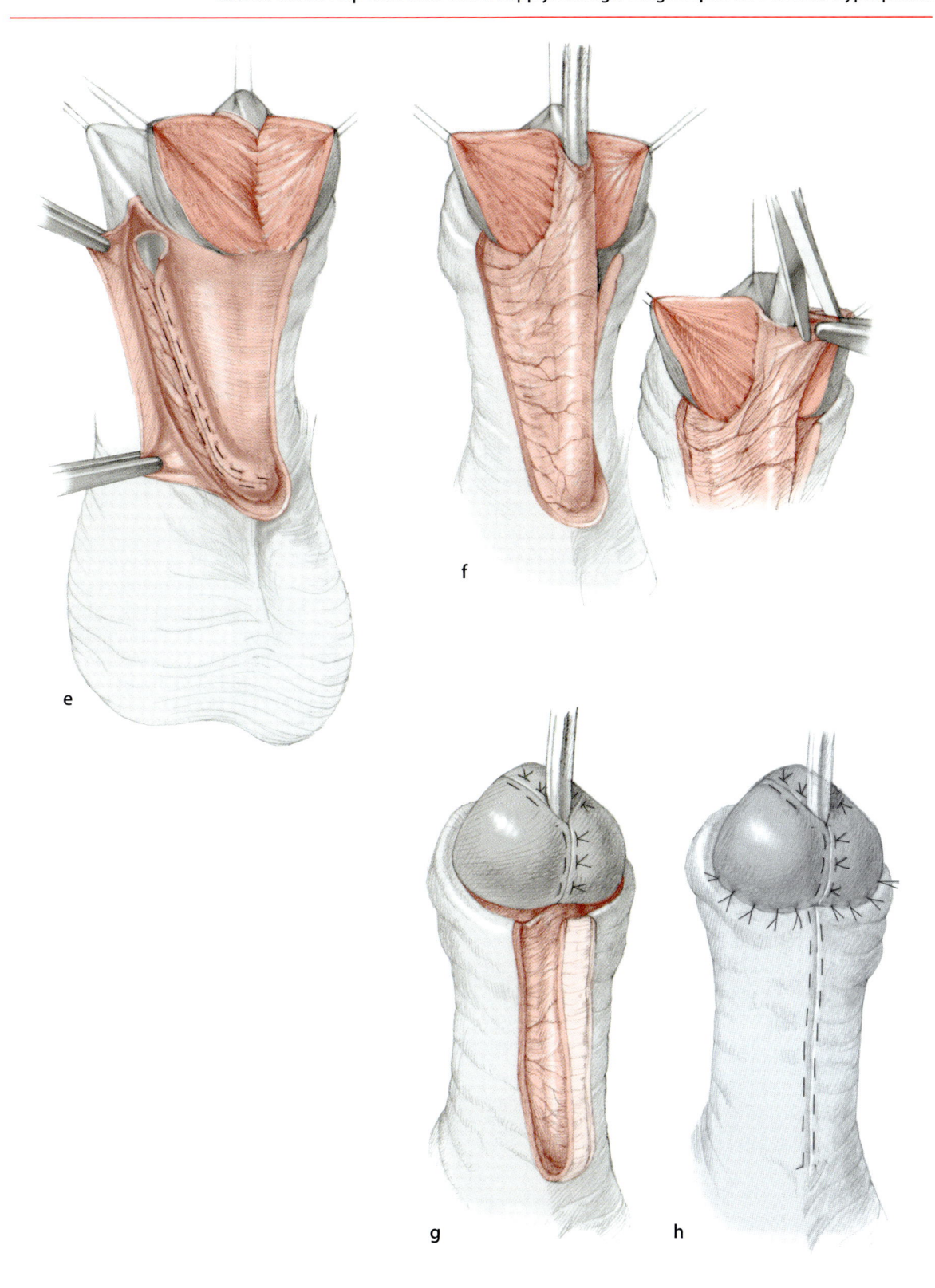

Fig. 21.1a–h. Steps of lateral-based (LB) flap technique for single stage repair of proximal hypospadias. **a, b** Y-shaped deep incision of the glans; **c** chordectomy; **d** outline skin incision and flap mobilisation; **e** formation of the neourethra; **f** glanulomeatoplasty; **g** protective intermediate layer; **h** skin closure

glans whatever the position of the hypospadiac meatus (Fig. 21.1d).

The skin incision is carried completely around the meatus, leaving a small cuff of skin (to wrap around the catheter). The meatus is freed proximally, using extreme care, from any fibrous attachment. This area is very vascular and meticulous haemostasis is important. The adjacent penile skin is elevated (rather than the flap to preserve the vascular areolar tissue with the flap). This is carried the same way as in transverse preputial island flap. This mobilisation should continue into the dorsum of the penis and down to the root of the penis to avoid any degree of penile torsion.

Step 5: Formation of the Neourethra

The skin strip and proximal cuff are tubed around a 10-F Nelaton catheter inside the urethra. The author prefers to use Vicryl 6-0 on a cutting needle. Suturing is carried out from proximal to distal in a subcuticular continuous manner. Several reinforcing interrupted stitches are usually inserted to form a watertight tube (Fig. 21.1e).

Step 6: Glanulomeatoplasty

The neomeatus is then constructed by suturing the terminal end of the neourethra to the central V of the cut edges of the glans. A final slit-like meatus is obtained by making another V at the neourethra. Then, the glanular wings are wrapped around the neourethra and approximated in the midline. On completion, a meatus of near normal width and appearance is created at the tip of a conical-shaped glans. The long anastomotic contact between the neomeatus and the glans created by the Y glanuloplasty is of utmost importance to create a large meatus, thus avoiding postoperative meatal stenosis (Fig. 21.1f).

Step 7: Protective Intermediate Layer

The vascular areolar subcutaneous tissue layer is then used to provide a complete covering for the neourethra (Fig. 21.1g)

Step 8: Skin Closure

Byars flaps are then fashioned to provide ventral skin coverage. This is achieved by making a dorsal midline incision. The skin is closed in the midline using 6-0 Vicryl in a continuous transverse mattress through-and-through manner. This helps to simulate the normal ventral median skin raphe (Fig. 21.1h).

Step 9: Formation of Penoscrotal Angle

If needed, a Z-plasty is performed at the penoscrotal junction. This helps to simulate the normal penoscrotal angle. Penoscrotal transposition, if present, can be corrected at this time by mobilising and suturing the scrotal tissues ventral to the corpus spongiosum with Z-plasty to create the penoscrotal junction.

Step 10: Insertion of a Percutaneous Suprapubic Cystostomy Catheter

At this stage, the intraurethral Nelaton catheter is removed and urinary diversion is accomplished by means of a percutaneous suprapubic cystostomy catheter (10 F). The cystocath is usually left in position for 10–14 days. Tetracycline ointment is applied and haemostasis is achieved by compression dressing for 12–24 h. Afterwards, the wound is left exposed.

Summary of Important Technical Points ▶ Deep Y-shaped incision of the glans helps to obtain a terminal, near normal looking glans and meatus. Subcuticular suturing of the neourethra allows for proper coaptation of the edges. Both ends of the neourethra are spatulated to avoid stricture formation. Careful dissection of the flap maintains dual blood supply. Proper mobilisation of the flap and its dorsal subcutaneous pedicle is important to avoid penile shaft torsion.

The presence of a protective intermediate layer (subcutaneous vascular areolar layer) minimises complications. Z-plasty helps to simulate the normal penoscrotal angle. No catheter is left inside the urethra in order to decrease irritation and infection. The dressing is removed in less than 24 h. Urinary diversion is maintained by a percutaneous suprapubic cystostomy catheter for 10–14 days.

Results

During a 6 year period, 49 patients with severe hypospadias underwent treatment using the new technique. The follow-up period ranged from 6 months to 6 years (mean 39 months). Results are considered satisfactory when the boy achieves a glanular meatus, single forward stream, unimpeded voiding, good cosmetic results and there is no need for secondary surgery (Fig. 21.2, pp. 214, 215). Satisfactory results were achieved in 43 (88%) of the 49 patients. Complications occurred in six patients. Five patients developed urethrocutaneous fistula, occurring mostly at the coronal sulcus. Four fistulae responded to simple closure and the fifth one was secondary to meatal stenosis and required Y-V glanuloplasty in addition for fistula closure. Distal glanular disruption occurred in one patient; however, the urethroplasty remained intact.

A minimal degree of rotation occurred in three patients early in the course of this study. However, this did not require further surgery and was avoided later on by adequate mobilisation of the vascular areolar flap. During this study and follow-up period, there was no instance of urethral diverticulum, stricture, meatal retraction or breakdown of the neourethra.

Comments

The author has used the lateral meatal-based flap as routine in any form of proximal hypospadias where a Y-V modified Mathieu procedure could not be applied. It has been used successfully in six "re-do" patients, including one patient who was already circumcised.

Discussion

Proximal types of hypospadias have always constituted a major challenge: they are very difficult to treat, more vulnerable to complications and have a higher incidence of failure. Unfortunately, the complications cannot be treated conservatively; secondary surgery is almost always required. As a result, most surgeons in the past advised staged repair for correction of this difficult and challenging problem (Greenfield et al. 1994).

In the past two decades, however, great progress has been made both in the basic understanding of this deformity and in its surgical repair, which has culminated in the discipline aptly termed hypospadiology (Duckett and Baskin 1996). In 1941, Humby wrote, in a prophetic foreword: "If, however, one could succeed in remodeling the urethra in one operation, the gain would be manifest". This now seems to be a reality. The current success is attributable to many factors, including delicate tissue handling, basic principles of plastic surgery and excellent fine instruments.

The first preputial flap was dsecribed by Van Hook in 1896. However, vascularised pedicle flap repairs dominated in the 1970s due to the work of innovative hypospadiologists such as Hodgson, Asopa and Duckett. In the course of time, however, pedicle flaps have a complication rate of 10–20%, and neourethral stricture or urethral diverticulum have been repeatedly documented with these types of repair (Duckett 1993).

In 1983 Koyanagi et al. introduced a technique for hypospadias repair which used parameatal-based flaps that extend distally around the distal shaft to incorporate the inner layer of the prepuce. Koyanagi's operation theoretically appeared to provide an ideal treatment for severe proximal hypospadias. However, in Koyanagi's large series of 70 patients 47% required secondary surgery (Koyanagi 1994). In a series of patients reported by Glassberg et al. in 1998, a secondary operation was required in 50% of those who underwent this technique. This high complication rate was attributed to inadequacy of blood supply to the neourethral flaps. This may be the result of excess mobilisation of the skin flaps from their lateral and dorsal blood supply (rendering the flap, which is several centimetres long, dependent entirely on the blood supply coming from the region of the urethral meatus). Furthermore, the presence of two anastomoses (dorsal and ventral) increased the risk of fistula formation. In the attempt to improve the results of this technique many modifications have been made, such as the yoke repair for hypospadias (Snow and Cartwright 1994) and the modification of Koyanagi's technique by Emir et al. (2000).

In this chapter a simple technique is reported that permits one-stage repair of posterior and severe hypospadias with a low complication rate and satisfactory functional and cosmetic results. It is well known that the key to successful hypospadias repair with a minimal complication rate is to ensure a good blood supply to the flap used for urethroplasty. In the present study, this was achieved by designing a lateral meatal-based skin flap which enjoys a dual blood supply from the preputial vascular pedicle and the parameatal tissue. The viability and good vascularity of the skin flap is confirmed by the fact that the neourethra has never broken down or stenosed in any of our patients.

One technical advantage of the procedure described here is the presence of a single longitudinal suture line in the urethroplasty. This helps to minimise the incidence of complications and increases the success rate. Furthermore, this single suture line is covered with a second protective layer of well-vascularised subcutaneous dartos tissue. Torsion of the penile shaft is avoidable through proper mobilisation of the flap and its dorsal subcutaneous pedicle.

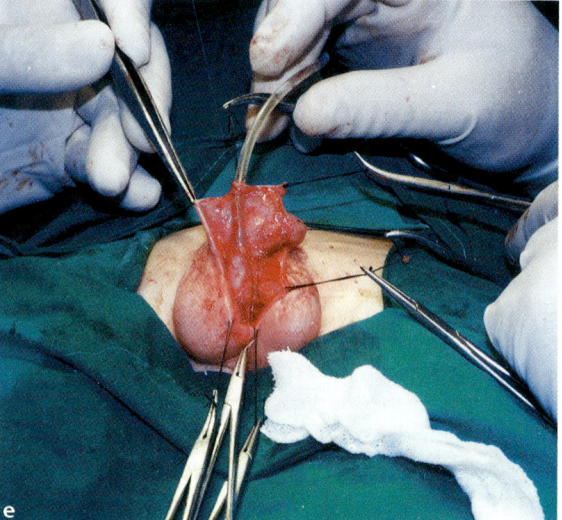

Fig. 21.2a–i. Lateral-based (LB) flap technique in a 1-year-old boy. **a** Preoperative; **b** after chordee excision; **c–e** after tubularisation of lateral-based flap; **f–i** see p. 215

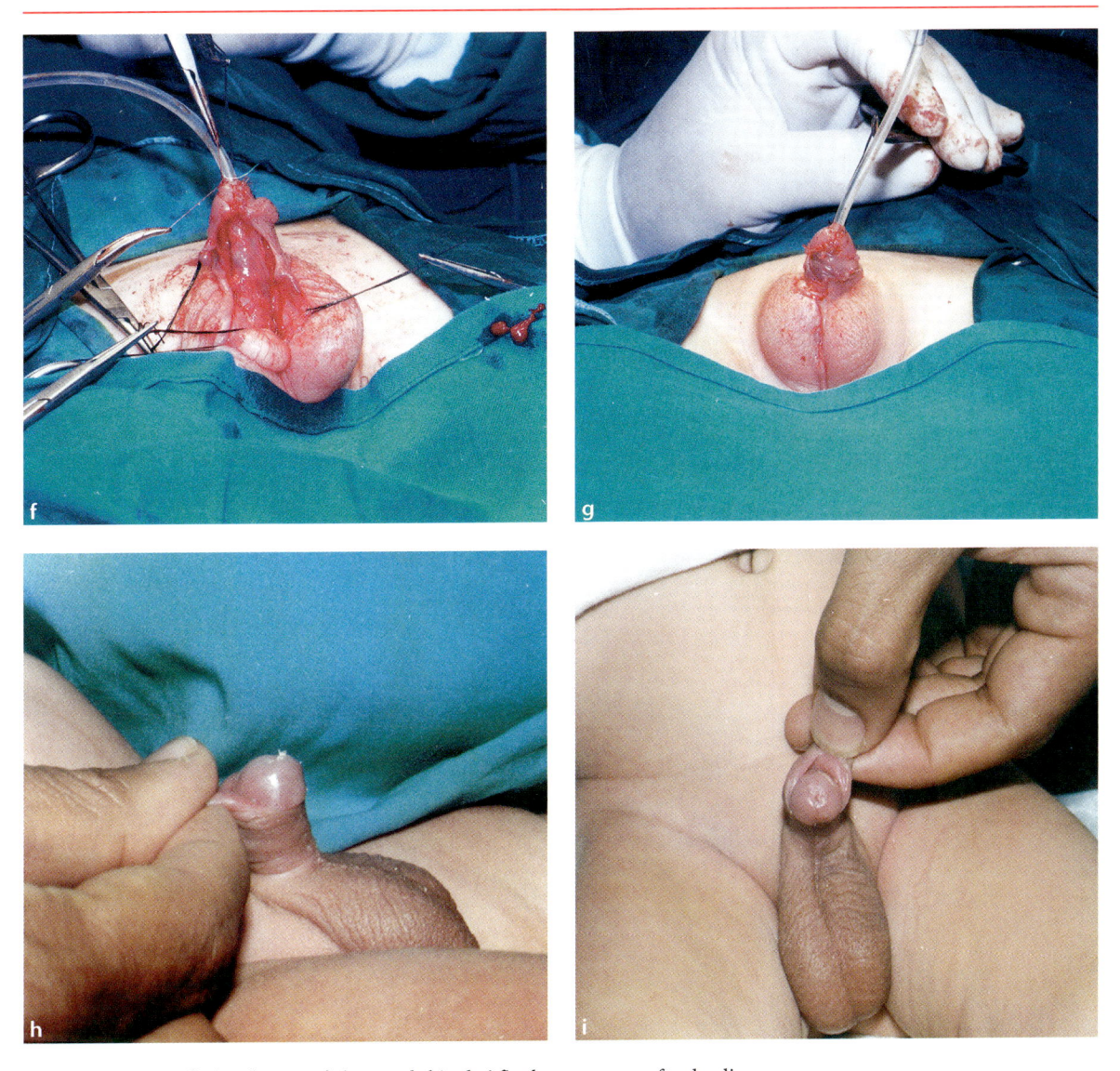

Fig. 21.2 (*contiuned*). **f, g** closure of glans and skin; **h, i** final appearance after healing

Another point in this study which deserves special comment, is the way in which the neomeatus is constructed. The use of Y glanuloplasty and creation of a long suture anastomotic connection between the urethral meatus and the glans results in a large apical meatus. Also, the excision of a small V from the apex of the neomeatus helps to achieve a terminal slit-like meatus. This decreases the risk of postoperative meatal stenosis, which is usually a major contributing factor in anastomotic failure or repair breakdown.

The lateral-based (LB) skin flap is not a totally new method of repair. It is based on, and is a natural development of, many well-established procedures such as those of Broadbent et al. (1961), DesPrez and colleagues (1961), Hinderer (1971), Koyanagi et al. (1983), Snow and Cartwright (1994) and Joseph (1995).

Broadbent et al. (1961) described a single-stage repair by using a buried skin strip based on the parameatal tissue and its blood supply. DesPrez et al., in the same year, described a similar technique using a full-thickness skin strip from the ventral shaft of the penis, extending it outward onto the inner surface of the prepuce. However, DesPrez, in his study on 65 patients during a 10-year period, reported that one third of the patients developed a fistula that necessitated a secondary procedure.

The results of the lateral meatal-based flap have been satisfactory from the cosmetic and functional point of view. This technique may offer patients with proximal and severe forms of hypospadias a good chance of a single-stage operation with a high success rate (over 88%) and minimal complications. However, a longer follow-up period is necessary to reach a final conclusion.

References

Broadbent TR, Woolf RM, Toksu E: Hypospadias: one-stage repair. Plast Reconstr Surg. 1961; 27:154.

DesPrez JD, Persky L, Kiehn CL: A one-stage repair of hypospadias by island-flap technique. Plast Reconstr Surg. 1961; 28:405.

Duckett JW: Hypospadias. In: Webster G, Kirby R, King L, Goldwasser B (eds): Reconstructive urology, vol 2, chap 54. Blackwell Scientific, Boston, 1993; pp 763–780.

Duckett JW, Baskin LS: Hypospadias. In: Gillenwater JY, Grayhack JT, Howards SS, Duckett JW (eds): Adult and pediatric urology, 3rd edn. Mosby-Year Book, St Louis, 1996.

Emir H, Jayanthi VR, Nitahara K, et al: Modification of the Koyanagi technique for the single stage repair of proximal hypospadias. J Urol. 2000; 164:973–976.

Glassberg K, Hansbrough F, Horowitz M: The Koyanagi-Nonomura 1-stage bucket repair of severe hypospadias with and without penoscrotal transposition. J Urol. 1998; 160:1104.

Greenfield SP, Sadler BT, Wan J: Two stage repair for severe hypospadias. J Urol. 1994; 152:498.

Hinderer U: New one-stage repair of hypospadias (technique of penis tunnelization). In: Hueston JT (ed): Transactions of the 5th International Congress of Plastic And Reconstructive Surgery. Butterworth, Stoneham, Mass, 1971; pp 283–305.

Humby G: A one-stage operation for hypospadias. Br J Surg. 1941; 29:84–92.

Joseph VT: Concept in surgical technique of one-stage hypospadias correction. Br J Urol. 1995; 76:504–509.

Koyanagi T, Matsuno T, Nonomura K, et al: Complete repair of severe penoscrotal hypospadias in 1 stage: experience with urethral mobilization, wing-flap-flipping urethroplasty and 'glanulomeatoplasty'. J Urol. 1983; 130:1150–1154.

Koyanagi T, Nonomura K, Yamashita T, et al: One-stage repair of hypospadias: is there no simple method universally applicable to all types of hypospadias? J Urol. 1994; 152: 1232.

Snow BW, Cartwright PC: The yoke hypospadias repair. J Pediatr Surg. 1994; 29:557–560.

Van Hook WV: A new operation for hypospadias. Ann Surg. 1896; 23:378.

Grafts for One-Stage Repair

Seif Asheiry, Ahmed T. Hadidi

The use of vascularised local penile or preputial skin has been the mainstay of hypospadias repair for a long time. If the reconstruction fails, for whatever reason, these precious commodities are irretrievably lost and further reconstruction necessitates the recruitment of new tissue from elsewhere, generally in the form of a free-graft.

Nove-Josserand, in 1897, started the school of urethroplasty utilizing the free inlay graft. A free full-thickness skin graft should be used in preference to split-thickness grafts because the former have better growth characteristics in children (Young and Benjamin 1949). Devine and Horton (1961) and Hendren and Horton (1988) had excellent results using the inner preputial skin after defattening. However, these results were not duplicated by other surgeons in a uniform manner (Vyas et al. 1987; Rober et al. 1990). It must be kept in mind that the free graft requires revascularisation. The free graft must be able to survive by imbibition for the first 48 h. Inosculation follows on days 2–4. For this to be successful, the recipient site must be well vascularised and immobilised in the postoperative period. Great care should be taken to obtain excellent skin cover to allow the graft a well-vascularised bed (Duckett and Baskin 1996).

A wide variety of options has been explored. Extragenital skin from the groin, the inner arm, or the postauricular area has been used with varying success (Webster et al. 1984). However, a widespread concern is that free graft skin is associated with fibrosis and contracture over many years. The use of bladder mucosa was therefore embraced enthusiastically in the 1980s, particularly in view of its free availability and its compatibility with urine (Hendren and Reda 1986; Mollard et al. 1989). The complication rate proved to be very high, however, partially because of metaplasia and stenosis when the mucosa was exposed to air at the tip of the penis (Ransley et al. 1987a, b; Keating et al. 1990). Such problems were compounded by the thin and relatively weak nature of the mucosa itself, resulting in ballooning of the reconstructed urethra with only the mildest degree of distal obstruction.

In this chapter, the three most popular techniques (i.e. preputial skin graft, buccal mucosa and bladder mucosa) will be described in detail. Whatever technique is used, the preoperative preparation and postoperative management are the same.

Preputial Skin Graft

Devine and Horton (1961, 1977) first reported the use of the free preputial graft in hypospadias surgery. Since this initial report, the application of the free preputial graft with pedicle flap has been extended, and onlay free grafts are currently being performed as frequently as the tubularised repairs. The technique was well described by Scherz (1999):

> A circumferential incision is made approximately 0.5 cm proximal to the corona, beginning dorsally, and the incision is carried ventrally down to the native meatus. After the shaft skin is completely dissected proximally to the penile base, chordee is assessed with an artificial erection. If chordee can be corrected with preservation of the urethral plate, as is often possible using dorsal plication, then an onlay free graft is used. However, when it becomes necessary to divide the urethral plate to straighten the penis, a tubularised free graft is constructed.
>
> The graft is harvested from the inner face of the prepuce by first unfolding the prepuce and then amputating the appropriately sized graft, which has been pre-measured (Fig. 22.1a). The graft is prepared by excising the subcutaneous tissue to create a thin, full-thickness strip of skin. This step is most easily done by pinning the skin strip to a board to stretch it out. To construct the free graft tube, the skin strip is tubularized over a 10 French red rubber catheter using a combination of interrupted and running 7-0 polyglycolic acid (PGA) sutures (Fig. 22.1b). The proximal end of the tube is left open as spatulation. The catheter is removed and replaced with an 8 French silicone Foley. The native urethra is spatulated, and the Foley is introduced into the bladder. The balloon is inflated, and the catheter is left indwelling. The proximal end of the graft is anastomosed to the native urethra with

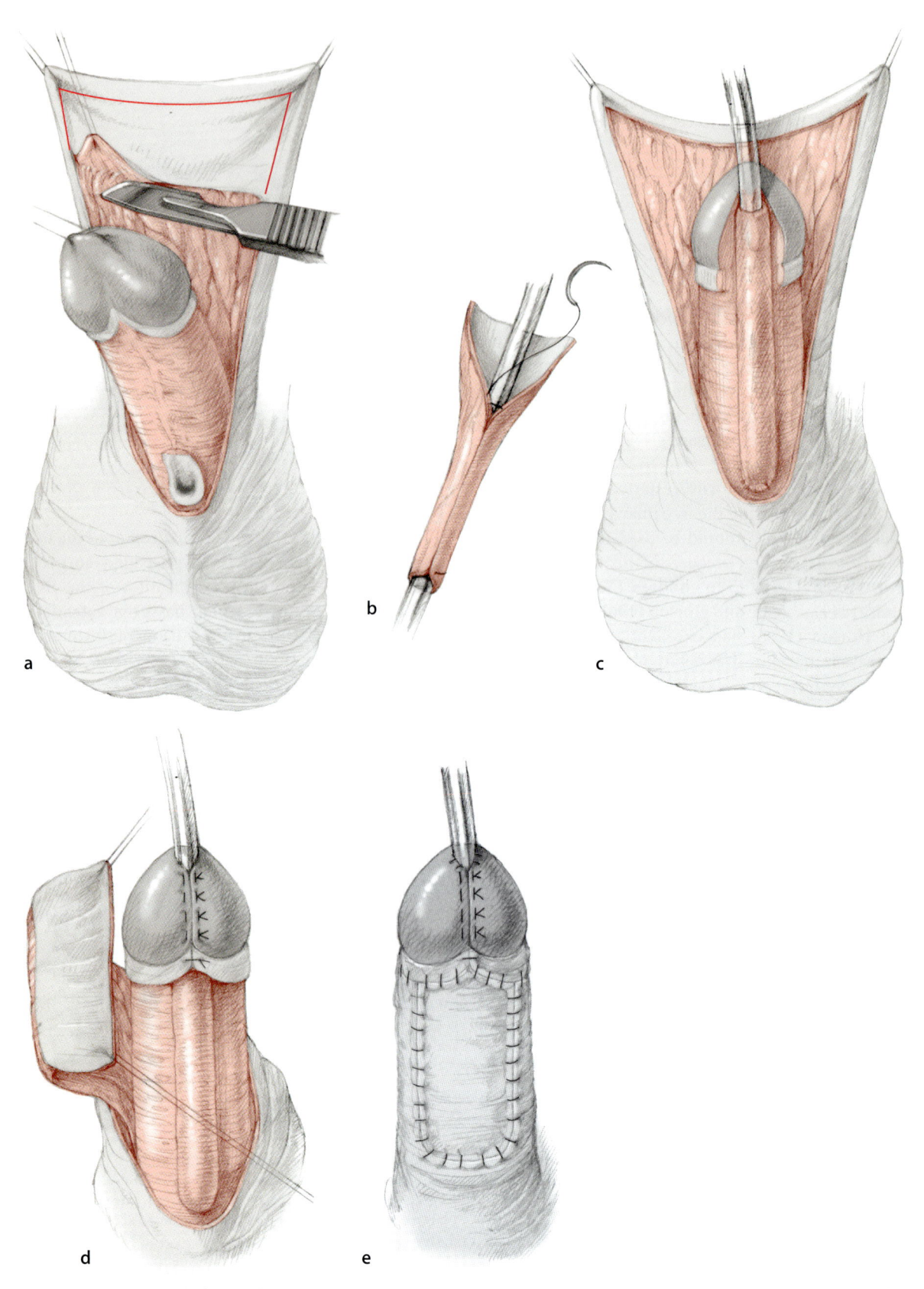

Fig. 22.1a–e. Preputial skin graft. **a** Elevation of the inner preputial skin. The graft is harvested. **b** The graft is tubularised over a 10-F catheter. **c** The glans is split and the graft is anastomosed at both ends. **d** The dorsal subcutaneous flap is developed. **e** The protective intermediate layer is transformed ventrally and sutured in to cover the skin graft

interrupted 7-0 PGA suture. The tube is constructed and anastomosed so that the seam of the neourethra is positioned against the corpora cavernosa. The glans is then split, and the distal end of the neourethra is anastomosed to the glans at the glans tip, also with interrupted 7-0 PGA (Fig. 22.1c). The glans wings are brought together ventrally with several deep 5-0 PGA sutures, and the glans epithelium is closed and the remainder of the meatus secured with 7-0 PGA. Several additional 7-0 PGA sutures are used to tack down the graft to the corpora cavernosa.

The outer face of the prepuce is then used to cover the ventral skin defect by fashioning the pedicle flap. An incision is made through the dermis of the outer prepuce at the approximate level of the corona. This distal skin is mobilized on its vascular pedicle by dissecting the more proximal dorsal skin from the subcutaneous tissue and continuing the dissection to the base of the penis (Fig. 22.1d). The distal strip of dorsal skin that now sits on this vascular pedicle can be transposed ventrally by either rotating the flap or bringing the glans through a buttonhole in the vascular pedicle in an avascular space. The latter technique may result in less penile torsion. The pedicle is secured over the graft with interrupted 7-0 PGA, which is also used as skin sutures for the remainder of the repair. Finally, the ventral skin of the pedicle flap is trimmed to fit, and the resurfacing of the shaft is completed (Fig. 22.1e). A Tegaderm and silicone prosthetic foam dressing is applied. Both are left in place for 1 week, with the patient immobilized.

When the urethral plate is preserved and an onlay free graft is used to reconstruct the urethra, the graft is sutured to the native urethra with interrupted 7-0 PGA sutures at the meatus, and each lateral border is anastomosed with a running subcuticular 7-0 PGA suture. Distally, we have used the Barcat balanic groove technique to advance the neourethra farther distally to achieve an improved cosmetic appearance.

The conditions necessary to ensure successful free graft survival were enumerated by Devine and Horton (1977). These include having a well-vascularized host bed, rapid onset of imbibition, close apposition of the graft to the host bed, immobilization of the graft, and rapid onset of inosculation. In imbibition, the graft absorbs nutrients from the host bed, and this phase lasts approximately 48 h. Inosculation involves reestablishment of vascularization to the graft by anastomosis of the exposed vessels of the host bed with the vessels of the graft. This phase is usually complete by 96 h.

Another possible reason for the good success of free graft with preputial flap may be the result of improved inosculation because the graft is sandwiched between two well-vascularized beds. The vascular pedicle also covers the repair, and this is a well-accepted technique in reducing the rate of fistula formation.

The use of the free graft repair may be relatively contraindicated when chordee is severe and a tunica vaginalis or dermal graft is required to bridge the defect created by incision of the tunica albuginea to accomplish penile straightening. In this situation, the host bed may be unsatisfactory to support imbibition and inosculation. Patients who have had previous failed hypospadias repairs may similarly have an unsatisfactory host bed and blood supply to allow graft survival.

Buccal Mucosa Graft

Humby was the first to propose and report the use of buccal mucosa for hypospadias repair in 1941. However, the current enthusiasm for the technique was promoted by Duckett (1986). The technique clearly has a definitive role for complex urethral reconstruction, and indeed, the short-term success is so encouraging that the threshold for its use is becoming lower all the time, to the point where primary buccal graft surgery may be appropriate in some circumstances when skin resources are limited, allowing their preservation for good vascularized coverage of the penile shaft.

Buccal mucosa lines the vestibule of the mouth, which is the space between the teeth and the cheek inside the mouth. A cut section of the cheek consists, from inside out, of mucosa (epithelium), submucosa (lamina propria), musculosa (buccinator muscle), subcutaneous fat and fascia (vessels and nerves) and the skin. The function of the buccal mucosa is a direct result of its structure. A tight spinosum layer and pump-functioning cells of the superficial layer provide protection from the foreign substances placed in the oral cavity. Elastin and collagen without bony attachment give the buccal mucosa flexibility and the ability to distend and compress. A rapid turnover rate and highly vascularized lamina propria ensure quick healing after injury. The immune response is quickly aided by a lamina propria laden with lymphocytes and macrophages. Many surgeons, after harvesting the buccal mucosa graft, leave the donor area without closure, because in reality it is too large to close without disfigurement.

Manzoni and Ransley (1999) have vast experience with buccal mucosa grafts, extending to more than 100 cases with more than 5 years' follow-up. The following is their description of the operative technique:

> Buccal mucosa may be used as an onlay patch, as a complete mucosal tube, or in various ways combined with other free graft tissue (bladder mucosa) or vascularized skin. It may be harvested from the inner surface of the cheek or the inner surface of the upper or lower lip (Fig. 22.2). For a single strip of buccal mucosa for use as an onlay patch, the adult cheek provides up to 6 cm and the lip 4 cm at 12–15 mm of width. [Ransley did not recommend extending the strip through the angle of the mouth to combine both cheek and lip segments as this may cause significant contracture at the angle of the mouth.]
>
> The strips of buccal mucosa obtained cannot be tubularized lengthwise to create 6-cm tubes, because the width is insufficient. They can be folded lengthwise to provide shorter tubes of up to 3 cm and 2 cm,

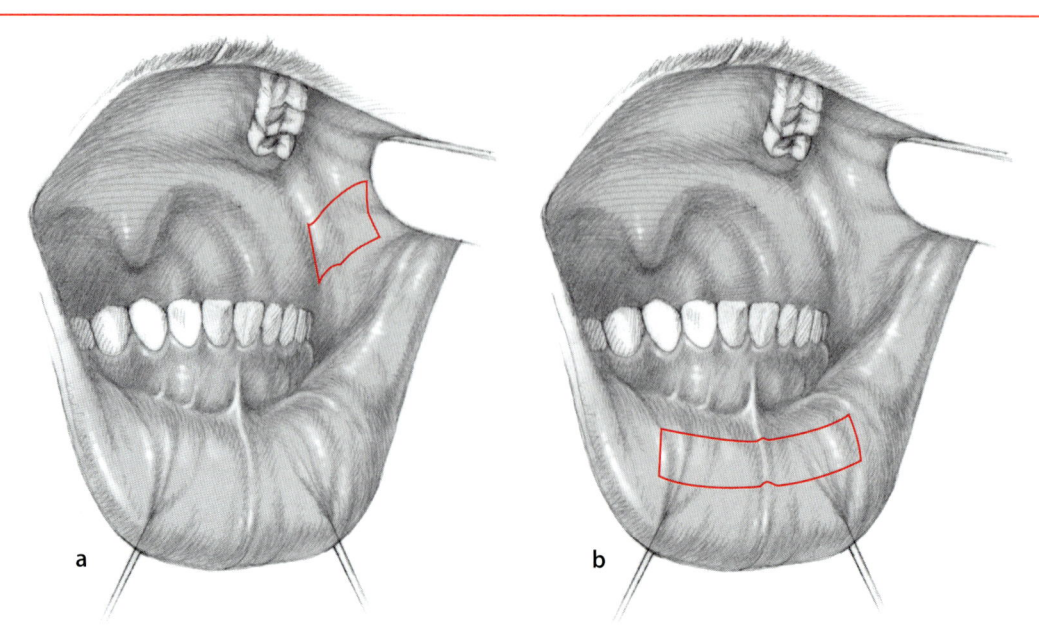

Fig. 22.2a, b. Harvesting of buccal mucosa

respectively, or a second graft of similar dimensions, can be applied to create a full-length cylinder of adequate diameter. When some vascularized preputial skin is available but is insufficient for tubularization, a strip may be usefully combined with buccal mucosa to form a compound neourethra. In very long urethral reconstructions, bladder mucosa may be used successfully for the proximal urethra, reserving buccal mucosa for the distal element and meatus.

Surgical Technique

For a right-handed surgeon standing on the right side of the patient, the lower lip and the left cheek are the most convenient donor sites. If the requirements for the buccal tissue are clear beforehand, the buccal mucosa may be obtained before commencing penile dissection to allow an elegant uninterrupted repair that benefits the penile tissue. Otherwise, the previous repair must be dismantled, the need for buccal mucosa assessed, and the graft obtained in midprocedure.

If a single strip of mucosa is required, the current preference is to use the left cheek as the mucosal layer because this site is thicker and more robust than the mucosa of the lip, and the donor site may be sutured. However, in terms of outcome, there is probably little difference between cheek and lip.

For cheek harvest, a suitable mouth retractor, such as the Boyle-Davis, with various sizes of tongue depressor blades, is very convenient. Additional stay sutures are placed on the mucocutaneous junction at the angle of the mouth. The parotid duct usually is easy to identify opposite the upper molars, and it may be cannulated with a short length of 3-0 nylon to identify it through the dissection and closure. The graft is outlined with a waterproof pen, and the submucosa infiltrated with 1% lignocaine containing 1:2000 epinephrine. After waiting for some minutes, the parallel upper and lower borders of the graft are incised. These incisions are then sharply angled to meet at the external limit near the angle of the mouth. One or two stay sutures are then placed to lift the graft toward the mouth cavity, and the mucosa is dissected away by sharp dissection. Buccinator muscle inserts directly into the mucosa, and careful dissection with a knife or sharp-pointed scissors is necessary to free the mucosa. Finally, the internal limit is incised and the graft is free. Diathermy usually is not needed, and the defect is closed with an absorbable 5-0 suture such as chromic catgut. No further local treatment is usually necessary, and patients may eat at once.

Lip harvest is simpler. A series of stay sutures is used to evert the lower lip and to protect the mucocutaneous junction. After epinephrine infiltration and the appropriate delay, the parallel incisions are made transversely, leaving the graft attached at either end. The mucosa (which is a little more delicate than the cheek and prone to tear) is elevated using fine tapered scissors in a manner similar to that used when creating a submucosal tunnel. Finally, the graft is released at either end and removed. The bare area is not sutured but may be packed with a temporary swab soaked in epinephrine until the end of the procedure. Healing is rapid and complete, and the scar is virtually invisible within 2 to 3 weeks.

The graft tissue is placed in a pot of normal saline for temporary storage while surgery in the mouth is completed. It is then pinned out, face down on a cork or Silastic block for preparation. Excess submucosal tissue and salivary glands are removed by sharp dissection. After a change of gloves, the graft may be deployed in various ways.

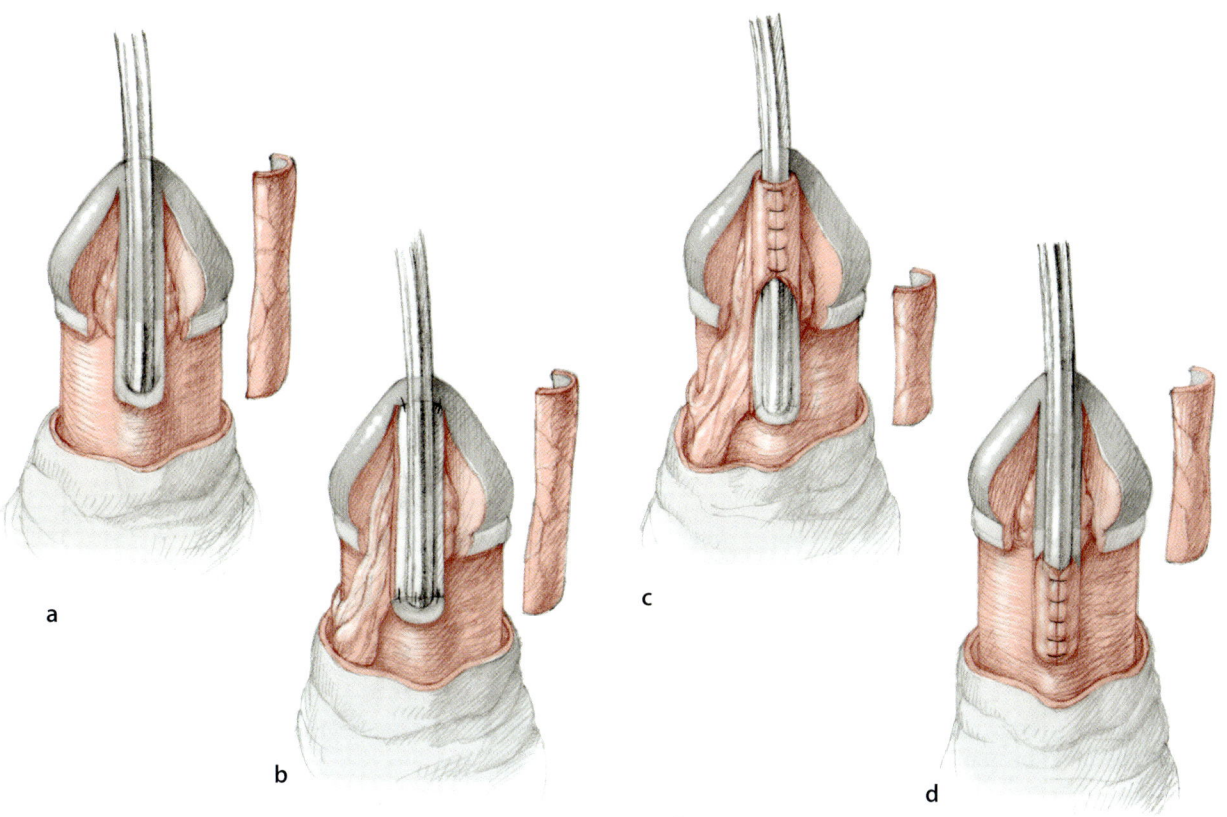

Fig. 22.3a–d. Some methods of urethral reconstruction using buccal mucosa

Onlay Patch

The urethral plate or previously reconstructed urethra is retained as a midline strip extending forward from the normal native urethra to the glans. This strip varies in width from a few millimeters to 1 cm. The native urethra is incised for at least 1 cm proximally to create a spatulated junction. The graft is trimmed to an appropriate length and width and anastomosed to the margins of the urethral strip using 6-0 or 7-0 polyglycolic acid sutures. Glans wings are wrapped around to provide a terminal meatus. A two-layer closure of well-vascularized penile skin is advised.

Tube Urethroplasty

Using either a folded graft or two segments of buccal mucosa as previously discussed, a mucosal tube is created of sufficient length to bridge the urethral defect. The proximal anastomosis is well spatulated, and glans wings are preferable to a tunnel for creation of the terminal meatus. Two-layer skin closure follows.

Compound Tube

A compound tube technique is valuable when some preputial skin remains after earlier surgery but is insufficient for tube urethroplasty on its own. The preputial skin strip is mobilized on its own vascular pedicle, and the buccal graft anastomosed to create the compound tube. This is placed in position on the ventral surface of the penis, with the vascularized skin lying against the corporal surface and the buccal mucosa lying superficially to be covered by a two-layer closure of penile skin (Fig. 22.3).

Clinical Experience and Results

Buccal mucosa is proving very satisfactory as a material for urethral reconstruction, particularly in hypospadias cripples who have undergone multiple previous procedures. It must be recognised that only short-term (5 years) follow-up has been reported. The frequency of meatal problems and urethral dilatation and ballooning is much less than with bladder mucosa.

It may be that growth factors within the mucosa promote rapid healing and that revascularisation occurs quickly because of the thin lamina propria and the originally highly vascular bed from which the buccal mucosa graft was taken.

Most surgeons experience indicate a secondary operation rate of approximately 20% (Manzoni and

Ransley 1999), mostly due to minor fistulas or the need for meatal revision. In difficult cases, preoperative testosterone treatment may improve the vascularity of the penile skin and thereby enhance the chances of success with a free graft technique.

Bladder Mucosal Grafts

The use of bladder mucosa for the repair of the urethra in hypospadias was first described by Memmelaar in 1947. He discussed the benefits of a one-stage hypospadias repair and the favorable characteristics of bladder mucosa in the reconstruction of the male urethra. Bladder mucosal grafts were used extensively in China in the late 1970s for one-stage hypospadias repairs. During the past decade, bladder mucosal grafts have been used rather extensively in one-stage repair of hypospadias and urethral stricture disease. Problems with stricture at the proximal anastomosis, along with fistulas and mucosal glanular protrusion, caused several investigators to devise ways of decreasing the complication rate. Duffy and associates (1988) used a tube of bladder mucosa combined with penile or preputial skin distally to avoid the mucosal protrusion problem. Other techniques have been described to decrease the incidence of mucosal protrusion and meatal stenosis by cutting the bladder mucosa flush with the glans or even undercutting the glans epithelium and invaginating it into the new meatus. When used as a free tube graft in the posterior or bulbar urethra for urethral stricture disease, bladder mucosa has been shown to work well.

Surgical Technique

Any prior failed tube graft tissue must be excised, and it may be necessary to freshen the proximal edge of the native meatus to reach well-vascularised tissue. Once the bed for the graft has been prepared and checked for good vascularity, the gap is then measured from the native meatus to the tip of the glans tunnel. Attention is then turned to the harvest of the bladder mucosal graft. The bladder is distended with saline so that it is palpable above the symphysis pubis. A Pfannenstiel incision is then performed to expose the underlying bladder. If the patient has had a previous suprapubic cystostomy, this site is avoided because of increased difficulty in obtaining a graft secondary to fibrosis. The detrusor muscle is then incised down to the underlying mucosa with a knife or blunt-tipped scissors. Once dissection reveals the bulging blue mucosa, further blunt dissection allows

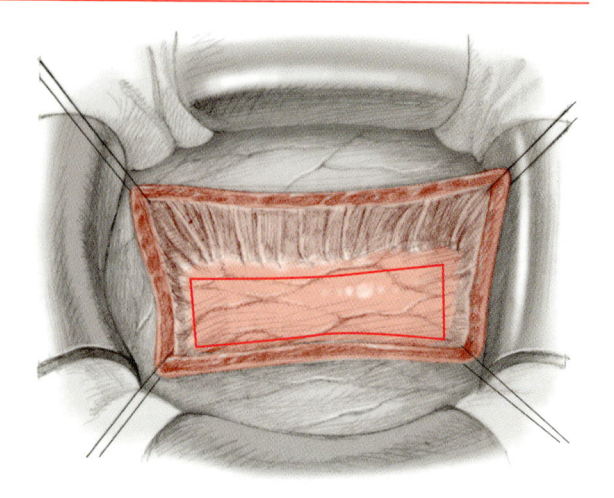

Fig. 22.4. Harvesting bladder mucosa for urethral reconstruction

separation of the detrusor muscle off the mucosa for a distance adequate to harvest the appropriate-sized graft. If the mucosa is inadvertently opened before obtaining an adequate graft, the bladder can be opened and the mucosa dissected off the detrusor (Fig. 22.4). However, this is much more tedious. Once an appropriate-sized area of bladder mucosa is exposed, it is marked with a sterile pencil, stay sutures of 7-0 polyglactin are placed at each corner, and the graft is harvested. A suprapubic cystostomy tube is placed, and the bladder is closed in one layer with no attempt to oppose the mucosa.

The bladder mucosal graft is then tubularised over an appropriate-sized catheter using a running, inverting 7-0 polyglactin suture with interrupted sutures on one end to facilitate size trimming of the tube graft without violating the running suture. Long grafts are augmented with a second layer of interrupted sutures. Tubularisation can be facilitated by placing the graft on a polystyrene needle board and immobilising it at the ends with 30-gauge needles. The graft is kept moist with cool normal saline until reimplantation. A wide, spatulated anastomosis is performed between the tube graft and recipient urethra with 6-0 or 7-0 running polyglactin suture. The graft suture line is placed dorsally against the corpora to avoid overlapping suture lines and thus decrease the chance of fistula formation. The graft can be anchored to the corpora at several points to decrease the risk that shear effect might compromise graft take. The distal end of the graft is then brought through the glans, and the bladder mucosa is cut flush with the glans edge while keeping the graft on stretch to avoid redundancy at the tip. The graft edge is then sutured to the glans with interrupted 6-0 or 7-0 polyglactin sutures. An appropriate urethral catheter or stent is placed for drainage, along with the suprapubic cystostomy tube (Malecot catheter). The graft is covered with at least two layers of well-vascularised tissue such as tunica vaginalis, including skin. Alternatively, bladder mucosa at the tip of the glans may be avoided by either tubularising the distal skin strip of the glans as described by King (1970) or combining the bladder mucosal graft with a strip of penile skin as described by Duffy and associates (1988). The penile or preputial skin may be closed using Byars flaps. The urethral and suprapubic catheters are connected to gravity drainage, and the penis is secured to the anterior abdominal wall with dressing to immobilise it and enhance graft take. In postpubertal patients, diazepam or oestrogen can be used to prevent erection in the postoperative period. The urethral catheter is removed on the 12th to 14th postoperative day, and the suprapubic tube capped. Once the voiding trial is deemed successful, the suprapubic catheter can be removed.

Results

In Keating and coworkers' (1990) extensive review of the literature related to bladder mucosa grafts, an overall complication rate of 40% was found. Two thirds of these complications were minor, with little or no treatment being deemed necessary. The majority of complications involve protrusion of the graft mucosa at the meatus with or without stricture. This troublesome complication has been dealt with in numerous ways, including cutting the graft flush at the glans tip, avoiding any redundancy. Others have proposed undercutting the glans epithelium and laying the edge into the distal anastomosis. Early and frequent dilatations of the neomeatus have also been proposed to help avoid stenosis. The problem with exposed bladder mucosa at the meatus is that it becomes hypertrophic, and metaplastic changes occur. Prevention of mucosal protrusion is the key to management. If mucosal protrusion or stenosis does occur, revision is necessary. Stricture at the proximal anastomosis or fistula can occur with free or vascularised flaps of all types. Urethral diverticulum of the graft tissue can occur if redundant tissue is not excised or distal obstruction is present. Stricture of the proximal or distal end of the graft may be treated with dilation or internal urethrotomy. Although bladder mucosa grafts have had a relatively high incidence of minor complications in the early postoperative period, they have succeeded well in the long run. Bladder mucosa is a good graft tissue for the urethra and has been shown by many investigators to work well.

Editorial Comments

The recent resurgence of interest in buccal mucosa has been fuelled because of its ease of harvest, thickened epithelium, and thin lamina propria when compared with bladder mucosa. Moreover, the fact that the bladder need not be opened makes the morbidity of surgery for buccal mucosal grafts less than that involved in obtaining bladder mucosa.

References

Devine CJ Jr, Horton CE: A one-stage hypospadias repair. J Urol. 1961; 85:166.

Devine CJ Jr, Horton CE: Hypospadias repair. J Urol. 1977; 118:188.

Duckett JW (quoted in Duckett et al): Proceedings of the Annual Meeting of the Society of Paediatric Urological Surgeons. Southampton, UK, 3 June 1986.

Duckett JW, Baskin LS: Hypospadias. In: Gillenwater JY, Grayhack JT, Howards SS, Duckett JW (eds): Adult and pediatric urology, 3rd edn. Mosby-Year Book, St Louis, 1996.

Duckett JW, Coplen D, Ewalt D, et al: Buccal mucosal urethral replacement. J Urol. 1995; 153:1660.

Duffy PG, Ransley PG, Malone PS, et al: Combined free autologous bladder mucosa/skin tube for urethral reconstruction: an update. Br J Urol. 1988; 61:505.

Hendren WH, Reda EF: Bladder mucosa graft for construction of male urethra. J. Pediatr Surg. 1986; 21:189.

Hendren WH, Horton CE Jr: Experience with one-stage repair of hypospadias and chordee using free graft of prepuce. J Urol 1988; 140:1259.

Humby GA: A one stage operation for hypospadias. Br J Surg. 1941; 29:84.

Keating MA, Cartwright PC, Duckett JW: Bladder mucosa in urethral reconstructions. J Urol. 1990; 144:827.

King LR: Hypospadias – a one stage repair without skin graft based on a new principle: chordee is sometimes produced by the skin alone. J Urol. 1970; 103:660-662

Manzoni GM, Ransley PG: Buccal mucosa graft for hypospadias. In: Ehrlich RM, Alter GJ (ed): Reconstructive and plastic surgery of the external genitalia: adult and pediatric. Saunders, Philadelphia, pp 121-125; 1999

Memmelaar J: Use of bladder mucosa in a one-stage repair of hypospadias. J Urol. 1947; 58:68.

Mollard P, Mouriquand P, Bringeon G, et al: Repair of hypospadias using bladder mucosal graft in 76 cases. J Urol. 1989; 142:1548.

Nove-Josserand G: Traitement de l'hypospadias; nouvelle method. Lyon Med. 1897; 85:198.

Ransley PG, Duffy PG, Oesch IL, et al: Autologous bladder mucosa graft for urethral substitution. Br J Urol. 1987a; 59:331.

Ransley PG, Duffy PG, Oesch IL, et al: The use of bladder mucosa and combined bladder mucosa/preputial skin grafts for urethral reconstruction. J Urol. 1987b; 138:1096.

Rober PE, Perlmutter AD, Reitelman C: Experience with 81 one-stage hypospadias/chordee repair using free-graft urethroplasties. J Urol 1990. 144:526.

Scherz H: Preputial graft in hypospadias. In: Ehrlich RM, Alter GJ (ed): Reconstructive and plastic surgery of the external genitalia: adult and pediatric. WB Saunders, Philadelphia, pp 83-86; 1999.

Vyas PR, Roth DR, Perlmutter AD: Experience with free grafts in urethral reconstruction. J Urol. 1987; 137:471.

Webster GD, Brown MW, Koefoot RJ Jr, et al.: Suboptimal results in full thickness skin graft urethroplasty using an extrapenile skin donor site. J Urol. 1984; 131:1082.

Young F, Benjamin W: Preschool-age repair of hypospadias with free inlay skin grafts. Surgery. 1949; 26:384.

23 Two-Stage Urethroplasty

Madan Samuel, Patrick G. Duffy

Free Full-Thickness Wolfe Graft

Introduction

The first recorded case of staged hypospadias repair was that by Nové-Josserand in 1897. However, Humby (1941) must be credited for his reference to the use of skin grafts and that of buccal mucosa in the reconstruction of the urethra. Cloutier (1962) described a modified Denis-Browne repair where the glans was split and lined with full-thickness Wolfe graft of preputial skin at the first stage, thereby allowing the neourethra to be advanced to the tip of the glans at the second stage. Various authors have introduced technical modifications of the use of full-thickness Wolfe skin graft since 1955 (Byars 1955; Nicolle 1976; Rabinovitch 1988; Turner-Warwick 1979; Webster et al. 1984; Zhong-Chu et al. 1981). It was Turner-Warwick in 1979 who used the two-stage urethroplasty for adult salvage surgery and produced impressive results. Subsequently, Rabinovitch and Bracka have resurrected the two-stage hypospadias repair and have popularised this technique not only for retrieving failed hypospadias repairs but also as an alternative technique for primary hypospadias (Bracka 1995a, b; Rabinovitch 1988).

Graft Material and Biology

The free-graft material initially thrives by imbibition (diffusion of nutrients between the donor and recipient sites) and this phase lasts for 48 h. During this period inosculation occurs where new blood vessels are formed to nourish the graft. The second phase of graft revascularisation occurs between day 2 and 4. Blood recirculation is re-established to the graft, and by day 4–5 lymphatic drainage is restored. Ideally, the donor material should allow these processes to occur efficiently, and this is helped by graft immobilisation for 7–10 days.

Full-Thickness Skin Free Graft (Wolfe)

The characteristics essential for long-term success of a free graft are efficient imbibition and inosculation, which ensures successful neovascularisation and graft uptake. Full-thickness skin from non-hair-bearing areas such as (in order of the authors' preference) inner preputial skin, penile shaft and post-auricular skin have been used with success. Groin and upper arm skin have also been successfully grafted.

Although full-thickness skin grafts have a high success rate for urethral reconstruction, there are related complications such as stricture formation, graft shrinkage, balanitis xerotica obliterans (BXO) and hypertrophic scar formation at the donor site (Bracka 1989, 1995a, b; Humby 1941; Snodgrass 1994). Moreover, preputial or penile shaft skin may not be available in patients in whom complications from previous surgery have resulted in paucity of usable adjacent skin or in those with severe reconstructive problems.

Buccal Mucosa Free Graft

Based on clinical experience the buccal mucosa is an ideal material for urethral reconstruction when there is a paucity of local skin. Studies on the healing of grafted buccal mucosa and underlying lamina propria suggest that a similar process occurs as in bladder mucosa graft, wherein the graft undergoes partial degeneration and desquamation, followed by complete epithelial regeneration from the basal layer (Duckett et al. 1995; Fairbanks et al. 1992; Ombrédanne 1932). This is in contrast to skin grafts, which maintain an intact epithelial layer throughout graft healing (Duckett et al. 1995; Fairbanks et al. 1992; Ombrédanne 1932). Hence the basal layer has the capability to regenerate the epithelium. The graft connective tissue is organised by 21 days. The buccal mucosa is probably similar to the bladder lamina propria and urothelium grafts in that it is unstable before complete epithelialisation, which occurs at 10–14 days, implying that the duration of graft stenting is critical and should be at least 7–10 days.

Immunohistochemistry using antibody to type IV collagen, which stains the basement membrane, has shown a vascular lamina propria, which allows efficient angiogenesis and inosculation between donor and recipient, explaining the excellent uptake of buccal mucosa (Dessanti et al. 1992; Duckett et al. 1995; Fairbanks et al. 1992). Imbibition is efficient due to the relative thinness of the lamina propria (Dessanti et al. 1992; Fairbanks et al. 1992).

There is abundance of healthy tissue, which can be harvested with ease from the inner cheeks. However, if a long strip of buccal mucosa is required it is preferable to harvest two strips, one from each cheek, and avoid crossing over the angle of the mouth to the lower lip. Long buccal mucosa graft harvested from the inner cheek to the lower lip usual results in scarring and deformity of the angle of the mouth. Due to the lack of luminal support of the corpus spongiosum, ballooning of the mucosal neourethra during voiding is a common occurrence. However, the elastin-rich connective tissue of the basement tissue of the buccal mucosa is relatively stiff and provides good scaffolding and prevents the occurrence of a diffuse diverticulum. Increased elastin infiltration of the buccal mucosa may explain its resilience and ease of harvest and suturing (Culp and McRoberts 1968; Dessanti et al. 1992). Buccal mucosa, unlike the bladder mucosa, does not have the propensity for prolapse. The neomeatus remains as a vertical slit, providing a good aesthetic appearance, and functionally there should be no urinary stream problems. Composite grafts of buccal mucosa and free skin graft, especially for the distal meatus, have shown improved results with regard to the adequacy of the neomeatus, good cosmesis by retaining the natural vertical glanular meatus configuration and a good-calibre, straight urinary flow in the forward direction. The main disadvantage of the buccal mucosa graft is the thick epithelial layer, which may explain its relative stiffness.

Bladder Mucosa

The bladder lamina propria and urothelium is well established as a mucosa free graft for single-stage hypospadias repair. The graft biology has been elucidated in the New Zealand white rabbit and dogs (Duckett et al. 1995; Ombrédanne 1932), and the urothelium is well suited for contact with urine (Byars 1955; Cloutier 1962; Dessanti et al. 1992; Johnson and Coleman 1998; Klijn et al. 2000; Turner-Warwick 1979). However, its use in a staged urethroplasty is not feasible as the bladder mucosa has the propensity to develop severe oedema on exposure to air. It is therefore not suitable for staged urethroplasty and there are no reports of its use in a two-stage hypospadias repair.

Operative Technique

Surgery is performed under general anaesthesia supplemented by a local bupivacaine caudal block. The authors do not use a tourniquet or infiltrate tissues with vasoconstrictors. The aspects of age of repair, magnification and psychological support have been detailed in other chapters.

First Stage

The first-stage is crucial as it lays the foundation for the performance of a straight, aesthetic and normally functioning penis in the second stage. This stage involves chordee correction, harvesting of the graft, laying down and anchoring of the graft and immobilisation of the graft by an appropriate dressing (Figs. 23.1, 23.2, 23.3, 23.4).

Degloving and Chordee Correction ▸ A Firlitt cuff is created and the penis is degloved. Dorsally the dissection is above Buck's fascia, and on the ventral aspect the urethral plate, the inelastic dysplastic Buck's fascia and the corpus spongiosum overlying the corpus cavernosa are excised (Fig. 23.1a). It is empirical that the glistening tunica albuginea of the corpora cavernosa is free of fibrous tissue. If necessary, the urethra may have to be mobilised (especially in "re-do" surgery for failed hypospadias surgery) by dissecting fibrous tissue and/or laterally diverging vascular spongy bands of aberrant corpus spongiosum laterally and dorsally. As a consequence the meatus may move to a proximal position. A ventral meatotomy is performed so that the meatus readily accepts a size 14/15 Clutton sound. Distally the incision in the glans is deepened to within 2–3 cm of the dorsal surface so as to facilitate a cleft in the glans. Glanular clefting must be deep enough to clearly visualise and demarcate the distal corpora cavernosa (Fig. 23.1b). This manoeuvre of clefting the glans is conducive to a satisfactory glandular reconstruction in the second stage. The dorsal limit of the incision at the tip of the glans corresponds to the dorsal aspect of the future external urethral meatus.

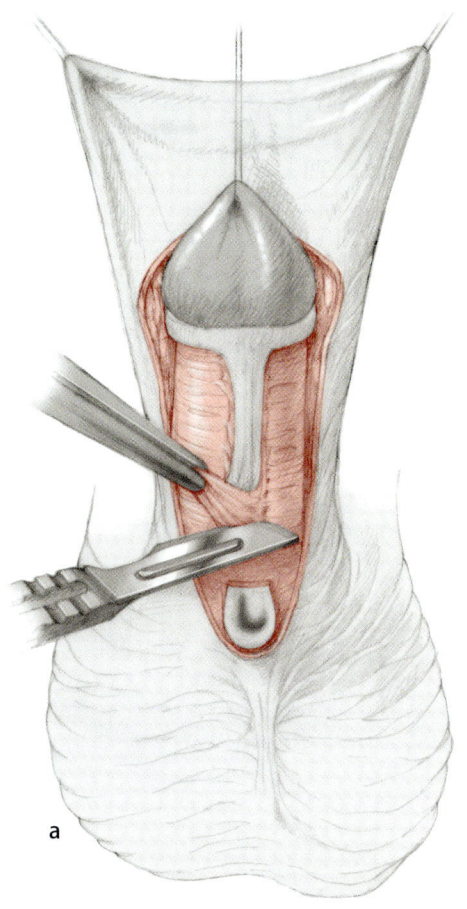

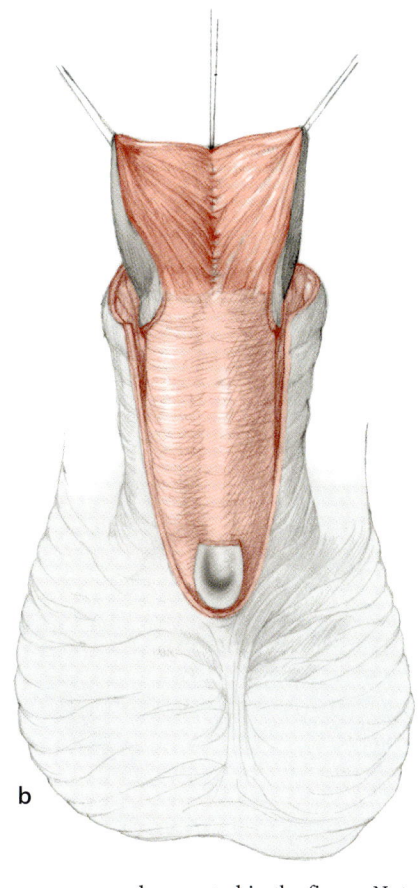

Fig. 23.1. a Proximal hypospadias. Excision of urethral plate and all fibrous tissue. **b** Ventrally, clefting of the glans should be deep enough to clearly visualise the distal ends of the corpora cavernosa as demarcated in the figure. Note all fibrous tissue is excised to leave a glistening tunica albuginea

The adequacy of chordee correction is then examined by means of an artificial erection (Fig. 23.2a–c). If there is persistence of penile chordee despite transecting the ventral tunica albuginea to gain further length, one of the various techniques of chordee correction is adopted as shown in Fig. 23.2b, c.

Harvesting of Graft ▶ A full-thickness inner preputial Wolfe skin graft of appropriate dimensions is harvested from the dorsal hooded foreskin. Obviously, if a large graft is necessary, the distal portion will either be preputial skin or composite grafts using a combination of inner preputial skin, postauricular skin and buccal mucosa. The inner prepuce is tacked down to a silicon block or wooden board, or alternatively the graft can be defatted over the back of a finger, to remove all surplus subcutaneous fat and alveolar tissue. This results in a thin translucent membrane (Fig. 23.5). The flexible nature of the inner prepuce allows ease of configuration of a short wide graft into the required length and width to cover the ventral defect. However, if the area is larger than the graft harvested, other skin donor sites can be used in conjunction with or instead of the prepuce. The other preferred site is the postauricular Wolfe graft, which is relatively thin, pliable and non-hairy and leaves an inconspicuous donor scar (Fig. 23.6). Buccal mucosa is a good urethral substitute due to its versatility and infrequency of complications, especially when BXO is a complication of previous repairs with skin grafts.

Buccal mucosa is harvested from the inner cheek or a combination of inner cheek and inner lip (Fig. 23.7). Stensen's duct, located below the second to third molar, should not be injured and the buccinator muscle should be left in situ, harvesting only the buccal mucosa and its lamina propria. Careful thinning of the graft is empirical, removing all fat and skeletal tissue inadvertently dissected from the inner cheek. Primary closure using polyglactin (5-0 or 6-0) is necessary for the defect in the inner cheek.

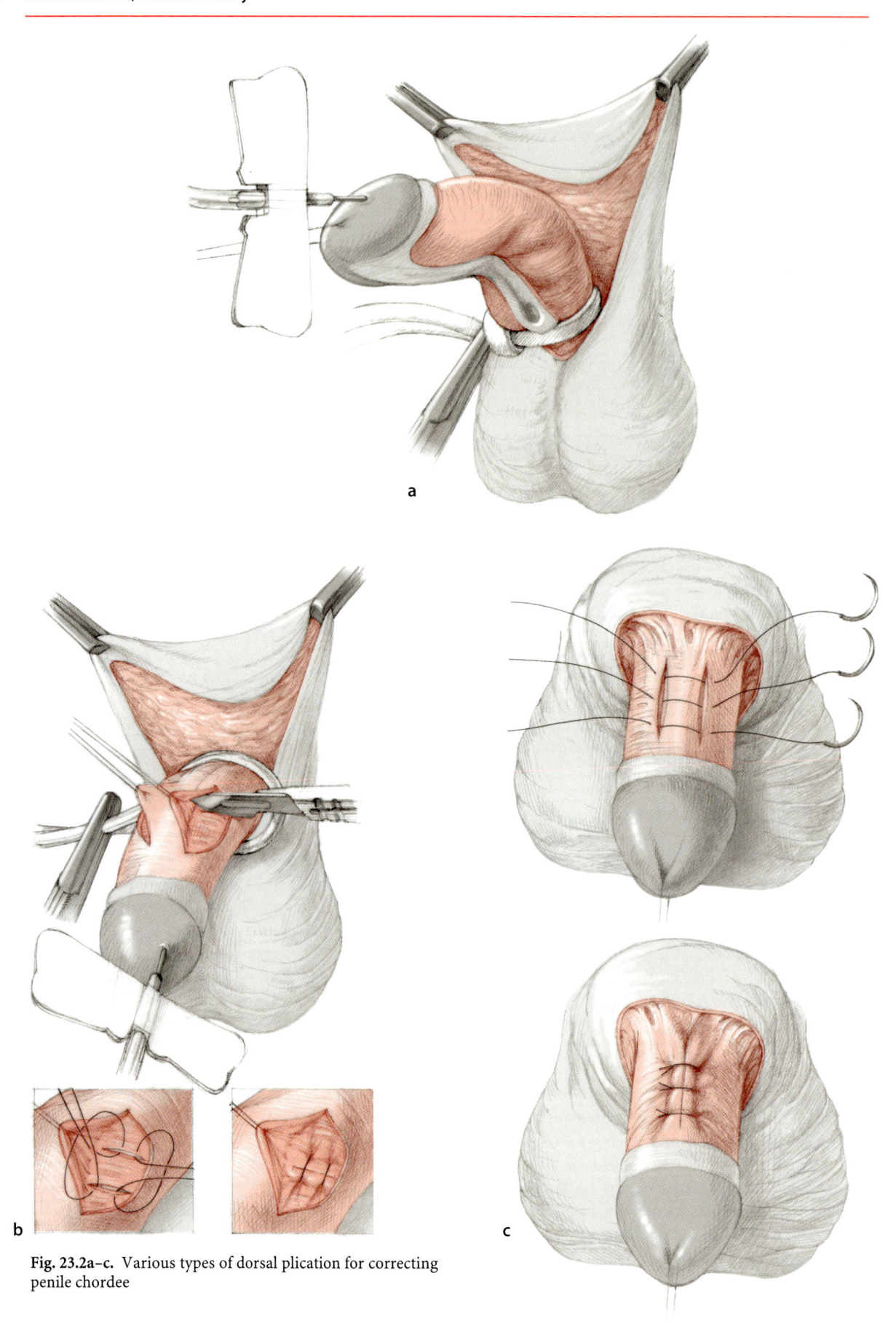

Fig. 23.2a–c. Various types of dorsal plication for correcting penile chordee

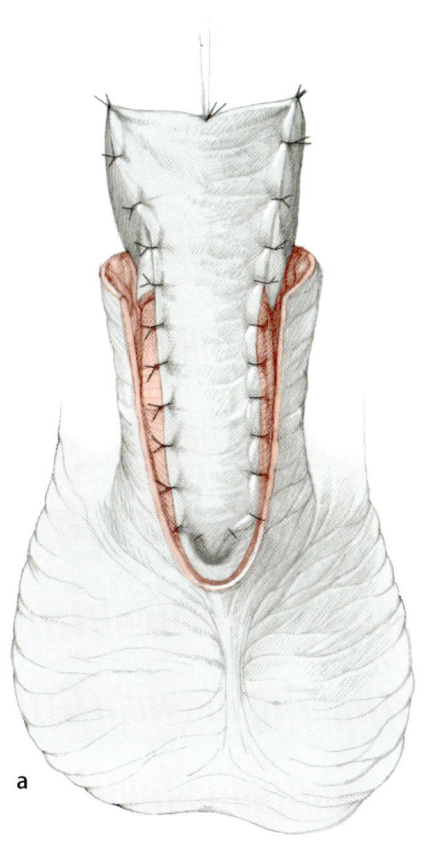

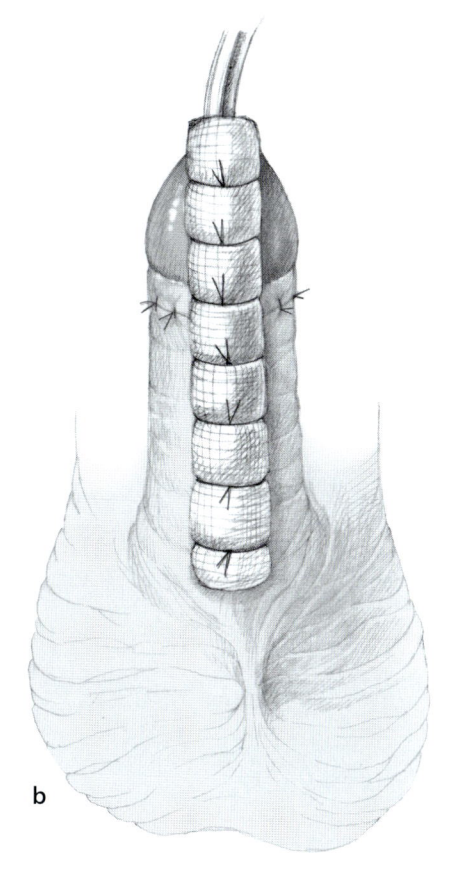

Fig. 23.3. a Wolfe skin graft accurately tailored to the defect with a V-shaped inset of the graft into the back wall of the urethral meatus. The dimensions of the graft should not be overgenerous; the graft should fit snugly into the ventral defect and should not heap up into folds. **b** Graft immobilised with a 'tie-over' pressure dressing prior to compressive foam dressing

However, if the graft is harvested from the inner lip, effective healing occurs by secondary intention without the need for primary closure.

Laying the Graft to the Graft Bed ▶ The glans is held apart by lateral stay sutures and the graft is accurately laid down with a V-shaped inset of the graft into the back wall of the urethral meatus to reduce the possibility of subsequent anastomotic stricture (◉ Figs. 23.3a, 23.8). The graft is then sutured to the margins of the graft bed by using interrupted 7-0 polydioxanone·(Ethicon, PDS II, Johnson & Johnson) monofilament absorbable suture. Tailoring of the graft to the recipient bed should be performed meticulously and all excess graft tissue trimmed so as to prevent an overgenerous graft. The graft should rest freely on the graft bed and should stretch out snugly without heaping into folds. If the graft is of significant length, a few midline-quilting sutures along the shaft will help to avoid shearing of the graft on the wound bed. Lastly, windows are created by either oblique incisions or by substantial pinpricks at regular intervals in the graft. This is essential to prevent haematoma and allow free drainage of oedema of the graft bed, i.e. recipient and donor site.

Immobilisation of the Graft ▶ An 8- or 10-Ch catheter is passed per urethram into the bladder. A roll of tulle-gras or Vaseline gauze of sufficient width and thickness is wound around the catheter so as to ensure that the edges of the glans are well separated. Two lateral stay sutures are used to make the first 'tie-over' and several looped 4-0 nylon sutures pick up the graft and the skin margins along with tunica of the shaft and are tied with knots in the midline. This firm "tie-over" dressing will hold the graft in place and prevent haematoma formation (◉ Fig. 23.3b). A conforming Cavi-care (Smith and Nephew, Hull, UK) foam dressing completed the first stage. Overnight hospital admission is advised for postoperative analgesia.

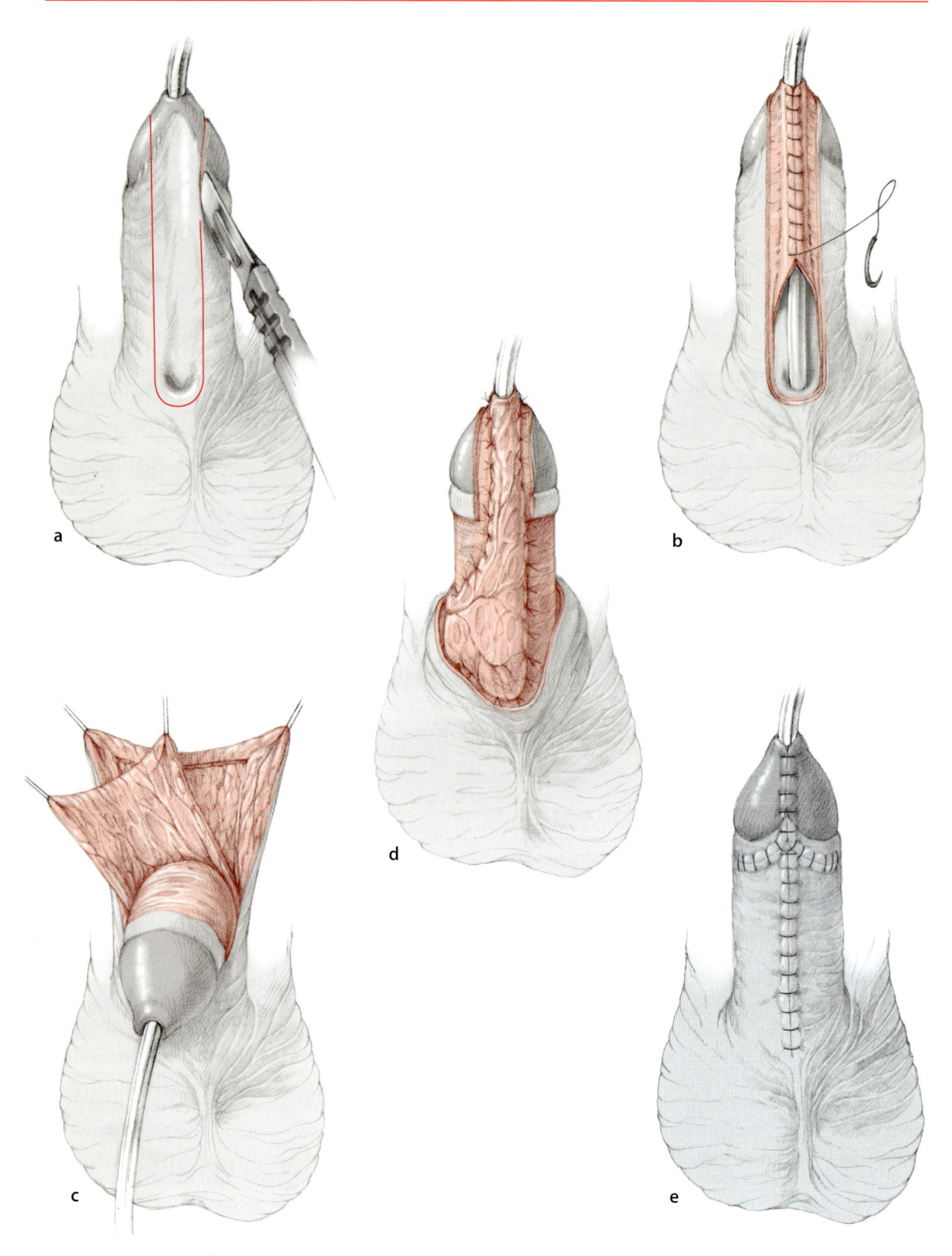

Fig. 23.4. a A U-shaped incision over the graft strip. **b** Shaft skin mobilised before tubing of the neourethra. **c** Harvesting of subcutaneous tissue on a vascularised pedicle for "waterproofing" (subcutaneous tissue harvested from the proximal penile shaft and scrotum). **d** Subcutaneous tissue harvested on its vascular pedicle from the penile shaft skin. **e** Penile skin transposed and completed repair of a circumcised penis

Two-Stage Urethroplasty   231

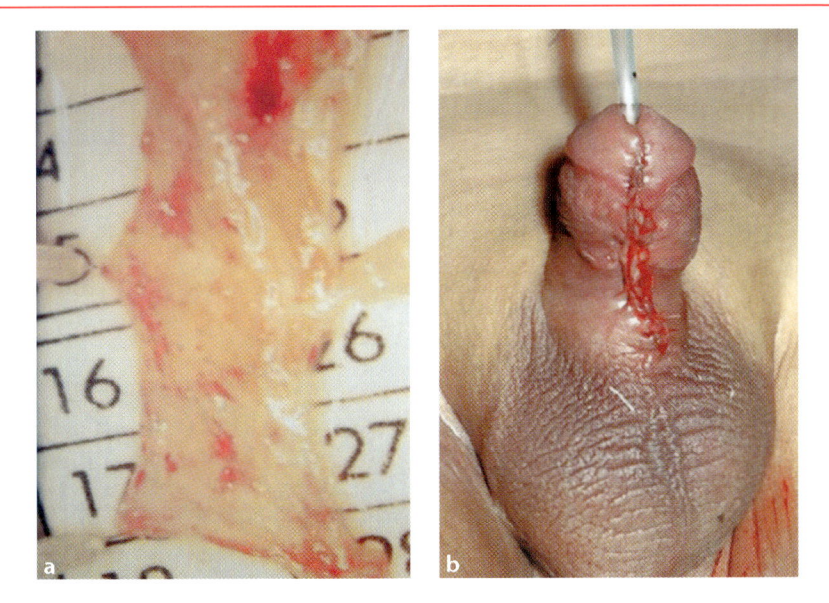

Fig. 23.5. **a** Thin translucent graft. **b** Completed two-stage urethroplasty

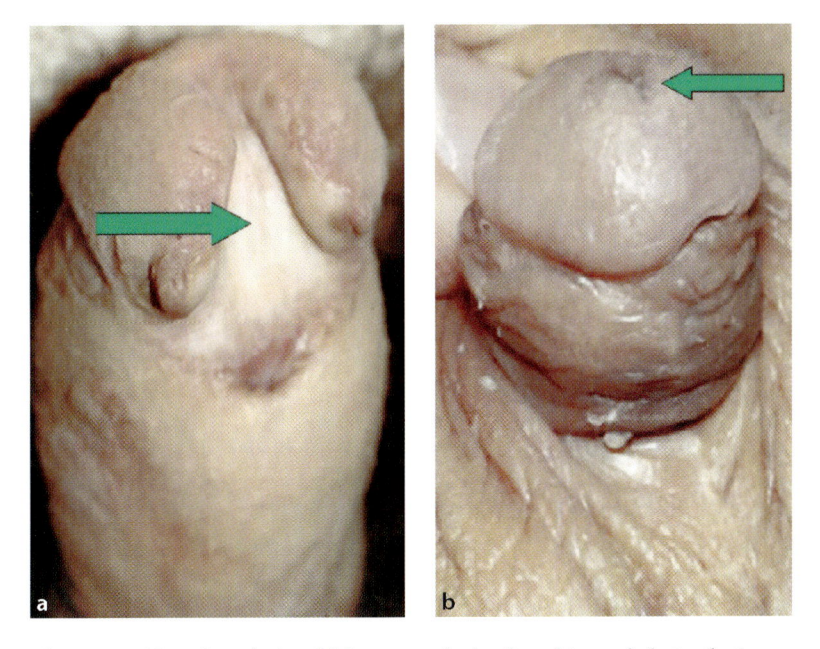

Fig. 23.6. **a** Note the relative thick post-auricular free skin graft. **b** Aesthetic-appearing penis following two-stage repair

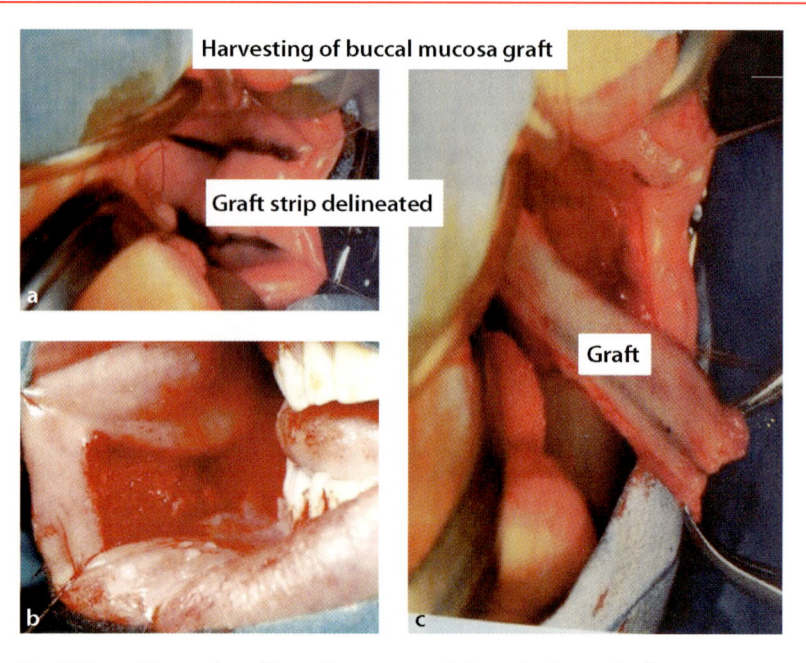

Fig. 23.7a–c. Harvesting of buccal mucosa graft from the inner cheek

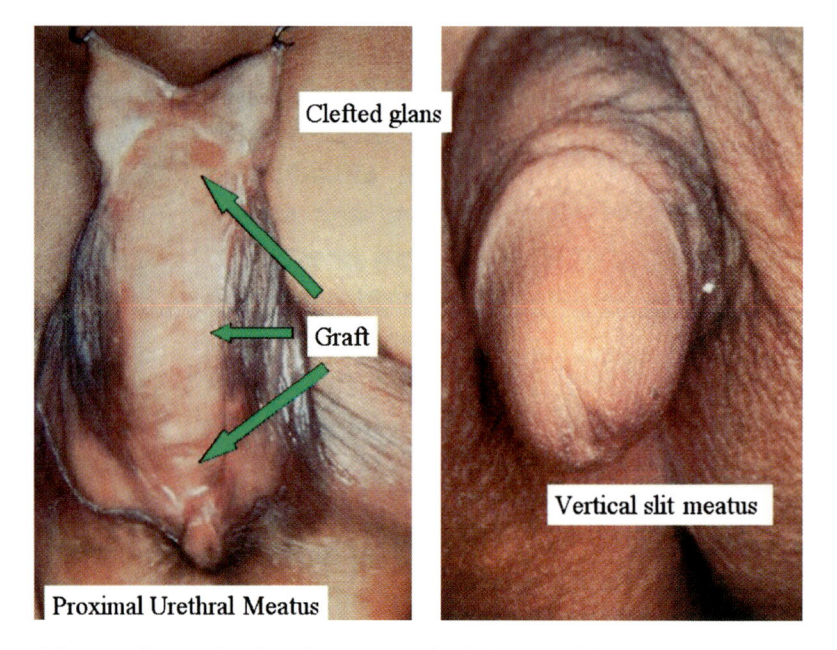

Fig. 23.8. Penoscrotal hypospadias. *Left:* After first stage. The distal end of the corpora cavernosa is clearly demarcated. Glans adequately clefted and skin graft is thin and well healed without folds. Note generous penile shaft skin. *Right:* Six months after the first stage, an aesthetic penis with a vertical slit meatus situated normally on the glans penis

The Cavi-care foam and tie-over dressing are removed along with the catheter under short general anaesthesia on the 10th day. The child is reviewed in the clinic 3 months postoperatively, and the second stage is planned approximately 6 months after the first operation.

Second Stage

A successful graft is smooth, well vascularised and the glans cleft sharply delineated (👁 Figs. 23.5, 23.8). A U-shaped strip of the grafted skin is marked from the ventral limit of the neoexternal urethral glanular meatus with the lower limits of the U skirting closely around the margin of the proximal urethral meatus (👁 Figs. 23.4a, b, 23.8). The size of the tubing should approximate the size of the existing urethra to ensure uniformity of the urethral calibre. The marked urethral strip should be 3 times the diameter of the catheter (8–10 Ch; circumference=π × diameter= approximately 3 times diameter). This is approximately 1.5 cm in a child and 2.5 cm in an adolescent. The marked ventral strip is incised and the subcoronal incision is extended around the dorsal aspect to allow the skin to be mobilised along Buck's fascia down to a level proximal to the ectopic meatus. The isolated graft strip is tubularised around an 8- or 10-Ch catheter without tension by either interrupted or continuous extraluminal inverting 7-0 PDS · monofilament absorbable suture starting at the neoexternal urethral meatus on the glans to the proximal old urethral meatus. Excess width of the graft is excised. A second "water-proofing" layer of proximally based flap of subcutaneous tissue is raised from the penile shaft skin to cover the neourethra. The base of the flap should be adequately mobilised so that it does not tether or twist the penis, and the flap should reach up into the glans split without tension. Alternatively, ventral cover can be achieved by turning up an anteriorly based flap of fascia from the midline scrotal septum. Such flaps, when required, can be configured to contain a vascularised island of midline scrotal skin. The water-proofing layer is anchored in place by 7-0 PDS sutures (👁 Fig. 23.4c, d). The glans wings are mobilised and a triangular wedge of glans tissue excised to obtain a secure glanular approximation. Glans closure is performed by interrupted box stitches using 7-0 PDS or it can be closed in two layers. It is desirable to remove all surplus subcutaneous tissue and excess skin to prevent a bulky unsightly penis. The skin is approximated, and compressive Cavi-care foam dressing completes the second-stage (👁 Fig. 23.4e). The dressing and catheter are removed on the ward on the 7th postoperative day and the child is reviewed in the outpatient clinic at 2 months.

Reconstruction of the Foreskin ▶ The authors prefer to perform a tidy circumcision as excellent cosmesis is achieved (👁 Fig. 23.8). Although a foreskin is often deemed aesthetically desirable in European society, in practice it is difficult to combine normal appearance with normal function. Techniques for preputial skin reconstruction as described by Kljin et al. (2000), or Johnson and Coleman (1998) can be performed to obtain retractile foreskins. The reconstructed foreskin should be retractile and supple so as not to hamper sexual activity in adolescence.

Catheters and Prevention of Erection ▶ Fine silicon catheter diversion per urethram is reliable, probably causes fewer bladder spasms, and is associated with fewer complications than suprapubic drainage. In younger children a dripping silicon stent into the nappy is efficient diversion. In older children and adolescents a urinary bag is required. Postoperative erections are not a significant problem in children, but in postpubertal and adolescent patients an erection is unpleasant and may damage the repair. Cyproterone acetate, 300 mg daily, is helpful in decreasing libido and spontaneous erections. It has a slow onset of action and hence must be started 10 days before surgery. Desipramine, 150 mg daily, has a rapid action and can be used as an adjunct to cyproterone acetate. Application of PR Freeze Spray (Crookes Healthcare, Nottingham, UK) can reverse unwanted erections in an acute situation.

Complications

First stage

To avoid complications and morbidity, attention to details during the first stage of the repair is paramount. Ischaemic necrosis of the graft can occur due to haematoma, rejection of the donor graft by the recipient bed due to an improperly prepared basal layer (the graft is not thinned appropriately and there is excess of subcutaneous or alveolar tissue), and poor graft healing primarily due to ischaemic rejection where the graft has not been sufficiently immobilised for neovascularisation to occur.

Second Stage

The complications published from 1985 to 2000 are summarised in Table 23.1. Following are the long-term complications of two-stage urethroplasty:

1. Urethrocutaneous Fistulae: The incidence of fistulae in the two-stage procedure from the published data is higher in re-do or salvage surgery (Bracka 1995a, b; Humby 1941). The fistula rate in salvage surgery was 10.5–26% versus 3–14% in primary two-stage urethroplasty (P=0.001) (Bracka 1995a, b; Humby 1941; Nové-Josserand 1897). This statistically significantly greater fistula rate for salvage two-stage urethroplasty may be due to the severity of the deformity, complications from recurrent previous redo hypospadias repairs and the type of graft used in the salvage operations. Use of the fibrotic in-situ surrounding skin as the tissue for a free graft in the first stage may contribute to the high incidence of fistulae formation. The use of buccal mucosa graft or composite graft using postauricular skin and buccal mucosa in the first stage may produce better results and lower the complication rate of fistulae and strictures. It is important not to select a graft site that may lead to hair bearing in the long term. It is also possible that a higher fistula rate is seen in the first years of hypospadias surgery as the frequency may be directly correlated with a learning curve. As the surgeon's experience grows, complications become fewer (Bracka 1995a, b; Humby 1941).
2. Strictures: The causes of postoperative urethral strictures are BXO, postoperative wound infection, urinary extravasation into the reconstructed tissue and, in a few cases, idiopathic. The majority of these strictures are amenable to dilatation, but in a few a tight stricture warrants urethral reconstruction. In such cases we recommend the use of buccal mucosal graft (Akporiaye et al. 1995).
3. Balanitis Xerotica Obliterans: BXO is the male genital form of lichen sclerosus et atrophicus. It commonly occurs in preputial and penile shaft skin grafts, while postauricular grafts fare better. There is a significant recurrence rate of BXO in all skin grafts irrespective of the donor site. If BXO occurs, it is advisable to abandon the Wolfe skin graft and reperform the two-stage urethroplasty using buccal mucosa (Akporiaye et al. 1995; Bracka 1989, 1995a, b).

Vascularised Preputial Skin Onlay Graft

Introduction

Bretteville in 1986 gave a comprehensive description of a two-stage urethroplasty, which was essentially a modification of the two-stage Cloutier procedure (Bretteville 1986; Cloutier 1962). The first-stage consisted of preputial onlay graft on a vascularised pedicle following a glans slit. Tubing of the neo-urethra occurs on the Denis Browne principle by 6 months (Browne 1949). The vascularised pedicled inner preputial onlay skin graft should provide a better quality skin than the free graft for the neo-urethra with reduced risk of graft failure or loss of skin compliance. This technique has lately been popularised by Moir and Stevenson with their modification, "the Dundee modification", in an attempt to produce a natural vertical slit meatus and overall superior cosmesis with a lower complication rate (Moir and Stevenson 1996).

Operative Technique (Dundee Modification of the Bretteville Procedure)

First Stage

Following release of chordee an inverted "lacrosse racquet" incision is then performed around the proximal hypospadiac meatus with the "handle" of the "racquet" forming the incision of the glans slit. The glans slit should be radical so as to clearly visualise the distal end of the corpora cavernosa. The proximal urethra should also be mobilised, especially the distal end of the hypospadiac meatus.

A 2-cm transverse incision is made on the inner surface of the dorsal prepuce close to its attachment to the corona. The longitudinal incisions are made extending up and onto the dorsal surface of the prepuce. The length of the vertical flap to be harvested from the inner preputial skin of 2 cm width, based on the superficial dorsal blood vessels, is determined by the severity of the hypospadias. The 2-cm wide flap raised from the inner surface of the dorsal prepuce is advanced ventrally between both halves of the slit glans and the tip is tailored around the proximal meatus with interrupted 7-0 PDS. As the flap is 2-cm wide the tip is 'gathered' during suturing to fit around the meatus. An 8- or 10-Ch catheter is passed per urethram into the bladder. The ventral skin and glans are closed over the flap, which will become the neo-urethra.

As the flap is sutured around the meatus and "gathered" it tends to form a tube (based on the Denis Browne principle). The tubing occurs along the whole length of the neourethral tube and most markedly around the proximal meatus where it is sutured. This tubing becomes more complete as the ventral skin and glans closure progresses distally. The flap must be 2 cm or more in width for the tubing to take place comfortably without the need for suturing. Closure of the ventral skin and glans is performed in three layers. Two inner layers of continuous 5-0 or 6-0 PDS sutures are inserted in the abundant subcuticular tissue. Interrupted horizontal mattress sutures of 6-0 PDS complete the repair. The ends of the subcuticular sutures are left long to secure a tie-over dressing of Jelonet and proflavin wool, which splints the wound.

The catheter is removed at 7 days and the child discharged home following a couple of comfortable voids. The tie-over dressing is removed at 2 weeks in the outpatient clinic.

Second Stage

A simple day-case procedure at 6 months completes the urethroplasty. The base of the flap is divided and inset around the neomeatus. The flap should be incised in an inverted 'V' so as to avoid a circular scar around the meatus, which may predispose to stenosis when it contracts.

Dundee Modification

The main difference in the Dundee modification is that the first stage includes the tubing and covering of the neourethra. The second stage becomes a simpler procedure of division of the base of the flap and meatoplasty. As a result the second stage is day-case surgery and saves a week of hospitalisation (Moir and Stevenson 1996).

Complications

In Moir and Stevenson's series of 40 patients, 70% had distal hypospadias (Moir and Stevenson 1996). Both Bretteville and Moir and Stevenson suggest that the urethroplasty is suitable for all degrees of hypospadias (Bretteville 1986; Moir and Stevenson 1996). This may be due to the fact that the length of the dorsal prepuce is equivalent to the length of the penis in children aged 16–36 months. The flap to be harvested can be extended as far proximally on to the outer preputial surface as required to form a neourethra even in severe proximal hypospadias. As the flap survives on a rich supply of superficial dorsal vessels, the quality of the skin for the neourethra should be superior to that of the free graft with reduced risk of graft failure or loss of skin compliance. The main complications reported by this technique are summarised in Table 23.1.

Table 23.1. Complications of two-stage urethroplasty (1985–2000)

Author and year	Fistula	Stricture
Free full-thickness Wolfe graft		
Rabinovitch (1988)	5/35 (14)	0
Bracka (1995a, b)	34/600 (5.7)	41/600 (7)
Johnson and Coleman (1998)	20/122 (16)	2/122 (2)
Bretteville (1986)	10/80 (12.5)	0
Moir and Stevenson (1996)	2/40 (5)	0

Percentages in parentheses.

Comments

For distal hypospadias tubularisation of the incised urethral plate (Snodgrass manoeuvre) or the MAVIS procedure provides a well-functioning and aesthetically pleasing penis (Boddy and Samuel 2000; Sanders et al. 1958). A one-stage procedure for proximal hypospadias is desirable but one may not achieve good function and cosmesis in all cases (Rabinovitch 1988).

References

Akporiaye L, Schlossberg S, Jordan G: Fossa navicularis reconstruction in surgical treatment of balanitis xerotica obliterans. J Urol. 1995; 153:372A.

Boddy S-A, Samuel M: Mathieu and 'V' incision sutured (M.A.V.I.S) results in a natural glanular meatus. J Pediatr Surg. 2000; 35:494–496.

Bracka A: A long-term view of hypospadias. Br J Plast Surg. 1989; 42:251–255.

Bracka A: Hypospadias repair: the two-stage alternative. Br J Urol. 1995a; 76 [Suppl 3]: 31–41.

Bracka A: A versatile two-stage hypospadias repair. Br J Plast Surg. 1995b; 48:345–352.

Bretteville G: Hypospadias: simple, safe and complete correction in two stages. Ann Plast Surg. 1986; 17:526–531.

Browne D: An operation for hypospadias. Proc R Soc Med. 1949; 41:466–470.

Byars LT: A technique for consistently satisfactory repair of hypospadias. Surg Gynecol Obstet. 1955; 100:184–190.

Cloutier A: A method for hypospadias repair. Plast Reconstr Surg. 1962; 30:368–373.

Culp OS, McRoberts JW: Hypospadias. In: Alken CE, Dix VW, Goodwin WE, et al (eds): Encyclopaedia of urology. Springer, Berlin Heidelberg New York, pp 11307–11344; 1968.

Dessanti A, Rigamonti W, Merulla V, et al: Autologous buccal mucosa graft for hypospadias repair: an initial report. J Urol. 1992; 147:1081–1084.

Duckett J, Coplen D, Ewalt D, et al: Buccal mucosa in urethral reconstruction. J Urol. 1995; 153:1660–1663.

Fairbanks JL, Sheldon CA, Khoury AE, et al: Free bladder mucosal graft biology: unique engraftment characteristics in rabbits. J Urol. 1992; 148:663–666.

Humby G: A one-stage operation for hypospadias. Br J Surg. 1941; 29:84–92.

Johnson D, Coleman DJ: The selective use of a single-stage and a two-stage technique for hypospadias correction in 157 consecutive cases with the aim of normal appearance and function. Br J Plast Surg. 1998; 51:195–201.

Klijn AJ, Dik P, de Jong TPVM: Results of preputial reconstruction in 77 boys for distal hypospadias. J Urol. 2000; 165:1255–1257.

Moir GC, Stevenson JH: A modified Bretteville technique for hypospadias. Br J Plast Surg. 1996; 49:223–227.

Nicolle F: Improved repairs in 100 cases of penile hypospadias. Br J Plast Surg. 1976; 29:150–157.

Nové-Josserand G: Traitement de l'hypospadias; nouvelle méthode. Lyon Med. 1897; 85:198.

Ombrédanne L: Précis clinique et opération de chirurgie infantile. Masson, Paris, p 851; 1932.

Rabinovitch HH: Experience with a modification of the Cloutier technique for hypospadias repair. J Urol. 1988; 139:1017–1019.

Sanders AR, Schein CJ, Orkin LA: Total mucosal denudation of the canine bladder: experimental observations and clinical implications. Final report. J Urol. 1958; 79:63–68.

Snodgrass W: Tubularized incised plate urethroplasty for distal hypospadias. J Urol. 1994; 151:464–468.

Turner-Warwick R: Observations upon techniques for reconstruction of the urethral meatus, the hypospadiac glans deformity, and the penile urethra. Urol Clin North Am. 1979; 6:643–655.

Webster GD, Brown MW, Koefoot RJ, et al: Suboptimal results in full thickness skin graft urethroplasty using an extrapenile skin donor site. J Urol. 1984; 131:1082–1083.

Zhong-Chu L, Yu-Hen Z, Ya-Xiong S, et al: One-stage urethroplasty for hypospadias using a tube constructed with bladder mucosa–a new procedure. Urol Clin North Am. 1981; 8:457–462.

Protective Intermediate Layer

Ahmed T. Hadidi

24

In 1973, Horton et al. estimated the incidence of fistula following hypospadias surgery to range between 15% and 45%. In 1996, Duckett and Baskin estimated the incidence to be between 10% and 15%. In the new millennium, the accepted rate of fistula in distal hypospadias is less than 5%.

One of the most important factors in reducing the incidence of fistula and other complications of hypospadias repair was the introduction of a protective intermediate layer between the neourethra and the skin layer. In an interesting article, Telfer et al. in 1998 reported their experience with a two-stage procedure. Between 1988 and 1993, they had fistulae in 14 out of 22 patients (i.e. a fistula rate of 63%). Between 1994 and 1997, they had a fistula in one out of 22 patients (fistula rate of 4.5%). They stressed that the only change in technique was the introduction of a waterproofing intermediate layer.

Durham Smith was the first to describe the introduction of an intermediate or interposition layer between the neourethra and the cutaneous suture in 1973. Since then a variety of different methods of waterproofing in different types of hypospadias have been published and each author has reported a lower fistula rate which they attribute to the intermediate layer. Snow and Cartwright (1999) showed that using tunica vaginalis has reduced the fistula rate from 20% to 8%. If this was associated with the use of the operative microscope, the fistula rate was 0%.

Types of interposition waterproofing layer include The following (Fig. 24.1):
- Durham Smith (1973) reported skin de-epithelialisation and double breasting.
- Snow (1986) described the use of a tunica vaginalis wrap from the testicular coverings.
- Retik et al. (1988) was the first to use a dorsal subcutaneous flap from the prepuce.
- Motiwala (1993) described the use of a dartos flap from the scrotum
- Yamataka et al. (1998) reported the use of an external spermatic fascia flap.

Skin De-epithelialisation

Durham Smith (1973) described de-epithelialisation of a strip of skin 5 mm wide on one side of the skin edges. This provides a raw surface of deep dermis. This is achieved by cutting two or three fine longitudinal strips with a pair of small curved-on-the-flat scissors. The medial edge of the shaved flap is brought across the neourethra and sutured to fascial tissue beneath the other flap. The latter is then sutured to the edge of the de-epithelialised strip (double breasting). Belman (1988, 1994) reported improved results using this technique.

The Tunica Vaginalis Flap

Snow (1986) described the use of tunica vaginalis to prevent fistula in hypospadias surgery. In 1999, Snow and Cartwright wrote the following:

> Tunica vaginalis may be easily obtained during almost any type of hypospadias repair without risk to the newly created urethra. As with all hypospadias surgery, the chordee is generally corrected and the urethroplasty performed according to the surgeon's preference. If the surgeon has chosen a pedicle-type hypospadias repair in which the pedicle wraps around one side of the phallus, the testicle opposite the pedicle wrap is chosen. This way, if either the neourethra pedicle or the tunica vaginalis pedicle exerts any pulling forces on the penis, they oppose and thereby neutralize each other. If the hypospadias procedure does not include a pedicle, the surgeon may chose either testicle to begin the tunica vaginalis procurement. At the base of the penis, where the penis has been degloved, two small retractors are placed. The assistant gently elevates the testicle into view at the penoscrotal junction between the retractors. The scrotal attachments to the tunica vaginalis and testicle are separated, and the testicle and tunica vaginalis can be easily delivered into the wound. Dissection of the filmy attachments along the spermatic cord is completed to the extent that is visible. The tunica vaginalis is opened distally over the testicle near

238   Ahmed T. Hadidi

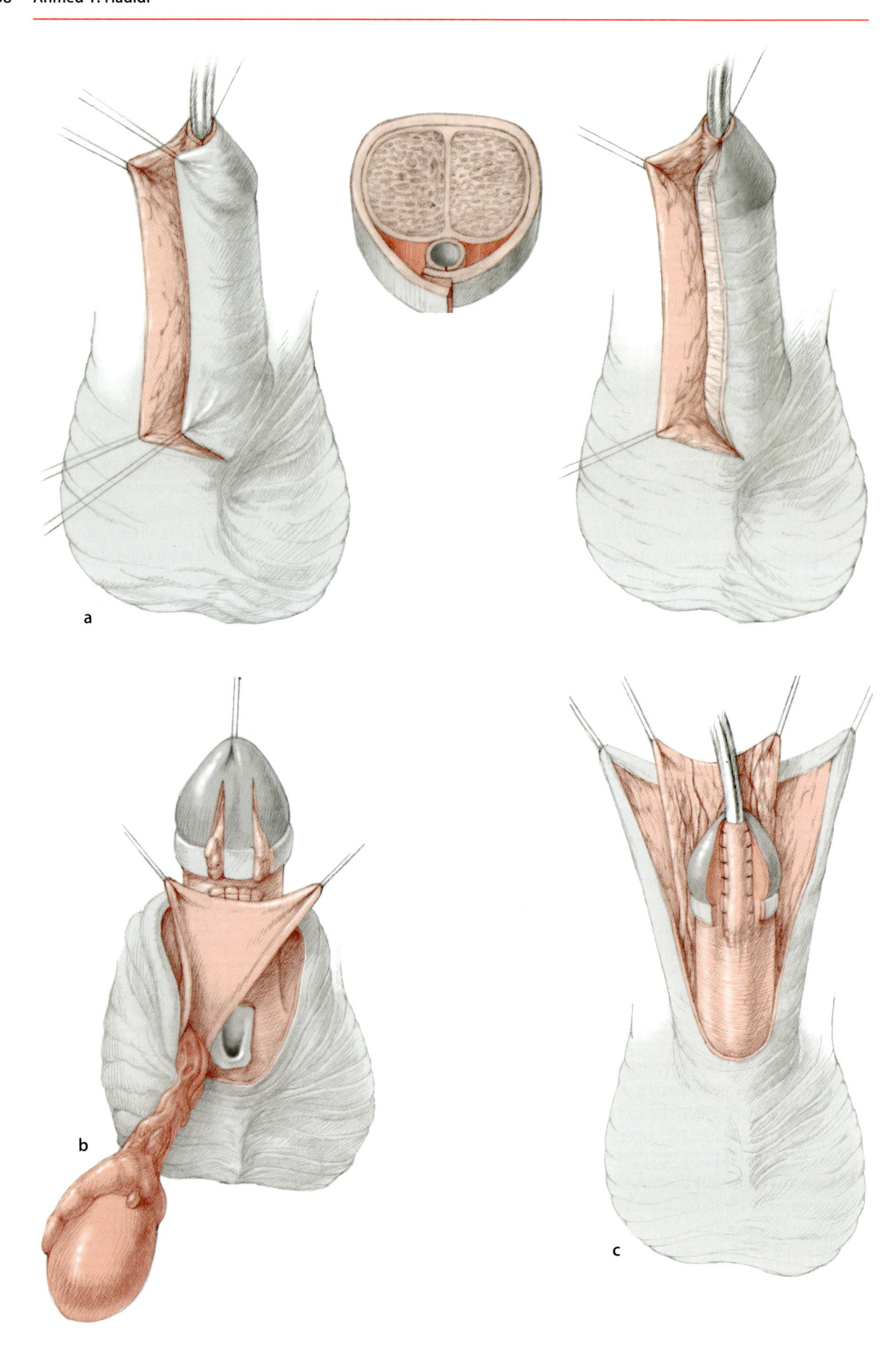

a

b

c

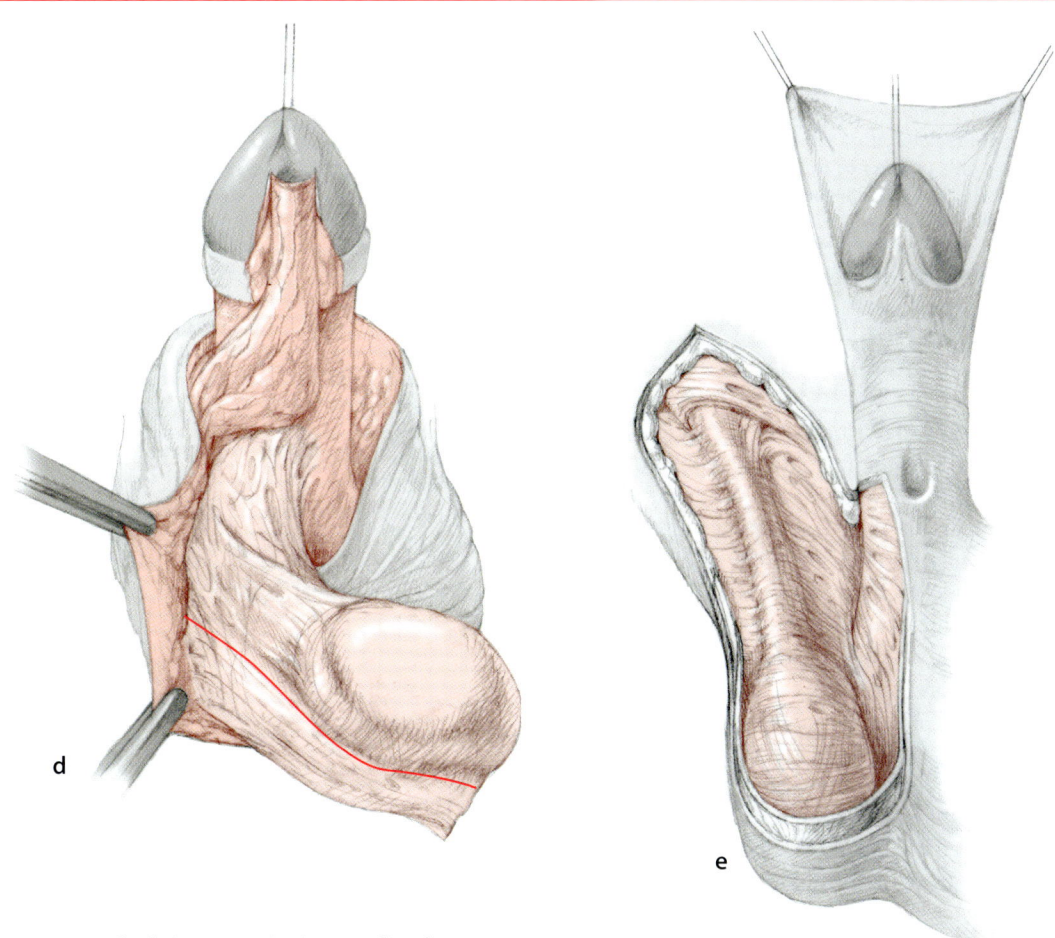

Fig. 24.1a–e. Methods for protective intermediate layer

the junction of the tunica vaginalis and epididymis, and the testicle is brought forth. Traction sutures are placed on the lateral edges of the tunica vaginalis, and incisions are made a few milimeters from the edge of the epididymis on either side. Proximal to the testicle, a transverse incision through the tunica vaginalis only is then made. This is similar to the dissection of the processus vaginalis from the spermatic cord during an orchiopexy at the proximal end of the spermatic cord. In some cases, the tunica vaginalis is generous and easily covers the penis without separating additional tunica vaginalis from the spermatic cord. In this situation, incisions parallel to the spermatic cord suffice. In the usual circumstance, with the proximal transverse tunica vaginalis incision made, careful dissection elevates the tunica vaginalis from the spermatic cord. This dissection is carried out parallel to the spermatic cord toward the superficial inguinal ring as far as vision and retraction allow, taking care to leave all of the surrounding tissue and cremaster fibers with the pedicle to ensure its rich blood supply. Length of the pedicle is seldom a problem, and extensive dissection is not regularly needed. As elevation of the tunica vaginalis takes place, the spermatic cord often seems to emanate from a sleeve of this pedicle. To allow the testicle to be replaced in the scrotum, the lateral margin of this sleeve may need a longitudinal incision to allow the tunica vaginalis to move medially and the testicle and spermatic cord to fall laterally. The incision is made laterally to preserve as much blood supply to the pedicle of the tunica vaginalis as possible. Once the dissection is completed, haemostasis is obtained with the electrocautery and the testicle is replaced into the scrotum in its natural position.

With the neourethra in place, the penis is ready to be covered with the tunica vaginalis like a blanket. It has not made a difference which side of the tunica vaginalis is placed toward the neourethra, and we prefer to place the shiny visceral surface toward the neourethra. Fine absorbable sutures are used longitudinally to suture the tunica vaginalis parallel and lateral to the dorsal neurovascular bundle. The flap, now sutured into place on the lateral aspect of the penis, is drawn across the ventral aspect of the penis to the other side, and a matching longitudinal closure is accomplished. This blankets the neourethra. If a glans-tunneling technique was used during the hypospadias repair, the tunica vaginalis may be passed distally through the glans channel with the neourethra or it may be tacked as far into the glans channel as possible, because coronal fistulas are among the most common that develop. If the neourethra has a pedicle, care should be taken not to confine the pedicle too tightly. It is seldom a problem. When this step is completed, the penis is covered on two thirds to three fourths of its circumference with a blanket of tunica vaginalis from one dorsal neurovascular bundle margin to the other and to the tip of the neourethra ventrally. The skin closure of the surgeon's preference can then be accomplished with ease. There are no special dressing requirements for the penis or scrotum in regard to the tunica vaginalis use. The familiar dressing and postoperative care that the surgeon customarily uses will suffice.

The Dorsal Subcutaneous Flap

In 1988, Retik et al. described the use of a dorsal subcutaneous flap from the foreskin to waterproof both free graft and meatal-based repairs. They published a 7-year follow-up of their experience with meatal-based repairs in 1994 (Retik et al. 1994). The technique is very simple. If circumcision is done at the same time, the circumcision incision is marked on the inner layer of prepuce. Then the inner layer is excised with sharp scissors, revealing the deep subcutaneous layer. This layer is mobilised from the dorsum of the penis, taking care to preserve the dorsal neurovascular bundle. The outer layer of the foreskin is separated from the subcutaneous layer and circumcision is completed. The flap of subcutaneous tissue is mobilised and brought around to the ventral surface. It needs to be sufficiently released in order to avoid the possibility of causing torsion of the penis.

The author has mobilised this dorsal subcutaneous vascular flap in many patients without having to do circumcision. This can be achieved by making a 1-cm longitudinal incision at the anterior border of the prepuce to reveal the subcutaneous vascular flap. Then, with sharp scissors, mobilise the subcutaneous flap without damaging the preputial skin. This can be of help in case the parents request reconstruction of the prepuce later on.

It is worth mentioning that the dorsal subcutaneous layer is a very important step in the Snodgrass tubularised incised plate technique (TIP).

The Dartos Flap

In 1993 Motiwala described the use of a dartos flap as an aid to urethral reconstruction. Churchill et al., in 1996, reported their experience in eight patients who underwent urethral reconstruction without a single fistula. They recommended the use of a dartos flap in secondary proximal hypospadias and complex urethral repair. According to their description:

The penile incision is extended along the median raphe to the mid scrotum. The dartos layer is dissected from the posterolateral surface of either testicle and isolated on a pedicle at the penoscrotal junction. The pedicle is approximately 1 cm. wide in infants and 2 cm. wide in a 10-year-old child. When dissection is maintained in the proper plane, the tunica vaginalis surrounding the testicles and skin of the scrotum are well preserved. The testicle is covered by visceral and parietal layers of tunica vaginalis, and the internal spermatic, cremasteric and external spermatic fasciae. Since the scrotum consists of skin and the dartos tunic comprises smooth muscle and fascia, care is required to maintain dissection away from the scrotal skin. Thus, all tissue between the testis and scrotal skin is not mobilised.

The flap contains vessels with fibroadipose tissue and resembles an omental flap. It is approximately 1 mm. thick and it does not result in difficult penile skin or glans closure. There is no need for epinephrine and bleeding is minimal. The dartos flap is long enough to reach the distal glans with no tension. The flap is tacked to the subcutaneous tissue of the ventral penile shaft lateral to the sides of the urethral repair. Scrotal orchiopexy is performed to fix the testicle on the side from which the dartos flap was isolated. Skin coverage is completed.

We have raised dartos flaps in patients who underwent inguinal or scrotal orchiopexy and in those with ambiguous genitalia. It is simple to isolate and exists in both scrotal compartments. It is distinct from the scrotal skin, or the visceral or parietal layers of the tunica vaginalis. Since the dartos flap can be raised from either side of the scrotum, it may also be used on more than one occasion should the need arise. It is well vascularised with small branches from the superficial and deep external pudendal branches of the femoral artery, the superficial perineal branch of the internal pudendal artery and the cremasteric branch from the inferior epigastric artery. These branches are from the internal and external iliac arterial trees and, thus, they are more reliable than a flap based on a single end artery. The dartos flap is mobile since its base is at the penoscrotal junction and we have also achieved good results with primary penoscrotal hypospadias repair. The dual blood supply, mobility, simplicity and availability of the dartos flap make it useful for the urethral reconstruction. Limitation of the dartos flap include the need for a peno-scrotal incision, and so it is not suitable for distal urethroplasty.

External Spermatic Fascia Flap

In 1998, Yamataka et al. described the use of external spermatic fascia (ESF) to protect against fistula and recurrence following hypospadias repair. The ESF is the outer layer of the coverings of the spermatic cord. It is the continuation of the innominate fascia covering the external oblique aponeurosis.

Fibrin Sealants

In 1992 Kinahan and Johnson reported their experience on the use of Tisseel in hypospadias repair. However, it may still be too early to reach any conclusions regarding the role of fibrin sealants in hypospadias surgery.

References

Belman AB: De-epithelialized skin flap coverage in hypospadias repair. J Urol. 1988; 140:1273–1276.
Belman AB: The de-epithelialized flap and its influence on hypospadias repair. J Urol. 1994; 152:2332–2334.
Churchill BM, van Savage JG, Khoury AE, et al: The dartos flap as an adjunct in preventing urethrocutanous fistulas in repeat hypospadias surgery. J Urol. 1996; 156:2047–2049.
Duckett JW, Baskin LS: Hypospadias. In: Gillenwater JY, Grayhack JT, Howards SS, Duckett JW (eds): Adult and pediatric urology, 3rd edn. Mosby-Year Book, St Louis, 1996.
Horton CE, Devine CJ, Baran N: Pictorial history of hypospadias repair techniques. In: Horton CE (ed): Plastic and reconstructive surgery of the genital area. Little Brown, Boston, pp 237–248; 1973.
Kinahan TJ, Johnson HW: Tisseel in hypospadias repair. Can J Surg. 1992; 35:75.
Motiwala HG: Dartos flap: an aid to urethral reconstruction. Br J Urol. 1993; 72:260.
Retik AB, Keating M, Mandell J: Complications of hypospadias repair. Urol Clin North Am. 1988; 15:223–236.
Retik AB, Mandell J, Bauer SB, et al: Meatal based hypospadias repair with the use of a dorsal subcutaneous flap to prevent urethrocutaneous fistula. J Urol. 1994; 152: 1229–1231.
Smith ED: A de-epithelialised overlap flap technique in the repair of hypospadias. Br J Plast Surg. 1973; 26:106–114.
Snow BW: Use of tunica vaginalis to prevent fistulas in hypospadias surgery. J Urol. 1986; 136:861–863.
Snow BW, Cartwright PC: Tunica vaginalis wrap. In: Ehrlich RM, Alter GJ (eds): Reconstructive and plastic surgery of the external genitalia. Saunders, Philadelphia, pp 109–112; 1999.
Telfer JRC, Quaba AA, Kwai Ben I, et al: An investigation into the role of waterproofing in a two-stage hypospadias repair. Br J Plast Surg. 1998; 51:542–546.
Yamataka A, Ando K, Lane G, et al: Pedicled external spermatic fascia for urethroplasty in hypospadias and closure of urethrocuteneous fistula. J Pediatr Surg. 1998; 33:1788–1789.

Procedures to Improve the Appearance of the Meatus and Glans

25

Ahmed T. Hadidi, Mahmoud Zaher

The ultimate goal of hypospadias repair is to have a near-normal looking penis, functionally and cosmetically. Until 30 years ago, normal appearance of the meatus and the glans was considered a luxury or a secondary issue. Many surgeons were reluctant to operate on patients with distal glanular hypospadias as most of those boys were able to function normally. With modern sophisticated technology, however, most surgeons are now only satisfied when they achieve a near-normal appearing penis for the majority of their patients.

As with every organ in the body, there is a lot of variation as regards the normal appearance of the penis. However, the normal glans is conical with a centrally located meatus. The lips of the meatus are smooth and sharp-edged, forming a vertical slit; the urethra is centrally placed within the glans, and the terminal urethra immediately proximal to the meatus, the so-called fossa navicularis, has a larger diameter which extends deep into the glans (Turner-Warwick 1979) (👁 Fig. 25.1).

Despite growing interest in the final postoperative appearance of the meatus and glans, there seems to be no clear detailed description or classification of the hypospadiac glans. This kind of classification may be important to standardise the different types of hypospadiac glans anomalies and evaluate the suitable methods of repair. Patients with hypospadias have an abnormal looking globular glans with a variable degree of clefting and urethral plate projection. The author, based on experience with more than 2,500 patients with hypospadias, proposes the classification of hypospadiac glans into three main groups (👁 Fig. 25.2):

1. Cleft glans. There is a deep groove in the middle of the glans with proper clefting; the urethral plate is narrow and projects to the tip of the glans. An example is "megameatus intact prepuce" hypospadias. Some form of Thiersch–Duplay, pyramid repair, Y-V glanuloplasty or TIP procedure may be employed with good results.

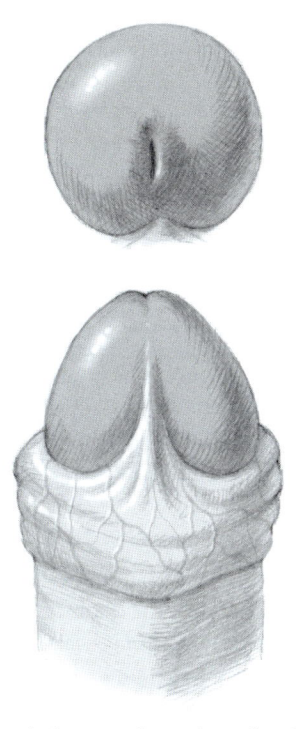

Fig. 25.1. Normal glans configuration. The glans is conical with a centrally located meatus. A normal meatus is vertical and slit like

2. Incomplete cleft glans. There is a variable degree of glans split, a shallow glanular groove and a variable degree of urethral plate projection. If the meatus is mobile, MAGPI or Y-V glanuloplasty procedure may give good results.
3. Flat glans. The urethral plate ends short of the glans penis; no glanular groove. There may be a variable degree of chordee, especially in proximal forms of hypospadias. Generous glans splitting is required to achieve good cosmetic and functional results. Y-V glanuloplasty usually gives good results.

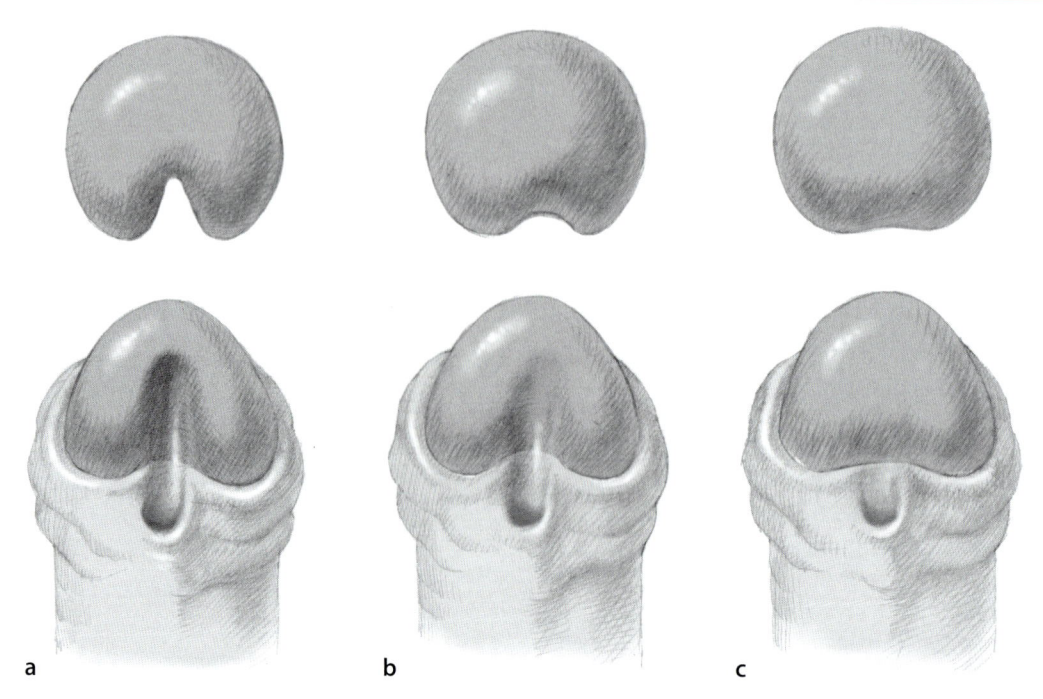

Fig. 25.2a–c. Hypospadiac glans configuration. The glans is globular in shape. The glans may be cleft, incompletely cleft or flat. The meatus is oval or circular. **a** *Cleft glans*. There is a deep groove in the middle of the glans with proper clefting; the urethral plate is narrow and projects to the tip of the glans. **b** *Incomplete cleft glans*. There is a variable degree of glans split, a shallow glanular groove and a variable degree of urethral plate projection. **c** *Flat glans*. The urethral plate ends short of the glans penis; no glanular groove. There may be a variable degree of chordee, especially in proximal forms of hypospadias

For decades, surgeons were very reluctant to operate on the glans penis. Understandably so, for the glans is the most sensitive part of the penis and probably they were concerned about glanular scarring, that may be ugly and even painful.

Clinical experience has shown that the glans penis is a very forgiving tissue. It is richly vascularised and heals quickly with nearly no scarring at all. Recognition of this resulted in the evolution of glans dissection. It has become also clear that it is not enough simply to tunnel the neourethra through the glans. Instead, one has to create a generous space for the neourethra to avoid subsequent stricture formation.

The following review shows the gradual historical development of techniques for glanuloplasty and meatoplasty (Fig. 25.3, pp. 246, 247):

Tunnelling, Canalisation, Coring and Wing Rotation ▶
Dieffenbach (1838), pierced the glans to the normal urethra and allowed a cannula to remain in position until epithelialisation occurred; this was not successful. Russell (1900) described the glans channel technique to deliver the urethra to the apex of the glans. This method was used for many years. Bevan (1917) reported a technique involving creation of a proximal penile flap that was converted into a urethral tube and was pulled through a tunnel in the glans. Davis (1940), Ricketson (1958), and Hendren (1981) all channelled a full-thickness skin tube through the glans.

Devine and Horton (1961) and Mustarde (1965) popularised the glans channel procedure and included a dorsal V flap with the glans channel. This led to triangularisation and then carving out of the interior to produce a generous tunnel.

Duckett (1981b), combined the glans channel technique with the creation of a vascularised island flap neo-urethra. This technique requires a generous channel through the glans tissue, allowing the vascularised skin flap to be placed through the glans without compression of the blood supply.

For 500 years, surgeons recommended canalisation, tunnelling or coring. These three methods are essentially the same with progressively larger channels, and glans stenosis was usually the end result.

Wing rotation may be used to mobilise the glanular wings and wrap them around the neourethra (Chap. 16.1).

Glans Split or Kippering ▶ The glans split has been used in various reports to move the meatus to the apex (Beck 1917; Humby 1941; Barcat 1973; Cronin and Guthrie 1973; Turner-Warwick 1979; Bracka 1995a, b).

Meatoplasty and Glanuloplasty Incorporated ▶ Duckett, in 1981, described the "meatal advancement and glanuloplasty incorporated" (MAGPI) procedure (Duckett 1981b). The two basic elements of MAGPI are meatoplasty and glanuloplasty. Meatoplasty comprises a generous longitudinal incision that is closed in a Heineke–Mikulicz style of transverse closure. Glanuloplasty is achieved by placing a stitch on the ventral meatal edge and approximating the glanular skin by three vertical mattress sutures. However, Hastie and coworkers (1989) reported a high incidence of partial meatal regression in their patients following the MAGPI procedure. Arap and colleagues (1984) modified the MAGPI technique by using two sutures instead of one. Decter, in 1991, described an "M inverted V" technique featuring an M-shaped incision and deepithelialisation of the tissue within the confines of that incision. A stitch is placed on the ventral lip of the meatus and is pulled toward the distal end of the penis. This reconfigures the M-shaped incision into an inverted V.

Urethral Plate Hinging ▶ Rich et al. (1989) described a urethral plate incision (hinging) as a modification of the Mathieu repair to improve the cosmetic outcome of the neomeatus. This helps to achieve a slit-like vertical meatus.

Tubularised Incised Plate ▶ Snodgrass (1994) extended the concept of urethral plate hinging by incising the whole urethral plate in the midline from the hypospadiac meatus distally. This helps in tubularisation of the plate (tubularised incised plate or TIP technique).

Y-V Glanuloplasty ▶ Hadidi, writing in 1996, described the Y-V glanuloplasty as a modification of the Mathieu technique (Mathieu 1932) to achieve a terminal meatus and a near-normal looking glans penis. This technique modifies the Y-V principle to increase the circumference of the urethral meatus by at least 1 cm. The use of Y-V glanuloplasty for distal hypospadias repair is described in detail in Chap. 14.2. The technique was very useful in most single-stage repairs for proximal hypospadias, e.g. the onlay flap (Elder et al. 1987), the Thiersch–Duplay U-shaped flap (Thiersch 1869; Duplay 1880), the lateral-based flap (Hadidi 2003), the Snodgrass procedure and transverse preputial island flap urethroplasty. The details of the technique are described later in this chapter.

Mathieu and V Incision Sutured Technique ▶ Boddy and Samuel (2000), described the "Mathieu and V incision sutured" (MAVIS) technique. They stated that the resulting meatus was a vertical slit. In this technique a "V" incision is made and excised at the apex of the parameatal-based flap. Then each side of the "V" is sutured to the glanular wings.

Y-V Glanuloplasty

Surgical Technique

Y-V glanuloplasty is performed in three steps (◉ Fig. 25.4, p. 248).

Step 1: Y-shaped Incision of the Glans

A Y-shaped incision is outlined on the glans. The centre of the Y is just below the tip of the glans and where the tip of the neo-meatus will be located. The two short upper limbs of the Y are 0.5 cm long and the angle between them is 60°. The long vertical limb of the Y extends down the whole length of the glans penis to the coronary sulcus (similar to urethral plate incision or hinging). The Y-shaped incision is made deep and results in three flaps, one small upper (median) and two large lateral flaps.

The three flaps are elevated and a core of soft tissue is excised from the bed of each flap to create a space for the neourethra.

In techniques that preserve the urethral plate, such as the onlay, Snodgrass or Thiersch–Duplay procedures, the upper small median flap is advanced forward and sutured to the raw surface created. The situation is different in techniques that reconstruct a complete tube-like transverse preputial island flap, lateral based flap, Koyanagi repair or yoke repair. In those techniques, the upper small median flap is sutured to the upper dorsal end of tube repairs (similar to the Devine V flap).

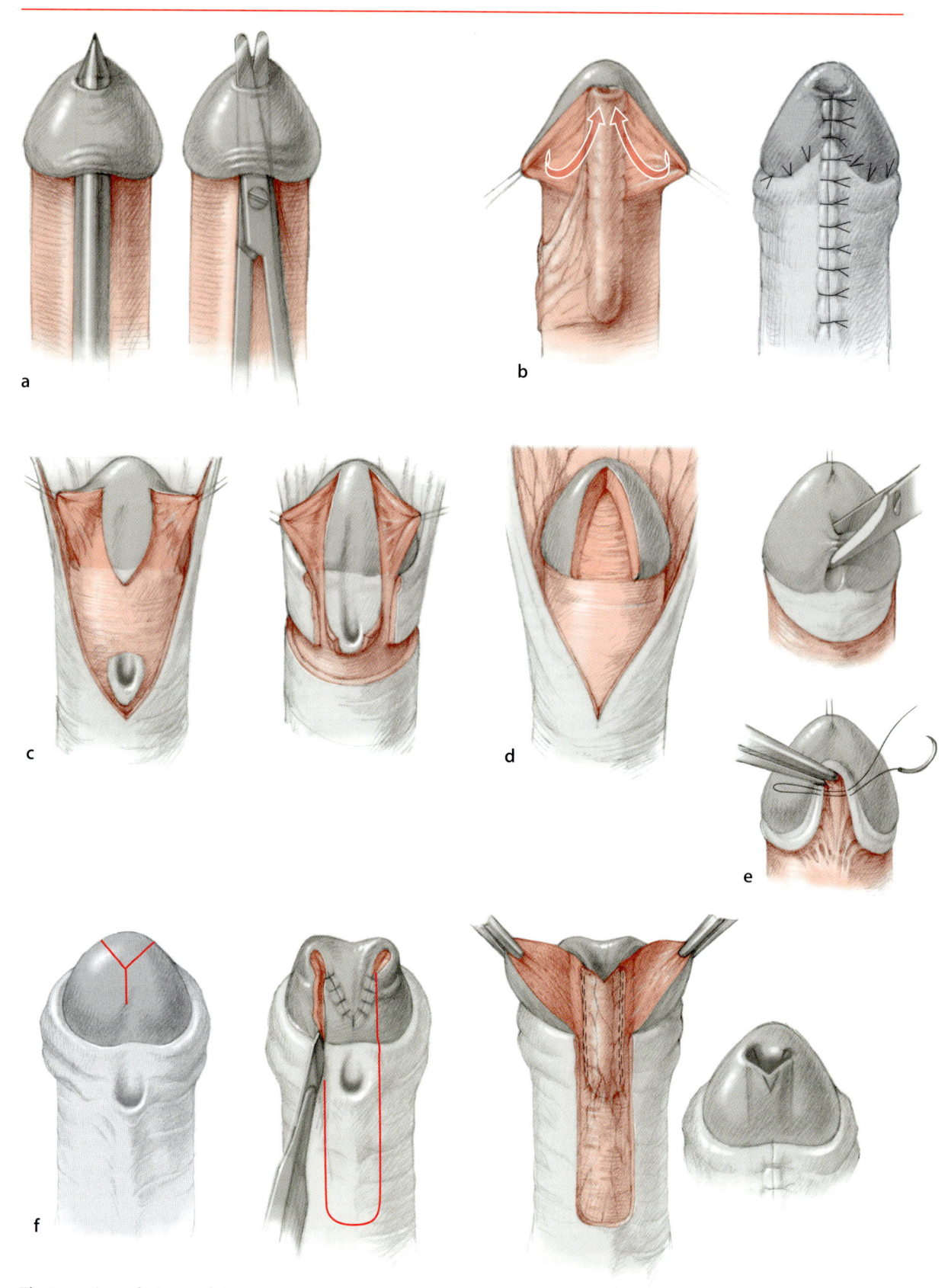

Fig. 25.3a–i. Techniques of glanuloplasty. **a** Glans tunnelling, canalisation or coring. **b** Wing rotation. **c** Glans V in the posterior wall by Devine and Horton (1961), Mustarde (1965). **d** Glans splitting or kippering has been used for 1000 years. **e** MAGPI (Duckett 1981b). **f** Y-V glanuloplasty (Hadidi 1996). **g–i** see p. 247

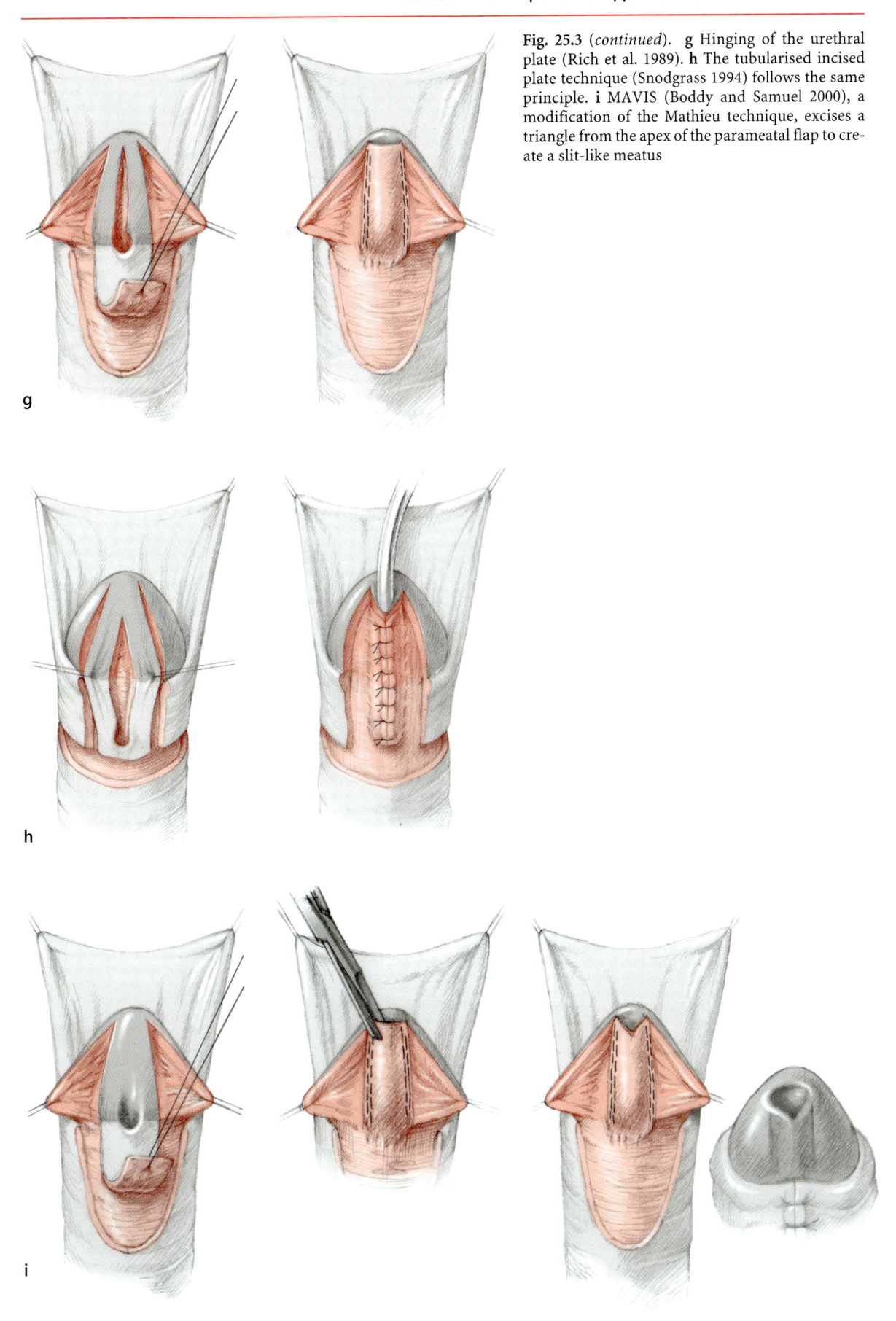

Procedures to Improve the Appearance of the Meatus and Glans 247

Fig. 25.3 (*continued*). **g** Hinging of the urethral plate (Rich et al. 1989). **h** The tubularised incised plate technique (Snodgrass 1994) follows the same principle. **i** MAVIS (Boddy and Samuel 2000), a modification of the Mathieu technique, excises a triangle from the apex of the parameatal flap to create a slit-like meatus

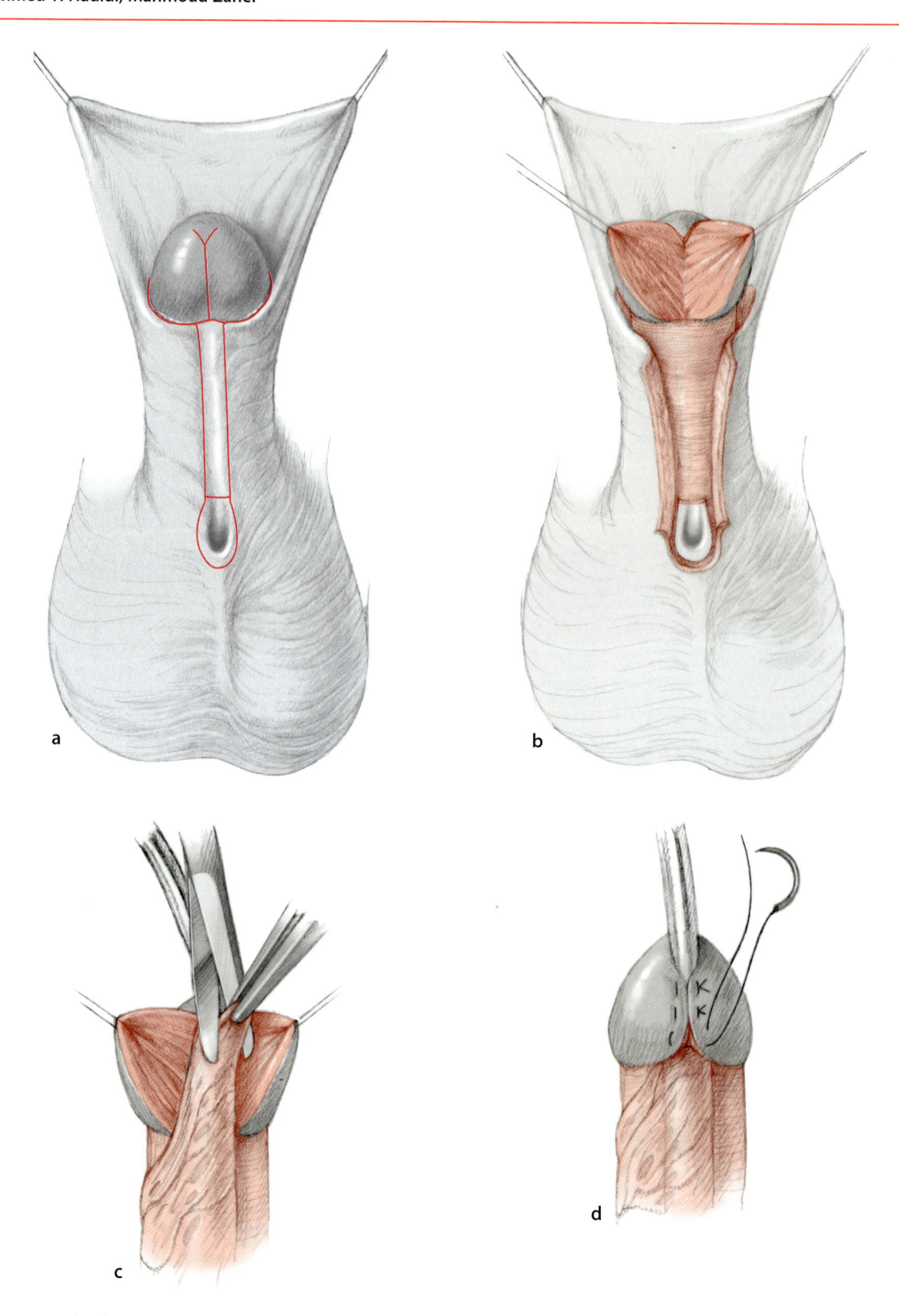

Fig. 25.4a–d. The technique of Y-V glanuloplasty in procedures that excise the urethral plate with the chordee. **a** Deep Y-shaped incision of the glans. **b** Three flaps result: a small upper flap and two large lateral glanular wings. After creating a space for the neourethra, the small upper flap is advanced proximally to widen the meatus. **c** A "V" is excised from the tip of the neourethra to create a slit-like meatus. **d** Glanuloplasty (the glanular flaps are wrapped around the neourethra) and meatoplasty (the upper edges of the glanular wings are sutured to the tip of the neourethra)

Step 2: V Excision of the Tip of the Neourethra

After reconstruction of the neourethra using whatever technique the surgeon prefers, a small V is excised from the ventral tip of the neourethra. The excision of the V achieves two targets: (1) a wider meatus and (2) a slit-like meatus.

Step 3: Glanuloplasty and Meatoplasty

The two large lateral glanular wings are wrapped around the neourethra with a catheter (10 F) inside and are sutured together using three transverse mattress sutures of Vicryl 6-0.

Meatoplasty is performed by suturing the upper edge of each of the two glanular wings to the upper edge of the neourethra that has become longer after excising the V. This helps to have a slit-like meatus.

This method was employed in 569 children with hypospadias during the 10-year period from January 1992 to July 2002. Three hundred and eighty-four boys had distal penile hypospadias, 79 had mid or proximal penile hypospadias and 106 had recurrent hypospadias. For socioeconomic and cultural reasons, their ages at presentation ranged from 3 months to 6 years. Surgery was performed shortly after referral to the author. The technique was employed in combination with the Mathieu procedure, onlay flap, lateral-based (LB) flap, transverse preputial island flap and Duplay urethroplasty.

The majority of patients with distal penile hypospadias were discharged on the same day, after voiding (as day cases). The remaining boys (with suprapubic cystostomy catheter) stayed for 5–14 days according to the site of the original urethral opening and the social condition of the family. The follow-up period ranged from 6 months to 10 years.

Results and Complications

Five hundred and forty six of the 569 patients had satisfactory results with an adequate terminal meatus in a near-normal looking glans penis. Three patients early in the series, before the technique was mastered, developed stenosis due to the use of smaller Nelaton catheters and inadequate dissection. The complication rate for the distal hypospadias group was 2% and for the proximal group, 12%. Apart from the three patients with meatal stenosis, no boys required urethral dilatation or calibration.

These data suggest that Y-V glanuloplasty can be performed in almost any case of hypospadias in combination with most standard techniques of hypospadias repair to provide a terminal meatus in a near-normal looking glans penis with minimal complications.

References

Arap S, Mitre AI, DeGores GM: Modified meatal advancement and glanduloplasty repair of distal hypospadias. J Urol. 1984; 131:1140.

Barcat J: Current concepts of treatment. In: Horton CE (ed): Plastic and reconstructive surgery of the genital area. Little Brown, Boston, pp 249–263; 1973.

Beck C: Hypospadias and its treatment. Surg Gynecol Obstet. 1917; 24:511.

Bevan AD: A new operation for hypospadias. JAMA. 1917; 68:1032.

Boddy SA, Samuel M: A natural glanular meatus after "Mathieu and V incision sutured" MAVIS. BJU Int. 2000; 86:394–397.

Bracka A: A versatile two-stage hypospadias repair. Br J Plast Surg. 1995a; 48:345–352.

Bracka A: Hypospadias repair: the two-stage alternative. Br J Urol. 1995b; 76 [Suppl 3]:31–41.

Cronin TD, Guthrie TH: Method of Cronin and Guthrie of hypospadias repair. In: Horton CE (ed): Plastic and reconstructive surgery of the genital area. Little Brown, Boston, pp 302–314; 1973.

Davis DM: The pedicle tube graft in the surgical treatment of hypospadias in the male. Surg Gynecol Obstet. 1940; 71:790.

Decter RM: M inverted V glansplasty: a procedure for distal hypospadias. J Urol. 1991; 146:641.

Devine CJ Jr, Horton CE: A one-stage hypospadias repair. J Urol. 1961; 85:166.

Dieffenbach JF: The simple canalization method. In: Dictionnaire encyclopedique de medecine. Biblioteque Nationale de Paris, France; 1838.

Duckett JW: Transverse preputial island-flap technique for repair of severe hypospadias. Urol Clin North Am 1980a; 7:423.

Duckett JW: MAGPI (meatal advancement and glanuloplasty): a procedure for subcoronal hypospadias. Urol Clin North Am. 1981b; 8:513.

Duplay S: Sur le traitement chirurgical de l'hypospadias et de l'epispadias. Arch Gen Med. 1880; 145:527.

Elder JS, Duckett JW, Snyder HM: Onlay island flap in the repair of mid-and distal penile hypospadias without chordee. J Urol. 1987; 138:376.

Hadidi AT: Y-V Glanuloplasty: a new modification in the surgery of hypospadias. Kasr El Aini Med J. 1996; 2:223–233.

Hadidi AT: Lateral based flap with dual blood supply: a single stage repair for proximal hypospadias. Egypt J Plast Reconstr Surg. 2003; 27 (3).

Hastie KJ, Deshpande SS, Moisey CU: Long-term follow-up of the MAGPI operation for distal hypospadias. Br J Urol. 1989; 63:320–322.

Hendren WH: The Belt-Fuqua for repair of hypospadias. Urol Clin North Am. 1981; 8:431.

Humby G: A one stage operation for hypospadias. Br J Surg. 1941; 29:84.

Mathieu P: Traitment en un temps de l'hypospadias balanique et juxta-balanique. J Chir (Paris). 1932; 39:481.

Mustarde JC: One-stage correction of distal hypospadias and other people's fistulae. Br J Plast Surg. 1965; 18:413–422.

Rich MA, Keating MA, Snyder HM, et al: "Hinging" the urethral plate in hypospadias meatoplasty. J Urol. 1989; 142:1551.

Ricketson G: A method of repair of hypospadias. Am J Surg. 1958; 95:279.

Russell RH: Operation for severe hypospadias. Br Med J. 1900; 2:1432.

Snodgrass W: Tubularized incised plate urethroplasty for distal hypospadias. J Urol. 1994; 151:464–465.

Thiersch C: Ueber die Entstehungsweise und operative Behandlung der Epispadie. Arch Heilkd. 1869; 10:20.

Turner-Warwick R: Observations upon techniques for reconstruction of the urethral meatus, the hypospadiac glans deformity and the penile urethra. Urol Clin North Am. 1979; 6:643.

Penoscrotal Transposition Associated With Hypospadias

Amir F. Azmy

The embryonic explanation for penoscrotal transposition associated with hypospadias is retraction in development of the pars phallica of the urogenital sinus, which is associated with delayed genital tubercle fusion in the midline. Labioscrotal folds fail to migrate caudally, or migrate only incompletely, and they remain fused anterior or lateral to the genital tubercle. In severe forms of prepenile scrotum, other anomalies, e.g. perineal hypospadias–absence of urinary tract, polycystic kidney and imperforate anus–may coexist.

The first published case of penoscrotal transposition was described by Broman in 1911. Forschall and Rickham (1956) reported repair in three stages: (1) straightening of the penis, (2) repair of the hypospadias; (3) later release of contracture. Campbell (1963) divided the scrotum, brought the penis forward and sutured the scrotum behind.

Bifid scrotum associated with proximal forms of hypospadias is the most common form and usually does not require surgical correction. However, more severe forms of malposition of the scrotum do occur, albeit rarely, and include prepenile scrotum, web scrotum and ectopic scrotum.

Penoscrotal transposition (Fig. 26.1) is probably the result of failure of caudal migration of the labioscrotal folds. In its severe form the penis may be barely visible until the scrotum is retracted laterally. Moderate to severe chordee is usually present. A long length of the urethra may be necessary for correction; this may be compromised by the lack of adequate foreskin and the staged repair may be preferable (Ehrlich and Scardino 1982). Mori and Ikoma, in 1986, suggested that a free bladder mucosal graft might be applied using tunica vaginalis for additional cover.

A planned two-stage repair should be considered, as the preputial skin is rarely sufficient to form the entire urethra during perineal hypospadias repair (Retik et al. 1994). In management of severe hypospadias with two-stage repair, the penis should be straightened and the skin brought to the ventral surface during the first stage. Urethral reconstruction is then fashioned 6 months later.

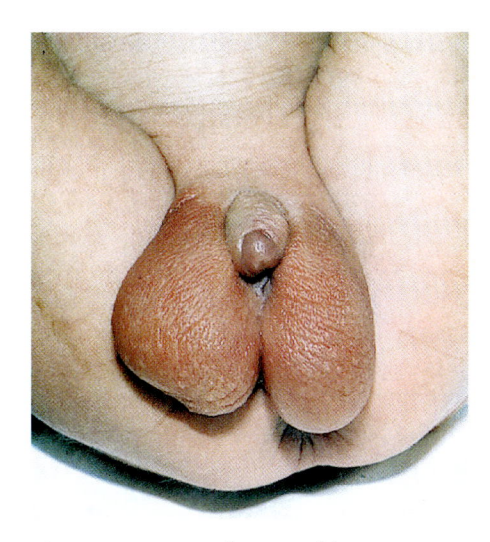

Fig. 26.1. Penoscrotal transposition

An incision is made 5 mm proximal to the meatus. The incision is carried laterally and around the scrotum to allow for mobilisation and the transposition of the scrotum downwards. A wide skin bridge connecting the midline dorsal penile skin with suprapubic skin is left undisturbed to ensure adequate blood supply. The new urethra is constructed and Byars flaps fashioned to cover the ventral surface. An alternative procedure is to use preputial full-thickness skin tube to form the urethra. Full-thickness skin graft can be combined with Thiersch–Duplay urethroplasty or transverse preputial island flap urethroplasty.

Scrotal procedures have been described for correction of penoscrotal transposition:

Campbell, writing in 1970, bisected the scrotum and sutured the two halves beneath the scrotum.

McIlvoy and Harris (1955) placed the penis anterior to the scrotum through a subcutaneous tunnel.

Glenn and Anderson (1973) performed simultaneous correction of penoscrotal transposition and repair of hypospadias. They completely mobilised the two halves of the scrotum as rotational advancement flaps with relocation of the scrotal compartment in a normal dependant position and constructed the neourethra at the same operation.

Ehrlich and Scardino's procedure is similar to the Glenn–Anderson technique, but with some modifications. They performed simultaneous chordectomy and scrotoplasty for incomplete scrotal transposition, chordee and perineal hypospadias. The initial stage was similar to the Glenn–Anderson technique; however, the incision differed in leaving a wide skin bridge connecting midline dorsal penile skin with suprapubic skin to preserve the vascularity of the penile shaft skin, and instead of carrying the incision distal to the original meatal position, the incision is made proximal to the meatus to allow formation of a Thiersch–Duplay skin tube. Ehrlich and Scardino elected to perform the correction in two stages and bring the meatus as far distally as possible, construct the ventral neourethra and cover it with Byars flaps; more foreskin was mobilised to facilitate completion of the neourethra at a second stage. They felt that simultaneous repair would allow part of the scrotal skin to integrate in the neo-urethra repair and the problem of hair growth might occur. Correction of penoscrotal transposition is shown in 👁 Fig. 26.2a–d.

Mori–Ikoma Technique

The incision for the Mori–Ikoma technique is an inverted omega around the scrotal skin and the base of the penis; closure of the flaps is in the form of a zeta (Mori and Ikoma 1986). The procedure is shown in 👁 Fig. 26.3a–c. The authors stated that the final results are better when scrotoplasty is performed after repair of hypospadias.

The penis is freed from the scrotum along the line shown in 👁 Fig. 26.3. The incision extends to the superior aspect of the scrotum to be swung inferomedially below the penis; chordee is extensively released, splitting the glans. Byars flaps are fashioned to cover the defect and extend to cover the split glans to create a distal urethra at the second stage. Diez-Garcia et al. (1995) reported on 10 boys treated during the period between 1992 and 1993 at an average age of 10 months; hypospadias was present in 9 of the patients. The Glenn–Anderson correction technique was used in 2 cases and the Ehrlich–Scardino technique in the others. Correction of the penoscrotal transposition was done during urethroplasty.

Shanberg–Rosenberg Technique

In the Shanberg–Rosenberg technique for treatment of partial transposition of the penis and scrotum with anterior urethral diverticulum in a child born with caudal regression syndrome, two flaps are cut, one with its base on the superior or pubic face and the other with its base on the inferior or scrotal face (Shanberg and Rosenberg 1989; Glassberg et al. 1998).

They reported their experience with the Koyanagi–Nonomura one-stage bucket repair of severe hypospadias with and without penoscrotal transposition. In 14 boys the age ranged from 10 to 20 months. Severe hypospadias and chordee were associated with the penoscrotal transposition in 8 cases. Shanberg and Rosenberg carried out simultaneous repair of the hypospadias and the penoscrotal transposition. In their technique, an initial circumferential incision around the corona is followed by a U-shaped incision with its base proximal to the meatus, extended approximately 8 mm proximal to the previously made coronal incision. This second incision is extended laterally and dorsally onto the dorsal hood parallel to and approximately 8 mm from the first incision, giving the appearance of a bucket. The urethral plate is preserved. When a "handle" is incised at 12 o'clock between the parallel coronal circumferential incisions it resembles a long Y. The urethral plate and attached strips are mobilised with the proximal urethra, the penis is degloved and the chordee is corrected. The medial edges of the two skin flaps are sutured to form the dorsum of the new urethra. The proximal urethra is formed by rolling the urethral plate, and sutures extend to roll the lateral edges of the skin flaps, completing the tubularisation. the glans is split in the midline for placement of the neourethra and the glanuloplasty is completed using a silicone tubing stent. The scrotal skin lying beside and cephalad to the penis is outlined, incised and tubularised. Byars flaps are fashioned and may be criss-crossed for ventral coverage.

Simultaneous repair of incomplete scrotal transposition, chordee and perineal hypospadias a skin bridge left in continuity with the pubic skin and penile sac is deemed essential to ensure adequate blood supply to the penile skin.

The largest series from a single institution, 53 patients, was published by Pike et al. (2001). The patients with penoscrotal transposition ranged in age from 1 day to 30 years. Thirteen per cent had a family history of penoscrotal transposition, one family showed inheritance in an X-linked recessive manner, 32% showed abnormalities in other organ systems, with the genitourinary system being affected most.

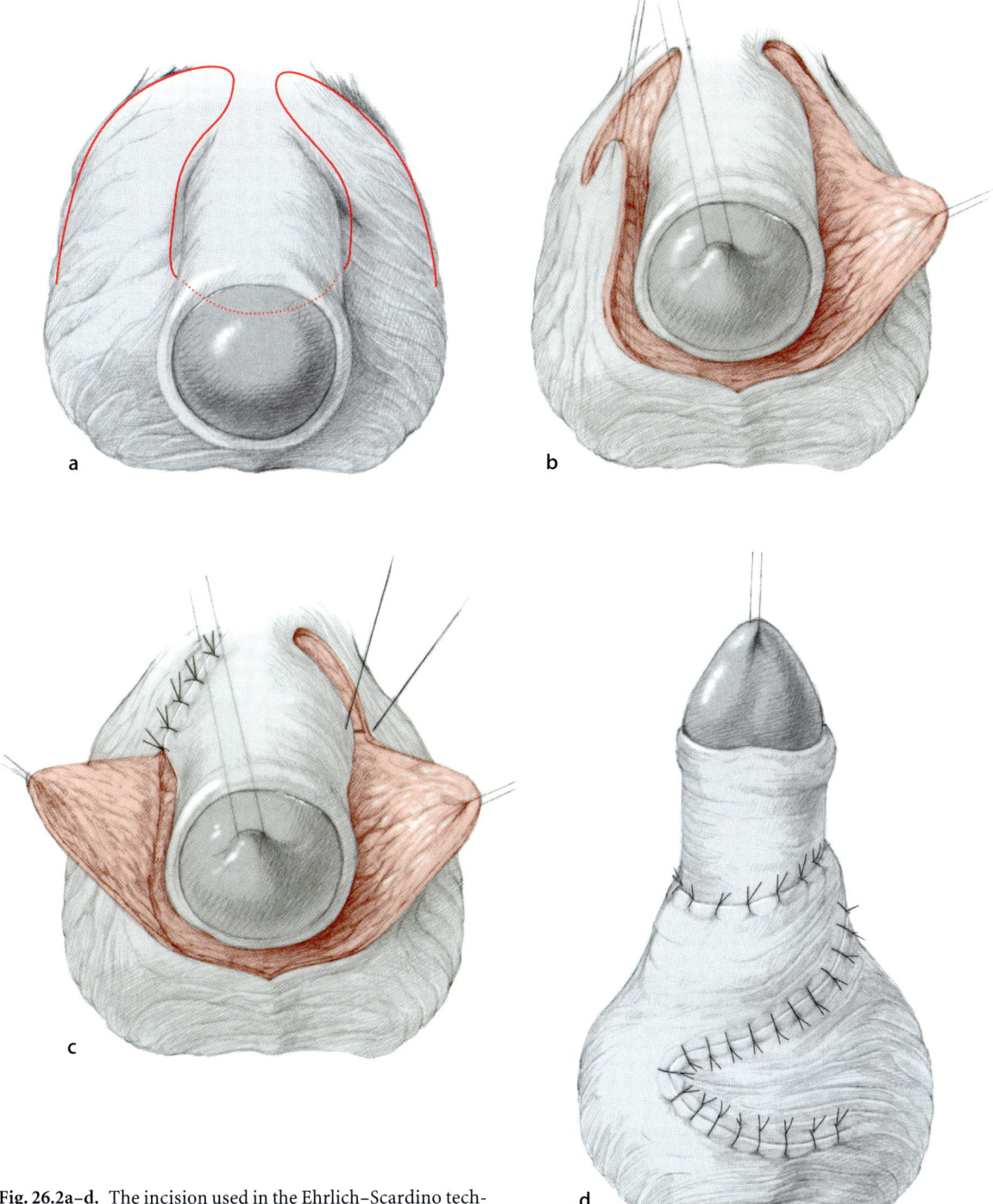

Fig. 26.2a–d. The incision used in the Ehrlich–Scardino technique

Fig. 26.3a–c. The incision used in the Mori–Ikoma technique

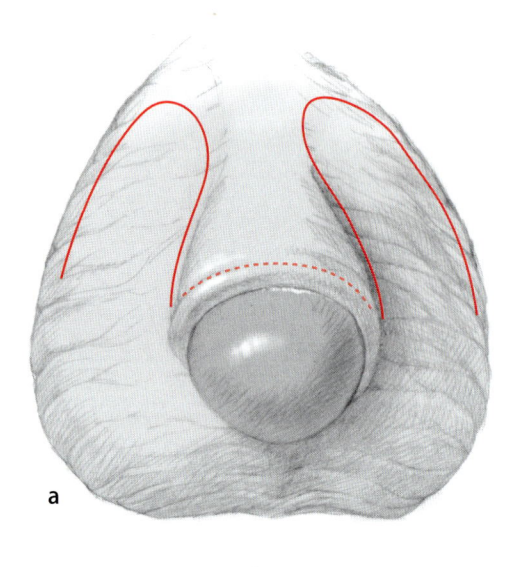

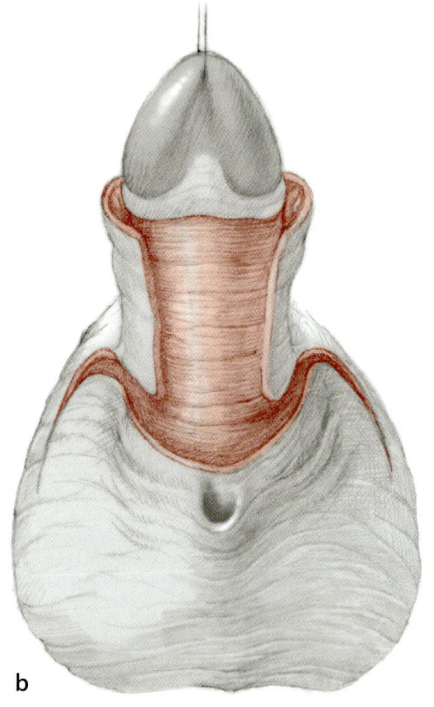

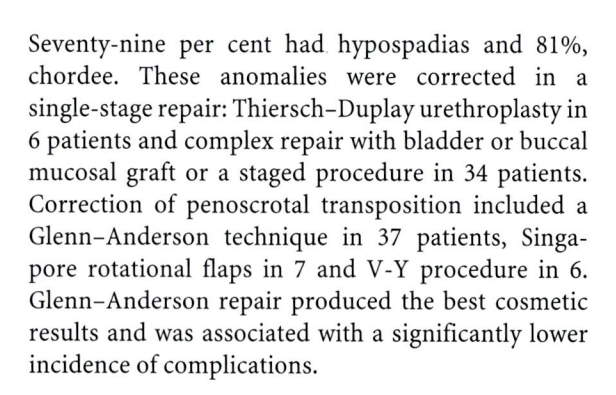

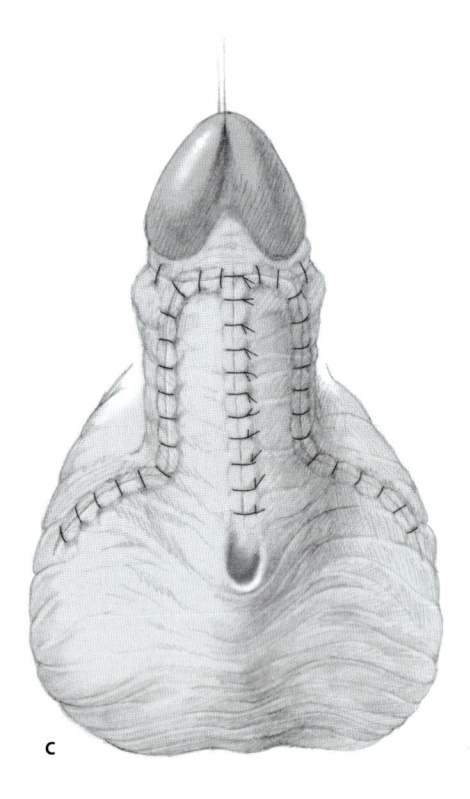

Seventy-nine per cent had hypospadias and 81%, chordee. These anomalies were corrected in a single-stage repair: Thiersch–Duplay urethroplasty in 6 patients and complex repair with bladder or buccal mucosal graft or a staged procedure in 34 patients. Correction of penoscrotal transposition included a Glenn–Anderson technique in 37 patients, Singapore rotational flaps in 7 and V-Y procedure in 6. Glenn–Anderson repair produced the best cosmetic results and was associated with a significantly lower incidence of complications.

Bifid Scrotum

Bifid scrotum may occur as an isolated anomaly, but often is associated with hypospadias. The anomaly is corrected by excision of midline strips of skin of each hemi-scrotum, approximation of external spermatic fascia and skin closed with interrupted stitches after ensuring haemostasis.

Penile Torsion

Penile torsion is a rotational deformity of the penis, usually in anticlockwise direction and commonly associated with hypospadias and chordee. The torsion is usually 90° (as shown in Fig. 26.1). Deviation of the median raphe without torsion may occur and is noted in 10% of newborns. The aetiology is not clear, but may be due to abnormal arrangement of penile skin during development. In minor forms and when the penis is straight there are no functional problems and there is no indication for correction. In severe forms, however, surgical correction is required, with complete degloving of the penile shaft and mobilisation of the base of the penis to remove fibrous bands responsible for the torsion. An anchoring stitch at the base of the penis may aid correction. The penile skin is resutured in a slightly overcorrected position (Azmy and Eckstein 1981).

References

Azmy A, Eckstein HB: Surgical correction of torsion of the penis. Br J Urol. 1981; 53:378–379.

Broman I: Normale und abnorme Entwicklung des Menschen: ein Hand- und Lehrbuch der Ontogenie and Teratologie, speziell für praktische Ärzte und Studierende der Medizin. Bergmann, Wiesbaden; 1911.

Campbell MF: Anomalies of the genital tract. In: Campbell MF, Harrison JH (eds): Urology, 2nd edn. Saunders, Philadelphia, p 1749; 1963.

Campbell MF: Anomalies of the genital tract. In: Campbell MF, Harrison JH (eds): Urology, 3rd edn. Saunders, Philadelphia, pp 1576–1577; 1970.

Diez-Garcia R, Banuelos A, Marin C, et al: Penoscrotal transposition. Eur J Pediatr Surg. 1995; 5:222–225.

Ehrlich RM, Scardino PT: Surgical correction of scrotal transposition and perineal hypospadias. J Pediatr Surg. 1982; 17:175–177.

Forshall E, Rickham PP: Transposition of penis and scrotum. Br J Urol. 1956; 28:250–252.

Glassberg KI, Hansborough F, Horowitz M: The Koyanagi-Nonomura 1 stage bucket repair of severe hypospadias with and without penoscrotal transposition. J Urol. 1998; 160:1104.

Glenn JF, Anderson EE: Surgical correction of incomplete penoscrotal transposition. J Urol. 1973; 110:603–605.

McIlvoy DB, Harris HS: Transposition of the penis and scrotum: case report J Urol. 1955; 73:540–543.

Mori Y, Ikoma F: Surgical correction of incomplete penoscrotal transposition associated with hypospadias. J Pediatr Surg. 1986; 21:46–48.

Pike LA, Rathburn SR, Husmann DA, et al: Penoscrotal transposition: review of 53 patients. J Urol. 2001; 166:1865–1868.

Retik AB, Mandell J, Bauer SB, et al: Meatal based hypospadias repair with the use of dorsal subcutaneous flap to prevent urethrocutaneous fistula. J Urol. 1994; 152:1229.

Shanberg AM, Rosenberg MT: Partial transposition of the penis and scrotum with anterior urethral diverticulum in a child born with the caudal regression syndrome. J Urol. 1989; 142:1060–1062.

Flaps Versus Grafts

Ahmed T. Hadidi

27.1

Continued clinical experience shows that no single type of urethroplasty is uniformly applicable to all types of hypospadias. Surgeons involved in hypospadias treatment should be able to offer a variety of technical solutions to the gamut of anatomical variations usually encountered. Surgeons who master one technique of repair or who plan to operate only on distal hypospadias are not acting in their patients' best interests. This chapter evaluates the role of different flaps and grafts in the management of hypospadias.

Flaps

Flaps used in hypospadias repair may be meatal-based [e.g. Mathieu, Mustarde and Barcat (Chap. 14), yoke (Chap. 20), Koyanagi (Chap. 19), lateral-based flap with double blood supply (Chap. 21)] or urethral plate-based [Thiersch Duplay (Chap. 13), Denis Browne (Chap. 27.2), Snodgrass (Chap. 15)].

Common pedicled flaps are usually based on preputial vessels and include Hodgson's flap, onlay island flap, transverse preputial island flap (Chap. 16) and Asopa's double-faced island flap (Chap. 18).

Vascularised fascial flaps have recently become popular. They help to provide a protective intermediate layer and minimise complications. Common examples are tunica vaginalis flap, preputial subcutaneous flap and dartos flap. The current routine use of these vascularised fascial flaps has significantly improved the results of hypospadias repair and reduced the incidence of complications to less than 5% in distal hypospadias repair (Snow 1986; Snow et al. 1995).

Grafts

Grafts commonly used in hypospadias repair include preputial skin (full thickness or partial thickness), abdominal skin (full thickness or dermal grafts following chordee excision), bladder mucosa and, currently, buccal mucosa (Chap. 22)

In Chap. 7, the basic principles, advantages and disadvantages of flaps and grafts were discussed. A simple practical maxim was mentioned: "A graft is a non-living tissue that you try to bring to life and a flap is a living tissue that you try not to bring to death". This is perhaps somewhat biased but nevertheless conforms to the basic principles of plastic surgery.

Duckett (1981b) believed that flap repair has an advantage over grafts since the normal blood supply to the tissues is intact. This again conforms to plastic surgery principles.

Many studies evaluated the results of different techniques in the management of proximal hypospadias (Kaplan 1988; Kumar and Harris 1994; Sommerlad 1975; Svensson and Berg 1983). However, in an excellent study, Powell et al. (2000) compared the results of flaps and grafts in the management of proximal hypospadias. In this retrospective investigation they reviewed the records of 142 patients who had undergone proximal hypospadias repair between 1981 and 1997. The techniques used in the repair were transverse preputial island flaps used as a tube or onlay and preputial skin grafts used as a tube or onlay. One surgeon operated on 93 patients (65%). Tube urethroplasty was the routine technique in the earlier years of the study (1980s) and onlay was the preferred technique in later years (1990s). Two thirds of the study group (95 patients) had the repair performed using grafts. Two thirds of the grafts were done as a tube (61 vs 34 patients). In the flap group (47 patients), 27 patients had a tube flap and 20 had an onlay flap. The authors concluded that there was no significant difference in the complication rates of flaps and grafts used to repair proximal hypospadias. However, in the graft group, there was a significantly higher proximal stricture rate when a tube rather than an onlay was used. The study also raised a very important issue, namely that a significant number of complications (67%) presented more than 1 year after surgery.

Table 27.1.1. Complication rates (*% comp.*) for tubed flaps and tubed grafts

Tubed flaps		Tubed grafts	
Study	% Comp.	Study	% Comp.
Powell et al. (2000)	33%	Powell et al. (2000)	34%
Monfort et al. (1983)	42%	Hendren and Crooks (1980)	8.9%
Bondonnay et al. (1984)	19.5%	De Sy and Oosterlinck (1981)	27%
Barraza et al. (1987)	56%	Redman (1983)	30%
Sauvage et al. (1987)	31%	Shapiro (1984)	20%
Harris and Jeffery (1989)	24%	Vyas et al. (1987)	39.4%
Hollowell et al. (1990)	15%	Rober et al. (1990)	50%
Rickwood and Anderson (1991)	28%		
Kass and Bolong (1990)	4.4%		
Wacksman (1986)	11%		

Table 27.1.2. Complication rates (*% comp.*) for onlay flaps and onlay grafts

Onlay flaps		Onlay grafts	
Study	% Comp.	Study	% Comp.
Powell et al. (2000)	30%	Powell et al. (2000)	29%
Elder et al. (1987)	6%	Vyas et al. (1987)	39.4%
Baskin et al. (1994)	8.6%	Rober et al. (1990)	38%

Table 27.1.1 shows the complication rate of tubed flaps and tubed grafts in different series, while Table 27.1.2 shows the complication rate of onlay repairs. The data in the two tables permit no definite conclusions. The retrospective studies were reported at different times, and different suture materials and suture techniques were used. The surgeons had different levels of experience, and selection criteria may have differed. Also, the follow-up period varied from one study to another.

There are other factors that need to be addressed when comparing flaps and grafts. These factors include single- or two-stage repair, the ease or difficulty of flap or graft preparation, the required period of hospitalisation, the duration and degree of mobilisation, the method of urinary diversion, if needed, the comfort of the child (hip spica in case of grafts; Cilento et al. 1997) and the degree of inconvenience to the family.

Further prospective multicentre studies involving a large number of patients using standardised operation techniques, suturing techniques and materials, with a follow-up period of at least 5 years, are needed to permit definite conclusions.

References

Barraza MA, Roth DR, Terry WJ, et al: One-stage reconstruction of moderately severe hypospadias. J Urol. 1987; 137:714.

Baskin LS, Duckett JW, Ueoka K, et al: Changing concepts of hypospadias curvature lead to more onlay island flap procedures. J Urol. 1994; 151:191.

Bondonnay JM, Barthaburu D, Vergnes P: L'Hypospadias balanique et penien. Les elements de la malformation; implicatins therapeutiques et resultats. A partir de l'etude de cent trent-cinq dossiers. Ann Urol (Paris). 1984; 18:21.

Cilento BG, Stock JA, Kaplan GW: Pantaloon spica cast: an effective method for postoperative immobilization after free graft hypospadias repair. J Urol. 1997; 157:1882.

De Sy WA, Oosterlinck W: One-stage hypospadias repair by free full-thickness skin graft and island flap techniques. Urol Clin North Am. 1981; 8:491.

Duckett JW: MAGPI (meatoplasty and glanuloplasty): a procedure for subcoronal hypospadias. Urol Clin North Am. 1981a; 8:513.

Duckett JW: The island flap technique for hypospadias repair. Urol Clin North Am. 1981b; 8:503.

Elder JS, Duckett JW, Snyder HM: Onlay island flap in the repair of mid and distal penile hypospadias without chordee. J Urol. 1987; 138:376.

Harris DL, Jeffery RS: One-stage repair of hypospadias using split preputial flaps (Harris). The first 100 patients treated. Br J Urol. 1989; 63:401.

Hendren WH, Crooks KK: Tubed free skin graft for construction of male urethra. J Urol. 1980; 123:858.

Hollowell JG, Keating MA, Snyder HM, et al: Preservation of the urethral plate in hypospadias repair: extended applications and further experience with the onlay island flap urethroplasty. J Urol. 1990; 143:98.

Kaplan GW: Repair of proximal hypospadias using a preputial free graft for neourethral construction and preputial pedicle flap for ventral skin coverage. J Urol. 1988; 140:1270.

Kass EJ, Bolong D: Single stage hypospadias reconstruction without fistula. J Urol. 1990; 144:520.

Kumar MV, Harris DL: A long-term review of hypospadias repaired by split preputial flap technique (Harris). Br J Plast Surg. 1994; 47:236.

Monfort G, Jean P, Lacoste M: Correction des hypospadias posterieurs en un temps par lambeau pedicule transversal (intervention de Duckett). A propos de 50 observations. Chir Pediatr. 1983; 24:71.

Powell CR, Mcaleer I, Alagiri M, et al: Comparison of flaps versus grafts in proximal hypospadias surgery. J Urol. 2000; 163:1286–1289.

Redman JF: Experience with 60 consecutive hypospadias repairs using the Horton-Devine techniques. J Urol. 1983; 129:115.

Rickwood AM, Anderson PA: One stage hypospadias repair: experience of 367 cases. Br J Urol. 1991; 67:424.

Rober PE, Perlmutter AD, Reitelman C: Experience with 81 1-stage hypospadias/chordee repairs with free graft urethroplasties. J Urol. 1990; 144:526.

Sauvage P, Rougeron G, Bientz J, et al: L'utilisation du lambeau preputial transverse pedicule dans la chirurgie de l'hypospadias. A propos de 100 cas. Chir Pediatr. 1987; 28:220.

Shapiro SR: Complications of hypospadias repair. J Urol. 1984; 131:518.

Snow BW: Use of tunica vaginalis to prevent fistulas in hypospadias surgery. J Urol. 1986; 136:861.

Snow BW, Cartwright PC, Unger K: Tunica vaginalis blanket wrap to prevent urethrocutaneous fistulas: an eight-year experience. J Urol. 1995; 153:472–473.

Sommerlad BC: A long-term follow-up of hypospadias patients. Br J Plast Surg. 1975; 28:324–330.

Svensson J, Berg R: Micturition studies and sexual function in operated hypospadias. Br J Urol. 1983; 55:422–426.

Vyas PR, Roth DR, Perlmutter AD: Experience with free grafts in urethral reconstruction. J Urol. 1987; 137:471.

Wacksman J: Use of the Hodgson XX (modified Asopa) procedure to correct hypospadias with chordee: surgical technique and results. J Urol. 1986; 136:1264.

Single Stage Versus Two Stage Repair

Ahmed T. Hadidi

27.2

Opinions about the best operative technique for patients with hypospadias have varied, evolving with time. Until the 1960s, the accepted methods for surgical management of hypospadias involved a two-stage approach. The most popular techniques were those of Thiersch (1869) and Duplay (1880), modified and popularised by Byars (1955), and that of Nove-Josserand (1897), subsequently adapted and popularised by Bracka (1995a, b), Denis Browne (1949), whose technique was modified by Durham Smith (1973), and Cecil and Culp (Cecil 1946; Culp 1966).

In 1941 T. Higgins wrote, in a prophetic foreword: "If, however, one could succeed in remodeling the urethra in one operation, the gain would be manifest" (Humby 1941).

The first one-stage repair was performed "by mistake" by Russell of Melbourne in 1900. Humby (1941), Broadbent et al. (1961), Devine and Horton (1961) and DesPrez et al. (1961) were instrumental in popularising the one-stage approach for the correction of hypospadias. Work by Standoli (1979) and Duckett (1980), in which the preputial skin was used in a vascularized fashion for correction, further extended the use of one-stage repairs. By 1988, it was being suggested that all primary hypospadias should be repaired with a single-stage approach (Sadove et al. 1988).

Clearly, the most important issue is to achieve a straight penis with a slit-like meatus at the tip of a normal-looking glans penis. How is this best achieved; in one stage or two? One-stage procedures are undoubtedly attractive, desirable and popular. They are associated with a shorter hospital stay and are more convenient for both patient and surgeon alike. However, some surgeons still favour two-stage repair. They base their argument on two points:

Firstly, they argue that most one-stage methods have their technical limitations; thus, a specialized surgeon needs to master a number of unrelated repairs and has to be capable of the decision making that goes with them. On the other hand, some two-stage procedures may be adapted for most deformities. Although this is true, most hypospadiologists agree that there is no place for the "occasional" hypospadias surgeon in the correction of so-called "minor" hypospadias. Surgeons should have a detailed understanding of the various concepts and surgical techniques and maintain a clinical workload that is sufficient to obtain consistently good results.

The other point of argument is that the circumferential meatus that results from some of the one-stage procedures is more liable to stenosis and puckering. Advocates of two-stage repair believe that the quality of the end results is better both psychologically and sexually than with one-stage procedures. This may be true for the older techniques of repair. However, with modern techniques and particularly for distal forms of hypospadias (70–80%), it is possible to achieve a terminal slit-like meatus with one-stage repair and to keep the complication rate down to 5–10% (Retik et al. 1994b; Borer and Retik 1999; Hadidi 1996; Hadidi et al. 2003).

On the other hand, using a two-stage repair, in more than 500 cases, Durham Smith (1981) reduced his incidence of fistula formation to less than 3%. Similarly, Greenfield and colleagues (1994) reported a urethral fistula rate of 2.5% with a two-stage modified Belt–Fuqua repair for severe hypospadias with chordee.

As in other areas of surgical correction, however, a unified approach for all patients is not always possible. Surgical treatment, in order to be most effective, needs to be individualized. For distal hypospadias, the general concept is to perform a single-stage repair (Borer and Retik 1999). The most popular techniques are Y-V modified Mathieu (Chap. 14.2), MAGPI (Chap. 11) and Snodgrass tubularized incised plate (TIP) urethroplasty (Chap. 15). However, few surgeons still recommend two-stage repair in all patients (Bracka 1995a, b, Chap. 23).

Approximately 20% of patients with hypospadias have a proximal defect. The majority of those can be treated with a one-stage repair. The most popular techniques are the onlay island flap (Chap. 16.1),

Transverse preputial island flap (Chap. 16.2), Koyanagi (Chap. 19), Yoke (Chap. 20) and lateral based flap (Chap. 21). For a subset of patients with scrotal or perineal hypospadias, a small phallus and severe chordee, a two-stage repair may be preferable. These patients, if treated with a one-stage repair, usually need a composite graft. Some centres reported unsatisfactory experience with the operative results in such patients managed with a one-stage repair (Retik et al. 1994a; Kroovand and Perlmutter 1980; Greenfield et al. 1994; Bracka 1995a, b).

In conclusion, a small proportion of patients, namely those with severe proximal hypospadias, chordee and a small phallus, may benefit from a two-stage procedure. In such children, a two-stage repair may offer a better cosmetic outcome and a lower complication rate than a one-stage repair with a free, vascularized or composite graft.

The Thiersch–Duplay and the Denis Browne technique are described in the following. Bracka's modification of the Nove-Josserand technique was described in Chap. 23.

Thiersch–Duplay Technique as Modified by Byars and Durham Smith

First Stage

In the first stage, a circumferential incision is made proximal to the coronal sulcus, the chordee is excised, and the penile shaft is degloved (Fig. 27.2.1). Failure to create a straight phallus is one of the avoidable complications of hypospadias surgery. Penile straightening and full removal of chordee must be confirmed by means of the artificial erection test. After securely placing an elastic band at the base of the penis, or using perineal compression, normal saline is injected with a 25-gauge butterfly needle placed in one corporeal body to fill the entire organ. This identifies any restraining fibrous bands that remain. Several tests may be necessary to ensure complete excision. If the penis remains bent despite resection of all chordee, an alternative approach may be needed, such as insertion of a dermal or tunica vaginalis graft into the shaft, or dorsal plication.

When it has been ascertained that the penis is straight, the glans is prepared. The glans is either divided deeply in the midline to the tip or, if the mucosal groove is deep, this is preserved and incisions are made just lateral to the groove on each side (Fig. 27.2.1c). The dorsal foreskin is unfolded carefully and divided in the midline (Fig. 27.2.1d). The most distal portion of the foreskin is rotated into the glanular cleft and sutured to the mucosa of the glans with interrupted sutures of 6-0 chromic catgut. A midline closure is performed, and the midline sutures catch a small portion of Buck's fascia. This eliminates dead space and helps to create a groove in preparation for the second stage (Fig. 27.2.1e). The bladder is drained with an 8-F Silastic Foley catheter for approximately 5–7 days.

Second Stage

The second stage of the procedure is carried out 6–12 months later, when the tissues have usually softened sufficiently and healing is complete. The previously transferred preputial skin is used to reconstruct the glans and urethra. A 16-mm-diameter strip is measured, extending to the tip of the glans (Fig. 27.2.1f). The strip is tubularized with a running subcuticular stitch of 6-0 Vicryl all the way to the tip of the glans (Fig. 27.2.1g). Suture-line tension is reduced before closing this layer by generous mobilization and undermining of adjacent tissues. A urine-tight anastomosis is made and inverted toward the lumen whenever possible. Eversion of suture lines increases periurethral reaction, which contributes to both urine leakage and potential fistula or diverticulum formation. The new urethra must be wide enough to avoid strictures.

Skin Closure ▶ The lateral skin edges are mobilized, and the remaining tissue is closed over the repair in at least two layers. A strip of skin (3–5 mm wide) is then de-epithelialised on one side to provide a raw surface of deep dermis (Fig. 27.2.1h, i). This is achieved by cutting two or three fine longitudinal strips with a pair of small "curved-on" scissors. The medial edge of the shaved flap is brought across the buried urethroplasty and sutured to fascial tissue beneath the other flap (double breasting) (Fig. 27.2.1 j, k). The skin closure is meticulously performed with nylon without strangulation to allow for the expected postoperative swelling. Penoscrotal transposition, if present, is usually repaired during this stage. A penile nerve block is used routinely.

Fig. 27.2.1a–k. Thiersch–Duplay two-stage repair of hypospadias. **a–e** *First stage*: **a** A circumferential incision is made proximal to the coronal sulcus. **b** The chordee is excised, and the penile shaft is degloved. **c** The glans is divided deeply in the midline to the tip. **d** The dorsal foreskin is unfolded carefully and divided in the midline. **e–k** see pp. 264, 265

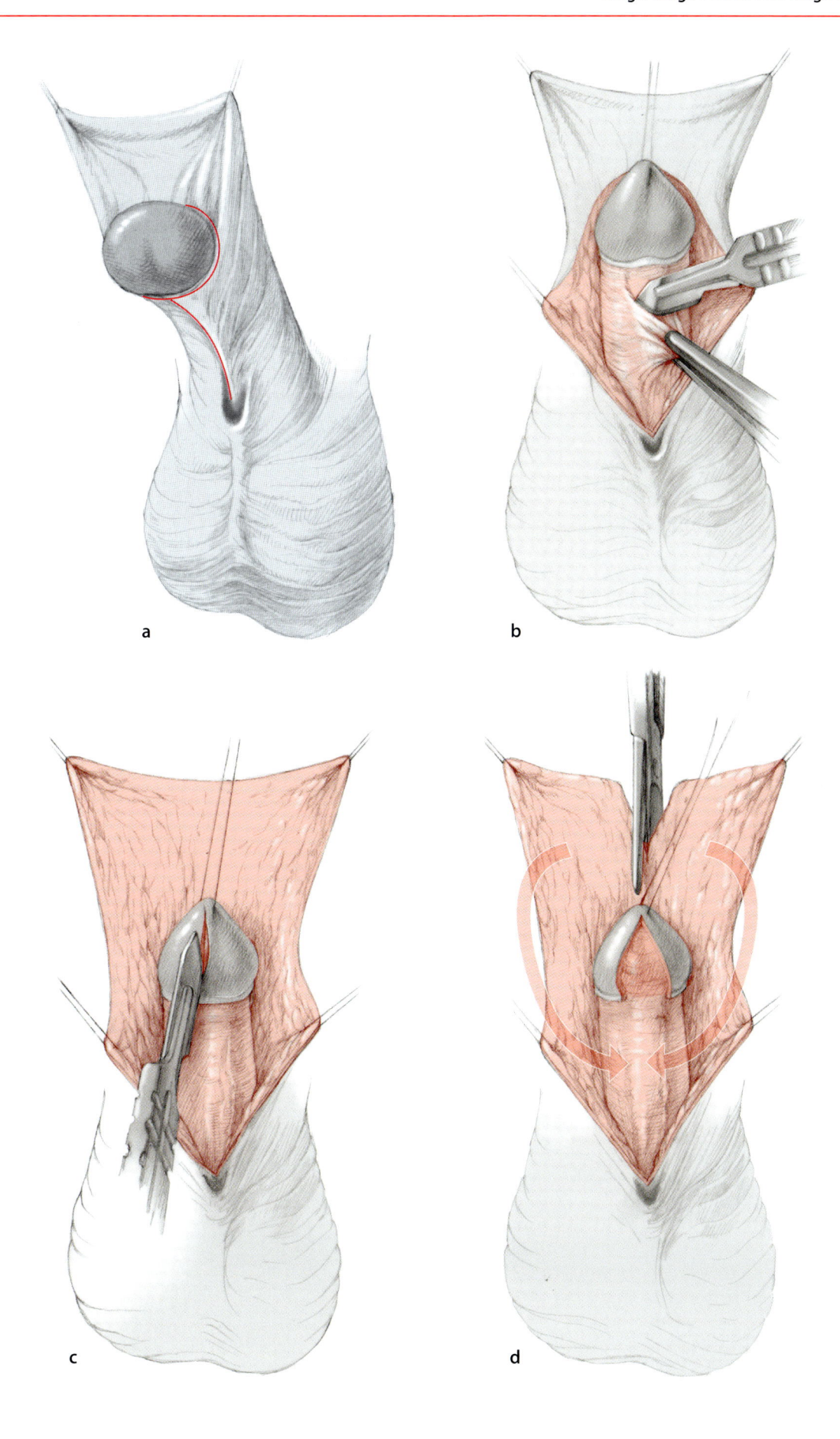

Single Stage Versus Two Stage Repair   263

a

b

c

d

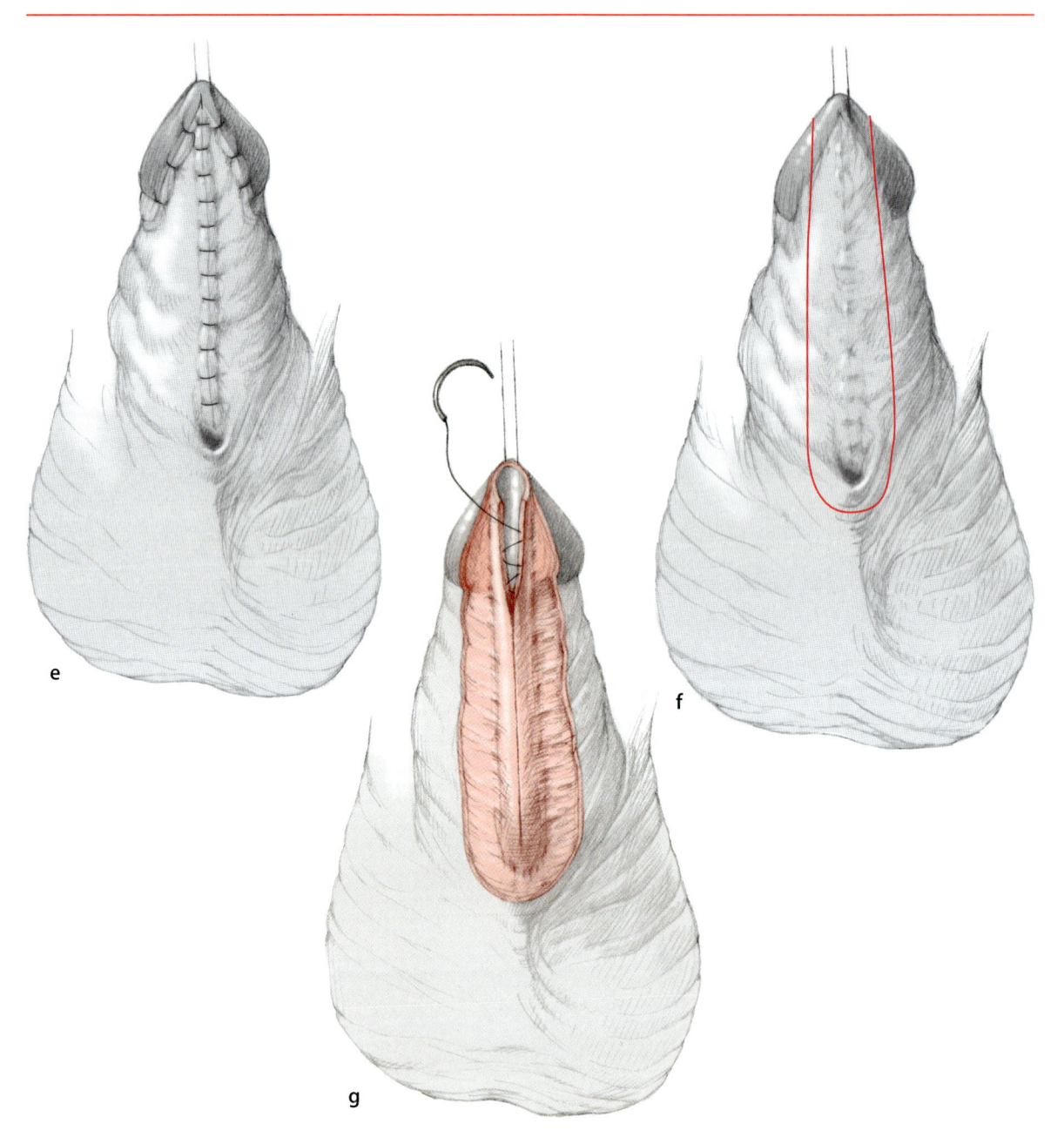

Fig. 27.2.1 (*continued*) **e** A midline closure is performed, and the midline sutures catch a small portion of Buck's fascia. **f–k** *Second stage*: **f** A 16-mm-diameter strip is measured, extending to the tip of the glans. **g** The strip is tubularised with a running subcuticular stitch of 6-0 Vicryl all the way to the tip of the glans. **h–k** see p. 265

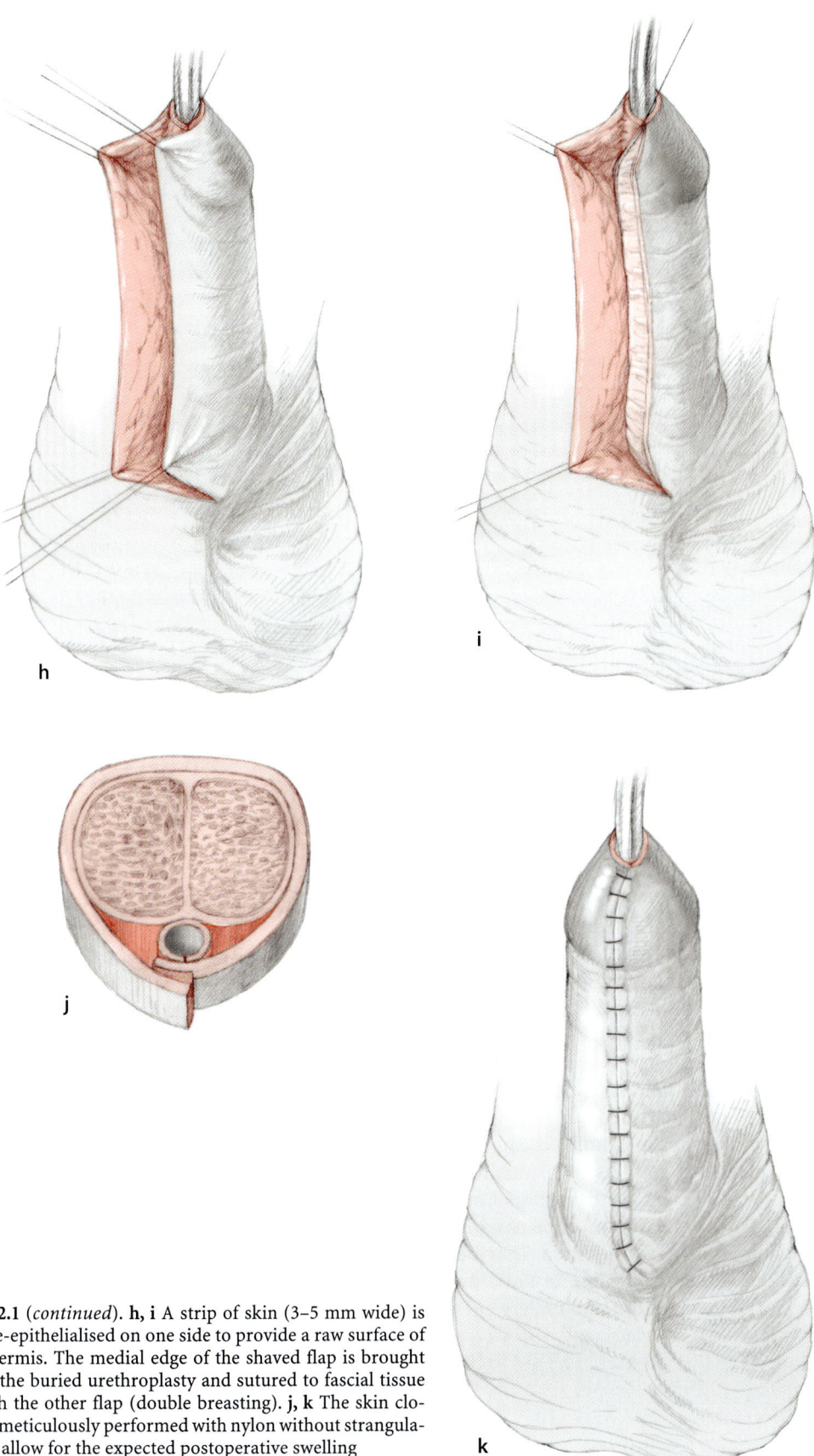

Fig. 27.2.1 (*continued*). **h, i** A strip of skin (3–5 mm wide) is then de-epithelialised on one side to provide a raw surface of deep dermis. The medial edge of the shaved flap is brought across the buried urethroplasty and sutured to fascial tissue beneath the other flap (double breasting). **j, k** The skin closure is meticulously performed with nylon without strangulation to allow for the expected postoperative swelling

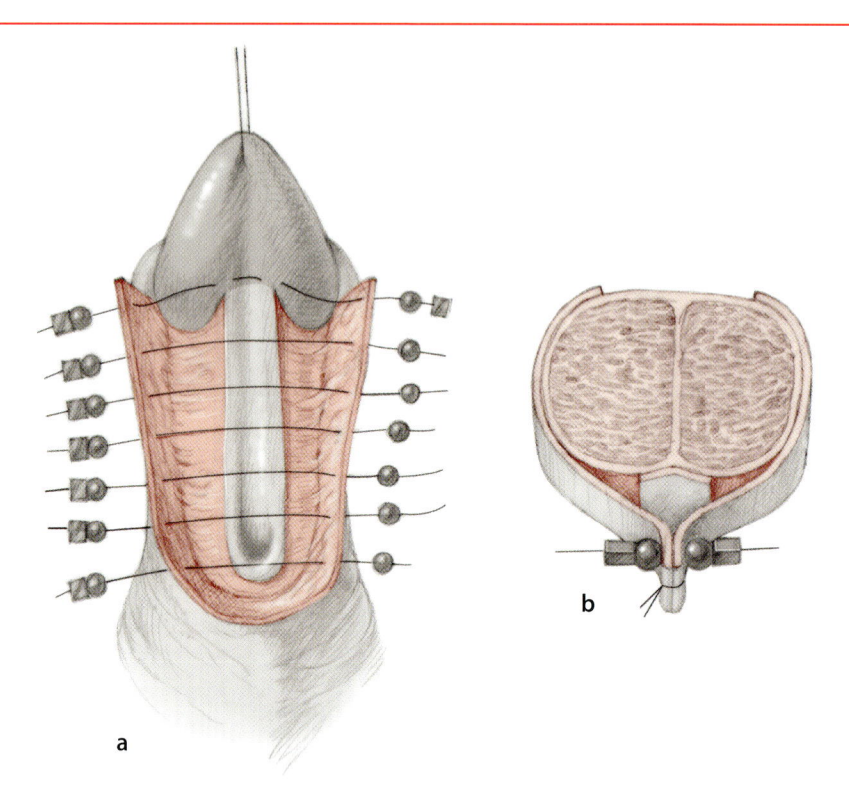

Fig. 27.2.2a, b. Denis Browne technique, second stage. Lateral skin flaps are approximated over the midline longitudinal strip of skin, which remains attached to the ventral surface of the penis. No catheter is placed over the buried strip of skin on the penis

Results

In 1994, Retik et al. reviewed their experience with two-stage hypospadias repair. From 1986 to 1993, they treated 1,437 children with hypospadias. Of those, 58 patients (4%) had scrotal or perineal hypospadias with severe chordee and a small phallus, often resistant to testosterone therapy, which was administered preoperatively as an ointment or parenterally. Those patients underwent a two-stage surgical repair. The use of added subcutaneous tissue or tunica vaginalis (Snow 1986) over the neourethra in several instances achieved the goal of nonoverlapping suture lines and may have offered increased vascularity. The penile nerve block and transparent biomembrane dressing allowed for early postoperative mobilization. The authors reported excellent functional and cosmetic results. In their series, only 3 of 58 children (5%) developed a urethrocutaneous fistula. They believed that the final cosmetic outcome in these patients was superior to that in those who underwent a one-stage repair for less severe defects.

Denis Browne Technique

In the Denis Browne technique (Fig. 27.2.2), the first stage of surgery is as in the Thiersch–Duplay technique. The second stage is completed at about 4–5 years of age. At that time a perineal urethrostomy is performed and a peripheral incision is made around a midline strip of skin on the ventral shaft of the penis, extending from the urethral meatus to the inferior portion of the glans. A small triangle of glans is denuded on each side of the midline. By combining wide undermining and a dorsal relaxing incision, lateral skin flaps can then be approximated over the midline longitudinal strip of skin, which remains attached to the ventral surface of the penis. No catheter is placed over the buried strip of skin on the penis. The perineal catheter is usually removed on the 10th postoperative day, thus allowing the perineal fistula to heal spontaneously.

Several points of surgical technique are important in this operation. First, an adequate urethral opening must be provided and the first-stage meatotomy is essential in most cases. Second, the dorsal longitudinal relaxing incision on the shaft of the penis must not extend past the base of the penis onto the abdominal wall. Incisions on the shaft of the penis heal with wide, flat, pliable scar unless they encroach upon the abdominal wall. At this point, a hypertrophied, keloid-like scar will commonly occur and may cause a disappointing result. Third, the longitudinal strip of skin which is buried must be wide enough to allow circumferential growth of an adequate, new urethra. This may vary with the size of the patient, but should never be less than 1 cm in width, even in a child. In an adult, this should measure 1.5 cm or more. Fourth, to prevent stenosis at this site during healing, the incision should extend well around the tube at the distal end of the normal urethra, leaving a circumferential cuff of normal skin measuring 4–6 mm in all directions. Fifth, the incisions made on the glans penis should extend distally as far as possible to elongate the urethra. This entire technique is simplified by bringing as much tissue as possible to the distal ventral surface of the penis and glans during the first stage of repair. Sixth, tension-relieving sutures should be used when the lateral flaps are brought over the buried strip of skin. Browne secured these sutures with glass beads and crimped metal sleeves so that if necessary the sutures could be loosened from time to time as oedema occurred.

Results

The Denis Browne operation, while probably the most popular method to correct hypospadias in the 1950s and 1960s, was not perfect. Culp (1959) reported a series of complications requiring reoperation in 22–44% of all cases in which the Denis Browne technique had been used. Most authors reported a 10–30% incidence of fistula formation. The usual complications of this operation consist of fistula formation, retrogression of the urethral meatus from the tip and, occasionally, stricture formation. This technique is constructed on sound principles and will produce consistent results when meticulous technique is utilized. Sir Denis Browne considered any modification of his original procedure to be the cause of fistulas and failure. It is important that the relaxing sutures should not be left in place too long. The glass beads should allow at least 0.5 cm of suture free on each side at the time of application, and the beads should be broken and removed if oedema begins to bury them in the skin. Culp (1959) modified this procedure by tying nylon mattress sutures over longitudinal bolsters of rubber tubing to cut down on necrosis of the skin caused by the small pressure points of the sutures. All sutures should be removed in 7 days.

References

Borer JG, Retik AB: Current trends in hypospadias repair. Urol Clin North Am. 1999; 26:15–37.

Bracka A: A versatile two-stage hypospadias repair. Br J Plast Surg. 1995a; 48:345–352.

Bracka A: Hypospadias repair: the two-stage alternative. Br J Urol. 1995b; 76 [Suppl 3]:31–41.

Broadbent TR, Woolf RM, Toksu EA: Hypospadias, one stage repair. Plast Reconstr Surg. 1961; 27:154–159.

Browne D: An operation for hypospadias. Proc R Soc Med. 1949; 41:466–468.

Byars LT: Technique for consistently satisfactory repair of hypospadias. Surg Gynecol Obstet. 1955; 100:184.

Cecil AB: Repair of hypospadias and urethral fistula. J Urol. 1946; 56:237–242.

Culp OS: Experiences with 200 hypospadiacs: evolution of a theraputic plan. Surg Clin North Am. 1959; 39:1007.

Culp OS: Struggles and triumphs with hypospadias and associated anomalies. Review of 400 cases. J Urol. 1966; 96:339–355.

DesPrez JD, Persky L, Kiehn Cl: A one-stage repair of hypospadias by island-flap technique. Plast Reconstr Surg. 1961; 28:405.

Devine CJ Jr, Horton CE: A one stage hypospadias, one stage repair. Plast Reconstr Surg. 1961; 26:164.

Duckett JW: Transverse preputial island-flap technique for repair of severe hypospadias. Urol Clin North Am. 1980; 7:423.

Duplay S: Sur le traitment chirurgical de l'hypospadias et l'epispadias. Arch Gen Med. 1880; 5:257.

Greenfield SP, Sadler BT, Wan J: Two-stage repair for severe hypospadias. J Urol. 1994; 152:498.

Hadidi AT: Y-V Glanuloplasty: a new modification in the surgery of hypospadias. Kasr EL Aini Med J. 1996; 2:223–233.

Hadidi A, Abdaal N, Kaddah S: Hypospadias repair: is stenting important. Kasr El Aini J Surg. 2003; 4 (2):3–8.

Humby G: A one stage operation for hypospadias. Br J Surg. 1941; 29:84.

Kroovand RL, Perlmutter AD: Extended urethroplasty in hypospadias. Urol Clin North Am. 1980; 7:431.

Nove-Josserand G: Traitement de l'hypospadias; nouvelle method. Lyon Med. 1897; 85:198.

Retik AB, Bauer SB, Mandell J, et al: Management of severe hypospadias with a 2-stage repair. J Urol. 1994a; 152: 749–751.

Retik AB, Mandell J, Bauer SB, et al: Meatal based hypospadias repair with the use of a dorsal subcutaneous flap o prevent urethrocutaneous fistula. J Urol. 1994b; 152:1229.

Russell RH: Operation for severe hypospadias. Br Med J. 1990; 2:1432.

Sadove RC, Horton CE, McRoberts JW: The new era of hypospadias surgery. Clin Plast Surg. 1988; 15:354.

Smith ED: A de-epithelialised overlap flap technique in the repair of hypospadias. Br J Plast Surg. 1973; 26:106–114.

Smith ED: Durham Smith repair of hypospadias. Urol Clin North Am. 1981; 8:451–455.

Snow BW: Use of tunica vaginalis to prevent fistulas in hypospadias surgery. J Urol. 1986; 136:861.

Standoli L: Correzione dell ipospadias in tempo unico: technica della uretroplastica con lembo ad isola preputiale. Ital Chir Pediatr. 1979; 21:82.

Thiersch C: On the origin and operative treatment of epispadias. Arch Heilkd. 1869; 10:20.

Stenting Versus No Stenting

27.3

Ahmed T. Hadidi

Many one-stage repairs for hypospadias have been developed in the past 25 years. The complication rate has remained stable at approximately 10% despite the use of optical magnification, fine instruments, meticulous haemostasis and broad-spectrum antibiotics (Mitchell and Kulb 1986).

Inherent to all hypospadias repairs has been the use of a bladder drainage catheter or a stent, the purpose of which has been to provide temporary urinary diversion, permit the repair to become watertight, immobilize the suture line, drain the neourethra, reduce tissue reaction and provide patient comfort. On the other hand, disadvantages of catheter drainage or stenting include the length of hospital stay (4–8 days), decreased patient mobility, bladder spasms, and increased potential for infection. Other complications include migration into the bladder and mechanical catheter problems that may create inadequate drainage and even result in pressure ischaemia of the neourethra (Rabinowitz 1987).

Urinary diversion following hypospadias surgery has gone through different stages: perineal urethrostomy, open suprapubic cystostomy, percutaneous suprapubic cystostomy, intraurethral catheter drainage of the bladder and urethral stenting short of the bladder.

Although Mathieu (1932) in his first description of his wonderful technique in the *Archives des Maladies du Rein*, did not leave a catheter, catheter drainage to divert urine has been considered necessary to allow for healing of the suture line so that it may become watertight. A catheter helps to immobilize and drain the neourethra. Catheter drainage and/or urinary diversion has been recommended for 2–14 days (Wacksman 1981; Kim and Hendren 1981; Gonzales et al. 1983; Devine et al. 1988; Man et al. 1986; Snodgrass et al. 1996). An informal hand-raising poll at the 1995 AAP Section on Urology Meeting suggested that most paediatric urologists do stent their non-MAGPI repairs (Freedman 1999).

In 1986, Mitchell and Kulb described the use of a silicon urethral splint instead of a bladder drainage catheter. They suggested deroofing the silicon stent. Thus, the stent would expand and contract according to the degree of oedema. Yet, it permits voiding and drainage of the neourethra and even catheterisation should thus be unnecessary.

Rabinowitz, writing in 1987, reported outpatient catheterless Mathieu repair for distal hypospadias in 59 boys, with an excellent cosmetic and functional outcome and few complications. He concluded that urinary diversion was unnecessary.

In 1993 Wheeler and colleagues, in a retrospective study, compared a group of 10 boys with a bladder stent following Mathieu repair with another group of 11 boys without a stent following the same procedure. There was no statistical difference in outcome or in complications. Thus, they supported Rabinowitz' conclusion that stenting is not mandatory in Mathieu repair.

In 1994, Buson et al. reported their experience with Mathieu repair for distal hypospadias in a non-random study that included 65 patients with stents and 37 patients without stents. They reported a statistically significant difference ($p<0.05$) between the group with stents (complication rate 4.6%) and the group without stenting (18.9%). They concluded that "the use of a multiperforated silicone urethral stent is advantageous for the Mathieu operation".

In 1996 Hakim et al., in a multicentre retrospective study, reviewed 336 boys who had undergone Mathieu repair for distal hypospadias. There were 114 patients with stents and 222 boys without stents. Interestingly, there were no instances of urinary retention in the unstented group, including those patients who received caudal anaesthesia. They found that the complication rate in the stented group (2.21%) was not statistically significantly lower than that in the non-stented group (3.6%; $p=0.756$). They suggested that "successful Mathieu hypospadias repair is independent of the use of a stent".

In 1997 Demirbilek and Atayurt, in a non-random study of 105 consecutive patients with different types of hypospadias, compared suprapubic diversion and transurethral drainage with stenting. In addition to the fact that it was a non-random study, they used a transurethral stent for 2 days even in the group where they did suprapubic drainage. A third drawback was the use of a suprapubic diversion in 28 cases of Mathieu repair for distal hypospadias. Many surgeons might consider this an unnecessarily invasive procedure. However, they concluded from their study that "the incidence of complications with transurethral stenting (26.5%) was significantly higher than with supra-pubic drainage (10.7%; $p<0.05$)". They also recommended "the use of supra-pubic diversion in all hypospadias repair because it provides lower complication rates and is more comfortable for children during the post-operative period". Using a suprapubic drainage in distal hypospadias repair goes a little too far.

Several large series support the performance of distal penile hypospadias repair without the use of a urethral stent (Borer and Retik 1999). In one large series of Mathieu repairs with limited use of urethral stents, there were no urethrocutaneous fistulas (Retik et al. 1994).

Recently, successful stent-free hypospadias repair has been reported using the Snodgrass modification (Steckler and Zaontz 1997).

Hadidi et al. (2003) conducted a prospective randomised study to evaluate the role of stenting in hypospadias. The study included 100 suffering from different degrees of hypospadias. The operations were performed by a single surgeon (A.H.) who was notified only at the end of the operation whether to insert a stent or not. The incidence of complications in the form of failure of repair, fistula formation or meatal stenosis was higher in group B with stenting (10%) than in group A without stenting (2%). The difference in complication rate was not statistically significant ($p=0.092$). However, the incidence of morbidity in the form of oedema, stent block or urinary retention was statistically significantly higher in group B with stenting (44%) than in group A without stenting (18%; $p=0.005$).

Because hypospadias repair is a surface operation that does not violate a body cavity, it lends itself readily to the outpatient setting. As such, there is no place for a complex postoperative regimen that restricts the child's mobility or interferes with the parents' general care of the child (Burbige and Connor 1999).

References

Borer JG, Retik AB: Current trends in hypospadias repair. Urol Clin North Am. 1999; 26:15.

Burbige KA, Connor JP: Postoperative management of hypospadias. In: Ehrlich RM, Alter GJ (eds) Reconstructive and plastic surgery of the external genitalia, adult and pediatrics, 1st edn, chap 33. Saunders, Philadelphia, p 163, 1999.

Buson H, Smiley D, Reinberg Y, et al: Distal hypospadias repair without stents: is it better? J Urol. 1994; 151:1059.

Demirbilek S, Atayurt HF: One-stage hypospadias repair with stent or suprapubic diversion: which is better? J Pediatr Surg. 1997; 32:1711–1712.

Devine CJJR, Horton CE, Gilbert DA, et al: Hypospadias. In: Mustarde JC, Jackson IT (eds): Plastic surgery in infancy and childhood, 3rd edn, chap 31. Churchill Livingstone, Edinburgh, pp 493–509; 1988.

Freedman AL: Dressings, stents and tubes. In: Ehrlich RM, Alter GJ (eds) Reconstructive and plastic surgery of the external genitalia, adult and pediatrics, 1st edn, chap 32. Saunders, Philadelphia, pp 159–162; 1999.

Gonzales ET Jr, Veeraraghavan KA, Delaune J: The management of distal hypospadias with meatal-based, vascularized flaps. J Urol. 1983; 129:119.

Hadidi A, Abdaal N, Kaddah S: Hypospadias repair: is stenting important? Kasr El Aini J Surg. 2003; 4(2):3–8.

Hakim S, Merguerian PA, Rainowitz R, et al: Outcome analysis of the modified Mathieu hypospadias repair: comparison of stented and unstented repair. J Urol. 1996; 156:836.

Kim SH, Hendren WH: Repair of mild hypospadias. J Pediatr Surg. 1981; 16:806.

Man DWK, Vorderwark JS, Ransley PG: Experience with single stage hypospadias reconstruction. J Pediatr Surg. 1986; 21:338.

Mathieu P: Traitement en un temps de l'hypospadias balanique et juxta-balanique. J Chir (Paris). 1932; 39:481.

Mitchell ME, Kulb TB: Hypospadias repair without a bladder drainage catheter. J Urol. 1986; 135:321.

Rabinowitz R: Outpatient catheterless modified Mathieu hypospadias repair. J Urol. 1987; 138:1074.

Retik AB, Mandell J, Bauer SB, et al: Meatal based hypospadias repair with the use of a dorsal subcutaneous flap to prevent urethrocutaneous fistula. J Urol. 1994; 152: 1229.

Snodgrass W, Koyle M, Manzoni G, et al: Tubularized incised plate hypospadias repair: results of a multicenter experience. J Urol. 1996; 156:839.

Steckler RE, Zaontz MR: Stent-free Thiersch-Duplay hypospadias repair with the Snodgrass modification. J Urol. 1997; 158:1178.

Wacksman J: Modification of the one-stage flip-flap procedure to repair distal penile hypospadias. Urol Clin North Am. 1981; 8:527.

Wheeler RA, Malone PS, Griffiths DM, et al: The Mathieu operation: is a urethral stent mandatory? Br J Urol. 1993; 71:492.

Dressing Versus No Dressing

Ahmed T. Hadidi

How important is the use of dressings in hypospadias surgery? Cromie and Bellinger (1981) gave a questionnaire to 45 hypospadias surgeons in the USA: "…85 to 95 percent felt the dressing was of importance. Its major effect is manifested by immobilisation of the penis and prevention of oedema. The ideal dressing would be supple and immobile, but generally a firm-immobile dressing is acceptable". Most individuals responding to the questionnaire felt that the dressing should not be changed and that it was unrelated to the occurrence of skin slough or infection. Most dressings were left in place for more than 3 days, and immobilisation with close attention to postoperative oedema was strongly recommended by the respondents.

If we review the process of wound healing, "within hours after the wound is closed, the wound space fills with an inflammatory exudate. Epidermal cells at the edges of the wound begin to divide and migrate across the wound surface. By 48 hours after closure, deeper structures are completely sealed from the external environment. Dressings over closed wounds should be removed on the third or fourth postoperative day. Dressings should be removed earlier if they are wet because soaked dressings increase bacterial contamination of the wound" (Mulvihill and Pellegrini 1994).

Dressings following hypospadias surgery are likely to become wet from four different sources; urine dripping through the urethra (even if diversion is used), exudate from wound edges, soiling following bowel movements (if permeable or semi-permeable dressings are used) and skin sweating, especially if impermeable dressings are used.

Understandably, dressing limits the degree of edema postoperatively. However, dressing may also decrease blood flow to the penis carrying oxygen, nutrients, inflammatory cells, chemotactic substances and growth factors which are important for healing. Surgeons are usually concerned that edema may be that severe to cut through the repair and stitches. In practice, the author has only experienced this in cases of severe infection. Otherwise, edema is unlikely to cut through the stitches.

If the use of a dressing is indeed important, as held by the many surgeons who advocate it, what is the best kind of dressing? Unfortunately, the ideal dressing for hypospadias repair remains elusive, to judge by the many varieties of dressing currently in use (Redman and Smith 1974; Tan and Reid 1990).

Reviewing the type of hypospadias dressings described in the literature, a great diversity becomes apparent with regard to the degree of concealment and the type of material and technique used. Horton et al. (1980) are strong advocates of unconcealing dressing. Falkowski and Firlit (1980) favoured the totally concealing type of dressing. However, the partially concealing dressing is the most popular type and has many variations. W. Campbell (1980, personal communication), wrapped the penis with elastic foam and passed a small intestinal straight needle transversely through the glans, resting it on top of the foam dressing. Another variation is the use of a styrofoam cup placed over the standard partially concealing dressing; this is secured by the use of the glandular traction stitch, which is then taped to the sides of the cup. Falkowski and Firlit described the X-shaped elastic dressing in 1980. Silicon foam dressings became very popular after they were first described by De Sy and Oosterlink (1982). Currently, many surgeons use simple methods of fixation such as Tegaderm (Freedman 1999), Opsite spray (Tan and Reid 1990) or Dermolite II tape (Redman 1991). Duckett (1996) recommended the use of Tegaderm for 48 h in distal forms of hypospadias and for 72 h in other types of hypospadias surgery with urinary diversion.

In 1965, Hermann published a report of a study in which all dressings from clean wounds were removed on the 2nd postoperative day with no evidence of an increased incidence of wound sepsis:

> What then is the explanation of our observation that postoperative dressings may be removed from a wound healing per primum on the second day, without increasing the incidence of infection? The answer must lie in the fact that wound edges, carefully approximated, are sufficiently sealed by coagulum and overlying epithelial regrowth to resist contamination. Of additional importance, it would seem, is the fact that an exposed wound is a dry wound and few bacteria retain their vitality on a dry surface.

Howells and Young (1966) progressed one step further and introduced the concept of completely undressed surgical wounds. They reported 105 widely varied surgical cases in which, after careful closure of the incision, the patient's gown was simply pulled down over the wound. The frequency of wound infection was 4%, comparable with the incidence of infection in clean wounds.

Law and Ellis randomised 170 consecutive patients undergoing either inguinal hernia repair or high saphenous ligation to one of three surgical options: a dry dressing of gauze, a polyurethane film dressing (Opsite) and immediate exposure. There was no difference in dressing comfort or dressing preference among the different groups, and the quality of the final scar was also not different. There was, however, a higher infection rate in the polyurethane (Opsite) group, although the difference did not attain statistical significance. This was probably due to the moist environment beneath the dressing (Law and Ellis 1987).

In hypospadias surgery, the main purpose of a dressing is to immobilise the penis, minimise oedema and prevent haematoma formation (Gaylis et al. 1989).

Van Savage et al., in 2000, conducted a randomised prospective study of dressing versus no dressing for hypospadias repair. They showed that the success rate for hypospadias surgery that preserves the urethral plate is independent of dressing usage. They concluded that dressings may not be indicated for all types of hypospadias repairs.

In 2001 McLorie et al., in a prospective study, evaluated the role of dressing in hypospadias repair. They showed that the surgical outcome and rate of complications were not compromised without a postoperative dressing. They concluded that "An absent dressing simplified postoperative ambulatory parent delivered home care". They recommended that dressings should be omitted from routine use after hypospadias repair.

Hadidi et al. (2003) conducted a prospective randomised study to assess the role of dressings in hypospadias surgery. The study concluded that repair of hypospadias without a dressing offers statistically significantly better results than when using a dressing ($p=0.014$). This may confirm Hermann's idea that "an exposed wound is a dry wound and few bacteria retain their vitality on a dry surface" (Hermann 1965). The study suggested that the higher incidence of complications in the dressing group may be due to the fact that the wound inevitably becomes wet due to the four potential sources, i.e. urine, ooze, sweat and stools.

References

Cromie WJ, Bellinger MF: Hypospadias dressings and diversions. Urol Clin North Am. 1981; 8:545.

De Sy WA, Oosterlink W: Silicone foam elastomer: a significant improvement in postoperative penile dressing. J Urol. 1982; 128:39.

Duckett JW: Hypospadias. In: Gillenwater JY, Grayhack JT, Howards SS, Duckett JW (eds): Adult and pediatric urology, 3rd edn, chap 55. Mosby Year Book, St Louis, pp 2549–2589; 1996.

Falkowski WS, Firlit CF: Hypospadias surgery: the X-shaped elastic dressing. J Urol. 1980; 123:904.

Freedman AL: Dressings, stents and tubes. In: Ehrlich RM, Alter GJ (eds) Reconstructive and plastic surgery of the external genitalia: adult and pediatrics, 1st edn, chap 32. Saunders, Philadelphia, pp 159–162; 1999.

Gaylis FD, Zaontz MR, Dalton D, et al: Silicone foam dressing for penis after reconstructive pediatric surgery. Urology. 1989; 33:296–299.

Hadidi A, Abdaal N, Kaddah S: Hypospadias repair: Is dressing important? Kasr El Aini J Surg. 2003; 4 (1):37–44.

Hermann RE: Early exposure in the management of the postoperative wound. Surg Gynecol Obstet. 1965; 120:503.

Horton CE, Devine CJ, Graham JK:. Fistulas of the penile urethra. Plast Reconstr Surg. 1980; 66:407.

Howells CH, Young HB: A study of completely undressed surgical wounds. Br J Surg. 1966; 53:436.

Law NW, Ellis H: Exposure of the wound – a safe economy in the NHS. Postgrad Med J. 1987; 63:27.

McLorie G, Joyner B, Herz D, et al: A prospective randomized clinical trial to evaluate methods of postoperative care of hypospadias. J Urol. 2001; 165:1669–1672.

Mulvihill SJ, Pellegrini CA: Current surgical diagnosis and treatment, 10th edn, chap 3 (Way LW, ed). Lange, Connecticut, p. 16; 1994.

Redman JF: A dressing technique that faciltates outpatient hypospadias surgery. Urology. 1991; 37:248–250.

Redman JF, Smith JP: Surgical dressing for hypospadias repair. Urology. 1974; 4:739–740.

Tan KK, Reid CD: A simple penile dressing following hypospadias surgery. Br J Plast Surg. 1990; 43:628–629.

Van Savage JG, Palanca LG, Slaughenhoupt BL: A prospective randomized trial of dressings versus no dressings for hypospadias repair. J Urol. 2000; 164:981–983.

Complications and Late Sequelae

Hypospadias Surgery

Early Complications

Ahmed T. Hadidi, Wael El-Saied

Infection

Every effort should be made to prevent wound infection. Separation of the foreskin adherent to the glans and removal of desquamated epithelial debris should be performed under anaesthesia prior to skin preparation. When the patient is postpubertal, skin preparation should be undertaken several days before surgery with thrice-daily cleansing.

Wound infection is a rare problem in hypospadias repair, especially in the prepubertal patient. As long as good viability of tissue is maintained, infection should be a minor problem.

Prophylactic antibiotics are of little value in avoiding wound infections in hypospadias surgery. Postoperatively, however, trimethoprim-sulfa or nitrofurantoin suppression may be helpful to prevent cystitis, particularly if the tube is left to drain openly into the diaper (Montagnino et al. 1988; Sugar and Firlit 1989).

In general, drains are not employed except when a skin graft or buccal mucosal graft is used. In such cases, a vacuum suction drain is created by placing a scalp vein needle into the vacuum tube while the tubing from the needle is placed under the skin. This helps keep the graft adherent to the overlying skin. Drains should be removed as soon as their purpose has been served, in order to keep the skin in continuity with the graft (24–48 h) (Duckett and Baskin 1996).

Meatal Stenosis

The meatus can become stenotic through crusting, oedema, or synechiae. Leaving a stent in place may help to avoid these complications.

If a stent is not left in place, baths twice daily, after which the parents place an ophthalmic ointment tube nozzle into the urethral meatus, will suffice. Gentle bougienage with a straight sound in initial follow-up visits also assists in meatal patency.

Loss of Skin Flaps

Poor wound healing is due primarily to ischaemic flaps. Appropriate care during the procedure should avoid this problem. If skin flap loss occurs over a well-vascularised island-flap neourethra, healing can occur after the sloughed skin is gone. If a free-graft technique has been used, a sloughed skin flap over the neourethra will jeopardise the entire procedure (Duckett and Baskin 1996).

Oedema

Oedema occurs after most hypospadias repairs and can be diminished by means of a compression dressing.

Oedema within the urethra may compromise healing if a urethral stent is too large. A compressible stent was described by Mitchell and Kulb (1986).

Haemorrhage

Intraoperative haemorrhage can, at times, be troublesome. With careful attention to the control of bleeding by judicious use of point-tip cautery or bipolar diathermy it can be kept to a minimum. Tourniquets or cutaneous infiltrations with dilute concentrations of epinephrine can be helpful but they should not replace careful technique (Duckett and Baskin 1996). Postoperative bleeding is controlled by the application of a compressive dressing (Murphy 2000). Evacuation of a haematoma is not usually necessary unless a free graft is used.

Erection

In the postpubertal patient, postoperative erections can be a significant problem. Various medications and procedures have been tried with little success.

The best of these is amyl nitrite pulvules (Duckett and Baskin 1996).

Retrusive Meatus

Occasionally, a meatus heals in such a way that it retracts and deflects the urinary stream downward. This problem is more common in older types of hypospadias repair. It may be corrected by a Mustarde-type flap and glans channel, or a Mathieu flip-flap procedure. However, long-term results with these as secondary procedures are not good (Secrest et al. 1993).

Bladder Spasm

When a catheter is left inside the bladder postoperatively for urinary diversion, bladder spasms may occur and are sometimes very troublesome. Oxybutynin chloride suspension may be helpful (Keating and Rich 1999). Valium 1–2 mg given orally or intramuscularly has been found helpful to relieve bladder spasms.

Catheter Blockage

Another problem that was common in the postoperative period in the past was catheter blockage. The catheter may be blocked with urinary crusts or blood clots. This is less common nowadays with the use of silastic catheters and deroofed stents. If it occurs, however, it can be very troublesome and will necessitate catheter removal. The patient may be left to void spontaneously, need another fine catheter inserted or require insertion of a percutaneous cystocath into the bladder.

References

Duckett JW, Baskin LS: Hypospadias. In: Gillenwater JY, Grayhack JT, Howards SS, Duckett JW (eds): Adult and pediatric urology, 3rd edn. Mosby-Year Book, St. Louis. pp 2549–2589; 1996.

Keating MA, Rich MA: Onlay and tubularised preputial island flaps. In Ehrlich RM, Alter GJ (eds) Reconstructive and plastic surgery of the external genitalia: adult and pediatrics. Saunders, Philadelphia, p 77; 1999.

Mitchell ME, Kulb TB: Hypospadias repair without a bladder drainage catheter. J Urol. 1986; 135:321.

Montagnino BA, Gonzales ET Jr, Roth DR: Open catheter drainage after urethral surgery. J Urol. 1988; 140:1250.

Murphy JP: Hypospadias: In: Ashcraft KW, Murphy JP, Sharp RJ et al (eds): Pediatric surgery, 3rd edn. Saunders, Philadelphia, p 763–782; 2000.

Secrest CL, Jordan GH, Winslow BH, et al: Repair of complications of hypospadias surgery. J Urol. 1993; 150:1415.

Sugar EC, Firlit CF: Urinary prophylaxis and postoperative care of children at home with an indwelling catheter after hypospadias repair. Urology. 1989; 32:418.

Fistula Repair

28.2

Ahmed T. Hadidi

There is no surgery without complications. Barry O'Donell of Dublin famously commented: "Three statements I never believed in my life: of course I love you, darling, the cheque is in the mail and I never had a complication or a fistula after hypospadias repair". A fistula is defined as a tract connecting two epithelial surfaces, and a sinus is a tract leading to an epithelial surface. Urethrocutaneous fistula is the most common complication in hypospadias surgery.

Incidence of Fistula Formation

The incidence of fistula formation has decreased gradually in the past two decades. In 1973, Horton and Devine estimated the incidence of fistula following hypospadias surgery to range between 15% and 45%. In 1984, Shapiro found a urethral fistula rate of 6.25% (11 cases) in a series of 176 hypospadias repairs including the MAGPI, flip-flap, island, and free-graft techniques. In 1996, Duckett and Baskin estimated the incidence to be between 10% and 15%. Nowadays, the incidence of urethrocutaneous fistula can be used to judge the success of hypospadias repair. Some procedures are more prone to fistula formation than others. For example, in an extensive review of hypospadias repairs in 1990, Durham Smith noted that the fistula rate for the meatoplasty and glanuloplasty (MAGPI) procedure ranged from 0.5% to 10%, whereas the rate for flip-flap repairs varied from 2.2% to 35% and that for island pedicle tubed repairs from 4% to 33%. Free-graft tubed repairs encountered even higher fistula rates of 15–50%. Urethral advancement for distal hypospadias repair has a variable incidence of fistula, from less than 1% to 16.7%. It has not been widely used because of the risk of urethral devascularisation with extensive mobilisation (Shapiro 1999). For the megameatus variety of hypospadias, the pyramid procedure has a reported fistula rate of less than 5%.

Using a two-stage repair, in more than 500 cases, Durham Smith (1981) reduced his incidence of fistula formation to less than 3%. Similarly, Greenfield and colleagues reported a urethral fistula rate of 2.5% with a two-stage modified Belt–Fuqua repair for severe hypospadias with chordee.

Causes of Fistula Formation

Many factors that may cause a high incidence of fistula formation. The most common reasons are technical and avoidable. They include rough tissue handling, the use of poorly vascularised tissues in repair, the use of very thin or fibrotic epithelium or skin, the type and size of suture material (e.g. PDS inside the urethra or non-absorbable material), the suturing technique, infection and distal stenosis.

Fistula Prevention

In distal hypospadias, a fistula rate of less than 5% is now to be expected (Belman 1994a). The numerous factors that have accounted for this lower incidence of fistula formation today are listed in Table 28.2.1. Better and finer suture materials are available today with greater tensile strength and less reactivity, in-

Table 28.2.1. Factors related to a lower incidence of urethral fistula formation

1. Technical points	Type of suture
	Fine instruments
	Magnification
2. Type of repair	Onlay island flap
	Mathieu procedure
	Lateral based flap
3. Protective intermediate layer	De-epithelialised skin
	Tunica vaginalis
	Dartos flap
	Dorsal subcutaneous flap
	External spermatic fascia
4. ? No intra urethral stenting	
5. ? No dressing	

cluding 6-0 to 7-0 polyglactin (Vicryl) and polyglycolic acid (Dexon). These sutures can be used on the skin (7-0 PDS, 6-0 and 7-0 polyglactin and polyglycolic acid) as well as internally. PDS should not be used in the urethra (subcuticular is satisfactory) because it may react with urine and fistula may result (El Mahrouky et al. 1987). Plastic surgical principles such as microvascular instruments and delicate tissue handling are now used by most hypospadias surgeons. Vascularised island pedicle flaps are preferred in the various repairs and their modifications. De-epithelialised flaps were first described by Smith in 1973. The principle was applied by Belman (1994) to the island pedicle procedures, with only one fistula in 32 onlay repairs. Hill and colleagues (1993) used the de-epithelialised flap to improve results of the pyramid procedure. Most surgeons use either the microscope or 3.5× optical magnification. Multiple layer closure has a major role in lowering the incidence of fistula formation. The additional layer may be obtained from either the fascia underlying the Mathieu flap, the fascia underlying the preputial skin(dorsal subcutaneous flap) or a tunica vaginalis wrap. Using the dorsal subcutaneous flap. Retik and associates (1994) performed 204 meatal-based flap hypospadias repairs without a urethrocutaneous fistula. Snow and coworkers (1995) used the tunica vaginalis blanket wrap for five different hypospadias repair procedures in 89 patients. The fistula rate decreased from 20% to 9% when microscope magnification was combined with the tunica vaginalis blanket wrap.

Intraurethral catheters and stents may have an important role in fistula formation. In a prospective comparative study in Cairo University, the role of stenting and catheterisation has been evaluated. The study included 100 patients divided randomly into a silicone stent group and a no stenting group. Although the difference was not statistically significant, the incidence of complications and fistula formation was higher in the stented group (Hadidi et al. 2003a).

However, if the surgeon prefers to use catheters or stents, non-reactive silicone stents or catheters are better employed. A stent or catheter one size smaller than the urethra should be selected to permit voiding around the tube should it become plugged or should bladder spasms occur.

Another major factor is the use of different types of dressings. In a comparative prospective study in Cairo University, the role of dressing has been evaluated. The study concluded that dressings in general statistically increase the incidence of complications and fistula formation in hypospadias repair (Hadidi et al. 2003b). Other authors showed that dressings should be omitted from routine use after hypospadias repair (van Savage et al. 2000; McLorie et al. 2001). For those surgeons who still prefer to use dressings, modern hypospadias dressings with materials such as Duoderm (ConvaTec, Bristol-Myers Squibb) or silicone foam have also aided in reducing the incidence of fistula.

Types and Sites of Fistula

The urethrocutaneous fistula encountered after hypospadias repair may be single and simple or it may be multiple and complicated. Simple tiny fistulas may occur even when experienced surgeons use good, delicate techniques. They may occur anywhere along the neourethra and even with urethral advancement (devascularisation). However, common sites include the site of the original meatus, at the corona or the glans penis. Fistulas at the corona and the glans are more difficult to treat and have a higher incidence of recurrence.

Multiple and complicated fistulas are less common; they may occur due to technical factors such as ischaemia, infection and distal stenosis.

Treatment of Fistula

Following fistula formation there may be inflammation and/or urine extravasation and urethral tissues quickly become oedematous and friable. There is little point in attempting to close a newly formed fistula by means of secondary sutures, and in fact further inflammation will inevitably result in a larger fistulous opening (Horton and Devine 1973). Recently, some surgeons have recommended the use of fibrin glue to aid the healing of a freshly formed fistula. The results are not promising as yet.

The classic management after fistula appearance is to insert a Foley catheter into the bladder for 10–14 days and give appropriate antibiotics until tissue induration and inflammation disappears. However, it is possible that fistulas which heal in this way would have healed in any case, without a catheter. In fact, the catheter (even a silicon one) may cause irritation that diminishes the chances of spontaneous healing.

Once a fistula has formed, it is recommended that no surgical repair be considered for 6–12 months. This is the minimum time required for complete wound healing and to allow for full resolution of scar tissue.

Before attempting any repair of a fistula, it is important to recognise the presence of a urethral diverticulum or distal urethral stricture, because any such structure leads to recurrence of the fistula. Accordingly, the distal urethra must be examined for evidence of obstruction by cystoscopy, retrograde urethrography, or urethral calibration. Any obstruction found has to be corrected simultaneously with the fistula repair. If stenosis is present at the level of the meatus, a midline meatotomy or a Y-V plasty as described in Chap. 25 is recommended to correct the meatal stenosis.

The next step is to identify the site of the fistula and to exclude any further fistulas. I prefer to insert a catheter or the nozzle of a syringe with diluted Betadine® into the meatus and inject the Betadine into the urethra. This has the advantage of identifying any additional fistulas and tracing the fistulous tract.

One has to carry out extensive débridement and elaborate excision of the fistulous tract down to healthy thin urethral tissue–usually. The fistulous tract is fibrous and has what can be called a "cornu" at the junction between the healthy urethra and the rest of the tract (Fig. 28.2.1). Most surgeons are reluctant to perform extensive débridement and excision of the fistulous tract for fear of making a small fistula larger. This may in fact increase the incidence of recurrence. Sometimes, the fistulous tract goes a long way before opening into the skin and there may be multiple tiny tracts that are not seen except during elaborate dissection. I feel it is very important to dissect and separate widely between the urethra and the overlying skin all around the fistula.

The same principles that apply to hypospadias repair apply to fistula closure (Chap. 8). Delicate instruments are required. Healthy tissue should be incorporated in the repair at all times. Magnification is important. The type of repair depends on the size and location of the fistula. For a small fistula, simple transverse approximation of healthy urethral tissue is often possible. A running subcuticular inverting suture of 7-0 Vicryl is used to close the urethral edges. Some surgeons prefer to irrigate the urethra with proximal compression to ensure watertight closure, although it is not really necessary. A protective intermediate layer plays an important part in avoiding recurrence. The details of the different intermediate layer techniques are discussed in Chap. 24. I personally use dorsal subcutaneous fascia, if it is available. The skin is closed in the usual fashion. No stent or catheter is left inside the urethra (Duckett et al.1982).

A fistula near the glans with thin skin distally can be repaired by connecting the skin between the meatus and the fistula. The defect then is closed using the Mathieu technique to cover over the new subglanular meatus. In this technique, either a ventral or an oblique or lateral strip of skin can be used to cover over the meatus as in the classic Mathieu procedure. In the case of a large fistula, a meatal-based flap or a flap based on an island pedicle of skin as an onlay island flap usually gives good results. Some surgeons are happy to use buccal mucosal grafts for repair of fistula and have reported good results (Nahas and Nahas 1994). However, most reserve grafts such as buccal mucosa, bladder mucosa or extragenital skin for repair of strictures. As with the flip-flap or island pedicle repairs, a second layer of subcutaneous tissue is necessary to cover the edges of the flap or onlay patch. Skin cover is accomplished by means of a rotation flap from either the lateral skin or the scrotum.

For multiple fistulas, a single-stage procedure is still a valid option. Two-stage procedures may be reserved for recurrent fistula where there is a deficiency of adequate healthy local tissue. The fistulas are converted into one large fistula. Figures 28.2.2 and 28.2.3 show the different possible techniques for fistula closure and skin cover. Figure 28.2.4 shows a patient with multiple fistulas. Meticulous attention to layered closure is essential, and the risk of fistula reformation is substantially lower when local well-vascularised skin is used. With all of these repairs, tension on suture lines must be avoided and narrowing of the urethral lumen must be prevented.

Fistulas may recur because of errors in technique. Contributing factors include inadequate layers of closure, ischaemic tissue, and overlapping suture lines. Infection, tension such as is created by oedema or haemorrhage, pressure of dressings and occlusion of catheters with urinary extravasation all contribute to fistula recurrence. The difficulty of fistula closure

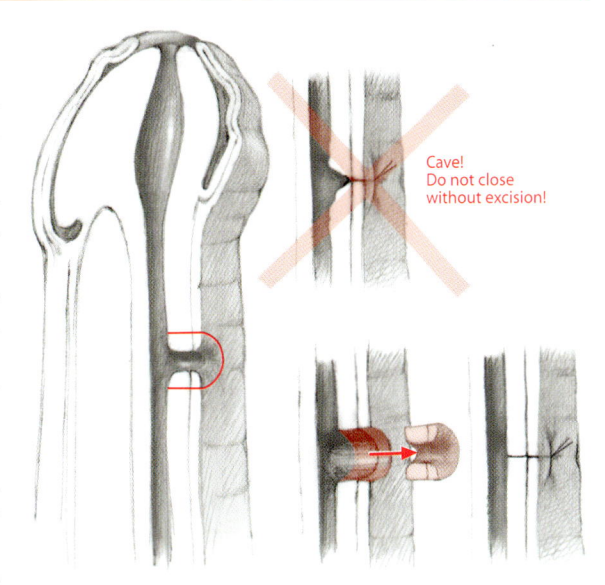

Fig. 28.2.1. Excision of the fistula cornu is crucial for repair. If it is not excised, there is an increased chance of recurrence

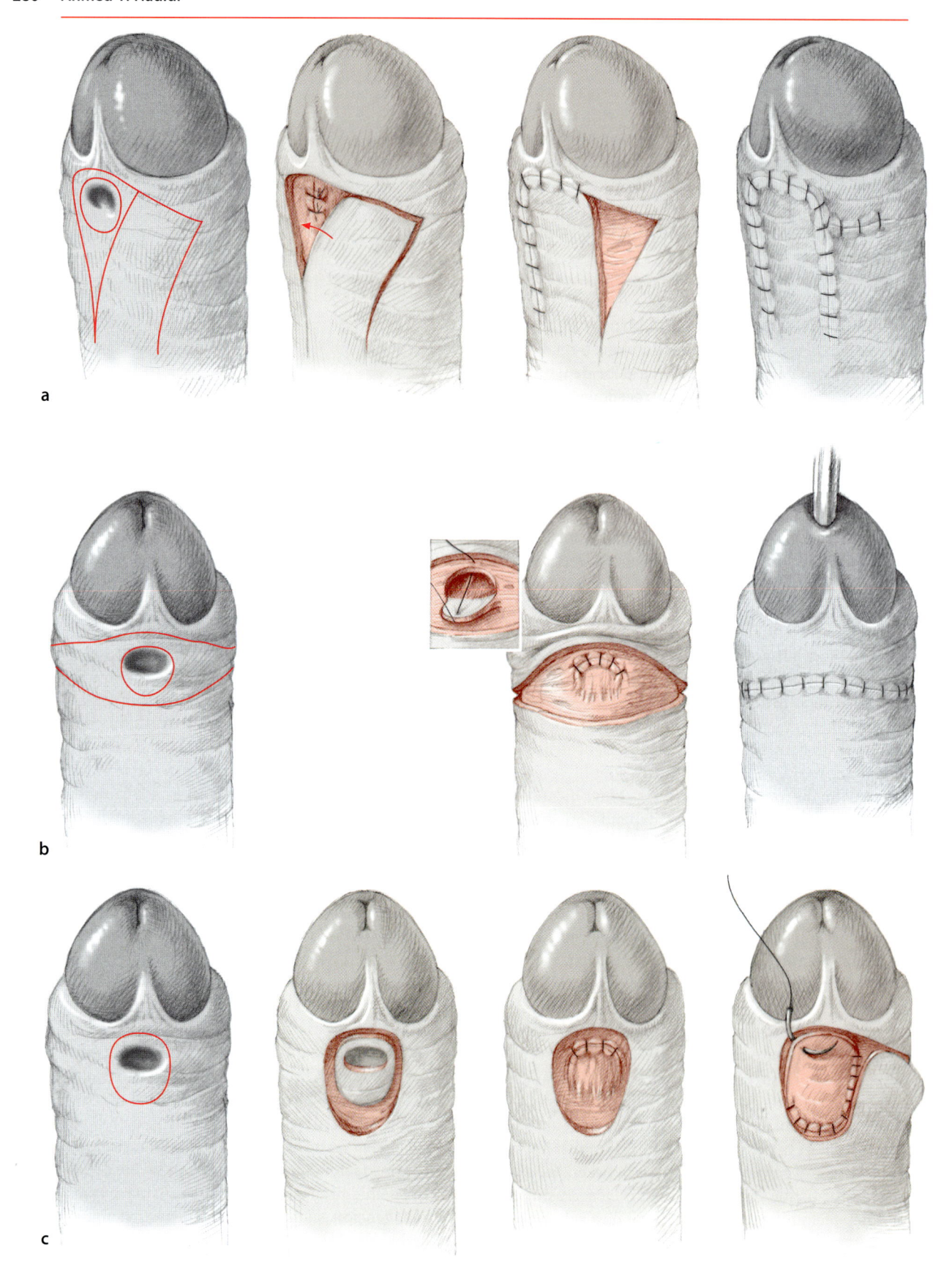

Fig. 28.2.2. a–c Different methods of fistula repair

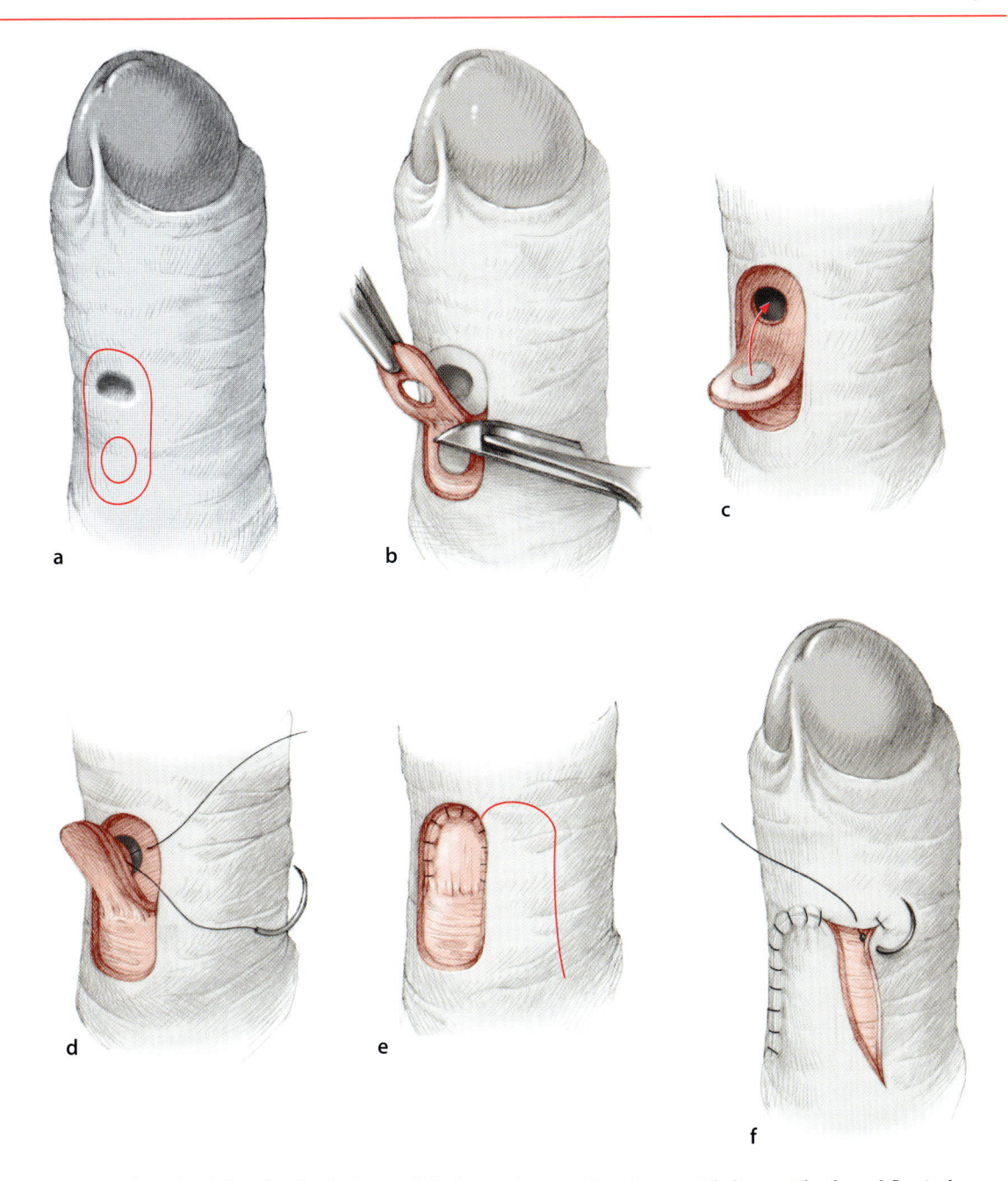

Fig. 28.2.3. a Outline of incisions for fistula closure. **b** Epithelium is removed from all areas except the central "plug" that is to be used to resurface the urethra. **c** Elevation of the dermal flap carrying the "epidermal plug." **d** The epidermal plug is sutured to the uroepithelium. **e** The dermal flap is then sutured to subcutaneous tissues. **f** Skin closure can be accomplished in many ways, e.g. with flaps or by simple straight-line approximation

should not be underestimated. Nevertheless, most fistulas can be repaired on an outpatient basis. Careful attention to detail and technique results in ultimate closure of nearly all fistulas.

Suture tracks (or sinuses) occur when epithelium grows along skin sutures before they dissolve or are removed postoperatively. These sinuses subsequently fill with desquamated keratin, producing unsightly marks. The likelihood that wound closure will leave suture tracks depends upon a variety of factors, including the size and composition of suture materials and the host conditions influencing wound healing.

During hypospadias repair the skin is closed using absorbable sutures, typically chromic catgut or Vicryl. According to the individual surgeon's preference, interrupted or continuous, simple or mattress sutures

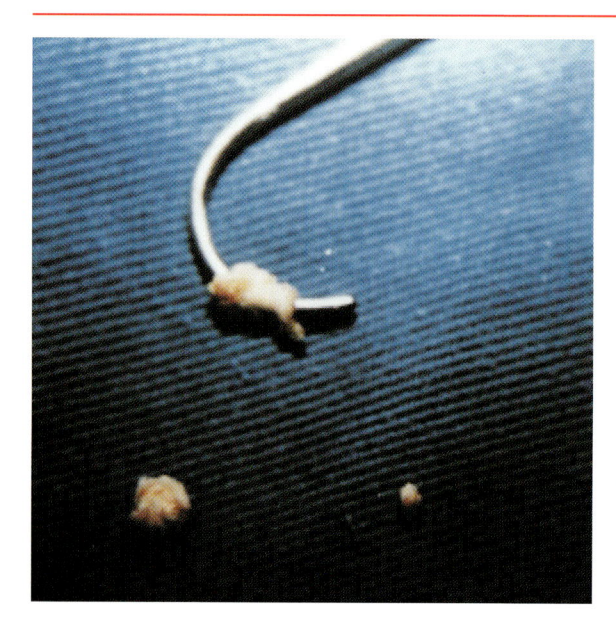

Fig. 28.2.4. A patient with multiple fistulas

of either 6-0 or 7-0 chromic catgut, Vicryl, polyglycolic acid or PDS are commonly used. Bartone et al. (1988) compared wound healing with catgut, polyglycolic acid and PDS in baboon foreskins and reported that catgut incited the least inflammation and was the most rapidly absorbed. Because tracks develop by epithelial growth along sutures, it is reasonable that longer-lasting materials may be more likely to produce tracks.

In 1999, Snodgrass wrote an excellent article about suture tracks following hypospadias repair. He reported a 43% incidence of suture tracks, which occurred exclusively on the ventral penile shaft, never involving the glans or the dorsal aspect of the circumcision. These tracks had not been detected during similar evaluations at a mean of 8 (3–18) months after surgery. Snodgrass recommended the use of modified Byars flaps, 6-0 chromic catgut and placing all shaft sutures subcuticularly.

References

Bartone FF, Adickes ED: Chitosan: effects on wound healing in urogenital tissue: preliminary report. J Urol. 1988; 140(pt 2): 1134–1137.
Belman AB: Editorial comment. J Urol. 1994a; 152:1237.
Belman AB: The de-epithelialized flap and its influence on hypospadias repair. J Urol. 1994b; 152:2332–2334.
Duckett JW, Baskin LS: Hypospadias. In: Gillenwater JY, Grayhack JT, Howards SS, Duckett JW (eds): Adult and pediatric urology, 3rd edn. Mosby-Year Book, St Louis. pp 2549–2589; 1996.
Duckett JW, Caldamone AA, Snyder HM: Hypospadias fistula repair without diversion (abstract 11). Proceedings of the Annual Meeting of the American Academy of Pediatrics, New York, Oct 1982, pp 23–28.
El-Mahrouky A, McElhaney J, Bartone FF, et al: In vitro comparison of the properties of polydioxanone, polyglycolic acid and catgut sutures in sterile and infected urine. J. Urol. 1987; 138:913–915.
Greenfield SP, Sadler PT, Wan J: Two stage repair for severe hypospadias. J Urol. 1994; 152:498–501.
Hadidi A, Abdaal N, Kaddah S: Hypospadias repair: is stenting important? Kasr El Ainy J Surg. 2003a; 4(2)3–8.
Hadidi A, Abdaal N, Kaddah S: Hypospadias repair: is dressing important? Kasr El Ainy J Surg. 2003b; 4(1)37–44.
Hill GA, Wacksman J, Lewis AG: The modified pyramid hypospadias procedure: repair of megameatus and deep glandular groove variants. J Urol. 1993; 150:1208.
Horton CE, Devine CJ: Urethral fistula. In: Horton CE (ed): Plastic and reconstructive surgery of the genital area. Little, Brown & Co., Boston, pp 397–403; 1973.
McLorie G, Joyner B, Herz D, et al: A prospective randomized clinical trial to evaluate methods of postoperative care of hypospadias. J Urol. 2001; 165:1669–1672.
Nahas BW, Nahas WB: The use of buccal mucosa patch graft in the management of a large urethro-cutaneous fistula. Br J Urol.1994; 74:679–681.
Retik AB, Mandell J, Bauer SB, et al: Meatal based hypospadias repair with the use of a dorsal subcutaneous flap to prevent urethrocutaneous fistula. J Urol. 1994; 152:1229.
Shapiro SR: Complications of hypospadias repair. J Urol. 1984; 131:518.
Shapiro SR: Fistula repair. In: Ehrlich RM, Alter GJ (eds): Reconstructive and Plastic surgery of the external genitalia, adult and pediatric. Saunders, Philadelphia, pp 132–136, 1999.
Smith ED: A de-epithelialized overlap flap technique in the repair of hypospadias. Br J Plast Surg. 1973; 26:106–114.
Smith ED: Durham Smith repair of hypospadias. Urol Clin North Am. 1981, 8:451–455.
Smith ED: Hypospadias. In Ashcraft K (ed): Pediatric urology. Saunders, Philadelphia, pp 353–395; 1990.
Snodgrass W: Suture tracts after hypospadias surgery. BJU Int. 1999; 84:843
Snow BW, Cartwright PC, Unger K: Tunica vaginalis blanket wrapped to prevent urethrocutaneous fistula: an eight year experience. J Urol. 1995; 153:472.
Van Savage JG, Palanca LG, Slaughenhoupt BL: A prospective randomized trial of dressings versus no dressings for hypospadias repair. J Urol. 2000; 164:981–983.

Cecil–Culp Operation

Amir F. Azmy

Cecil in 1946 described an operation in which penile skin is used for urethroplasty and the newly formed urethra is buried in the scrotum, to be released 6 months later. This procedure is used when the penile skin is insufficient to cover the defect on the ventral part of the shaft and skin coverage can be obtained by burying the penis in the scrotum. The first stage of Cecil urethroplasty is to make an incision to allow tubularisation of the ventral penile skin; the neourethra is constructed over a catheter with interrupted sutures of fine Vicryl. The neourethra is buried in the scrotum. The glans is approximated to the scrotum with interrupted sutures, and the skin is closed with subcuticular sutures (Fig. 28.3.1). In the second stage of Cecil urethroplasty, incisions in the scrotum are joined at the neomeatus, the urethra is freed from the glans and scrotal dissection is carried out with a catheter in the urethra to allow orientation. A Z-plasty is fashioned at the penoscrotal junction, and the skin is closed with fine interrupted stitches (Fig. 28.3.2).

Culp, in 1966, reviewed cases repaired according to the Cecil urethroplasty procedure and added a modification of the technique for patients whose meatus lies on the penile shaft. The neourethra is constructed from the penis out to the glans tip over a catheter, a corresponding incision is made in the scrotum, some normal as well as reconstructed urethra is buried in the scrotum and the penoscrotal region is left free. Results have been improved with regard to prevention of urethrocutaneous fistula by using the Cecil–Culp technique; if fistula does occur, it tends to close spontaneously.

In a study of 75 patients operated on using a modified Cecil–Culp procedure (Kelalis et al. 1977; Glassman et al. 1980) only 3 developed fistulas, which closed spontaneously in each case, meatal stenosis occurred in 15% and spraying of the urinary stream in 20% of cases. The abnormal meatus after the first stage could be corrected during the second stage. Culp wrote in 1966 "Deliberate termination of the urethra on the base of the glans poses no functional limitations, extending the urethra to the tip of the glans is fraught and hazardous that more than offsets any added cosmetic effect".

Modifications

Marshall et al. (1979) reported a three-stage modification of Cecil–Culp urethroplasty and scrotoplasty for patients with penoscrotal hypospadias. During the first stage, chordee is released and the dorsal skin is brought to the ventral surface by the button-hole technique. In the second stage, the urethroplasty is performed and skin cover is achieved with scrotal flaps. During the third stage the repair is completed by the release of the penis from the scrotum. Figure 28.3.3 shows the steps of the second-stage procedure.

In the modification described by Marberger and Pauer (1981), the urethroplasty and skin coverage are performed in a one-stage operation. The preputial skin is mobilised on a vascular pedicle and rotated to cover the ventral surface of the penis. The steps of the procedure are shown in Fig. 28.3.4.

In conclusion, the Cecil–Culp procedure has been used with excellent results for repair of difficult urethrocutaneous fistula and complex cases of hypospadias where penile skin is in short supply.

References

Cecil AB: Repair of hypospadias and urethral fistula. J Urol. 1946; 56:237.

Culp OS: Struggles and triumphs with hypospadias and associated anomalies: review of 400 cases. J Urol. 1966; 96:339.

Glassman CN, Machlus BJ, Kelalis PP: Urethroplasty for hypospadias: long term results. Urol Clin North Am. 1980; 7:437.

Kelalis PP, Benson RC Jr, Culp OS: Complications of single and multistage operations for hypospadias. A comparative review. J Urol. 1977; 118:657.

Marberger H, Pauer W: Experience in hypospadias repair. Urol Clin North Am 1981; 8:403.

Marshall M Jr, Johnson SH III, Price SE Jr, et al: Cecil urethroplasty with concurrent scrotoplasty for repair of hypospadias. J Urol. 1979; 121:335.

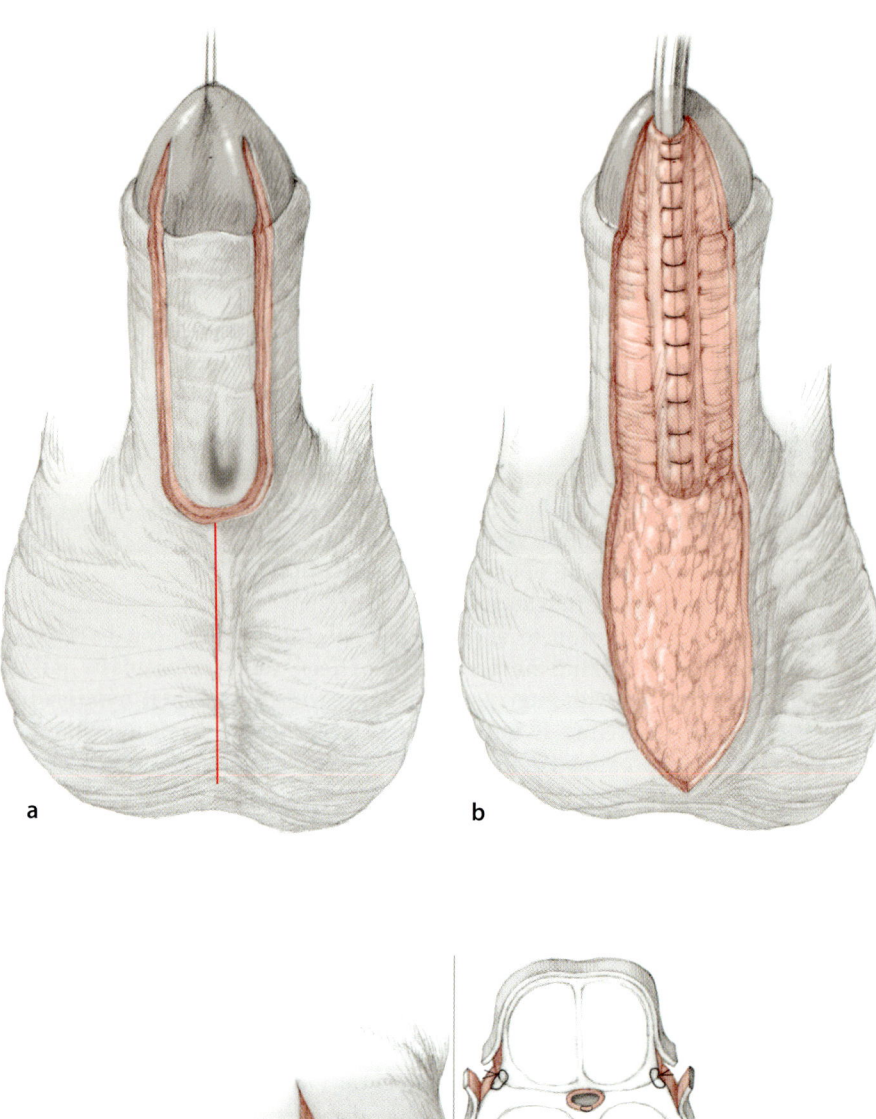

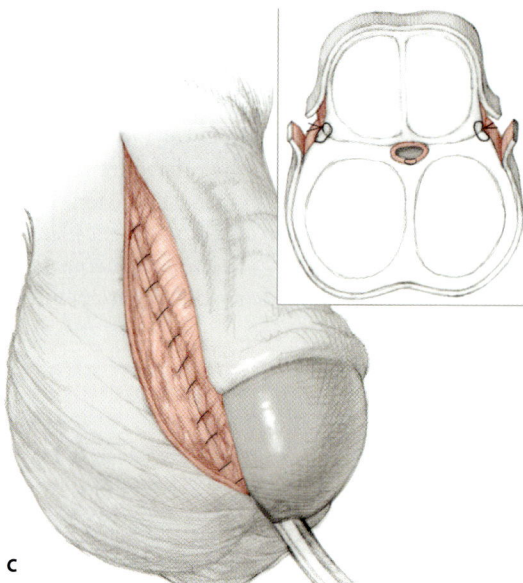

Fig. 28.3.1a–c. Steps of first stage. **a** Incision on the ventral skin to allow tubularisation. **b** Neourethra constructed around a catheter. **c** The neourethra buried in the scrotum

Cecil–Culp Operation 285

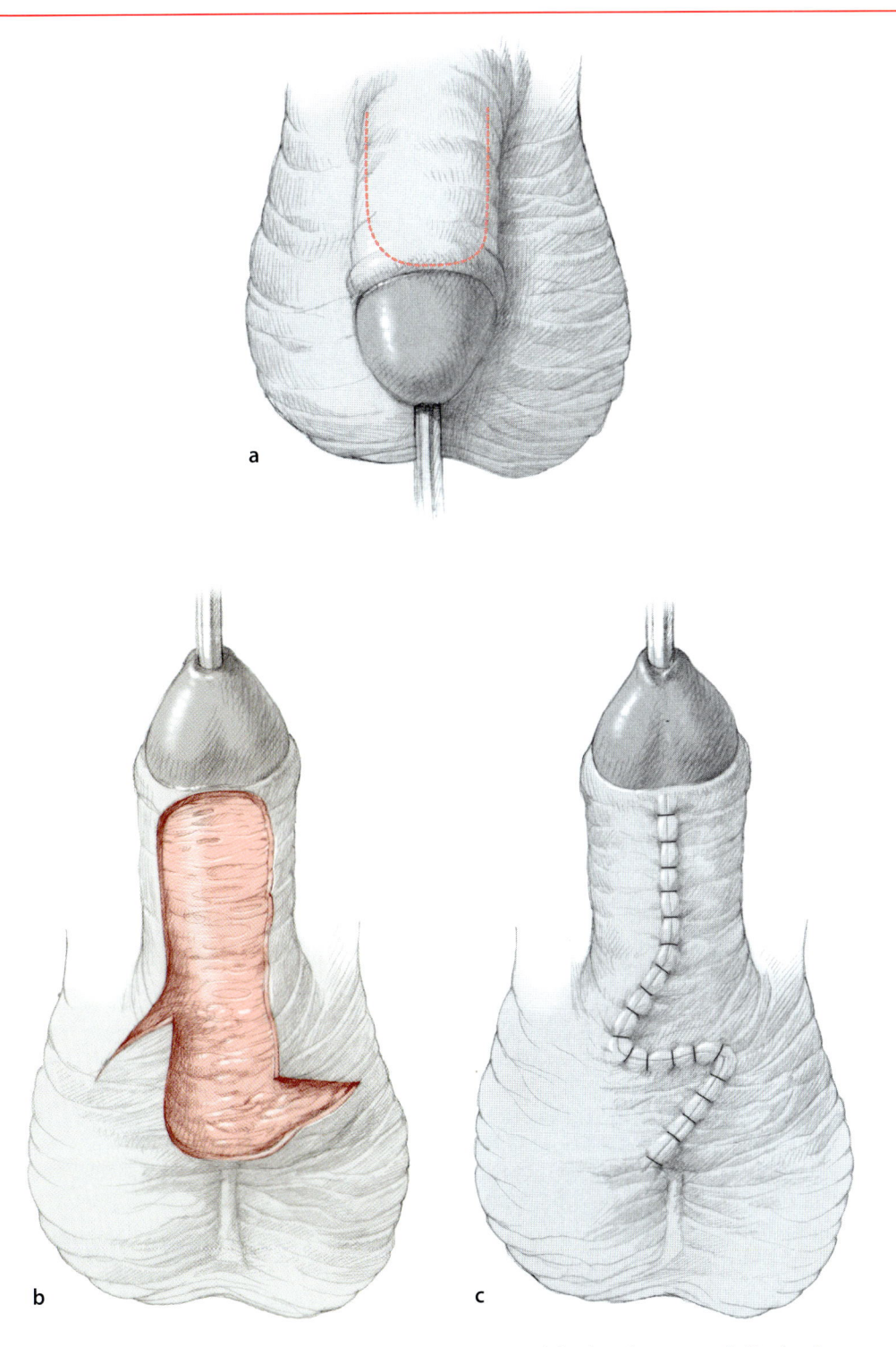

Fig. 28.3.2a–c. Steps of second stage. **a** Incision in scrotum joined at the meatus. **b** Urethra is separated from scrotum and Z-plasty at penoscrotal junction. **c** Skin closed

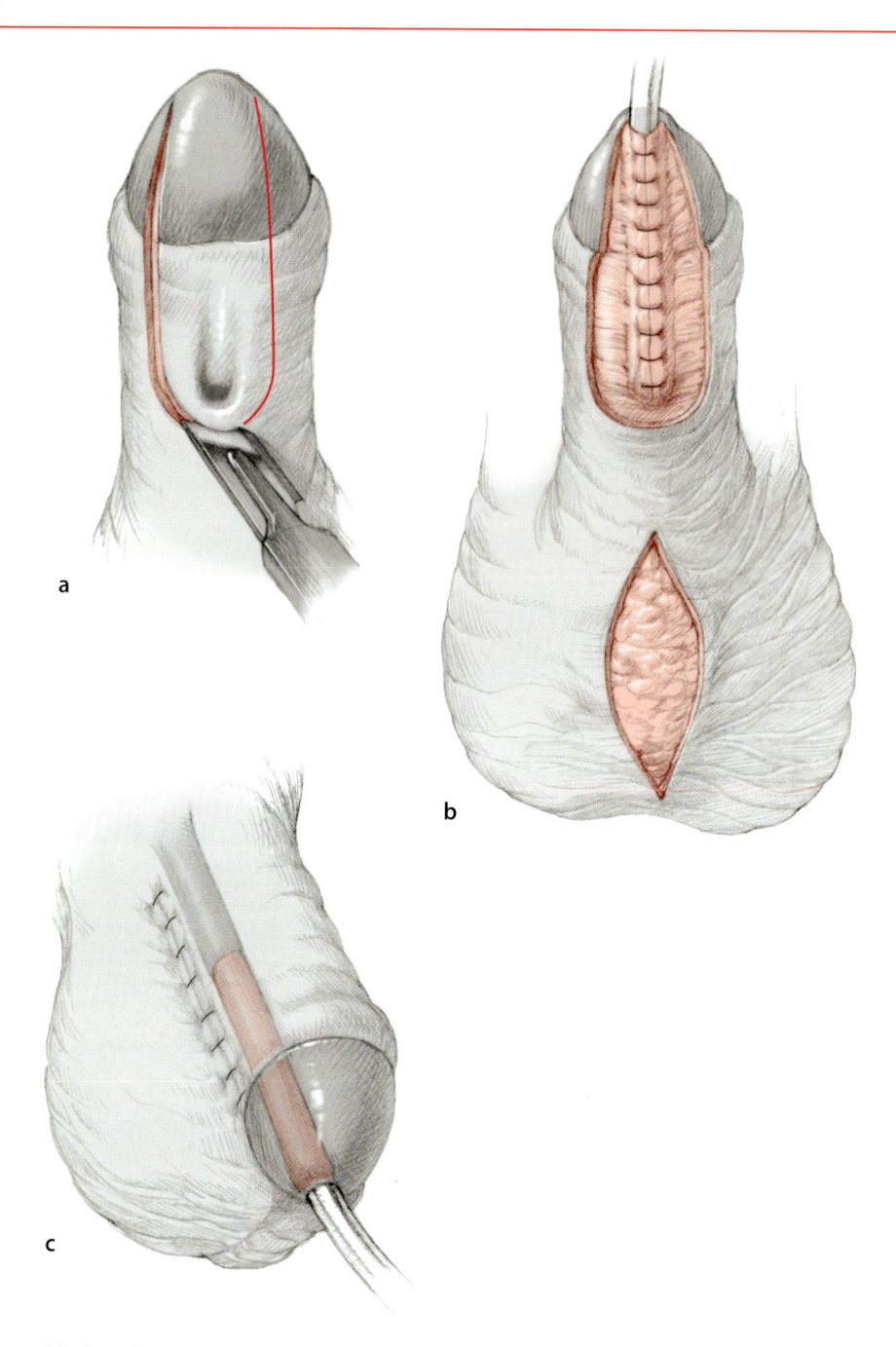

Fig. 28.3.3a–c. Modified Cecil urethroplasty (Marshall et al. 1979). **a** Incision to allow tubularisation. **b** Neourethra constructed around a catheter and a separate corresponding incision in the scrotum. **c** Part of normal and reconstructed urethra buried in scrotum

Cecil–Culp Operation 287

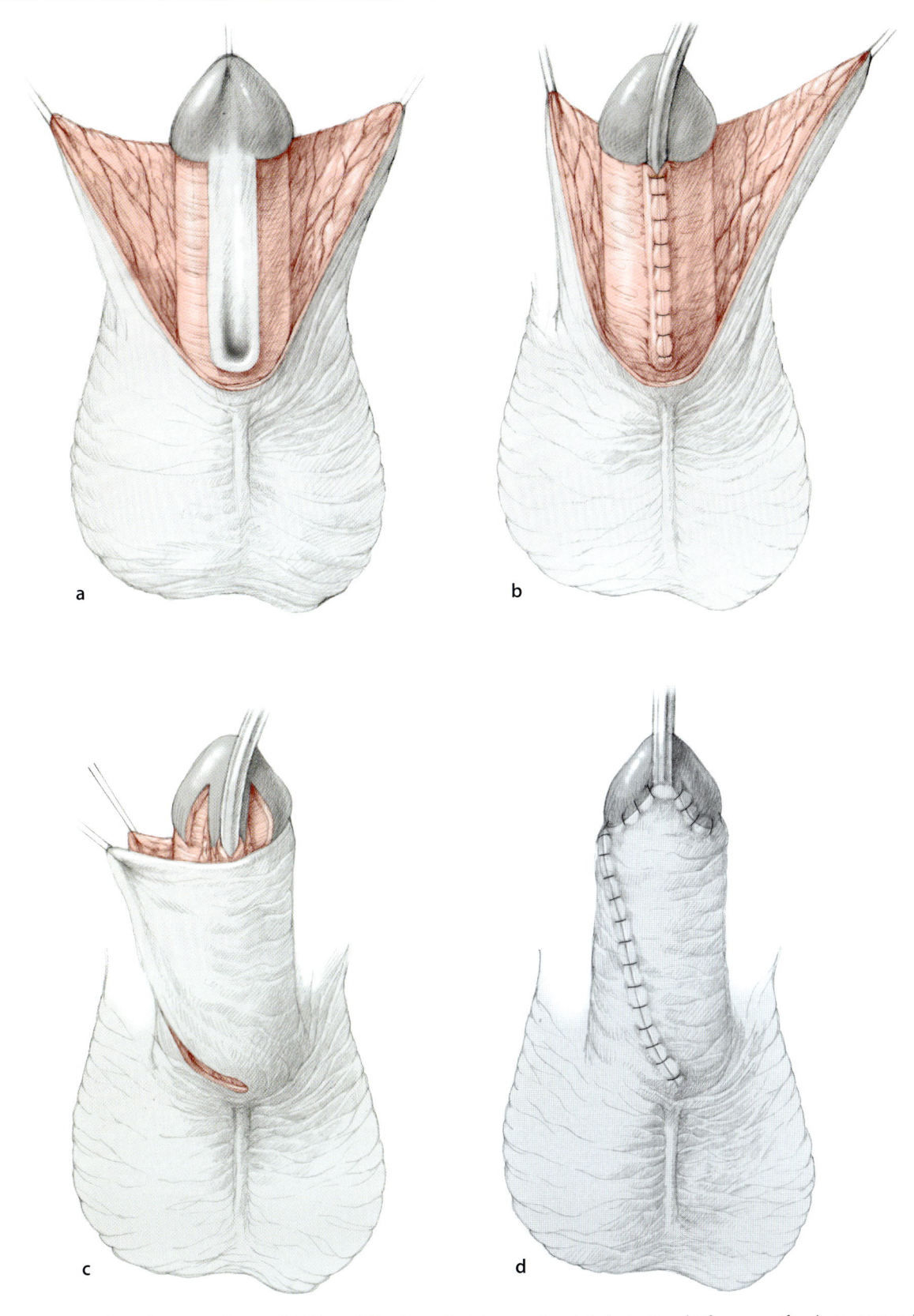

Fig. 28.3.4a–d. Marberger and Pauer (1981) modification. **a** Incision to allow tubularisation. **b** The neourethra is constructed, and preputial skin is mobilised in asymmetrical flaps to avoid overlapping suture lines. **c, d** Skin closure with interrupted sutures

Modified Cecil–Culp Technique for Repair of Urethrocutaneous Fistula

Christopher S. Cooper, Charles E. Hawtrey

Introduction and Patient Selection

Urethrocutaneous fistula is the most common complication of hypospadias repair (Kass and Bolong 1990; Joseph 1995). Several factors are significant in the development of fistulas, including distal obstruction, loss of vascularity of the neourethra and its flap, incomplete coverage of the neourethra, and infection.

Optical magnification, delicate tissue handling, and fine suture materials are thought to reduce the possibility of fistula formation. Other principles of hypospadias repair include the avoidance of overlapping suture lines and interposition of layers of well-vascularized tissue between suture lines. Multiple authors attribute decreased fistula formation to additional tissue coverage between the neourethra and the skin (Baskin et al. 1994; Cooper et al. 2001; Gearhart et al. 1992; Kass and Bolong 1990; Retik et al. 1994; Snow et al. 1995). Deficient penile skin often makes it difficult to obtain a subcutaneous flap for additional tissue coverage. Furthermore, the additional bulk of a subcutaneous pedicle flap in these patients can make creation of a tension-free closure difficult. A tight flap or skin closure may constrict the urethral repair and possibly induce local ischemia with an increased risk of recurrent fistula.

The modified Cecil–Culp repair for fistula utilizes the penile mobility to place the repair in a scrotal location. This ensures a well-covered suture line with vascularized tissue that is free of tension. Previous series have demonstrated a reduction or elimination of fistula with the use of the Cecil–Culp method for primary hypospadias repair (Culp 1966; Kelalis et al. 1977). We have successfully employed a modification of the Cecil–Culp technique in patients who had failed previous urethrocutaneous fistula closures and had limited local tissue with which to create a tension-free multilayered closure (Ehle et al. 2001). The disadvantage of this approach is the requirement of a secondary procedure; however, in patients with recurrent fistula despite multiple previous attempts at repair, the high success rate with the modified Cecil–Culp technique often outweighs the disadvantage of a second operation.

Preoperative Evaluation

Fistula repair should not be attempted for at least 6 months following previous penile surgery. A careful preoperative examination determines the likely technique of fistula repair; however, intraoperative findings may alter this plan and require the surgeon to be skilled in a variety of techniques for fistula correction. Each case of hypospadias fistula must be treated on an individual basis and the surgeon must assess the location of the fistula, the integrity and caliber of the glanulo-meatoplasty, the quality and amount of surrounding tissue, the amount of penile shaft skin, and the number of previous penile operations. Fistulas located in a subcoronal location frequently have little surrounding soft tissue with which to cover the fistula closure and often require a tissue flap or the modified Cecil–Culp technique to create a multilayered closure. Urethral calibration must be performed preoperatively or intraoperatively to assess the glanulo-meatoplasty since an uncorrected meatal stenosis results in increased urethral pressure with voiding and stresses the fistula repair. When there is minimal or deficient penile shaft skin, reapproximation of the skin over a multilayered fistula closure may result in excessive tension on the suture line or compression of the repair. In this case the modified Cecil–Culp technique provides coverage without tension or compression. Parents must be informed that the modified Cecil–Culp technique for fistula repair requires a brief second operation; however, parents of a child with a fistula are often relieved to know that there is a considerable likelihood that the child will void with a single stream as the surgical outcome.

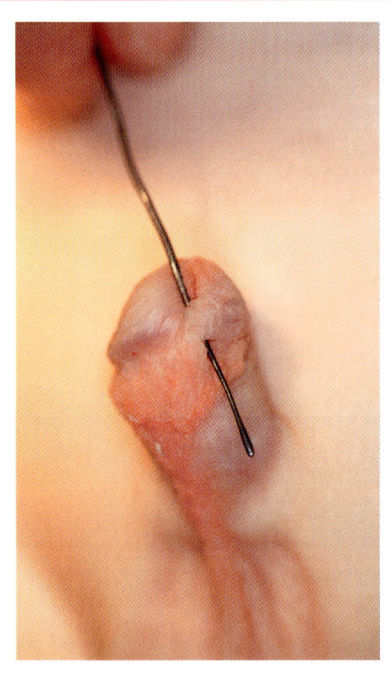

Fig. 28.4.1. Lacrimal duct probe demonstrating a recurrent fistula in subcoronal location

Operative Technique

Prior to fistula closure the urethra is assessed to rule out stenosis or diverticula (Fig. 28.4.1). The technique of fistula closure routinely involves an elliptical incision around the fistula tract. If the fistula is adjacent to the glans penis, infiltration with 1% lidocaine will facilitate separation of the fistula from the glans. The fistula tract is then excised, followed by approximation of the epithelial edges of the open urethra with fine absorbable suture (7-0 PDS or Vicryl). An attempt is made to invert the epithelial edge. A second layer of parallel mattress sutures is used to further invert and cover the epithelial closure toward the urethral lumen (Fig. 28.4.2). A midline skin incision in the scrotum is created and the dartos fascia is exposed for utilization as additional tissue coverage of the repair. This third layer of closure is accomplished by suturing the dartos to the subcutaneous subdermal tissue under the skin edge of the penile incision (Fig. 28.4.2b). These sutures are also absorbable, but are usually larger (6-0 PDS) in order to withstand the tensile forces between the penis and scrotum with erection or activity. Finally, the penile skin edges are sutured to the scrotal skin edges, completing a fourth layer of closure. The closure buries the urethra in the median raphe tissues of the scrotum and maintains a deep separation from the skin surface (Fig. 28.4.2c).

A urethral catheter or drip stent is routinely left in place for 1 week. The stent may prevent urethral obstruction secondary to edema, ensure luminal continuity until epithelialization and tensile strength is obtained in the healing wound, and prevent forceful (often painful) urination into periurethral tissues. If a stent is used, it should be sutured in place. We prefer to place these sutures through the inner portion of the meatus, which avoids unsightly glans scarring as a result of holding sutures transgressing the glanular epithelium.

The repair is performed on an outpatient basis. Postoperative pain is managed with acetaminophen with codeine elixir (0.5–1.0 mg/kg every 4 h). Bladder spasms, particularly during the first 72 h postoperatively, are managed with oxybutynin suspension (0.2 mg/kg every 8 h). Trimethoprim–sulfamethoxazole (0.5–1 tsp) is given once daily while the urethral stent remains indwelling.

The second stage of the operation is performed routinely 6 or more weeks following the first stage (Fig. 28.4.3). An intraoperative Foley catheter is used to delineate the course of the urethra and removed at the end of the procedure since the urethra is well healed. At this time the reapproximated skin edges are incised and the penile shaft is sharply freed from the scrotum, taking care to preserve the penile soft tissue and prevent transfer of scrotal skin to the phallus. Subcutaneous sutures are used to reapproximate the skin edges (Fig. 28.4.4). The skin closure completes repair and heals per primam.

Modifications of Original Technique

The Cecil technique was originally described as a two-stage operation for hypospadias repair (Cecil 1946). In 1966, Culp described a modification of the Cecil technique and demonstrated this technique's excellent results in preventing fistula formation when used for hypospadias repair (Culp 1966). The disadvantage of this technique for a primary repair is the requirement of two operations when most hypospadias repairs are successful with one. Modification of this technique for repair of hypospadias fistula as described above continues to require two operations; however, in a select group of boys with recurrent fistula and limited penile skin the high success rate justifies a two-stage procedure.

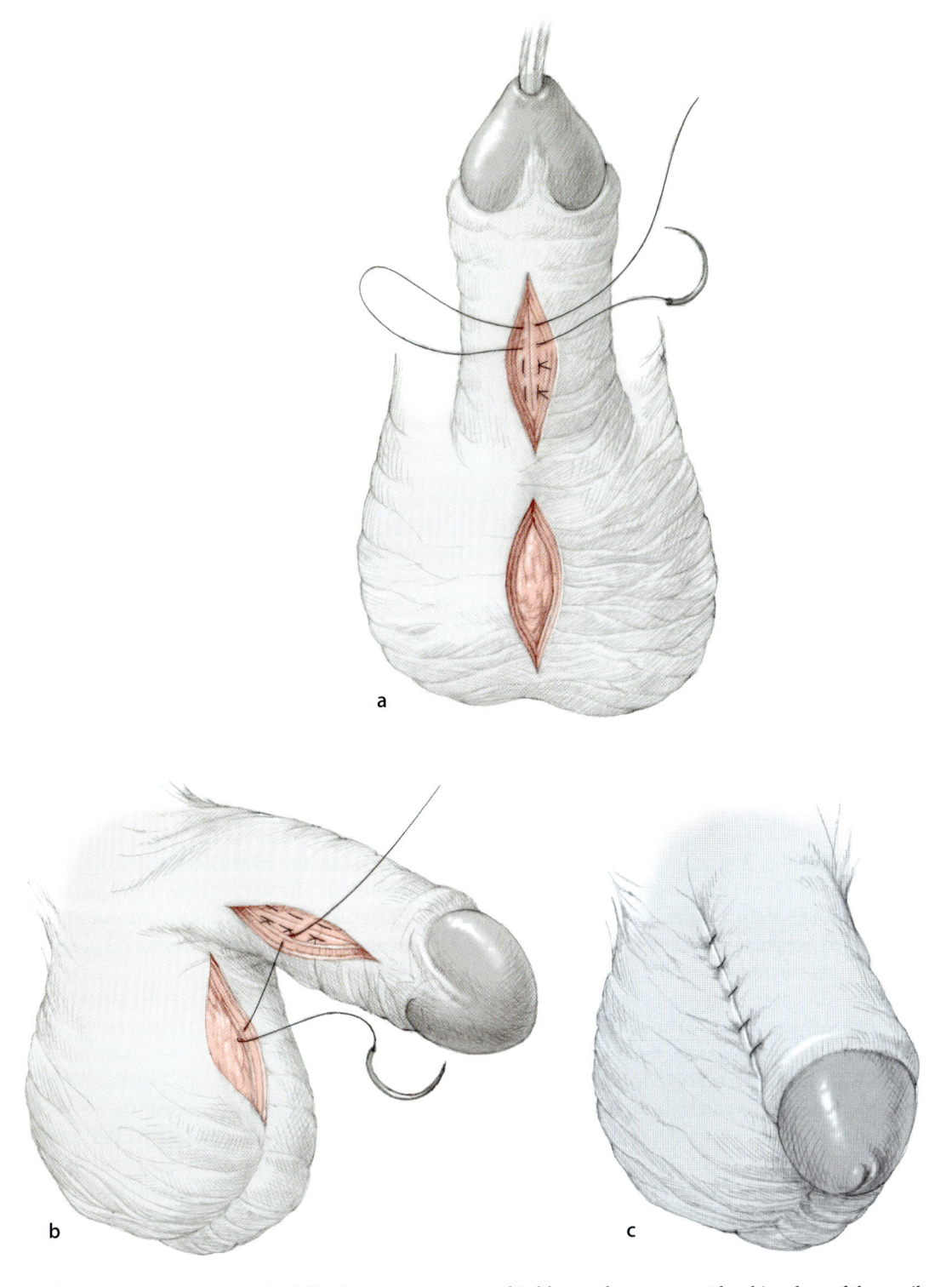

Fig. 28.4.2. a The edges of the urethral fistula are approximated and closed over with a second layer. **b** The scrotal dartos layer is approximated lateral to the urethra, providing a third layer of coverage. **c** The skin edges of the penile and scrotal incisions are approximated. Images from Ehle et al. (2001), Elsevier: reprinted with permission

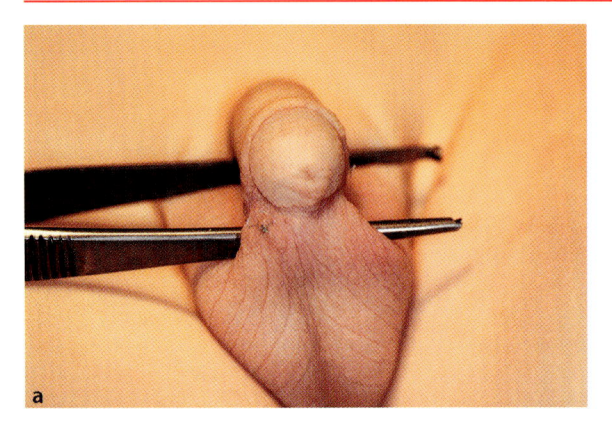

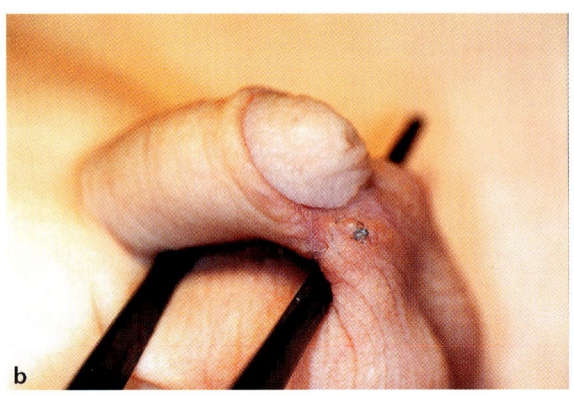

Fig. 28.4.3a, b. Preoperative images 8 weeks following first stage of the modified Cecil–Culp repair, demonstrating scrotal coverage of subcoronal repair

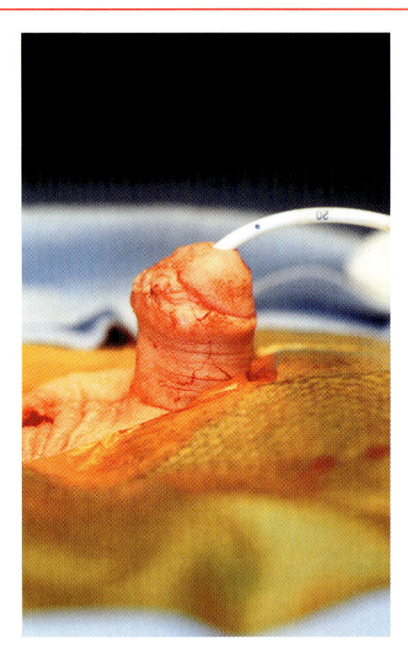

Fig. 28.4.4. Intraoperative image following release and closure of penile incision. Note that the scrotal incision requires closure and the catheter will be removed after the procedure

Results

The modified Cecil–Culp technique of hypospadias repair produced excellent results in a select group of boys with urethrocutaneous fistula (Ehle et al. 2001). In this series, 15 boys underwent repair with this technique over a 6-year period. The average age at the time of the first stage of fistula repair was 3.5±1.2 (range 1.8–6.0) years. The average time between the first and second stages was 10±3 (range 5–19) weeks. Eleven of the 15 boys had undergone prior fistula repair with urethral stents. Five boys had undergone one previous fistula repair, four had undergone two previous fistula repairs, and two had undergone three previous fistula repairs. All 11 boys with recurrent fistulas had recurrence at the primary site. The remaining four boys had deficient penile skin at the time of their first fistula repair by the Cecil technique. The majority had one fistula at the time of Cecil repair, including eight at the corona, four along the penile shaft, and three in a more proximal location. No patients had a recurrent fistula with a mean follow up of 21±19 (range 1–62) months. Despite these excellent results the modified Cecil–Culp method is rarely required. The patients we select for its use include those who have failed previous multiple fistula closures and those with limited penile skin at the time of their first fistula.

Complications

Complications with this procedure as with any urethrocutaneous fistula or hypospadias repair may include urinary tract infection, recurrent fistula, and urethral scarring. A complication unique to this technique is the potential transfer of scrotal hair follicles onto the penile shaft. There have been no cases of this in our follow-up, although only two patients have reached pubertal age. The authors are aware of others who have used finer suture (7-0 Vicryl) to approximate the penis to the scrotum and then had difficulty with disruption of the repair (unpublished data).

References

Baskin LS, Duckett JW, Ueoka K, et al: Changing concepts of hypospadias curvature lead to more onlay island flap procedures. J Urol. 1994; 151:191–196.

Cecil AB: Repair of hypospadias and urethral fistula. J Urol. 1946; 56:237–242.

Cooper CS, Noh PH, Snyder HM III: Preservation of urethral plate spongiosum: technique to reduce hypospadias fistulas. Urology. 2001; 57:351–354.

Culp OS: Struggles and triumphs with hypospadias and associated anomalies. Review of 400 cases. J Urol. 1966; 96:339–355.

Ehle JJ, Cooper CS, Peche WJ, et al: Application of the Cecil–Culp repair for treatment of urethrocutaneous fistulas after hypospadias surgery. Urology. 2001; 57:347–350.

Gearhart JP, Borland RN: Onlay island flap urethroplasty: variation on a theme. J Urol. 1992; 148:1507–1509.

Joseph VT: Concepts in the surgical technique of one-stage hypospadias correction. Br J Urol. 1995; 76:504–509.

Kass EJ, Bolong D: Single stage hypospadias reconstruction without fistula. J Urol. 1990; 144:520–522.

Kelalis PP, Benson RC Jr, Culp OS: Complications of single and multistage operations for hypospadias: a comparative review. Trans Am Assoc Genitourin Surg. 1977; 68:88–90.

Retik AB, Mandell J, Bauer SB, et al: Meatal based hypospadias repair with the use of a dorsal subcutaneous flap to prevent urethrocutaneous fistula. J Urol. 1994; 152:1229–1231.

Snow BW, Cartwright PC, Unger K: Tunica vaginalis blanket wrap to prevent urethrocutaneous fistula: an 8-year experience. J Urol. 1995; 153:472–473.

Meatal Stenosis and Urethral Strictures After Hypospadias Surgery

Pat Malone

Introduction

Urethral stricture and meatal stenosis are the second most common complication of hypospadias surgery, after urethrocutaneous fistula. It is difficult to determine the exact incidence of these complications, but in a textbook of paediatric surgery published in 1986 Belman presented a table drawing data from 21 publications (from 1974 to 1981) and the range was 0–22.7% (Belman 1986). In two more recent textbooks of paediatric urology, both published in 2001, Belman (2001) and Mouriquand and Mure (2001) devoted considerably less space to the complications of stricture and stenosis, with Mouriquand and Mure claiming that the incidence of stenosis had significantly decreased since surgeons were no longer employing circumferential anastomoses. This claim is supported by the work of Harris and Jeffrey (1989) and Kumar and Harris (1994), who reported a 9–31% incidence of early stricture when the inner preputial skin was tubularised as a one-stage repair. However, despite the reduction in the incidence of these complications, Duel et al. (1998) stated as recently as 1998 that stricture disease continued to be a significant complication of hypospadias reconstruction, with an incidence of symptomatic stricture at their institution of 6.5% in 582 patients.

There remains controversy as to how strictures should be diagnosed: symptomatically or with the routine use of uroflowmetry. Hamilton et al. (2000) reported the detection of previously unsuspected stenoses with the use of routine urinary flow rate measurements. Garibay et al. (1995) also studied the routine use of uroflowmetry following hypospadias repair and concluded that it was an important non-invasive tool and helped to detect significant asymptomatic strictures. These findings make the case for a more objective means of assessing the results of hypospadias surgery, as undiagnosed stenoses may have a detrimental effect on long-term bladder function and ultimately on the upper urinary tract. If a routine objective means of assessing hypospadias surgery were widely introduced, we might discover that stricture disease is more common than previously suspected (Table 29.1).

Table 29.1. Presenting features and means of assessment of meatal stenosis/urethral stricture

Presenting features
  Spraying stream
  Decreased stream
  Straining to void
  Urinary retention
  Dysuria
  Urinary tract infection
  Frequency/urgency
  Urinary incontinence
  Fistula
  Hypospadias breakdown
  Reduced urinary flow rate
Assessment of stricture
  Examination
  Uroflowmetry
  Postvoid ultrasound
  Urethrography
  Endoscopy

Aetiology and Prevention

Meatal Stenosis

Meatal stenosis is more common than urethral stricture and its incidence increased when the practice of placing the external urethral meatus at the tip of the glans was routinely adopted in hypospadias surgery. Duckett (1995) stated that the problem arose as a result of a circular anastomosis and recommended that a dart of glans tissue should be excised or an oblique anastomosis should be constructed to avoid the complication. Belman (1986) suggested that stenosis could be due to a tight glans closure and recommended that a glans tunnel of sufficient width should be created to readily accept the new urethra. There is no doubt that these manoeuvres helped to reduce the incidence of meatal stenosis and the subsequent use of onlay instead of tubularised flaps or grafts, helped to reduce it still further. The concern surrounding meatal stenosis increased again following the widespread adoption of the techniques of urethral tubularisation. When there was a deep glanular groove meatal stenosis was rarely reported as a problem but Elbakry (1999) reported a significant incidence of early stenosis when the incised urethral plate was used and recommended a 3 month period of daily meatal dilatation to avoid the complication. Elbakry (2002) also carried out a randomised controlled trial of patients undergoing tubularisation of the incised urethral plate and found a significant increase in stricture disease in patients not undergoing routine postoperative dilatation. Lorenzo and Snodgrass (2002) refuted the need for routine meatal dilatation and reported an incidence of meatal stenosis of 0.7% when no dilatation was employed. In the author's personal experience the incidence of meatal stenosis was 1.6% for the Snodgrass procedure, suggesting that routine meatal dilatation was unnecessary. The final and perhaps most serious cause of meatal stenosis detected on long-term follow-up following primary hypospadias repair is balanitis xerotica obliterans (BXO) (Kumar and Harris 1999). This is being recognised with increasing frequency as a cause of urethral stricture following hypospadias repair and will be dealt with in detail in the next section.

When bladder mucosa grafts were widely used for salvage hypospadias surgery, meatal problems, including stenosis, were commonly seen when the graft was brought to the tip of the glans (Keating et al. 1990). This problem has largely disappeared since buccal mucosa has replaced the use of bladder mucosa.

Urethral Stricture

Procedures that involved an end-to-end circumferential anastomosis led to stricture formation at the hypospadiac meatus. It was recommended that the anastomosis should be spatulated or triangulated, and although this probably minimised the problem, it still occurred. Garibray et al. (1995) reported that 5 out of 16 patients with a tubularised preputial island flap developed a stricture but no patient with an onlay preputial flap did. They concluded that meatal-based and onlay flap urethroplasties had a low risk for stricture formation but tubularised preputial flaps frequently developed anastomotic strictures. Mouriquand et al. (1995) also recommended avoiding of circular anastomoses to reduce the risk of stricture formation, and Bracka (1995) proposed a two-stage repair to produce a normal-appearing external meatus and to reduce the incidence of urethral stricture and meatal stenosis.

When pedicled flaps are used devascularisation is always a possible risk, and this can lead to scarring and urethral stenosis. This has led to the increased number of procedures employing some method of tubularising the native urethral plate, most of which are dealt with in other chapters of this text. When there is a deeply grooved and wide urethral plate stricture or stenosis is rarely a problem, but concern has been expressed that problems may arise when shallow and narrow urethral plates are tubularised using the Snodgrass technique (Holland and Smith 2000). Holland and Smith (2000) found that after tubularisation of the incised urethral plate, patients with a shallow urethral plate were more likely to have a neourethra calibre of 6 F or less. In addition they found that these boys had a higher incidence of meatal stenosis, and also, when the urethral plate was less than 8 mm wide, there was a higher incidence of urethral fistula. However, these results are disputed by Snodgrass (1999). He carried out urethral calibration, urethroscopy and uroflowmetry in 72 boys and failed to identify any evidence of neourethral stricture (Snodgrass 1999). In the author's personal experience stricture does not occur even when shallow and narrow incised urethral plates are tubularised. Regular dilation is not recommended.

BXO is now being increasingly recognised as a cause for late presenting urethral strictures following hypospadias repair. Kumar and Harris reported the first series in 1999, describing eight patients whose strictures presented between 1 and 16 years following their original surgery. Uemura et al. (2000) also described this problem in three patients, with symptoms developing 3 months to 6 years following surgery. BXO is a form of lichen sclerosus et atrophicus affecting the genital skin of the prepuce and glans. It has been widely recognised as a cause of phimosis and meatal stenosis (Bainbridge et al. 1994) and more recently has been recognised as a cause of anterior urethral stricture (Venn and Mundy 1998). It is not surprising, therefore, to see it as a cause of stricture following hypospadias repair, particularly when genital skin has been used.

Presentation and Assessment

Meatal stenosis and/or urethral stricture typically present symptomatically with voiding difficulties (that may be severe enough to progress to urinary retention), urinary tract infection and urinary inconti-

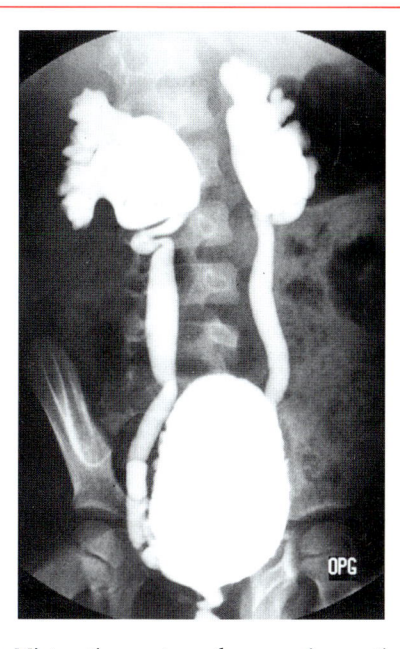

Fig. 29.1. Micturating cystourethrogram in a patient with a distal urethral stricture following hypospadias repair, demonstrating dilating bilateral vesicoureteral reflux

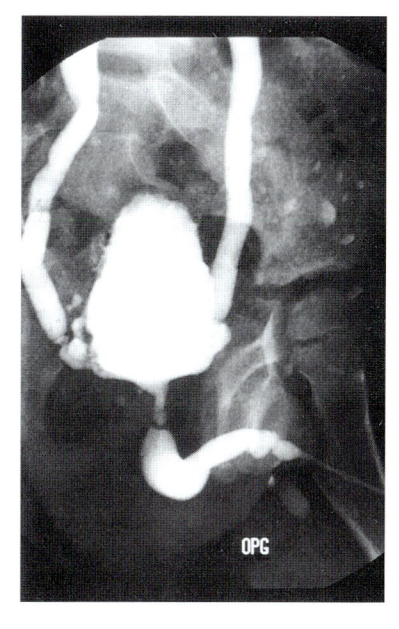

Fig. 29.2. Distal urethral stricture following hypospadias repair

nence as a result of acquired detrusor instability. In meatal stenosis the voiding problem usually consists of a thin spraying urinary stream that is difficult to direct. With urethral strictures the problem is usually a poor stream and the patient may have to strain to void. Dysuria may be a feature of both meatal stenosis and urethral stricture, and urinary retention may also occur in both. Dysuria should also raise the suspicion of urinary infection, which must be excluded with urine sampling. Infection arises as a result of poor bladder emptying which can progress to the development of large postvoid residual volumes. Detrusor instability develops under these conditions and this can then lead to vesicoureteric reflux, increasing the risk of infection and, more importantly, renal scarring (Fig. 29.1). Detrusor instability can also manifest itself with frequency, urgency and urge incontinence. In the series reported by Duel et al. (1998), the mean interval from initial surgery to presentation was 27 months (range 1 month to 12.5 years), but when presentation is delayed for years one should always suspect the presence of BXO (Kumar and Haris 1999; Uemura et al. 2000).

Severe stricturing may lead to early breakdown of the hypospadias repair or fistula formation. In a recent report by Shankar et al. (2002), meatal stenosis or urethral stricture was present in 8/109 (7.4%) of patients presenting with a fistula. Therefore, a stenosis should always be excluded, and if present treated, at the time of fistula repair. If there is extensive scarring and stricturing, severe chordee may also develop.

Meatal stenosis, breakdown of the repair and fistula formation are usually easily recognisable on clinical examination. Sometimes a meatal stenosis is not immediately obvious, as the narrowing may just be inside the meatus itself and will be diagnosed only if the meatus is opened and carefully examined. In the presence of a distal stenosis dilatation of the proximal urethra may occur during micturition and there may also be terminal dribbling. Therefore it is always valuable to watch the patient void. In the case of proximal urethral stricture there may be no physical signs.

In the absence of physical signs further assessment will be necessary. The least invasive form of assessment is uroflowmetry. There will frequently be a reduced flow rate, but it must be remembered that even in the presence of a severe narrowing there may be a normal flow, providing the bladder can generate sufficient pressure. It is worthwhile combining uroflowmetry with bladder scanning when the thickness of the bladder wall can be assessed and postvoid residuals measured. Urethrography or micturating cystourethrography (if infection has occurred) is also another useful means of assessing strictures (Fig. 29.2). Finally, it may be necessary to assess strictures under anaesthetic with urethroscopy and calibration before deciding on the best management.

Lastly, asymptomatic strictures may be detected with routine assessment using uroflowmetry. However, there continues to be controversy as to whether these strictures require treatment, although this is recommended by Garibay et al. (1995) and Hamilton et al. (2000). There is little doubt that patients with asymptomatic strictures require close follow-up to prevent the late sequelae of infection and incontinence.

Treatment

Meatal dilatation is always worth trying, as in most series some patients will require no further treatment (Belman 1986; Duel et al. 1998; Mouriquand et al. 1995). In the majority of patients, however, recurrent stenosis develops and the next step may be a dorsal urethrotomy or a formal meatotomy which can be carried out by performing a dorsal or ventral incision into the meatal ring and advancing the urethra distally. Kim and King (1992) suggested that conventional meatotomy was frequently complicated by recurrent meatal stenosis and recommended a V-shaped flap meatoplasty, with the flap raised from the dorsal aspect of the glans. If the meatal stenosis is thought to be secondary to BXO the use of topical steroids in conjunction with dilatation or meatotomy is reasonable, but if the BXO extends down the urethra recurrent stenosis is inevitable and more extensive surgery will be required (Depasquale et al. 2000).

The traditional treatment of urethral stricture disease has always started with dilatation or visual urethrotomy. However, for the majority of patients with strictures not related to hypospadias repair these approaches are palliative rather than curative (Andrich and Mundy 2000). Duel et al. (1998) reported similar findings managing strictures following hypospadias repair. In their series of 29 patients treated initially with dilatation or urethrotomy, 79% ultimately required urethroplasty. Therefore it may be worthwhile attempting a one-off urethrotomy with dilatation, but if the stricture recurs this management should be abandoned and an early urethroplasty should be performed.

There are numerous different approaches to urethroplasty for strictures following hypospadias repair. In the presence of extensive scarring and associated chordee there is little doubt that the best approach is the two-stage procedure popularised by Bracka (1995). In this approach all the scarred ventral tissue, including the urethra, is excised back to the normal urethra. A buccal mucosa graft (BMG) (Duckett et al. 1995) is laid on the raw area and secured with a tie-over dressing. Approximately 6 months later the graft is tubularised and the results, both in functional and cosmetic terms, are very satisfactory. It is possible to perform this buccal mucosal urethral replacement as a single-stage procedure, but the results are now generally recognised to be inferior to those achieved with the staged approach and the single-stage approach has largely been abandoned. Although Bracka would recommend the two-stage BMG for the majority of revisions, there are other single-stage procedures that offer very reasonable results.

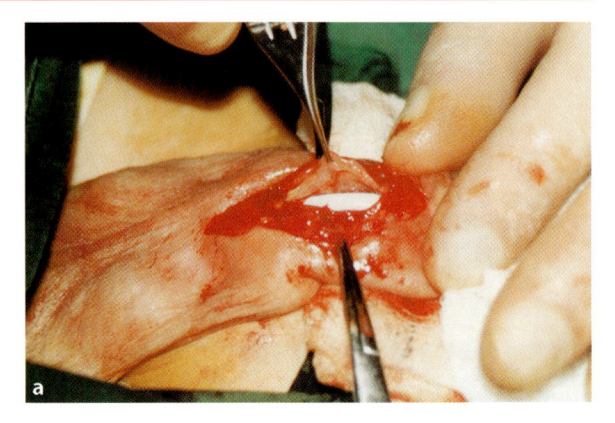

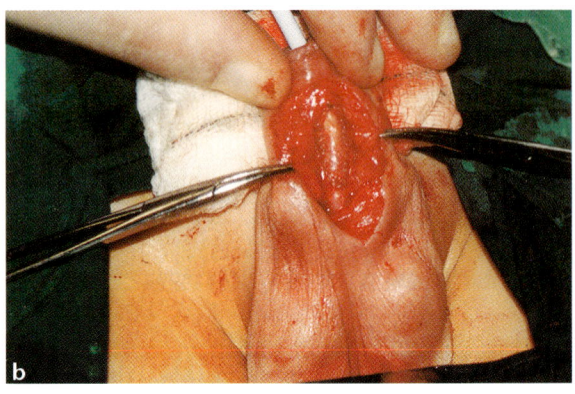

Fig. 29.3. a Urethral stricture laid open with ventral urethrotomy prior to buccal mucosa graft. **b** Buccal mucosa graft in place

For short strictures of the glanular or penile urethra there will usually be sufficient skin available to raise a local pedicled skin flap and lay it into the ventrally incised urethra as described by Orandi (1972) and Jordan (1987). Although the results of these approaches are satisfactory from the functional aspect the appearance of the external urethral meatus is usually not slit-like when glanular strictures are treated. If the stricture is long or if there is insufficient genital skin some form of free graft will be required. Postauricular Wolff grafts and bladder mucosa all had a period of popularity, but have now been almost entirely replaced by buccal mucosa. The stricture is laid open along its ventral wall and the graft is laid into the urethra (Fig. 29.3), and success rates are very good (Baskin and Duckett 1995). One of the problems with the ventral free graft is that it has to take its blood supply from the local penile skin, and if this is very scarred an increased incidence of graft failure may result. An alternative approach is to use a modification of the Snodgrass procedure as described by Hayes and Malone in 1999. The penis is degloved and the site of the urethral stricture is identified and mobilised. The urethra is opened longitudinally and an urethrotomy is performed on the dorsal wall of the urethra. This produces a dorsal defect down to the corpora and a BMG is laid into this gap (Fig. 29.4). This graft is immobilised by the corpora, and the blood supply is also better than it would be on the ventral aspect of the urethra, thus hopefully reducing the incidence of graft failure. Foley et al. (2000) reported the outcome of 13 such grafts and found only one graft failure, suggesting that this may be the best approach for grafting urethral strictures. Interestingly, similarly good results have been reported using dorsal grafting for acquired bulbar urethral strictures (Andrich and Mundy 2000; Barbagli et al. 1996).

For a stricture secondary to BXO some surgeons would suggest a trial of local steroid treatment. In their series Uemura et al. (2000) treated one patient with periurethral injections of triamcinolone and achieved a satisfactory outcome. However, the vast majority of BXO strictures will require surgical intervention. Surgery will involve total excision of the abnormal urethral tissue and replacement with a graft. Nongenital skin has been used but has been associated with significant rates of recurrence, and there is now universal acceptance that the graft material of choice is buccal mucosa and the surgery is best performed as a two-stage procedure (Depasquale et al. 2000; Kumar and Harris 1994; Uemura et al. 2000; Venn and Mundy 1998).

Conclusions

There is little doubt that the incidence of meatal stenosis and urethral stricture following hypospadias repair has decreased with the introduction of current operative techniques. However, it remains a serious complication when it does occur, as it may have a detrimental long-term effect on bladder function and, ultimately, renal function. The routine use of uroflowmetry after repair may be useful in detecting stricture disease before it becomes symptomatic. When a stricture is diagnosed one should always exclude BXO, which is increasingly being recognised. Dilatation and visual urethrotomy may be worth trying once, but if the stricture recurs some form of surgical intervention will be inevitable.

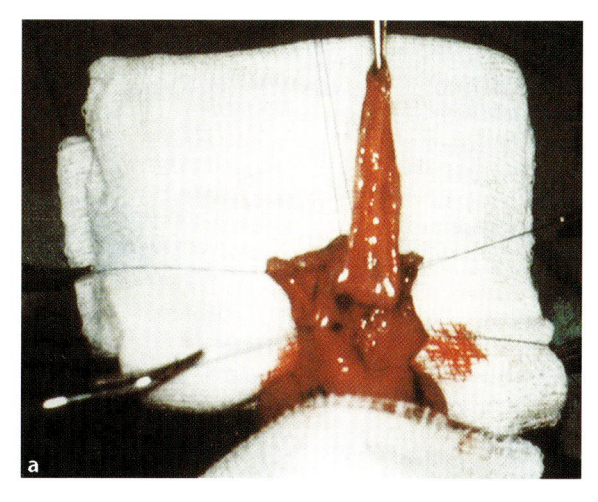

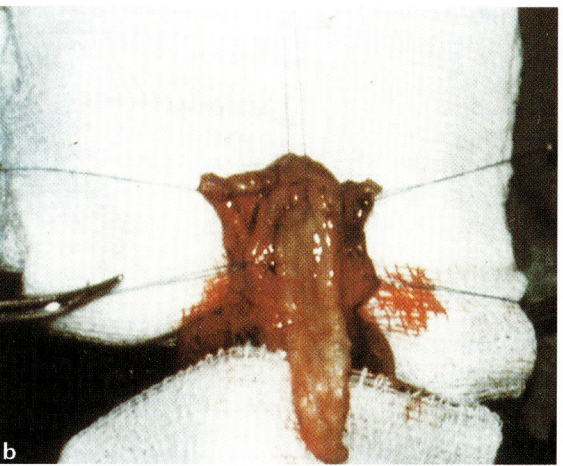

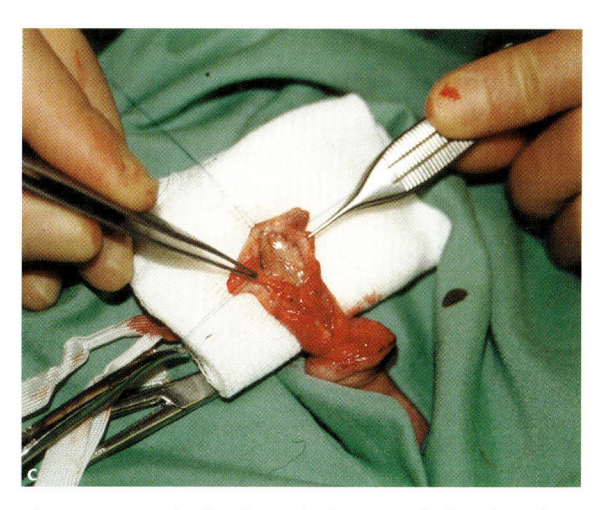

Fig. 29.4. a Urethral stricture laid open with dorsal urethrotomy and buccal mucosa graft partially in place. b Buccal mucosa graft being laid into dorsal defect. c Buccal mucosa graft completed prior to tubularisation. (Reproduced with permission from Hayes and Malone 1999, Fig. 1)

References

Andrich DE, Mundy AR: Urethral strictures and their surgical treatment. BJU Int. 2000; 86:571–580.

Bainbridge DR, Whitaker RH, Shepheard BGF: BXO and urinary obstruction. Br J Urol. 1994; 43:487–491.

Barbagli G, Selli C, Tosto A, et al: Dorsal free graft urethroplasty. J Urol. 1996; 155:123–126

Baskin LS, Duckett JW: Buccal mucosa grafts in hypospadias surgery. Br J Urol. 1995; 76 [Suppl 3]:23–30.

Belman AB: Hypospadias. In: Welch KJ, Randolph JG, Ravitch MM, O'Neill JA, Rowe MI (eds): Pediatric surgery, 4th edn. Year Book, Chicago, pp 1286–1302; 1986.

Belman AB: Hypospadias and chordee. In: King LR, Belman AB, Kramer SA (eds) Clinical pediatric urology, 4th edn. Dunitz, London, pp 1061–1092; 2001.

Bracka A: Hypospadias repair: the two-stage alternative. Br J Urol. 1995; 76 [Suppl 3]:31–41.

Depasquale I, Park AJ, Bracka A: The treatment of balanitis xerotica obliterans. BJU Int. 2000; 86:459–465.

Duckett JW: The current hype in hypospadiology. Br J Urol. 1995; 76 [Suppl 3]:1–7.

Duckett JW, Coplen D, Ewalt D, et al: Buccal mucosal urethral replacement. J Urol. 1995; 153:1660–1663.

Duel BP, Barthold JS, Gonzalez R: Management of urethral strictures after hypospadias repair. J Urol. 1998; 160:170–171.

Elbakry A: Tubularized-incised urethral plate urethroplasty: is regular dilatation necessary for success? BJU Int. 1999; 84:683–688.

Elbakry A: Further experience with the tubularized-incised urethral plate technique for hypospadias repair. BJU Int. 2002; 89:291–294.

Foley SJ, Denny A, Malone PS: Combined buccal mucosal grafting and Snodgrass technique for salvage hypospadias repairs: a promising alternative (abstract). BJU Int. 2000; 85 [Suppl 5]:46.

Garibay JT, Reid C, Gonzalez R: Functional evaluation of the results of hypospadias surgery with uroflowmetry. J Urol. 1995; 154:835–836.

Hamilton SA, Clinch PJ, Goodman PJ et al: The objective assessment of hypospadias repair (abstract). BJU Int. 2000; 85 [Suppl 5]:45–46.

Harris DL, Jeffrey RS: One-stage repair of hypospadias using split preputial flaps (Harris). Br J Urol. 1989; 63:401–407.

Hayes MC, Malone PS: The use of a dorsal buccal mucosal graft with urethral plate incision (Snodgrass) for hypospadias salvage. BJU Int. 1999; 83:508–509.

Holland AJA, Smith GHH: Effect of the depth and width of the urethral plate on tubularized incised urethral plate urethroplasty. J Urol. 2000; 164:489–491.

Jordan GH: Reconstruction of the fossa navicularis. J Urol. 1987; 138:102–104.

Keating MA, Cartwright PC, Duckett JW: Bladder mucosa in urethral reconstructions. J Urol. 1990; 44:827–834.

Kim KS, King LR: Method for correcting meatal stenosis after hypospadias repair. Urology. 1992; 39:545–546.

Kumar MVK, Harris DL: A long term review of hypospadias repaired by split preputial flap technique (Harris). Br J Plast Surg. 1994; 47:236–240.

Kumar MVK, Harris DL: Balanitis xerotica obliterans complicating hypospadias repair. Br J Plast Surg. 1999; 52:69–71.

Lorenzo AJ, Snodgrass WT: Regular dilatation is unnecessary after tubularized incised-plate hypospadias repair. BJU Int. 2002; 89:94–97.

Mouriquand PDE, Mure PY: Hypospadias. In: Gearhart JP, Mouriquand PDE, Rink R (eds) Pediatric urology. Saunders, Philadelphia, pp 713–728; 2001.

Mouriquand PDE, Persad R, Sharma S: Hypospadias repair: current principles and procedures. Br J Urol. 1995; 76 [Suppl 3]:9–22.

Orandi A: One stage urethroplasty: four year follow up. J Urol. 1972; 107:977–980.

Shankar KR, Losty PD, Hopper M, et al: Outcome of hypospadias fistula repair. BJU Int. 2002; 89:103–105.

Snodgrass W: Does tubularized incised urethral plate hypospadias repair create neourethral strictures? J Urol. 1999; 162:1159–1161.

Uemura S, Hutson JM, Woodward AA, et al: Balanitis xerotica obliterans with urethral stricture after hypospadias repair. Pediatr Surg Int. 2000; 16:144–145.

Venn SN, Mundy AR: Urethroplasty for balanitis xerotica obliterans. Br J Urol. 1998; 81:735–737.

Urethral Diverticula and Acquired Megalourethra

Paolo Caione, Simona Nappo

Urethral diverticula are less common complications than fistulas and stenoses after hypospadias repair. Diverticula are reported in 4–12% of patients after preputial island flap urethroplasty (Aigen et al. 1987; Castanon et al. 2000; Elder and Duckett 1987), but are extremely rare after meatal-based flap urethroplasty and after tubularised incised plate techniques (0–0.6%) according to De Badiola et al. (1991) and Kass and Chung (2000). In a review of 5 years' experience and 1,022 hypospadias repairs, Baskin reported diverticula to occur in 7% of the patients treated using the tubularised preputial island flap technique and in no case of onlay island flap procedure (Baskin et al. 1994). Elbakry observed diverticula in 4% of 74 preputial island tube urethroplasty (Elbakry 1999). De Badiola reported diverticula in 9% of 54 preputial island flap tubes, with only 3% occurring after a single-faced flap and 13% after double-faced flaps (de Badiola et al. 1991); in a more recent series, Gonzales reported a 5% incidence of diverticula among 18 cases of double onlay preputial island flap urethroplasty (Gonzales et al. 1996). Castanon reported an incidence of megaurethra of 4.9% in 42 patients who underwent the Duckett technique, and no case out of 38 onlay island flap procedures (Castanon et al. 2000).

Urethral diverticula are generally diagnosed at long-term follow-up, from a few months to several years after the urethroplasty, suggesting a process of gradual dilatation of the new urethra. The diagnosis is easy when ventral urethral "ballooning" of the anterior urethra is seen during voiding, followed by postvoid dribbling (Fig. 30.1a). When the diverticulum is associated with a distal urethral or meatal stenosis, weak stream and dysuria can be the presenting signs (Fig. 30.2a). Less often, haematuria, irritative voiding symptoms, urinary infections or urethral calculus formation are the principal complaints.

Voiding cystourethrography permits evaluation of the presence and the size of the diverticulum and, if present, a distal urethral stenosis or a tiny urethral fistula.

The majority of diverticula are located in the anterior, reconstructed urethra. When the dilatation involves the whole length of the neourethra, it has been termed "acquired megalourethra" by Aigen et al. (1987). Less often, if a proximal segment of the urethra with absent or hypoplastic corpus spongiosum is left in place during surgery, a diverticulum may appear in that tract, involving therefore the native urethra proximally to the anastomosis.

Concerning the causes of diverticula formation, distal urethral or meatal stenosis must always be ruled out. In the absence of distal obstruction, the most likely cause of urethral diverticulum is the creation of an excessively wide flap for the neourethra at the time of surgery. The characteristics of the flap used for the urethroplasty can also play a role. In double-faced flap urethroplasties, De Badiola reported a significant higher incidence of diverticula when the more elastic inner preputial layer was used for the urethroplasty (De Badiola et al. 1991). The subsequent use of the outer preputial layer for the urethroplasty and the inner layer for the coverage of the shaft resulted in a significant decrease in the incidence of this complication, according to De Badiola and Gonzales (de Badiola et al. 1991; Gonzales et al. 1996). An inadequate vascular supply or the lack of supportive periurethral tissue to prevent expansion of the neourethra are considered significant concurrent factors. A diverticulum can also result from urine extravasation at the site of the anastomosis, and therefore it may be associated with a urethral fistula.

According to Duckett, the prevention of urethral diverticula is straightforward and is based on the excision of all redundant tissue from the stretched flap at the time of initial surgery, in order to achieve a neourethra of adequate diameter (Duckett 1995). Prevention of local infection is also warranted.

When urethroplasty is performed for the correction of a urethral stenosis, reapproximation of the bulbocavernous muscle over the flap has been suggested (Mundy and Stephenson 1988) in order to increase the periurethral support. If a free skin patch

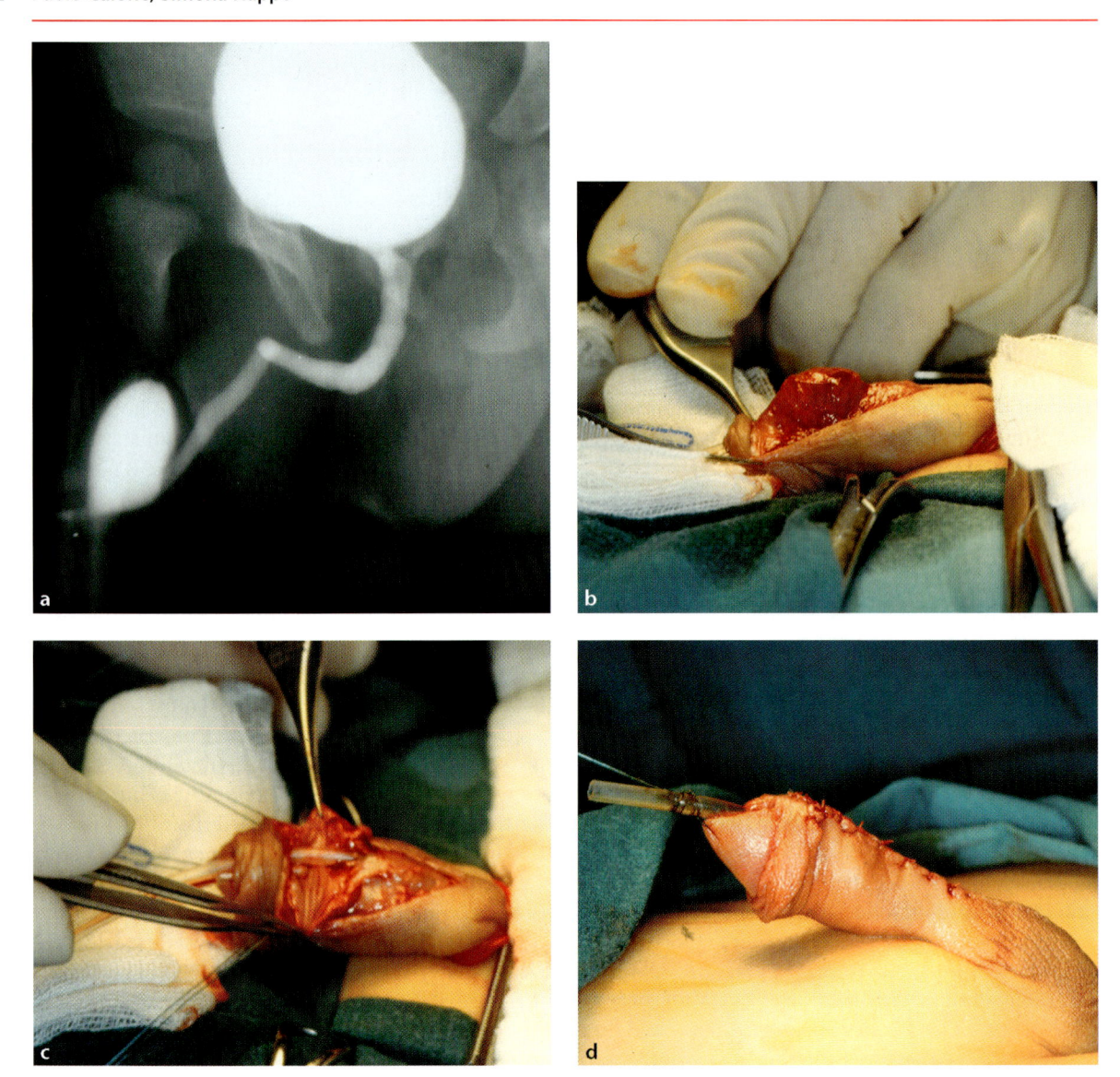

Fig. 30.1. a Voiding cystourethrogram showing a large diverticulum of the anterior urethra in a 4-year old-boy who underwent tubularised island flap urethroplasty at age 1 year. **b, c** (Same patient) Through a sagittal incision of the ventral penile aspect, the diverticulum walls are isolated and split in the sagittal plane. An 8-F catheter is positioned to rule out meatal or distal urethral stenosis. Excision of the diverticulum and Duplay urethroplasty are carried out, with a double-layer covering of periurethral and subcutaneous tissue (6-0 or 7-0 polyglycolic acid sutures). **d** A distal urethral stent may be left in place for 2–3 days postoperatively, using a soft silicone 8-F catheter fixed to the glans, to avoid dysuria

is necessary, suturing the skin graft dorsally rather than ventrally with subsequent fixation of the skin graft to the tunica albuginea of the corpora has been advocated by Lenzi, Barbagli and Stomaci, in order to avoid the development of a urethral diverticulum (Lenzi et al. 1984).

Urethral diverticula almost always require surgical correction. Relief of a distal obstruction, when present, by means of urethral dilatation, meatotomy and meatoplasty is of paramount importance for the ultimate outcome of surgery. The urethra must be inspected carefully for any microfistula which might otherwise be overlooked. In order to avoid overlapping suture lines, degloving of the penis, subsequent diverticulectomy and a "pants over vest" overlapping of the closed urethral defect with periurethral tissue has been advocated by Zaontz et al. (1989). Some technical points to respect in the surgical correction of urethral diverticula are presented in 👁 Figs. 30.1b–d and 30.2b–d. Aigen and al. recommended treating the acquired megalourethra in a fashion similar to that of primary megalourethra,

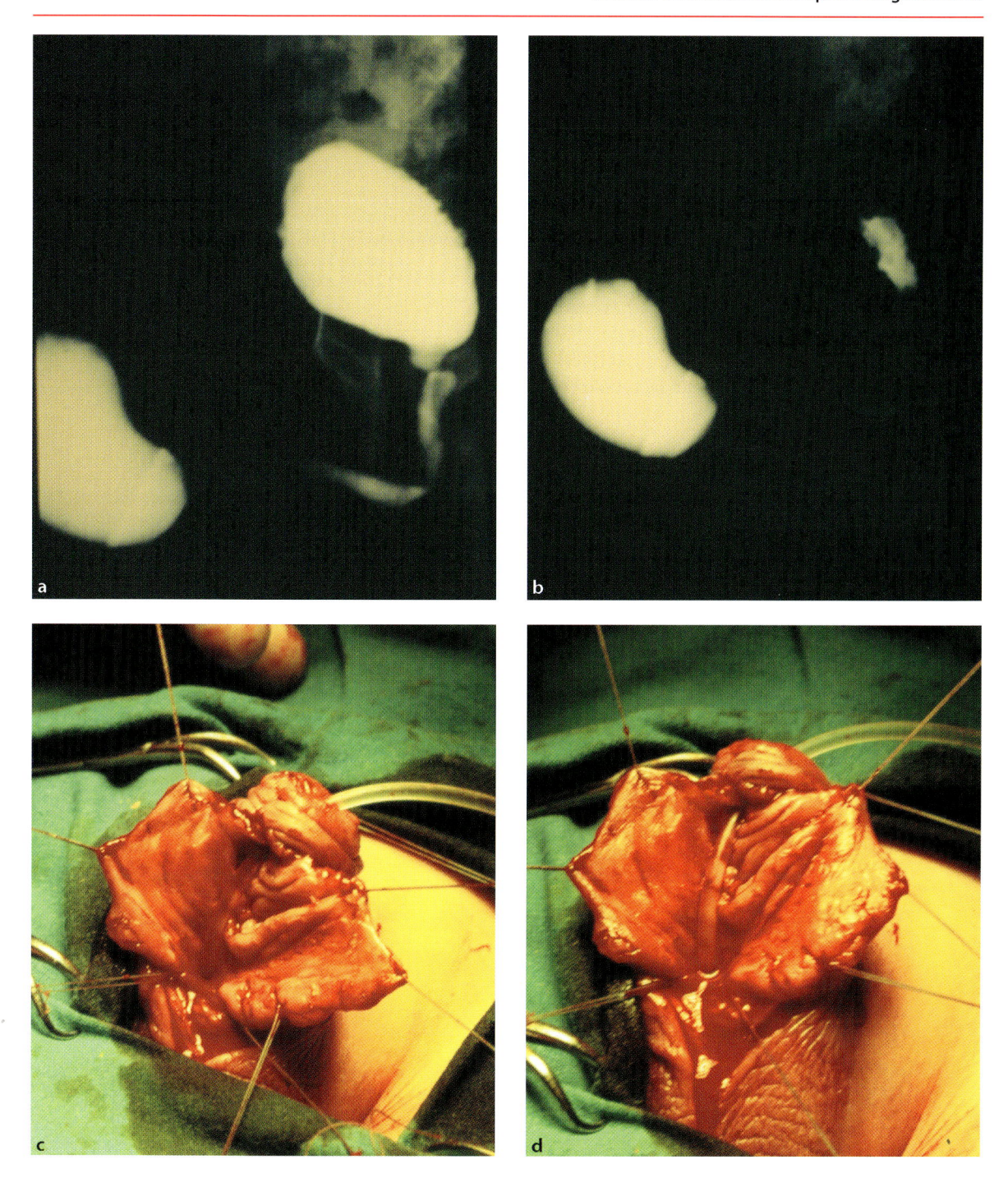

Fig. 30.2. a A huge anterior urethral diverticulum is seen ballooning on a voiding cystourethrogram obtained in a 6-year-old boy who had undergone hypospadias repair using dorsal preputial onlay graft. The diverticulum increases in volume during micturition, mimicking the volume of the bladder (on the right). Dribbling incontinence is present. **b–d** Intraoperative pictures of the case. After meatotomy and indwelling catheter, subcoronal incision and penile degloving are performed. Care must be taken, as the skin is often firmly adherent to the wall of the diverticulum. The diverticulum is divided sagittally. Two wings of tissue are prepared and rotated to augment the glanular urethra and the proximal anastomosis. Two-layer cover in double-breasted fashion is accomplished over the urethral suture

with a de-epithelialised layer to prevent both fistula formation and diverticulum recurrence (Aigen et al. 1987). Repair of the urethral diverticulum by plication has also been suggested, in order to preserve the urethral blood supply, avoid the urethral opening and fistula formation and guarantee adequate reinforcement of the ventral urethra (Heaton et al. 1994). The correction of any urethral diverticulum always demands an adequate and careful technique, since diverticulectomy can be followed by the same complications as hypospadias correction, e.g. urethral stenosis and fistula formation.

Recurrence of the diverticulum after surgical repair is also possible, if pathogenetic factors have not been eliminated.

References

Aigen AB, Khawand N, Skoog SJ, et al: Acquired megalourethra: an uncommon complication of the transverse preputial island flap urethroplasty. J Urol. 1987; 137:712–713.

Baskin LS, Duckett JW, Ueoka K, et al: Changing concepts of hypospadias curvature lead to more onlay flap procedures. J Urol. 1994; 151:191–196.

Castanon M, Munoz E, Carrasco R, et al: Treatment of proximal hypospadias with a tubularized island flap urethroplasty and the onlay technique: a comparative study. J Pediatr Surg. 2000; 35:1453–1455

De Badiola F, Anderson K, Gonzalez R: Hypospadias repair in an outpatient setting without proximal urinary diversion: experience with 113 urethroplasties. J Pediatr Surg. 1991; 26:461–465.

Duckett JW: The current hype in hypospadiology. Br J Urol. 1995; 76 [Suppl 3]:1-7.

Elbakry A: Complications of the preputial island flap tube urethroplasty. BJU Int. 1999; 84:89–94.

Elder JS, Duckett JW: Urethral reconstruction following an unsuccessful one-stage hypospadias repair. World J Urol. 1987; 5:16–19.

Gonzales R, Smith C, Denes ED: Double onlay preputial flap for proximal hypopspadias repair. J Urol. 1996; 156:832–834.

Heaton BW, Snow BW, Cartwright PC: Repair of urethral diverticulum by plication. Urology. 1994; 44:749–752.

Kass EJ, Chung AK: Glanuloplasty and in situ tubularization of the urethral plate: long-term follow-up. J Urol. 2000; 164:991–993.

Lenzi R, Barbagli G, Stomaci N: One stage skin-graft urethroplasty in anterior middle urethra: a new procedure. J Urol. 1984; 131:660–663.

Mundy AR, Stephenson TP: Pedicled preputial patch urethroplasty. Br J Urol. 1988; 61:48–52.

Zaontz MR, Kaplan WE, Maizels M: Surgical correction of anterior urethral diverticula after hypospadias repair in children. Urology. 1989; 33:40–42.

Management of Failed Hypospadias Repairs

31

Pierre Mouriquand, Pierre-Yves Mure, Smart Zeidan, Thomas Gelas

Introduction

The very large number of procedures described for repairing hypospadias and the very meagre data available on long-term follow-up of these operations are striking evidence of the difficulty of this surgery. The surgeon's criteria of success may differ quite significantly from the patient's criteria of satisfaction, as shown in Mureau's studies (Mureau et al. 1996).

If most surgeons consider a straight penis with no redundant skin, regular scars, and an apical urethral meatus with a "good" urine stream as a satisfactory result, evaluation of the results is often very subjective, with a lack of accurate, unbiased and standardised criteria. Several attempts have been made to judge the long-term outcome of this surgery but none have achieved a consensus (Baskin 2001).

The most important question that one needs to address is why hypospadias surgery can fail. The answers are multiple. Some failures may come from the surgeon's inexperience, others from the procedure's inadequacy, and yet others from the failure of the patient's tissues to heal properly, and very often it is a mixture of all three! However good we are, most of us will experience a complication rate for hypospadias surgery of around 20%, with a range from 5% to 70% depending on the procedure used and the surgeon's honesty.

Various complications may be seen. Bad cosmetic results with skin blobs, irregular scars and redundant ventral skin (Figs. 31.1, 31.2) are the most common complications, although poorly recognised by surgeons; urethral fistulas (Fig. 31.3) are also very frequent, often situated at the base of the glans (corona) and often lateralised. The temptation to simply close the hole without understanding the failure mechanisms is dangerous and often leads to recurrence of the fistula or even worse (Rickwood 1997). Proximal urethral strictures have become rarer with the development of onlay urethroplasties, which avoid circular anastomosis, but they represent the most severe com-

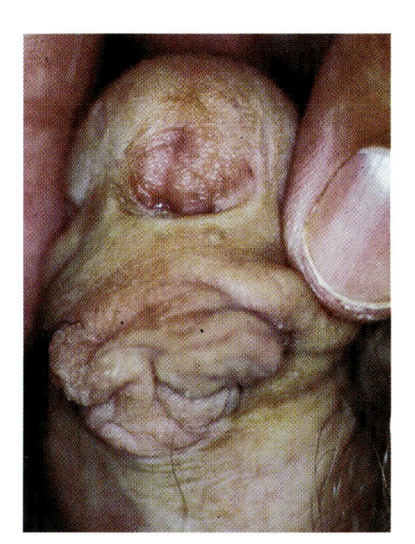

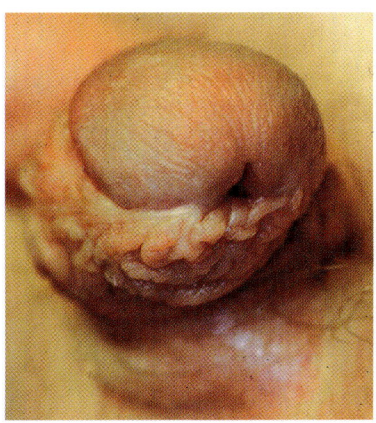

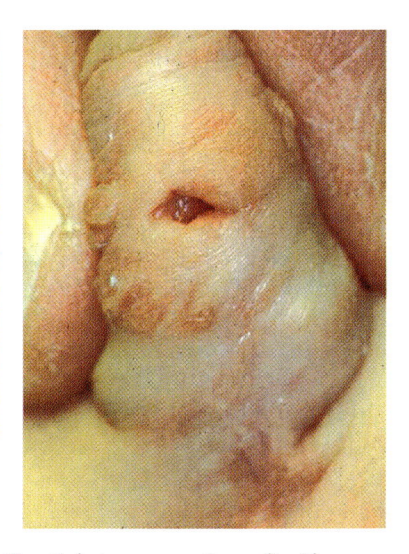

Fig. 31.1 (*left*). A "hypospadias cripple" with a glans ventral dehiscence and redundant ventral skin

Fig. 31.2 (*middle*). Unsatisfactory cosmetic result with a poor ventral aspect of the glans and redundant skin

Fig. 31.3 (*right*). Midshaft fistula

plications (Scherz et al. 1988), requiring full "re-do" operations, given that repeated urethral dilatations are poorly accepted by children and urethrotomy has a poor long-term outcome (Barbagli et al. 2001). Meatal strictures are still common and relatively easy to repair (Duel et al. 1998), although they can be associated with fistulas requiring a more extensive salvage procedure (El Bakry 2001). Other complications are more related to the procedure itself, such as urethral prolapse or urethrocoele (Figs. 31.4, 31.5) with bladder graft urethroplasty and onlay island flap urethroplasty; urethral stones with scrotal skin graft urethroplasty (Rogers et al. 1992); meatal retraction with the MAGPI procedure (Issa and Gearhart 1995); and balanitis xerotica obliterans (BXO) with urethroplasties using foreskin. Persistent or recurrent chordee raises the question of the long-term outcomes of the procedures aiming at straightening the penis. Finally, complete dehiscence of a urethral reconstruction is often linked to a local penile infection or to insufficient blood supplies of the tissues used to replace the missing urethra (Secrest et al. 1993).

The Principles of Hypospadias "Re-do" Surgery

Whatever the cause of the failed reconstruction, the principles of re-do surgery remain identical to those of the primary surgery. Re-do surgery includes three main steps (Mouriquand 1998, 2001; Mouriquand et al. 1995): (1) ascertainment and possible correction of penile chordee; (2) replacement of the defective urethra using either local well-vascularised tissues or free grafts (essentially buccal mucosa); (3) reconstruction of the ventral aspect of the penis (ventral radius), which includes meatoplasty, glanuloplasty, spongioplasty and shaft skin cover.

Ascertainment and Correction of Chordee

Scarred ventral tissues are often a cause of recurrent chordee, so degloving of the penis is the first step before checking the straightness of the corpora (Gittes and McLaughlin 1974). Although in primary cases lifting and preserving the urethral plate is a positive additional manoeuvre to correct the chordee (Baskin 1996b; Mollard et al. 1991; Mouriquand 1998, 2001; Mouriquand et al. 2001), in re-do cases the untethering of the urethral plate from the ventral aspect of the corpora really depends on the quality of this strip of mucosa. If it is well vascularised and not scarred, the urethral plate should be preserved and used as a

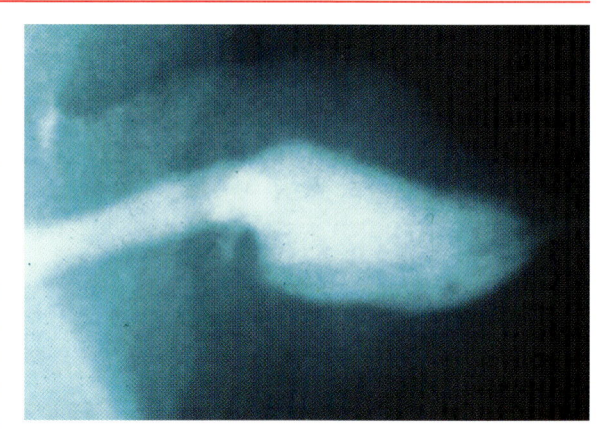

Fig. 31.4. Urethrocoele with a distal stenosis of the urethra (X-ray)

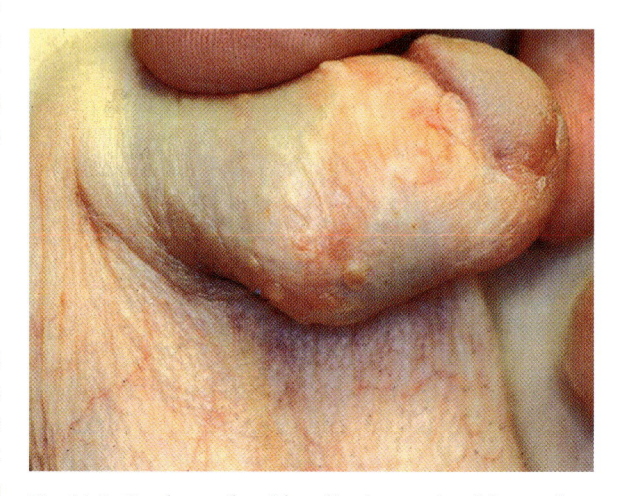

Fig. 31.5. Urethrocoele with a distal stenosis of the urethra. Same patient. Figures 1 to 5 are taken from an article published in *BJU International* (Mouriquand et al. 1995), with permission

mooring plate for the urethroplasty. In some cases, the urethral plate cannot be preserved and is better replaced by "fresh" tissues. If the ventral chordee persists after dissection of the ventral radius of the penis, corporeal plication is then indicated to shorten the dorsal aspect of the corpora (Baskin 1996a).

Repeated Urethroplasty

Once the penis is straight, one should consider redoing the missing urethra. This follows the same principles as in primary cases. If the urethral plate is healthy and wide enough, it can be re-tubularised following the Thiersch–Duplay technique (Duplay 1874; Thiersch 1869). If it is not wide enough it can be split longitudinally and then tubularised following the Snodgrass technique (Snodgrass 1994; Snodgrass and Lorenzo 2002a, b). If the length of urethra to reconstruct is short and if the distal urethra is healthy, full mobilisation of the urethra can be performed following Koff's technique (Koff 1981; Paparel et al. 2001). If the urethral plate is healthy but narrow, extra tissue must be found and laid onto the urethral plate (Mollard et al. 1991, 1994; Mouriquand et al. 1995; Mouriquand 1998, 2001; Paparel et al. 2001). It can either be pedicled preputial foreskin, if this is still available (Mollard et al. 1991), penile ventral skin (Mathieu 1932) or a rectangle of buccal mucosa (Baskin and Duckett 1995; Dessanti et al. 1992).

In rare cases, the urethral plate cannot be preserved and a full tube must be created to replace the missing urethra. It can either be a foreskin tube (Asopa et al. 1971; Duckett 1980, 1986) or a buccal tube (Andrich and Munday 2001). This type of reconstruction requires circular anastomosis and therefore exposes the child to a higher risk of urethral stricture.

Reconstruction of the Ventral Radius of the Penis

Once the missing urethra has been replaced, it is highly advisable to cover the neourethra using surrounding penile tissues, which are mobilised cautiously in order to preserve their blood supply (Churchill et al. 1996). In many cases, the two lateral pillars of distal spongiosum can be mobilised and sutured over the neourethra (spongioplasty) (Zaidi et al. 1997). The meatus, ventral aspect of the glans and skin shaft are reconstituted following the same principles as in primary cases.

Preoperative Care

In re-do surgery as well as in some severe primary cases, preoperative hormonal stimulation (Gearhart and Jeffs 1987) is advisable in order to increase the "healing abilities" of the tissues and to increase the size of the penis. Three main treatments can be proposed prior to surgery: β-HCG stimulation, which has a limited action, testosterone injections, which may expose the child to early bone maturation, or local application of dihydrotestosterone, which seems a safe option with limited systemic side effects. Growth hormone has also been tested in hypospadiac patients but this clinical trial has not been validated yet (personal data).

Postoperative Care and Follow-up

Each surgeon has his or her own habits, and there is certainly no magic recipe in the postoperative period (Mouriquand et al. 1995; Mouriquand 1998, 2001). Penile dressing is important to keep the penis still, avoid penile swelling, reduce postoperative discomfort and avoid trauma. We favour the so-called daisy dressing, where the penis is wrapped with a mesh of Mepitel (which does not stick to the wound) and with an elastic bandage maintained by an Elastoplast dressing. As we do not use any coagulation during the procedure, this type of dressing allows slight haemostatic compression. It is removed or changed on the 4th postoperative day.

Urinary drainage varies considerably from one centre to another. We keep a transurethral catheter for 4 days for Mathieu, Thiersch–Duplay and Snodgrass procedures, whereas we maintain a catheter in place up to 10 days for onlay urethroplasties, buccal graft urethroplasties and Asopa–Duckett tubes. Some surgeons favour suprapubic catheters alone or in combination with a transurethral catheter.

The antibiotic treatment is also extremely variable. Some keep it going for the whole duration of catheterisation, while others add metronidazole if a free graft is used, as the risk of anaerobic infections is then higher.

The Various Techniques of Re-do Urethroplasty

The Salvage Mathieu Procedure

In distal urethral breakdowns or in fistulas located at the coronal level, a Mathieu urethroplasty is a safe procedure if the penile skin proximal to the ectopic meatus is healthy (Mathieu 1932; Wheeler and Malone 1993; Retik et al. 1994a). Two parallel incisions are made on either side of the urethral plate up to the tip of the glans and deep down to the corpora cavernosa. The incision line delimits a perimeatal-based skin flap that is folded over and sutured to the edges of the urethral plate. The lateral wings of the glans are generously dissected from the corpora cavernosa. The rest of the procedure follows the recommendations given earlier. Distal strictures are rare (1%) and the fistula rate is low, around 5%. Minevich et al. (1999) reported a 1.5% reoperation rate with the Mathieu procedure in 202 cases with no stricture over a period of 5 years. The half-moon-shaped meatus is sometimes disappointing, but an extensive dissection of the two wings of the glans allows a nice glanuloplasty

(Mouriquand et al. 1995; Mouriquand 1998, 2001). The overall results remain good, although it is likely that very little blood supply irrigates the perimeatal skin flap and the Mathieu procedure should be considered almost as a free skin graft urethroplasty.

Koff Urethral Mobilisation

When the urethral gap to bridge is short (<2 cm), full penile mobilisation is an elegant way to bring the meatus to the apex of the glans without introducing non-urethral tissue into the urethra. The fistula rate is very low, as there is no proper urethroplasty, but in our series we encountered several meatal stenoses (19.2%), probably due to distal urethral ischaemia.

In Koff's technique (Koff 1981), the whole urethra is detached from the anterior aspect of the corpora cavernosa and then moved forward to bring its opening to the tip of the glans. A gain of urethral length of 5–15 mm is possible using this technique. More length can be obtained if a more proximal freeing of the urethra is achieved using the Turner–Warwick procedure (Warwick et al. 1997).

Thiersch–Duplay/Snodgrass Urethroplasty

Rolling the urethral plate and covering the reconstructed urethra by the two wings of the glans is a possibility if the urethral plate is healthy and if the glans groove is deep enough. The urethral plate is freed with two vertical incisions following its edges. The two glans wings are deeply dissected laterally. The urethral plate is then rolled around a urethral catheter using fine resorbable suture (6-0 to 7-0 polydioxanone or polyglactin) (Duplay 1874; Thiersch 1869). The Snodgrass procedure is an alternative when the distal urethral plate is too narrow to be rolled. A longitudinal midline incision (open urethrotomy) is made on the urethral plate, which is then rolled around a urethral catheter, leaving a raw area inside the urethra, which one hopes is subsequently epithelialised (Snodgrass 1994).

In a recent publication, Snodgrass (2002a) reported the results of his technique for proximal hypospadias with a mean follow-up of 9 months. Subsequent urethral calibration was needed in 48% of cases, urethroscopy in 39%; 33% had complications. The supple appearance of the urethral plate was an important factor in the overall success rate. Re-do hypospadias using the Snodgrass procedure is possible as long as the urethral plate looks healthy (Shanberg et al. 2001; Snodgrass and Lorenzo 2002b).

Onlay Island Flap Urethroplasty

A pedicled flap of preputial mucosa is harvested on the dorsal aspect of the penis and transferred to its ventral side (Duckett 1980, 1986; Mollard et al. 1991; Mollard and Castagnola 1994). The urethral plate is used as a mooring plate and constitutes the roof of the neourethra. The pedicled rectangle of preputial mucosa is stitched along the edges of the urethral plate using fine resorbable sutures. In many re-do cases the foreskin is no longer available and therefore buccal graft urethroplasty is favoured.

In the 92 cases of Mollard's series (Mollard and Castagnola 1994), 15 presented complications. Elbakry (1999) reported an overall complication rate of 42% in 74 patients: 5 (7%) had a urethral breakdown, 17 (23%) a urethrocutaneous fistula, 7 (9%) had urethral strictures and 3 (4%) urethral diverticula.

The Asopa–Duckett Tube

As mentioned above, in some cases the urethral plate cannot be preserved as it is too scarred. Complete replacement of the missing urethra is then necessary using the technique of Asopa and Duckett (Asopa et al. 1971; Duckett 1980). If the foreskin remains available a tube is constituted with a rectangle of pedicled preputial mucosa; if not, a free graft of buccal mucosa is favoured. The tube of foreskin or buccal mucosa is interposed between the ectopic meatus and the apex of the glans.

The complication rate of these techniques varies between 3.7% (El-Kasaby et al. 1986) and 69% (Parsons and Abercombie 1984) in the literature. Duckett himself reported a complication rate varying between 9% and 15% (Duckett 1986).

Bladder Mucosa Graft Urethroplasty

Substitution of the missing urethra has always been a major issue in hypospadiology. Skin was favoured for decades, with a high complication rate mainly comprising severe strictures. In the mid-1980s, urethral substitution using bladder mucosa was resuscitated following the original description by Mammelaar in 1947, as it appeared logical to replace the missing urethra with an urothelial segment.

A rectangle of bladder mucosa was harvested from the anterior aspect of the bladder (Fig. 31.6). It was made into a tube (Fig. 31.7) and interposed between the ectopic meatus and the tip of the glans (Fig. 31.8).

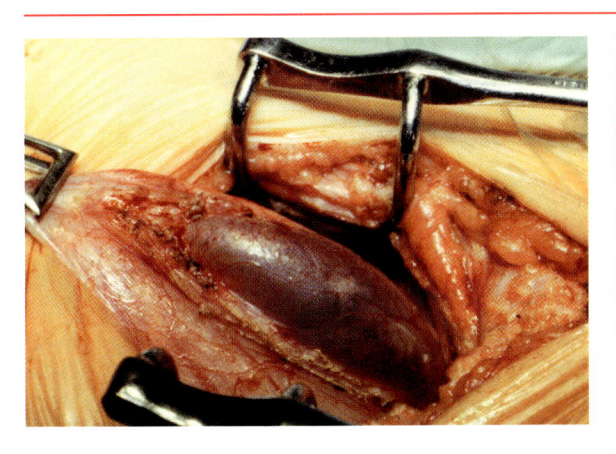

Fig. 31.6. Bladder mucosa after incision of the detrusor muscle

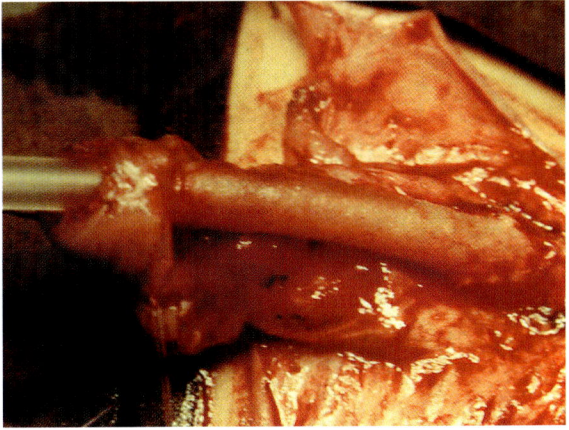

Fig. 31.8. The bladder mucosal tube is inserted between the ectopic meatus and the tip of the glans. We express our special thanks to Professor P. Mollard for Figs. 6–8

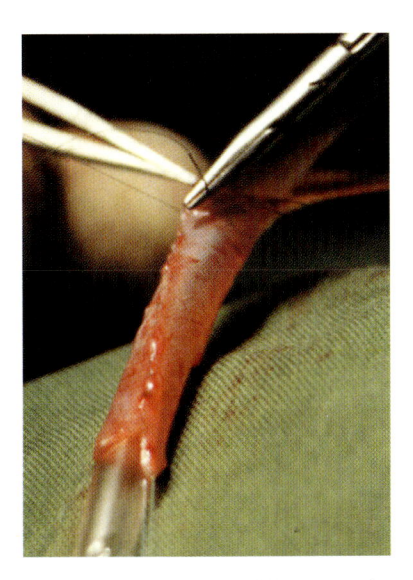

Fig. 31.7. Tubularisation of the bladder mucosal graft

After a phase of enthusiasm for this technique (Decter et al. 1988; Keating et al. 1990; King 1994; Koyle and Ehrlich 1987; Long-Cheng et al. 1995; Mollard et al. 1989), complications soon occurred, mainly urethral prolapse, sticking meatus and urethrocoele. Most patients who underwent this operation required a revision procedure. Ehrlich et al. (1989) reported 15.2% of severe complications and 42% of minor ones. Sixty-six per cent of Ransley's patients (Kinkead et al. 1994) required between one and nine additional procedures to treat complications. The most common complications were meatal stenosis and/or prolapse. The attempt to combine preputial skin with bladder mucosa (Ransley et al. 1987) to reduce the meatal problems did not appear satisfactory on a long-term basis.

Onlay bladder graft urethroplasties have never been reported and it is possible that results would have been better with the preservation of the urethral plate. With the description of buccal graft urethroplasties in the late 1980s, bladder graft urethroplasties went out of fashion.

Buccal Mucosa Graft Urethroplasty

In 1992 Dessanti et al., following Humby's original idea (Humby 1941), described urethral substitution using buccal mucosa. The main advantages of this technique is that buccal mucosa is abundant, easy to harvest and less elastic than bladder mucosa (Ahmed and Gough 1997; Burger et al. 1992; Duckett et al. 1995)

Two main sites are used to harvest buccal mucosa: the inner aspect of the lower lip or the inner aspect of the cheek (Eppley et al. 1997; Morey and McAnanich 1996). In that case the parotid duct must be first identified to avoid injury.

A solution of adrenalin (1:200,000) and lidocaine (1%) is used to lift the buccal mucosa and reduce bleeding. A rectangle of mucosa of variable length is lifted from the underlying tissues and harvested (Fig. 31.9). We do not suture the buccal site when the lower lip is used, in order to avoid the retractile scars that have been described. The cheek site can be sutured safely. It is important to incise the buccal mucosa at 2–3 mm from the lip edges and from the teeth to avoid retraction of the buccal scar. A Surgicel mesh is applied against the buccal site until the end of the procedure to stop the bleeding.

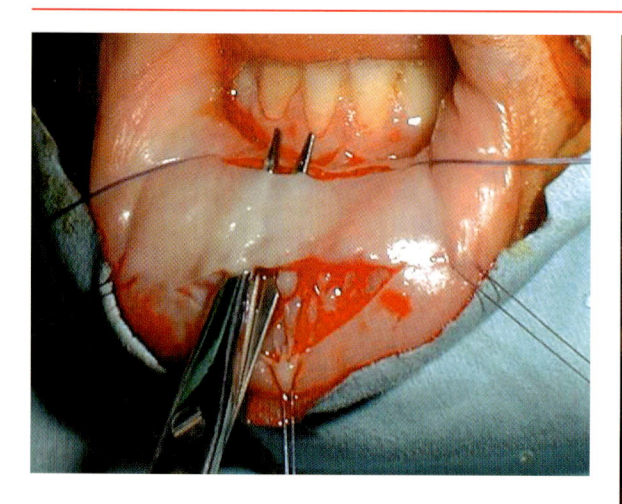

Fig. 31.9. A rectangle of buccal mucosa is harvested from the inner aspect of the lower lip

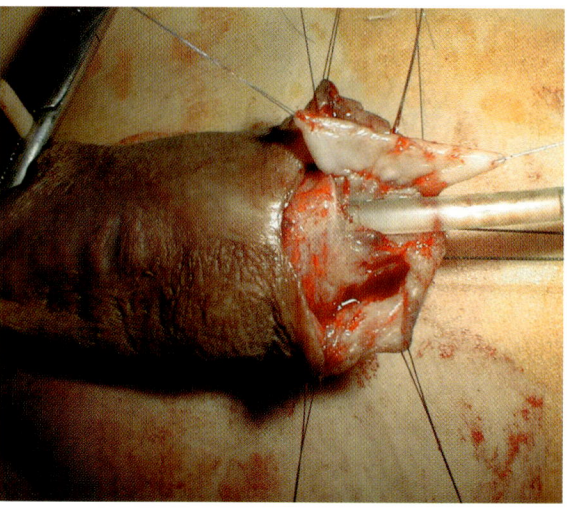

Fig. 31.11. The buccal mucosal graft is laid onto the preserved urethral plat

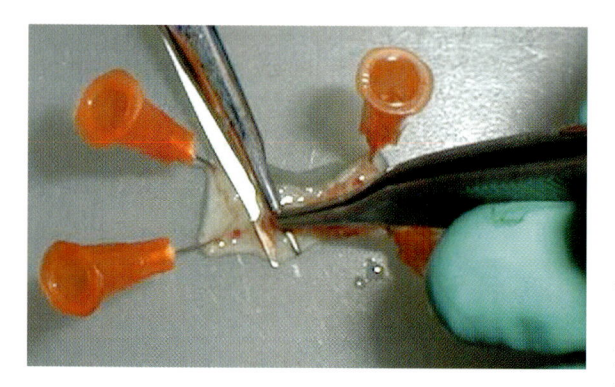

Fig. 31.10. The buccal graft is prepared by removing the globules of fat

Once harvested, the mucosal rectangle is prepared by removing the lobules of fat tissue with fine sharp scissors (Fig. 31.10). The rectangle of buccal mucosa is then sutured to the edges of the urethral plate using 6-0 or 7-0 resorbable sutures (Fig. 31.11), leaving a urethral catheter (usually size 8 for toddlers) in place for 10 days.

A first report from Great Ormond Street (Etker et al. 1993) in 1993 showed severe complications in about 25% of cases. In 2001, the group from Philadelphia (Mollard et al. 1989) reported complications in 17 of 30 patients (57%) including meatal stenosis (5), strictures (7), fistula (2), and breakdown (1), with a 5-year follow-up. The same group had better results with tubes than with patches, whereas others (Venn and Mundy 1998) seem to prefer patches. The results of onlay buccal urethroplasty in our last 15 cases (9 proximal, 6 midshaft/distal) showed 2 straightforward good results, 7 fistulas, 4 dehiscences, 1 stenosis, and 1 lost to view with a mean follow-up of 17 months. With a very high reoperation rate with single-stage onlay buccal urethroplasty (Metro et al. 2001), two-stage procedures using buccal mucosal graft might be a preferable option in the future.

Two-Stage Procedures

For decades multistage procedures were advocated for repair of hypospadias. The Denis Browne (1936) procedure using scrotal skin was one of the most popular. Unfortunately the long-term outcomes were poor, and most of these procedures were abandoned (Baskin and Duckett 1998).

In the late 1980s, Bracka (1995) resuscitated the Cloutier (1962) two-stage procedure. In the first stage the penis is straightened, the glans opened widely and the ventral radius of the penis is grafted with a free graft of preputial mucosa. A few weeks later, the graft is tubularised. The cosmetic results of this two-stage approach were very good, although the urethral stricture rate was high (7%), causing Bracka to change his technique and adopt buccal graft mucosa to reconstruct the urethra (Snodgrass 2002). Further evaluation is needed to assess the reliability of two-stage procedures using buccal mucosa (Filipas et al. 1999).

Two-stage procedures certainly remain a solid option in complex cases, as the results of one-stage procedures are disappointing (Greenfield et al. 1994; Rabinovitch 1988; Retik et al. 1994b).

Other Urethroplasties and Composite Urethroplasties

Skin urethroplasties have lost popularity in view of the very high complication rate, essentially urethral strictures. Onlays or patches seem preferable to tubes, which inevitably lead to bad results (Mundy 1995).

Free-graft preputial urethroplasties also have a high complication rate. Rober et al. (1990) reported 35 reoperations in 81 cases (43%): 28 (34%) for persistent fistula, 7 (9%) for stricture. Relocated penile skin can be a reasonable salvage option. The Toronto team (Jayanthi et al. 1994) reported their experience of pedicle flap salvage urethroplasties in 16 boys. Seven (43%) required no further treatment. Rickwood and Fearne (1997) reported 4 fistulas in 14 cases using the same technique.

Split-thickness skin graft urethroplasties associated with tunica vaginalis flaps for failed hypospadias repairs have also been described in complex re-do hypospadias repair (Ehrlich and Alter 1996; Shankar et al. 2002).

References

Ahmed S, Gough DCS: Buccal mucosal graft for secondary hypospadias repair and urethral replacement. BJU Int. 1997; 80:328–330.

Andrich DE, Mundy AR: Substitution urethroplasty with buccal mucosal-free grafts. J Urol. 2001; 165:1131–1134.

Asopa HS, Elhence EP, Atria SP, et al: One stage correction of penile hypospadias using a foreskin tube. A preliminary report. Int Surg. 1971; 55:435–440.

Barbagli G, Palminteri E, Lazzeri M, et al: Long-term outcome of urethroplasty after failed urethrotomy versus primary repair. J Urol. 2001; 165:1918–1919.

Baskin LS: Controversies in hypospadias surgery: penile curvature. Dial Pediatr Urol. 1996a; 19(7):1–8.

Baskin LS: Controversies in hypospadias surgery: the urethral plate. Dial Pediatr Urol. 1996b; 19(8):1–8.

Baskin LS: Hypospadias: a critical analysis of cosmetic outcomes using photography. BJU Int. 2001; 87:534–539.

Baskin LS, Duckett JW: Buccal mucosa grafts in hypospadias surgery. Br J Urol. 1995; 76 [Suppl 3]:23–30.

Baskin LS, Duckett JW: Hypospadias. In: Stringer MD, Mouriquand PDE, Oldham KT, Howard ER (eds) Pediatric surgery and urology: long term outcomes. Saunders, Philadelphia, pp. 559–567; 1998.

Bracka A: Hypospadias repair: the two-stage alternative. Br J Urol. 1995; 76 [Suppl 3]:31–41.

Browne D: An operation for hypospadias. Lancet. 1936; i:141–149.

Burger RA, Muller SC, El-Damanhoury H, et al: The buccal mucosa graft for urethral reconstruction: a preliminary report. J Urol. 1992; 147:662–664.

Churchill BM, Van Savage JG, Khoury AE, et al: The dartos flap as an adjunct in preventing urethrocutaneous fistulas in repeat hypospadias surgery. J Urol. 1996; 156:2047–2049.

Cloutier A: A method for hypospadias repair. Plast Reconstr Surg. 1962; 30:368–373.

Decter RM, Roth DR, Gonzales JR: Hypospadias repair by bladder mucosal graft: an initial report. J Urol. 1988; 140:1256–1258.

Dessanti A, Rigamonti W, Merulla V, et al: Autologous buccal mucosa graft for hypospadias repair: an initial report. J Urol. 1992; 147:1081–1084.

Duckett JW: Transverse preputial island flap technique for repair of severe hypospadias. Urol Clin North Am. 1980; 7:423–431.

Duckett JW: Hypospadias. In: Walsh PC, Gittes RF, Perlmutter AD, Stamey TA (eds): Campbell's urology. Saunders, Philadelphia, pp. 1987–1989; 1986.

Duckett JW, Coplen D, Ewalt D, et al: Buccal mucosal urethral replacement. J Urol. 1995; 153:1660–1663.

Duel BP, Barthold JS, Gonzales R: Management of urethral strictures after hypospadias repair. J Urol. 1998; 160:170–171.

Duplay S: De l'hypospade périnéo-scrotal et de son traitement chirurgical. Arch Gen Med. 1874; 1:613–657.

Ehrlich RM, Alter G: Split-thickness skin graft urethroplasty and tunica vaginalis flaps for failed hypospadias repairs. J Urol. 1996; 155:131–134.

Ehrlich RM, Reda EF, Koyle MA, et al: Complications of bladder mucosal graft. J Urol. 1989; 142:626–627.

Elbakry A: Complications of the preputial island flap-tube urethroplasty. BJU Int. 1999; 84:89–94.

Elbakry A: Management of urethrocutaneous fistula after hypospadias repair: 10 years' experience. BJU Int. 2001; 88:590–595.

El-Kasaby AW, El-Beialy H, El-Halaby R, et al: Urethroplasty using transverse penile island flap for hypospadias. J Urol. 1986; 136:643–644.

Eppley BL, Keating M, Rink R: A buccal mucosal harvesting technique for urethral reconstruction. J Urol. 1997; 157:1268–1270.

Etker AS, Duffy PG, Ransley PG: Buccal mucosa graft urethroplasty: the first 50 cases. Abstract of the British Association of Urological Surgeons 1993.

Filipas D, Fisch M, Fichtner J, et al: The histology and immunohistochemistry of free buccal mucosa and full-skin grafts after exposure to urine. BJU Int. 1999; 84:108–111.

Gearhart JP, Jeffs RD: The use of parenteral testosterone therapy in genital reconstructive surgery. J Urol. 1987; 138:1077–1078.

Gittes R, McLaughlin AP III: Injection technique to induce penile erection. Urology. 1974; 4:473–474.

Greenfield SP, Sadler BT, Wan J: Two-stage repair for severe hypospadias. J Urol. 1994; 152:498–501.

Humby G: One-stage operation for hypospadias. Br J Surg. 1941; 29:84.

Issa MM, Gearhart JP: The failed MAGPI: management and prevention. Br J Urol. 1989; 64:169–171.

Jayanthi VR, McLorie GA, Khoury AE, et al: Can previously relocated penile skin be successfully used for salvage hypospadias repair? J Urol. 1994; 152:740–743.

Keating MA, Cartwright PC, Duckett JW: Bladder mucosa in urethral reconstructions. J Urol. 1990; 144:827–834.

Kinkead TM, Borzi PA, Duffy PG, et al: Long-term follow-up of bladder mucosa graft for male urethral reconstruction. J Urol. 1994; 151:1056–1058.

King LR: Bladder mucosal grafts for severe hypospadias: a successful technique. J Urol. 1994; 152:2338–2340.

Koff SA: Mobilization of the urethra in the surgical treatment of hypospadias. J Urol. 1981; 125:394–397.

Koyle MA, Ehrlich RM: The bladder mucosal graft for urethral reconstruction. J Urol. 1987; 138:1093–1095.

Long-Cheng L, Xy Z, Si-Wei Z, et al: Experience of hypospadias using bladder mucosa in adolescents and adults. J Urol. 1995; 153:1117–1119.

Mammelaar J: Use of bladder mucosa in a one stage repair of hypospadias. J Urol. 1947; 58:68.

Mathieu P: Traitement en un temps de l'hypospade balanique et juxta-balanique. J Chir (Paris). 1932; 39:481–484.

Metro MJ, Hsi-Yang W, Snyder HM, et al: Buccal mucosal grafts: lessons learned from an 8-year experience. J Urol. 2001; 166:1459–1461.

Minevich E, Pecha BR, Wacksman J, et al: Mathieu hypospadias repair: experience in 202 patients. J Urol. 1999; 162:2141–2143.

Mollard P, Mouriquand P, Bringeon G, et al: Repair of hypospadias using a bladder mucosa graft in 76 cases. J Urol. 1989; 142:1548–1550.

Mollard P, Mouriquand P, Felfela T: Application of the onlay island flap urethroplasty to penile hypospadias with severe chordee. Br J Urol. 1991; 68:317–319.

Mollard P, Castagnola C: Hypospadias: the release of chordee without dividing the urethral plate and onlay island flap (92 cases). J Urol. 1994; 152:1238–1240.

Morey AF, McAninch JW: Technique of harvesting buccal mucosa for urethral reconstruction. J Urol. 1996; 155:1696–1697.

Mouriquand PDE, Persad R, Sharma S: Hypospadias repair: current principles and procedures. Br J Urol. 1995; 76 [Suppl 3]:9–22.

Mouriquand PDE: Hypospadias. In: Atwell JD (ed): Paediatric surgery. Arnold, London, pp. 603–616; 1998.

Mouriquand PDE, Mure PY: Hypospadias. In: Gearhart J, Rink R, Mouriquand P (eds) Pediatric urology. Saunders, Philadelphia, pp. 713–728; 2001.

Mundy AR: The long-term results of skin inlay urethroplasty. BJU Int. 1995; 75:59–61.

Mureau MAM, Slijper FME, Slob AK, et al: Satisfaction with penile appearance after hypospadias surgery: the patient and surgeon view. J Urol. 1996; 155:703–706.

Paparel P, Mure PY, Margarian M, et al: Approche actuelle de l'hypospade chez l'enfant. Prog Urol. 2001; 11:741–751.

Paparel P, Mure PY, Garignon C, et al: Translation uréthrale de Koff: a propos de 26 hypospades présentant une division distale du corps spongieux. Prog Urol. 2001; 11:1327–1330.

Parsons K, Abercrombie GF: Transverse preputial island flap neo-urethroplasty. Br J Urol. 1982; 54:745–747.

Rabinovitch HH: Experience with a modification of the Cloutier technique for hypospadias repair. J Urol. 1988; 139:1017–1019.

Ransley PG, Duffy PG, Oesch IL, et al: The use of bladder mucosa and combined bladder mucosa/preputial skin grafts for urethral reconstruction. J Urol. 1987; 138:1096–1099.

Retik AB, Mandell J, Bauer SB, et al: Meatal based hypospadias repair with the use of a dorsal subcutaneous flap to prevent urethrocutaneous fistula. J Urol. 1994a; 152:1229–1231.

Retik AB, Bauer SB, Mandell J, et al: Management of severe hypospadias with a 2-stage repair. J Urol. 1994b; 152:749–751.

Rickwood AMK: Hypospadias repairs. BJU Int. 1997; 79:662.

Rickwood AMK, Fearne C: Pedicled penile skin for hypospadias 'rescue'. Br JUrol. 1997; 80:145–146.

Rober PE, Perlmutter AD, Reitelman C: Experience with 81, 1-stage hypospadias/chordee repairs with free graft urethroplasties. J Urol. 1990; 144:526–529.

Rogers HS, McNicholas TA, Blandy JP: Long-term results of one-stage scrotal patch urethroplasty. Br J Urol. 1992; 69: 621–628.

Secrest CL, Jordan GH, Winslow BH, et al: Repair of the complications of hypospadias surgery. J Urol. 1993; 150:1415–1418.

Scherz HC, Kaplan GW, Packer MG, et al: Post-hypospadias repair urethral strictures: a review of 30 cases. J Urol. 1988; 140:1253–1255.

Shanberg AM, Sanderson K, Duel B: Re-operative hypospadias repair using the Snodgrass incised plate urethroplasty. BJU Int. 2001; 87:544–547.

Shankar KR, Losty PD, Hopper M, et al: Outcome of hypospadias fistula repair. BJU Int. 2002; 89:103–105.

Snodgrass W: Tubularized, incised plate urethroplasty for distal hypospadias. J Urol. 1994; 151:464–465.

Snodgrass WT, Lorenzo A: Tubularized incised-plate urethroplasty for proximal hypospadias. BJU Int. 2002a; 89:90–93.

Snodgrass WT, Lorenzo A: Tubularized incised-plate urethroplasty for hypospadias reoperation. BJU Int. 2002b; 89:98–100.

Snodgrass WT: Reoperative hypospadias: a spectrum of challenges. Dial Pediatr Urol. 2002; 25:1–8.

Snow BW: Use of tunica vaginalis to prevent fistulas in hypospadias surgery. J Urol. 1986; 136:861–863.

Snow BW, Cartwright PC, Unger K: Tunica vaginalis blanket wrap to prevent urethrocutaneous fistula: an 8-year experience. J Urol. 1995; 153:472–473.

Thiersch C: Über die Entstehungsweise and operative Behandlung des Epispadie. Arch Heilkd. 1869; 10:20–25.

Venn SN, Mundy AR: Early experience with the use of buccal mucosa for substitution urethroplasty. Br J Urol. 1998; 81:738–740.

Warwick RT, Parkhouse H, Chapple CR: Bulbar elongation anastomotic meatoplasty (BEAM) for subterminal and hypospadiac urethroplasty. J Urol. 1997; 158:1160–1167.

Wheeler R, Malone P: The role of the Mathieu repair as a salvage procedure. Br J Urol. 1993; 72:52–53.

Zaidi SZ, Hodapp J, Cuckow P, et al: Spongioplasty in hypospadias repair. Abstract of the British Association of Urological Surgeons, 1997.

The Long-Term Consequences of Hypospadias

32

Christopher Woodhouse

Introduction

The techniques for the correction of hypospadias have changed considerably over the past 40 years. Many of the principles were laid down more than 100 years ago, but a recent textbook chapter identified 212 named operations for hypospadias. Although many of these operations are only minor variations on previous themes, the rapid changes in fashion in children make critical long-term follow-up of adults very difficult. There seems no doubt that the surgical results have improved in the last century.

The operations that were performed on the children who now are adults and whose sexual function can be investigated are largely obsolete. It is perfectly possible to assess the sexual function of adults who have been operated for hypospadias, but it is almost impossible, without some control group, to judge the effect of the original diagnosis and surgical treatment.

In view of these difficulties, it seems reasonable to consider the surgical results separately from the sexual outcome.

Surgical Results

Appearance

Urologists are aware of the wide range of size and appearance of the penis. Its growth with age has been documented and a centile growth chart is available (Schonfeld 1943). The normal appearance has not been so well documented – like other human features there is a wide variation in that which is considered normal or beautiful.

It has been established, however, that the meatus is not always at the tip of the penis. Thirteen percent of apparently normal men have a hypospadiac meatus and in a further 32% it is in the middle third of the glans. Most of these men thought they were normal; all voided normally and had sexual intercourse (Fichtner et al. 1995). It could, therefore, be said that minor degrees of hypospadias, especially if there is no chordee, do not greatly matter to men or to their partners.

With this observation in mind, the results of surgery for distal hypospadias must be looked at very critically – if men can have a minor hypospadias without even recognising it, the surgical correction must be virtually complication-free. Such surgery can be achieved with complication rates as low as 5–10% (Caione et al. 1997; Kass and Chung 2000), though there are still reports of series with as few as 56% of men satisfied with the long-term outcome (Mor et al. 2000).

Although the large number of operations described might suggest that none is any good, there is evidence that long-term outcomes are improving. In a comparatively small series of adults followed for a mean of 27 years, 11 of 23 patients who had had a two-stage Denis Browne operation were satisfied compared with 13 of 15 who had had the single-stage Mathieu repair (Aho et al. 1997).

The cosmetic results of hypospadias surgery are entirely observer dependent. Surgeons reviewing their own results have a somewhat rosy view of the outcome. For example, in one personal series of 220 men reviewed at a mean age of 18.4 years, the surgeon reported a good outcome with all patients having a straight erection and a normal, formed urinary stream (Johanson and Avellan 1980). Unfortunately, further analysis of his data shows that 65% of the men still had a degree of hypospadias that would, by current standards, require correction.

When there is an independent review, a more realistic outcome is seen. Summerlad looked at 60 patients with apparently successful repairs operated on by his predecessors. He found that the meatus was rarely at the tip of the penis and 22% of the patients had chordee even when the penis was flaccid (Fig. 32.1). Almost none of the patients could void normally, and 16 of 60 could not stand to void into a toilet bowl (Summerlad 1975).

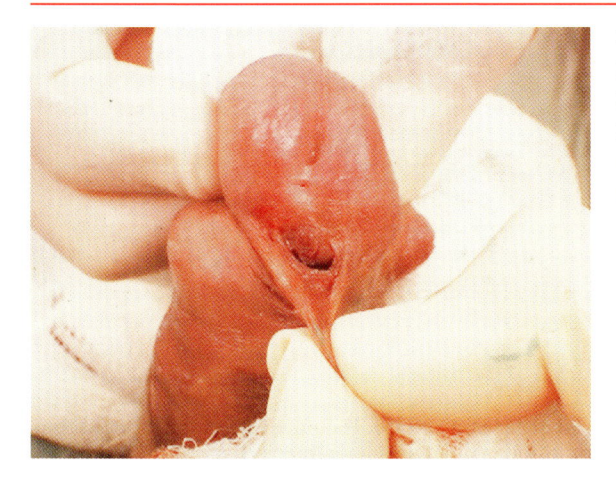

Fig. 32.1. Adult penis following a Denis Browne repair of hypospadias in childhood showing a patulous coronal meatus. Note the dimple on the glans which should have been the meatus

Table 32.1. The features of the Genital Perception Score described by Mureau et al. (1996). All features are scored, but they are divided here into surgically correctable and uncorrectable items

Correctable features	Uncorrectable features
Glans shape	Penile size
Position of meatus	Penile thickness
Scars	Glans size
Scrotum	
General appearance	

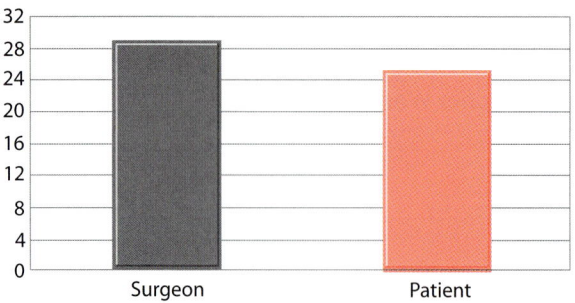

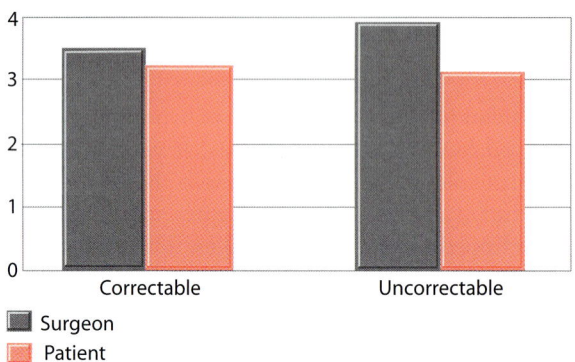

Fig. 32.2. *Above:* Histogram to show the Genital Perception Score for all eight features of the corrected hypospadiac penis by the surgeon and the patient. Maximum score is 32. The difference between the scores of the surgeon and the patient is significant with p=<0.001 (Mureau et al. 1996). *Below:* Mean scores (maximum score 4) for features of hypospadias that are correctable and those that are not correctable by surgery. It is seen that there is little difference between patient and surgeon for the correctable features

Recently, efforts have been made to establish scoring systems to allow more objective assessment of the outcome. A Hypospadias Objective Scoring Evaluation (HOSE) was applied to 20 children. It was found that a parent, two surgeons and a nurse could give a consistent and reproducible score (Holland et al. 2001). Unfortunately, the children, with a median age of 23 months, were too young to have an opinion.

Adult patients themselves have a gloomier view of the appearance. Up to 80% of adolescents are dissatisfied with their penile appearance, though only 38–44% are sufficiently displeased to want further surgery (Bracka 1989; Mureau et al. 1995). There is a difference in results depending on the attitude of the community to circumcision: in countries where childhood circumcision is routine, results are perceived to be better than in those where it is uncommon.

When there is a direct comparison between the opinions of the patient and the surgeon, there is almost no agreement. Mureau et al. (1996) introduced the helpful concept of the Genital Perception Score (GPS). Eight features of the penis are scored from 1 to 4, giving an overall range of 8 to 32, with the highest score being the best result (Table 32.1). This allows a numerical comparison between observers and helps to identify areas of concern for the patient. It is important to note, however, that three of the eight features were concerned with penile size, which cannot be altered by surgery.

The authors asked patients and their surgeons to give a GPS for the surgical result. Surgeons gave a mean score of 29.1 and the patients gave a mean of 25.1, a difference which is statistically significant (Fig. 32.2 above). For the uncorrectable, size-related features, the patients gave a mean satisfaction score of 3.1 (out of 4) while the surgeons gave a score of 3.9. For the features related to the surgical result the patients' score was 3.2 and the surgeons' was 3.5 (Fig. 32.2 below). Much of the dissatisfaction seems to have been related to the circumcised appearance in a society where circumcision is unusual and is perceived to shorten the penis (Mureau et al. 1996).

It seems likely, therefore, that surgeons can reliably correct those abnormal features of the hypospadiac penis that are amenable to reconstruction: chordee, the hooded prepuce (especially if the circumcised appearance is acceptable) and the position of the meatus. Features related to the size of the corpora or the glans are not correctable.

Voiding

In a public urinal young men like to void standing up through their opened flies. Inability to perform in this way is a serious social impediment. The stream must be well formed and directable, a goal that is most easily achieved with a slit-like terminal meatus. In some series up to 40% of patients have a stream that sprays. There is a trend to improvement in these gloomy figures with newer repairs, but voiding problems remain common in adults especially when compared with controls (👁 Fig. 32.3).

Fortunately, the results achieved in childhood seem to be maintained or may even improve. In a large series of patients of all ages up to 66 years, the proportion of men with a normal peak flow rate increased with age (👁 Fig. 32.4) (van der Werff et al. 1997). The implication of this finding is that the neourethra grows appropriately with age. The patients in this study seem to be a reasonable cross section of the hypospadias population, although 87% originally had a glanular or coronal meatus. Seventeen percent had a spraying stream. The results are particularly good as the more severe cases had the Byars–Denis Browne operation, which now is outmoded.

This effect of age may explain why flow rates in children with hypospadias before surgery have been recorded around the 5th centile with little improvement after surgery (Malyon et al. 1997).

With severe penoscrotal hypospadias it is particularly difficult to achieve normal voiding, and a spraying stream is found in the majority of operated men (Eberle et al. 1993). Flow rates are on the low side of normal, but in the biggest long-term follow-up only nine of 42 patients (21%) were at or below the 5th centile (Eberle et al. 1993).

All large series of hypospadias surgery record some strictures. As ever, there is a difficulty in defining just what constitutes a stricture. In the series of patients whose flow rates were measured (see above), all the patients had completed surgery and so, presumably, those with symptomatic strictures had had revision operations. There were 14 (of 175) patients who had a flow curve that "suggested distal urethral obstruction", but none was symptomatic. Urodynam-

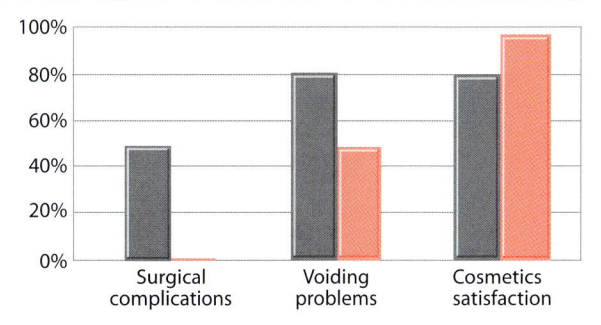

Fig. 32.3. This histogram compares the adult outcome of surgery for hypospadias (*grey bars*) and circumcision (*red bars*). Hypospadias patients have more complications and more voiding problems. Nonetheless, cosmetic satisfaction is nearly equal and 47% of circumcision patients have some voiding problems. The survey was done in Finland, where circumcision is rare. (Aho et al. 2000)

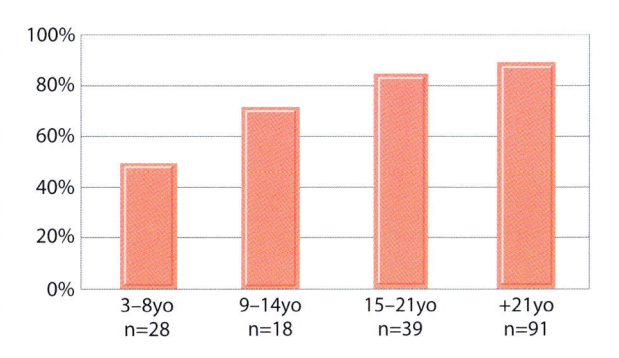

Fig. 32.4. Histogram to show the percentage of patients in each age group who had a valid flow rate between the 5th and 95th centiles for age. (van der Werff et al. 1997)

ic studies were not performed, so it is not known whether these patients had a functional obstruction (van der Werff et al. 1997).

In children, a significant stricture has been defined in terms of flow rate as a flat, plateau-like trace with a peak flow more than two standard deviations below the appropriate mean for age and surface area (Garibay et al. 1995). On this basis the authors found that 7 of 32 children had strictures, but only two were symptomatic. In a later paper from the same group, 38 strictures were identified, all of which were symptomatic and none was identified by flow rate alone, the incidence being 6.5% (Duel et al. 1998).

It would seem sensible, especially in view of the tendency for flow rates to improve with age, to accept symptomatic criteria as the basis for diagnosis.

Meatal or very distal strictures may be corrected by the Snodgrass procedure, but even this has a 15%

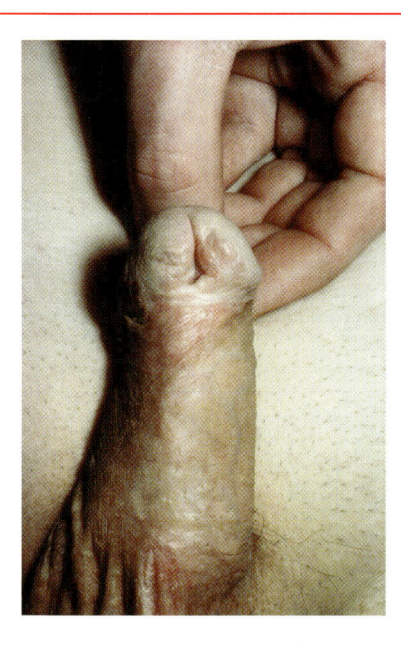

Fig. 32.5. Extensive balanitis xerotica obliterans of the glans and coronal meatus (*xerotica* means white)

complication rate (Shanberg et al. 2001). Minor proximal strictures will occasionally respond to internal urethrotomy, but most will require formal urethroplasty. More severe strictures always require urethroplasty. All of the techniques for stricture disease can be used, but the anastomotic urethroplasty seldom is possible. Patches, either of pedicled skin or of buccal mucosa, generally do well (Greenwell et al. 1999).

An unknown number of strictures develop late, often as a result of balanitis xerotica obliterans (BXO). This chronic fibrosing process is of unknown aetiology (Fig. 32.5). Once the urethra is affected, BXO progresses proximally to produce particularly severe strictures. It may be seen both in men who have had hypospadias repair and in those whose hypospadias has never been corrected. Indeed, in previously unoperated hypospadiacs, meatal stricture due to BXO is a relatively common reason for presentation to the surgeon. Because of the progressive nature of the condition, it is most important that all of the affected skin and urethra is excised before reconstruction. For this reason, single-stage operations usually fail and a two-stage operation is recommended (Venn and Mundy 1998; Kumar and Harris 1999). Some men who have never had hypospadias surgery and present with a BXO stricture may wish only to have the stricture excised, and decline urethroplasty when they learn of the extent of surgery that is needed. Other strictures are a part of the disastrous problem of the "hypospadias cripple".

Chordee

Hypospadias repairs currently in use put great emphasis on correction of chordee, recommending frequent intraoperative artificial erections to check that the penis is straight. Older repairs were much less successful in this regard and at long-term follow-up 20% of patients or more had residual chordee. As with strictures, it is very important to confirm that the man actually has significant symptoms from the chordee. The bend may be sufficient to prevent intercourse and therefore demand correction. There is also a group of men for whom the bent appearance, even if not a physical impediment to penetration, is an emotional cause of sexual dysfunction. It is interesting that in Summerlad's late review 13 patients were thought objectively to have chordee, of whom only eight had symptoms, while two of 47 complained of curvature that was not confirmed on examination (Summerlad 1975).

More recent series reporting on the current style of repair have much better results, especially with the use of artificial erections during surgery. Bracka (1989) reported an 18% incidence of chordee in adult follow-up. Whatever else may be said about current techniques of hypospadias repair, it is usually possible to correct the chordee.

Several late reviews report the presence of chordee either remote from the site of the hypospadias or, apparently, appearing many years after the original repair.

In a very careful study, Vandersteen and Husmann have shown that delayed onset or recurrent chordee are real entities. In a group of 34 men referred for alleged recurrent chordee, they identified 22 who appeared to have had adequate initial surgery, confirmed by intraoperative erection and reported absence of chordee during follow-up. All had had proximal, or even penoscrotal, chordee and had had a tubularised free-graft urethroplasty. The chordee developed during puberty between the ages of 12 and 18 years. The median age at presentation, a mean of 17 years after the original surgery, was 21 years. Although in two thirds of cases the urethra was shortened and fibrosed, its division did not correct the chordee in all cases. Disproportion of the corpora was present in 68% of men, with or without short urethra (Vandersteen and Husmann 1998). The cause of this late deterioration is unknown.

Residual chordee is a well-known and important cause of late morbidity. Even now many men are embarrassed to present themselves for treatment and sympathetic management is essential. The patient's description of the chordee is usually inadequate to

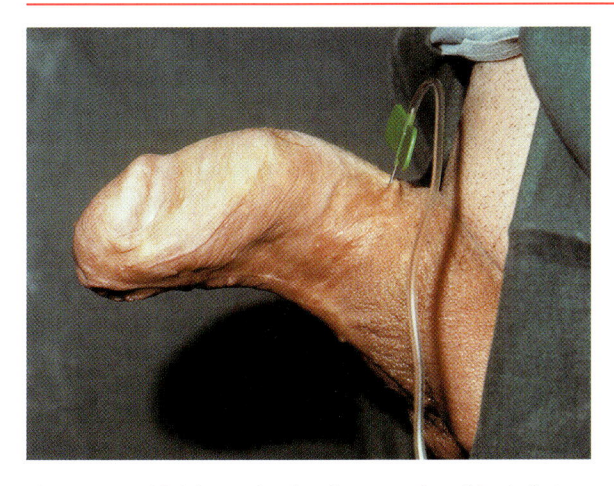

Fig. 32.6. Artificial erection has been produced by infusion. There is chordee more proximal than would have been expected from the relatively minor distal hypospadias

plan surgery. Sometimes a Polaroid photograph will be sufficient but I have found direct inspection of the erection to be invaluable. This can be achieved by injection of prostaglandin in the clinic. However, for an embarrassed patient with a difficult penile problem (often a hypospadias cripple), an erection under anaesthetic may be needed (Fig. 32.6). It is most important to induce the erection by infusion of the corpora under pressure without a tourniquet: the chordee is sometimes more proximal than the site of the original hypospadias and may be disguised by a tourniquet.

Several techniques are available for chordee correction. Nesbit's procedure has stood the test of time but does produce a little shortening of the penis. In the hypospadias cripple this may be a virtue as it makes the urethroplasty easier. When the chordee occurs in isolation, techniques to put a graft into the concave aspect of the corpora may be better. In Peyronie's disease, several tissues have been used (Gelbard et al. 1999). Experience in hypospadias is limited. Dermal grafts have been the most popular and have had promising results in children. It is recommended that the straightening is done first and urethroplasty left for a second-stage operation. Results up to 5 years are good but long-term results are lacking (Lindgren et al. 1998).

Sexual Function

Sexual Activity

Problems with sexual intercourse, both physical and emotional, have been reported. The "physical causes" include soft glans, poor ejaculation, tight skin and pain. "Emotional causes" are small size, poor appearance and the anxieties arising from the physical causes (Bracka 1989).

The difficulties in assessing these claims lie partly in the knowledge that similar problems are found in many adolescents (with or without genital anomalies) and partly in the fact that hypospadiac men appear to have intercourse in much the same way as everybody else. All reported series record that most men have sexual intercourse, even though the quality and quantity may be difficult to decipher from the data. Rates for successful intercourse range from 77% to 90% (Johanson and Avellan 1980; Bracka 1989; Kenawi 1976). Curiously, the frequency of sexual intercourse does not seem to be related to the success of the repair, though it is probably related to the degree of severity of the original hypospadias.

Nowhere in medicine is it more necessary to have control patients than in the assessment of adolescent sexual function. The greatest difficulty lies in the identification of a satisfactory control group to compare with the hypospadiac patient. Without controls it is impossible to know whether the myriad of sexual problems that have been identified are caused by the hypospadias. There is no group that mirrors all of the features of hypospadias, but infant circumcision, herniorrhaphy and appendicectomy have all been used.

Two studies have shown no difference in the number of sexual episodes or their perceived quality between hypospadiacs and controls (herniorrhaphy patients and circumcision patients respectively) (Mureau et al. 1995; Aho et al. 2000). This was despite the observation that the hypospadiacs had significantly more erection problems, such as curvature, shortness and pain, than the controls (Aho et al. 2000). There was no significant difference in the ages at which boys started masturbating, necking or having sexual intercourse. Hypospadiac men described themselves as more sexually inhibited than controls who had had a hernia repair (24% vs 1.8%) (Mureau et al. 1995).

The quality of sexual satisfaction may be different when the hypospadiac man has suffered complications, as there is a correlation between more complications, dissatisfaction with the surgical outcome and dissatisfaction with sexual performance (Aho et al. 1997). More complications are seen with the old Denis Browne operation, which is no longer used, and it may be reasonable to assume that the current surgical techniques with fewer complications may give a better sexual result.

When the components of male sexual function are analysed in more detail, differences from normal do appear. Chordee and other erectile deformities are more common than would be expected and, indeed, than in the control groups. In early series it seems that chordee was almost never corrected adequately in proximal hypospadias. Up to 60% of patients with penile hypospadias and all patients with scrotal and perineal hypospadias had chordee in Kenawi's series (Kenawi 1976).

Men with major complications in the surgical outcome often have physical difficulty with intercourse. Apart from chordee, tight scarred skin makes penetration painful and may even tear with intercourse. Matters may be worsened if BXO has developed.

In the patients with most severe hypospadias there is a considerable overlap with intersex abnormalities, especially androgen insensitivity syndromes. In one series of posterior hypospadias 13 of 42 men had a major intersex anomaly. All had severe hypospadias (usually perineo-scrotal) and micropenis (Eberle et al. 1993). None of the 13 patients had sperm in their ejaculate. Even with hypospadias as severe as this, intercourse still occurs. In a series of 19 patients born with ambiguous genitalia, subsequently determined to be caused by perineal hypospadias, it was reported that 63% had had intercourse. However, only four had a regular partner (Miller and Grant 1997). Less good figures were given in the series of Eberle et al.: although 25 of 42 reported satisfactory erections, masturbation and ejaculation, few had sexual intercourse. Nine of 42 were married and three had children, but only six had a stable relationship (Eberle et al. 1993).

Ejaculation

Ejaculation is a complex function. It begins with the formation of a bolus of semen in the prostatic urethra. The bolus is then expelled forcefully by the contraction of the prostatic urethral muscles against a closed bladder neck. Thus far, the hypospadiac male should be normal unless there is a major prostatic anomaly associated with intersexuality.

The next stage is the expulsion of the semen by the bulbospongiosus muscle. In very proximal hypospadias, this muscle is likely to be absent. It is, therefore, not surprising to find that ejaculation is unsatisfactory in 63% of severe hypospadiacs even though orgasm is normal in most (Miller and Grant 1997). Poor surgical results from the distal urethroplasty may cause a baggy urethra or even a diverticulum, further slowing the ejaculation. In more general reviews most authors state that ejaculation is normal though, by asking the right questions, Bracka (1989) found that 33% had "dribbling ejaculation" and 4% were dry.

Psychological Aspects of Intercourse

Emotional satisfaction with intercourse is particularly difficult to measure, and series without controls are valueless. Most teenagers, exploring their sexuality, have anxieties that are unrelated to any penile abnormality though a penis that is perceived to be abnormal may get the blame.

In terms of episodes of sexual activity, number of partners, sexual problems and libido there is no significant difference between hypospadiacs and controls (herniorrhaphy or circumcision patients) (Mureau et al. 1996; Aho et al. 2000). Similarly, there is little difference in the age of sexual debut compared with either controls or established community norms.

Penis size may be a cause of dissatisfaction. The hypospadiac penis is often said to be short. In part this may be because of the circumcised appearance, especially in countries where infant circumcision is unusual. However, where a formal measurement has been made, 20% of hypospadiac penises have been below the 10th centile. The finding is most marked in adolescents with four of seven being below the 10th centile (Fig. 32.7) (Mureau et al. 1996).

Penile size is a source of considerable anxiety in many adolescents. Limited research is available on the relationship of penile size to sexual satisfaction. My own work has shown that patients with micropenis and with epispadias have intercourse that is satisfactory to themselves, though the opinions of their partners have not been investigated (Woodhouse 1998). An investigation of women with multiple sexual partners has suggested that intercourse with an uncircumcised penis gives greater pleasure than a circumcised one (O'Hara and O'Hara 1999).

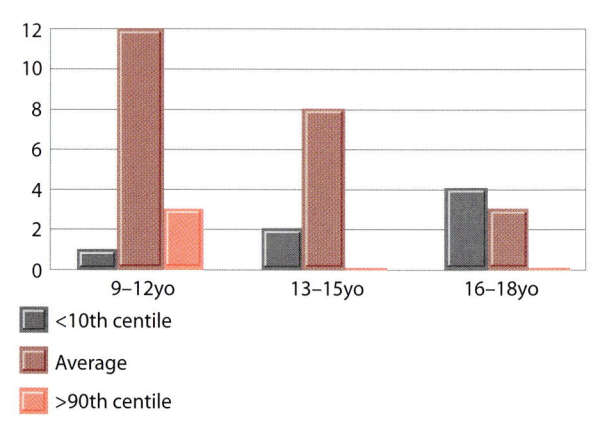

Fig. 32.7. Histogram to show the number of patients with stretched penile length by age compared to normal centiles. (Mureau et al. 1996)

As there is no realistic means of enlarging the penis in hypospadias, it seems wise to help the patient to make the best use of that which he has, rather than embark on futile surgery. If the comparative trials of Mureau et al. and Aho et al. are correct, hypospadiac boys are not greatly different from their peers in their sexual activity and enjoyment.

There is conflict over the effect of the success of the repair. Bracka (1989) made the interesting observation that those who were satisfied with the results of their repair had a sexual debut at a mean age of 15.6 years, while those who were dissatisfied had a debut at 19 years. On the other hand, it has been reported that in a group of boys whose "curative repair" was delayed beyond 12 years old, 50% had their sexual debut before the definitive surgery (Avellan 1976). It could be said that the experience of intercourse, acknowledged by the authors to be less satisfactory, drew attention to the shortcomings of the repair.

Endocrine Function in Hypospadias

In uncomplicated cases of hypospadias it seems likely that the sex hormones are normal. In Bracka's series, luteinising hormone (LH), follicular stimulating hormone (FSH) and testosterone were measured only in the first 100 patients because they were all normal in all cases (Bracka 1989).

There do seem to be some exceptions to this observation. In a series of 16 adults with mild hypospadias, the mean levels of LH and FSH were higher than in normals though not outside the normal range. Testosterone levels were normal. The means were distorted by five patients who had grossly abnormal values, but three of them were fertile (Gearhart et al. 1990). Low levels of 5-alpha reductase have been reported (Berg and Berg 1983b).

Fertility

It seems probable that boys with uncomplicated hypospadias are normally fertile. There have been no studies of a large cohort of hypospadiac patients. There is no excess of hypospadiacs in infertility clinics. In an apparently unselected group of 169 hypospadiac men, 50% were found to have a sperm count below 50 million/ml and 25% below 20 million/ml. More than half of those with the lowest sperm counts had associated anomalies such as undescended testes which might have accounted for the poor result (Bracka 1989). In a detailed study of 16 hypospadiacs, true oligo-astheno-teratozoospermia (OATS) was only found in the two patients with perineal hypospadias; low counts were seen in one of three with glanular and in two of six with penile hypospadias, but other parameters were normal. With two minor exceptions of slightly elevated LH, all the patients had normal hormone profiles (Zubowska et al. 1979).

Perineal hypospadias is frequently associated with other genital anomalies and intersex, and it is not surprising that a high incidence of azoospermia and abnormalities of the hypothalamic-gonadal axis is found (Eberle et al. 1993).

The inheritance of hypospadias is incompletely defined. It has been thought of as an autosomal recessive condition, but even this has been questioned by Harris and Beaty (1993), who suggest an autosomal dominant or codominant model. Whatever the mode of inheritance, the risk of hypospadias occurring in a brother or first-degree relative is 17–21% (Bauer et al. 1981; Stool et al. 1990).

There is some evidence that the incidence of hypospadias is increasing. Data can be confusing. There may be variations in reporting, as shown by the number of adult men found to have previously unrecognised hypospadias when presenting for prostatectomy (Fichtner et al. 1995). Rates appear to increase in some countries in some periods but not in others; for example, there appears to have been an increase in Norway and Denmark in the 1980s but not in Finland. The USA has reported a steady increase throughout the past 30 years, especially when the mother is over 35 years old (Toppari et al. 2001; Fisch et al. 2001).

The widespread use of assisted conception for infertility, especially intracytoplasmic sperm injection (ICSI), has been predicted, somewhat unscientifically, to be responsible for an increased risk of congenital anomalies. Such fears have been unfounded. In general the anomalies seen have been consistent with the maternal age and the number of multiple pregnancies. However, two studies have shown that there is a threefold increase in the risk of hypospadias for infants conceived by ICSI (Wennerholm et al. 2000; Aberg et al. 2001).

Psychological Consequences

There is much debate about the psychological consequences of hypospadias and, again, there is a great need for control patients in the analyses. The problem is the selection of the controls. In the studies quoted above, the control patients had had circumcision (Mureau et al. 1995) or a hernia repair (Aho et al. 2000). In the very extensive psychological reviews undertaken by Berg and Berg, the control patients had

had appendicectomies. Faults can obviously be found with all of these controls, none having undergone surgery on the same scale as hypospadiacs. On the other hand, there is no other condition that could be compared to hypospadias in terms of diagnosis and surgical trauma.

From the uncontrolled series, it seems that about 20% of adults remembered their surgery as traumatic. A third of men avoided changing their clothes in public (Summerlad 1975; Bracka 1989).

In the controlled studies, the main outcomes have been in sexual development, discussed above. There is no difference (from circumcision patients) in success in the military in Finland, where there is conscription, or in the number of men living with a partner (Aho et al. 2000). Similarly, there were no differences in IQ, general health or socio-economic background in the Swedish men reviewed by Berg and Berg. In the Dutch study, there was no evidence that hypospadiac men had less good psychosocial adjustment than the age-matched controls (Mureau et al. 1995).

In one study, however, hypospadiacs were found to be underachievers. Berg and Berg found that they had lower ego strength and poor utilisation of their mental resources. Their levels of hostility, general anxiety and castration anxiety were higher and they had lower self esteem than the control appendicectomy patients. In childhood the boys had been shy, timid, isolated and mobbed. As adults they showed neurotic (but not psychotic) disturbances and formed abnormal social and emotional relationships. They had less rewarding and less demanding jobs. Eventually, like the men in other studies, they did establish secure and long-lasting sexual partnerships. The outcome was not related to the original severity of the hypospadias (Berg and Berg 1983a,b; Berg et al. 1982, 1983).

These studies are open to some criticism, and the picture they paint is somewhat out of line with ordinary clinical observation. It appears that the authors anticipated psychological morbidity and set out to prove it. The majority of patients appear to have had a poor surgical result. Nonetheless, they are careful and detailed studies that cannot be dismissed out of hand. There is some corroborating evidence from similar (but less detailed) studies on severe hypospadiacs, though many of the patients had ambiguous genitalia or even Reifenstein's syndrome (Eberle et al. 1993; Miller and Grant 1997).

Hypospadias in Adults

An adult practice in hypospadias is likely to be small. In spite of the many shortcomings of the surgery in children already discussed, the vast majority of patients do achieve a satisfactory outcome in early childhood. In adult life there will be a few with late or incompletely corrected complications and some who, for a variety of reasons, have never undergone surgery.

Late Complications

The possible complications, occurring in isolation, have been considered above. Even when a patient has had a less than perfect result, he may not have sufficient trouble to want further surgery, although he may develop troublesome symptoms up to 50 years later (Flynn et al. 1980).

Patients with the most serious problems are often described as hypospadiac cripples (Fig. 32.8). Symptoms are, in varying degree, of chordee, fistula, stricture and sexual dysfunction. For the older repairs, there may be the added complications of a hair-bearing neourethra. From the surgical point of view, the urethra is usually too short, strictured and made of poor material. There is inadequate residual skin to make a comprehensive reconstruction. No specific type of initial repair is associated with this disaster. Characteristically, several operations will have been

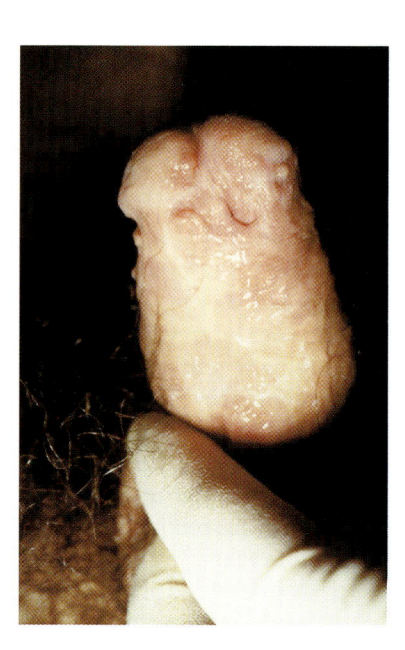

Fig. 32.8. Hypospadias cripple. The meatus is eccentric and coronal. The skin is tight and heavily scarred

performed in childhood, each seeming to change one problem for another.

Even in patients with an apparently reasonable repair, the use of hairy skin for the urethroplasty will always produce long-term complications. It is virtually impossible to depilate skin, if only because up to two thirds of follicles may not be growing a hair at the time of surgery and are thus invisible. A hairy urethra causes dysuria, infection, hair balls and stones. Although stones and hair can generally be removed endoscopically, the problem will always recur. If a man has a reasonable urethra, hair can be removed by self-instillation of the proprietary depilating agent Immac. This chemical is sterile and will dissolve urethral hair in 75% of cases within 10 min. The instillation must be made with a full bladder so that it can be washed out by voiding. Patients will have dysuria for 24 h after treatment (Bagshawe et al. 1980).

The principles for reconstruction in a hypospadias cripple were defined more than 20 years ago, and most surgeons will use at least two stages. The penis should be carefully examined at the beginning of the operation with an artificial erection. The remains of the neourethra and any poor-quality skin should be removed, the chordee corrected and the glans split to allow the later formation of a terminal slit-like urethra (Flynn et al. 1980; Stecker et al. 1981).

The destructive part of this first operation is relatively easy; the main mistake is to be too conservative. The reconstructive phase is much more difficult. By definition, there is a shortage of skin and some new skin must be brought in.

The use of a pedicled tube of scrotal skin was recommended by Flynn. The advantage is its ready availability so that a single-stage reconstruction is possible. The main drawback is the problem of hair, already discussed. The mid-line of the scrotum is relatively (but not completely) hairless. In his own series all of six hypospadiac cripples had a satisfactory result at 2- to 4-year follow-up. One had a minor hair problem resolved with Immac (Flynn et al. 1980). In spite of these good results, few surgeons still use scrotal skin.

For a two-stage urethroplasty, the techniques available for stricture disease are all appropriate. It is obviously important to move in enough skin to allow for the formation of the neourethra and to make up any deficit in that available for penile closure. Meshed split skin is popular in Europe. A graft of 0.1 mm thickness is cut with a compressed air-driven dermatome and then meshed. It is applied to the ventral aspect of the corpora to cover the defect from the excised urethra. The meshing allows free drainage of serum and is said to aid healing. The second stage is performed at least 8 weeks later. All of nine hypospadiac cripples were reported to have had a good result at 2–8 years of follow-up with this technique (Schreiter and Noll 1987). Unmeshed split skin may also be used but with less good results, only 6 of 11 patients having a good outcome (Burbige et al. 1984).

Full-thickness skin has been used for many years, but was probably popularised for hypospadias repair by Devine and Horton (1977). An adequate supply of non-hairy skin is usually available behind the ear. More recently, buccal mucosa, already popular for difficult hypospadias repairs in children, has been used for the two-stage reconstruction of the penis in hypospadiac cripples.

In general, the results of these types of urethroplasty are given without subdivision by aetiology, combining hypospadias cripples with stricture disease in general. As the results are reasonably good and patients with severe strictures have much the same tissue deficiencies (especially of spongiosum) as hypospadiacs, such combined reports are probably valid. In a series of 26 patients, 10 had hypospadias; 18 had postauricular Woolf grafts and 8 had buccal mucosa grafts. Eight required a revision of the first stage. Three years after the final surgery the re-stricture rate was 13% (Greenwell et al. 1999). In a later paper from the same group on 38 patients, none of whom had hypospadias, the surgical complication rate was 21% (8 patients) after the second stage (Joseph et al. 2002).

These results are the best available for hypospadias cripples. It is disappointing that so small an area of skin and so short a length of epithelialised tubing can cause so much trouble. My own experience has been less satisfactory and more in line with that reported from New York. In a group of 22 adult hypospadiac cripples having a wide variety of operations, there was a surgical complication rate of 64%. After "secondary surgery" 18 of the original 22 patients achieved a satisfactory outcome (Hensle et al. 2001). The patients generally end up with a good result, but I agree with the authors that men should be specifically warned of the high complication rate. In my experience some patients will decline reconstruction.

New Adult Patients

From time to time a man will present with hypospadias who has had no previous surgery. Most often BXO will have caused a stricture. Occasionally, a man will present with an unconnected symptom and the hypospadias will be a chance finding (Fig. 32.9). Even an uncomplicated hypospadiac meatus may not be large enough to accept a conventional cystoscope or resectoscope. The distal urethra is often fragile

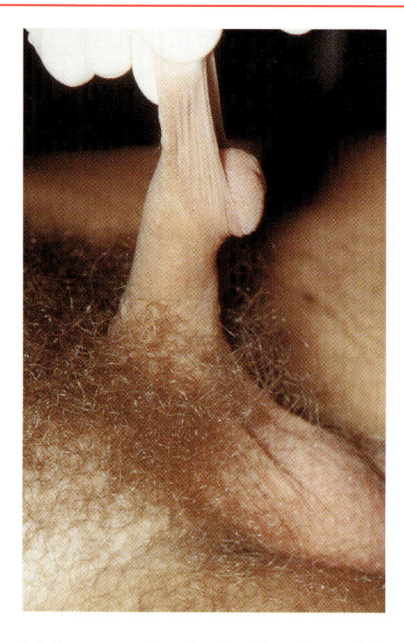

Fig. 32.9. Adult presenting for the first time with untreated hypospadias. The chordee was his main complaint

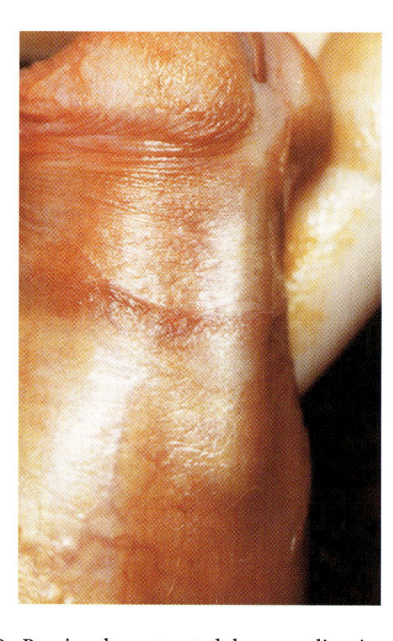

Fig. 32.10. Previously untreated hypospadias in an adult. There is a sound in the meatus which is just on the glans. Note the sound is bulging through the distal urethra which is made of very thin tissue with no surrounding corpus spongiosum

with no supporting corpus spongiosum and may easily be damaged by instrumentation (Fig. 32.10).

Before deciding on treatment, it is essential to establish what the patient hopes to achieve from surgery. With limited objectives, such as enlargement of the meatus, simple, local surgery will suffice.

For complete reconstruction, the same techniques may be used as in children. Unfortunately, the complication rate of around 33% is much higher than that seen in younger patients (Hensle et al. 2001). Wound healing seems to be slower, and the infection higher, than in children. Again, careful discussion with the patient about objectives and possible outcomes is essential.

References

Aberg A, Westbom L, Kallen B: Congenital malformations among infants whose mothers had gestational diabetes or pre-existing diabetes. Early Hum Dev. 2001; 61:85–95.

Aho MO, Tammela OKT, Tammela TLJ: Aspects of adult satisfaction with the result of surgery for hypospadias performed in childhood. Eur J Urol. 1997; 32:218–22.

Aho MO, Tammela OKT, Somppi EMJ, et al: A long term comparative follow up study of voiding, sexuality and satisfaction among men operated for hypospadias and phimosis during childhood. Eur J Urol. 2000;37:95–101.

Avellan L: Development of puberty, sexual debut and sexual function in hypospadiacs. Scand J Plast Reconstr Surg. 1976;10:29–34.

Bagshawe HA, Flynn JT, James AN, et al: The use of thioglycolic acid in hair bearing skin inlay urethroplasty. Br J Urol. 1980; 52:546–548.

Bauer SB, Retik AB, Colodny AH: Genetic aspects of hypospadias. Urol Clin North Am. 1981; 8:559–564.

Berg G, Berg R: Castration complex: evidence from men operated for hypospadias. Acta Psychiatr Scand. 1983a; 68: 143–153.

Berg R, Berg G: Penile malformations, gender identity and sexual orientation. Acta Psychiatr Scand. 1983b; 68:154–166.

Berg R, Berg G, Svensson J: Penile malformation and mental health: a controlled psychiatric study of men operated for hypospadias in childhood. Acta Psychiatr Scand. 1982; 66:398–416.

Berg G, Berg R, Edman G, et al: Androgens and personality in normal men and men operated for hypospadias in childhood. Acta Psychiatr Scand. 1983; 68:167–177.

Bracka AA: A long term view of hypospadias. Br J Plast Surg. 1989; 42:251–255.

Burbige KA, Hensle TW, Edgerton P: Extra genital split skin graft for urethral reconstruction. J Urol. 1984; 131:1137–1139.

Caione P, Capozza N, Lais A, et al: Long term results of distal urethral advancement glanuloplasty for distal hypospadias. J Urol. 1997; 158:1168–1171.

Devine CJ, Horton CE: Hypospadias repair. J Urol. 1977; 118:188–193.

Duel BP, Bartold JS, Gonzalez R: Management of urethral strictures after hypospadias repair. J Urol. 1998; 160: 170–171.

Eberle J, Uberreiter S, Radmyr C, et al: Posterior hypospadias: long term follow-up after reconstructive surgery in the male direction. J Urol. 1993; 150:1474–1477.

Fichtner J, Filipas D, Mottrie AM, et al: Analysis of meatal location in 500 men: wide variation questions the need for meatal advancement in all pediatric anterior hypospadias cases. J Urol. 1995; 154:833–834.

Fisch H, Golden RJ, Libersen GL, et al: Maternal age as a risk factor for hypospadias. J Urol. 2001; 165:934–936.

Flynn JT, Johnston SR, Blandy JP: The late sequelae of hypospadias repair. Br J Urol. 1980; 52:555–559.

Garibay JT, Reid C, Gonzalez R: Functional evaluation of the results of hypospadias surgery with uroflowmetry. J Urol. 1995; 154:835–836.

Gearhart JP, Donohue PA, Brown TR, et al: Endocrine evaluation of adults with mild hypospadias. J Urol. 1990; 144:274–277.

Gelbard MK: Correction of penile curvature using tunica albuginea plication, flaps and expansion with fascial grafts. In: Ehrlich RM, Alter GJ (eds) Reconstructive and plastic surgery of the external genitalia, 1st edn. Saunders, Philadelphia, 1999, pp 479–488.

Greenwell TJ, Venn SN, Mundy AR: Changing practice in anterior urethroplasty. BJU Int. 1999; 83:631–635.

Harris EL, Beaty TH: Segregation analysis of hypospadias: a re-analysis of published pedigree data. Am J Med Genet. 1993; 45:420–425.

Hensle TW, Tennenbaum SY, Reiley EA, et al: Hypospadias repair in adults: adventures and misadventures. J Urol. 2001; 165:77–79.

Holland AJA, Smith GHH, Ross FI, et al: HOSE: an objective scoring system for evaluating the results of hypospadias surgery. BJU Int. 2001; 88:255–258.

Johanson B, Avellan L: Hypospadias: a review of 299 cases operated 1957–1969. Scand J Plast Reconstr Surg. 1980; 14:259–267.

Joseph JV, Andrich DE, Leach CJ, et al: Urethroplasty for refractory anterior urethral stricture. J Urol. 2002; 167:127–129.

Kass EJ, Chung AK: Glanuloplasty and in situ tubularisation of the urethral plate: long term follow-up. J Urol. 2000; 164:991–993.

Kenawi MM: Sexual function in hypospadiacs. Br J Urol. 1976; 47:883–890.

Kumar MV, Harris DL: Balanitis xerotica obliterans complicating hypospadias repair. Br J Plast Surg. 1999; 52:69–71.

Lindgren BW, Reda E, Levitt S, et al: Single and multiple dermal grafts for the management of severe penile curvature. J Urol. 1998; 160:1128–1130.

Malyon AD, Boorman JG, Bowley N: Urinary flow rates in hypospadias. Br J Plast Surg. 1997; 50:530–535.

Miller MAW, Grant DB: Severe hypospadias with genital ambiguity: adult outcome after staged hypospadias repair. Br J Urol. 1997; 80:485–488.

Mor Y, Ramon J, Jonas P: Is only meatoplasty a legitimate surgical solution for extreme distal hypospadias? A long term follow up. BJU Int. 2000; 85:501–503.

Mureau MAM, Slijper FME, Nijman RJM, et al: Psychosexual adjustment of children and adolescents after different types of hypospadias repair: a norm related study. J Urol. 1995; 154:1902–1907.

Mureau MAM, Slijper FME, Slob AK, et al: Satisfaction with penile appearance after hypospadias surgery: the patient and surgeon view. J Urol. 1996; 155:703–706.

O'Hara K, O'Hara J: The effect of male circumcision on the sexual enjoyment of the female partner. BJU Int. 1999; 83 [Suppl 1]:79–84.

Schonfeld WA: Primary and secondary sexual characteristics. Am J Dis Child. 1943; 65:535–549.

Schreiter F, Noll F: Mesh graft urethroplasty. World J Urol. 1987; 5:41–46.

Shanberg AM, Sanderson K, Duel BP: Re-operative hypospadias repair using the Snodgrass incised urethral plate. BJU Int. 2001; 87:544–547.

Stecker JF, Horton CE, Devine CJ, et al: Hypospadias cripples. Urol Clin North Am. 1981; 8:539–544.

Stoll C, Alembik Y, Roth MP, et al: Genetic and environmental factors in hypospadias. J Med Genet. 1990; 27:559–563.

Summerlad BC: A long term follow up of hypospadias patients. Br J Plast Surg. 1975; 28:324–330.

Toppari J, Kaleva M, Virtanen HE: Trends in the incidence of cryptorchidism and hypospadias, and methodological limitations of registry based data. Hum Reprod Update. 2001; 7:282–286.

Van der Werff JF, Boeve E, Brusse CA, et al: Urodynamic evaluation of hypospadias repair. J Urol. 1997; 157:1344–1346.

Vandersteen DR, Husmann DA: Late onset recurrent penile chordee after successful correction at hypospadias repair. J Urol. 1998; 160:1131–1133.

Venn SN, Mundy AR: Urethroplasty for balanitis xerotica obliterans. Br J Urol. 1998;81:735–737.

Wennerholm U, Bergh C, Hamberger L, et al: Incidence of congenital malformations in children born after ICSI. Hum Reprod. 2000; 15:944–948.

Woodhouse CRJ: Sexual function in boys born with exstrophy, myelomeningocoele and micropenis. Urology. 1998; 52:3–11.

Zubowska J, Jankowska J, Kula K, et al: Clinical, hormonal and semiological data in adult men operated in childhood for hypospadias. Endokrynol Polska. 1979; 30:565–573.

Psychological Problems and Adjustment

Christina Del Priore, Kathleen McHugh, Sita Picton, Elizabeth Haldane

Introduction

Evidence-based research into psychological adaptation in physical disorder, in cosmetic challenge and in medical and surgical interventions in childhood is increasingly available and indicates the importance of sound early adjustment in the child and of continued psychological support across the changing phases of childhood if good psychological outcome is to result and if secondary psychological disorder is to be avoided. Good psychological adjustment includes self-esteem; capacity for emotional and behavioural regulation, for positive relationships and for skill development; peer integration; developmental progress; and eventual realisation of social and educational potential in adulthood. Secondary psychological disorder not only impacts on the psychosocial dimension but can create challenge to medical and surgical management including dialogue with parents, decision taking, adherence to treatment, functional rehabilitation and quality of life.

Despite increased risk of secondary disorder, psychological services for children with physical disorder are only sporadically available across the UK and are often used to cover many different medical disorders. Therefore, the clinical service availability for any specific condition may be limited unless there happens to have been local initiative. It has become increasingly clear to those working in the field that key indications for best practice for the very specific challenges of particular disorders such as hypospadias must be developed and that this can only be done by forging new expertise to supplement the widely established general skills in developmental psychology and pathology in childhood. The aims of service should include facilitation of coping, reduction of distress, reduced dependency including reduced postoperative stay, lowered levels of anxiety and pain, reduction of risk factor behaviour as well as specific interventions for pain and anxiety etc., and promotion of psychological and family well-being and the child's developmental progress and quality of life.

The biomedical correlates of psychological disorder secondary to physical disorder include severity of disorder and related functional effects, i.e. disruption of normal opportunity, course, visibility and stigma, need for intrusive and painful care and duration of events. Child correlates include gender and age at any event, temperament of child, child coping mechanisms and neurocognitive processes, access to experience and knowledge about development and disorder. Social ecological correlates include social economic status, family functioning, marital and parental adjustment, parenting practices and cognitive processes.

Specific Findings

Psychological Adjustment to Hypospadias

On the whole, morbidity in psychological outcome in hypospadias is found to be subtle rather than marked. Aho et al. (2000) conclude that even patients with a less than perfect technical result are able to live a satisfactory sexual life and succeed in life in general. Cracco et al. (1989) found their subjects to have a degree of psychological difficulty before and during surgery but to be without major pathology in school profession and sexuality spheres, relating this to high-quality surgery, brief convalescence and, importantly, the presence of preacquired positive attitudes. Sandberg et al. (1989) found that a history of hypospadias did not appear to have a lasting negative impact on the family but that surgery-related hospitalisations were correlated with poorer school performance. In another study, Sandberg et al. (2001) found that although few significant differences emerged between cases and controls, boys with hypospadias showed slightly lower social involvement in school and fewer externalising behavioural problems than controls; worse school performance was associated with poor cosmetic appearance of genitals, and greater surgical and hospital experiences were associated with increased internalising problems. Schultz et al. (1983), studying the timing of elective hypospadias repair, found that adults who had undergone repair as children had sexual difficulty despite erectile competence and generally occupied less independent professions than intelligence-matched cohorts. Schultz emphasised the importance of the role of the family in psychological outcome. Berg and colleagues found men operated on for hypospadias in childhood to be less secure in their maleness (Berg and Berg 1983a) and reported greater shyness, more anxiety and less stress tolerance (Berg et al. 1982). They also emphasised the need for psychological guidance for boys and their parents. Svensson et al. (1981) reported sexual debut of hypospadiacs to be delayed, but not first ejaculation. He found hypospadiacs to have a satisfactory sexual life but be restricted to fewer partners. He found early-operated hypospadiacs to have more infantile sexual identity and to have had more enuresis and shyness during childhood.

Childhood and Hypospadias

The psychological development of the child with hypospadias is affected by those common variables which affect all children, those pertaining to children with physical disorder and the requirement for medical and surgical intervention and those very specific to children with genital anomaly.

General principles for good psychological management of any child with a disorder involve minimum disruption of family, school and social life, maximum opportunity for calm informed empowerment through access to information, training and practical and emotional support. Clinicians need to be alert to risk factors and to comorbidities in either child or parent, including social disadvantage, parental psychopathology, parenting capabilities and coping styles, and extreme adverse attitudinal and belief systems in a parent or parents, in the nuclear family or in the cultural group. Cognitive or other disability in the child, extreme temperamental characteristics or sensitising past history in child or parent, and presence or absence of support within the parental partnership and the wider family should also be taken into account.

Chronic childhood illness is a well-recognised stressor for children and their families. Findings for specific disorders vary but the risk for adjustment disorder is estimated to be 1.5–3 times as high as for healthy peers (Thomson and Gustafson 1999). Chronic childhood conditions increase the risk of parental adjustment disorder. The emotional impact and the practical burden fall mainly on the mother. There is a significant increase in levels of distress compared with mothers of well children. The risk of adjustment difficulty is related to disorder severity but more strongly to illness length and degree of functional impairment.

It is important to be alert to the specific risks and protective factors for male children. There is a known greater incidence of psychological disorder in boys generally. There are specific interactive effects of social vulnerability and male status and a direct and indirect adverse effect on children from marital and partnership conflict. The number of single parents and changing male partnerships and the absence of the natural father in households is a source of concern. Children are known to be adversely affected by ambivalent relationships, by parental anxiety, by exposure to harsh and inconsistent discipline, by separation during attachment, by disruption of peer attachment and schooling, by exposure to fear and trauma and by poor communication, particularly in relation to the expression of feeling states and the development of reassuring and explanatory concepts.

There is evidence that the children who are at greatest risk of developing secondary psychological disorder are those with pre-existing disadvantage and vulnerability and poorly functioning families. Protective factors have to do with intelligence and with consistent calm and affectionate parenting. The presence of an accepting, affectionate and effective father is particularly important to boys.

Selfhood and Genital and Gender Awareness

The psychological concept of "self" has been demonstrated by Kagen (1981) to have taken considerable shape in the infant by 24–30 months, by which time the child demonstrates awareness of itself as an entity by using the terms "mine", "me do it" etc. Associated with this emerging sense of self is social shyness, a realisation of the impact of self on others, an awareness of social approbation, the child usually wishing to achieve approval and a sense of "intactness" as opposed to "the broken", a sense of "the good me" as opposed to "the bad me". At this time of life there is a clear development of the capacity for feelings of guilt. The establishment of trust in the goodness of self and others is vital to psychological health and is formed by calm, loving parenting in which the child's needs for comfort in physical or emotional distress are met. Children are sensitive to the feeling states of carers, and anxiety and mood states are known to be contagious. The sense of self-worth, of acceptance and belonging, starts to become established early in life and is formed through the child's experiences of parents' feelings, attitudes and behaviours toward the child.

The deep early sense of worth or non-worth, of intactness or lack of it, tends to persist in primitive form into adulthood. Alongside early awareness of self comes primitive but rapidly entrenching awareness of gender identity and vague awareness of how genitals are associated with this. Gender is an early, pervasive and powerful identity for the child. Genital awareness is much less important at this stage. The gender of the child is a primary identity factor for parents and for people generally. Awareness by the child of his gender is affected by parental attitudes to gender and to genitals. Some parents feel and convey a sense of shame in relation to the genital area. Other parents convey a sense of pride and confirmation of their own self-esteem in relation to well-formed genitals of a male child. The origin of this pride is attributable in part to the symbolic nature of the phallus and maleness. In such households the genital anomaly may be particularly distressing, genital malformation being a source of increased shame.

Awareness of genitals emerges for the child as part of the toilet training experience, which is not infrequently associated with a somewhat tense dialogue between parent and child, in which a connection between guilt and shame and genital area and function can be established. Parents who carry a prominent sense of shame in relation to genital areas of the body and those who have psychological difficulty with mess or dirt may have prominent difficulties in acceptance of toilet training problems.

Initially children are only vaguely curious about genital features and differences. Neutral curiosity moves across childhood with positive or negative values depending on experience and parental attitude. Initial awareness of genital difference should be slight in the child, but parental attitudes can have a prominent effect on the child's sense of self.

Modesty at exposure of the genital area, which emerges at the mid preschool period is not thought to be a wholly culturally based attitudinal development. Psychoanalytical thinkers describe anxiety in relation to the genitals and consequent castration fears during the oedipal phase, centring around the 5th or 6th year of life. Berg and Berg (1983b) interpreted their findings of higher anxiety and hostility levels, reduced self-esteem and reduced capacity for interpersonal relationships in hypospadiacs as evidence of castration anxiety and emphasised the importance of psychotherapeutic support. Anxiety is described in all children in relation to a sense of inferiority to adult, particularly male, sexual organs during this phase which is accompanied by a growing sense of the power of gender and of the sexual dynamic. The child before pubescence is unlikely, generally speaking, to be particularly interested in the exact appearance of the genital area. Having passed the toilet training stage with its interest in the genitals and the role in elimination, and not having until much later any real awareness or interest in the actual sexual function of the genitals, the child's surprised interest re genitals is part of his greater interest in where babies come from. The child at this stage is unlikely to be the subject of unfavourable comparisons by peers on those rare occasions on which exposure of genitals occurs, although mild curiosity might be present in children. However, despite these poorly defined concepts the child does develop an early and clear gender identity, and this identity is central to sense of self.

Genital body perception of hypospadias patients aged 9–18 years correlated positively with psychosocial functioning, albeit at low levels, in a study by Mureau et al. (1997). The same team (Mureau et al. 1995) found more negative genital appraisal in men operated on for hypospadias. They found severity of hypospadias negatively affected genital appraisal and that patient age at final operation correlated positively with sociosexual development.

Gender and Society

In society as a whole gender, and hence the genitalia as gender identifiers, is not only of biological importance but has very considerable social, cultural, political and religious importance. All societies have, or have had, significant gender-related legislative and other frameworks. The power axis in lineage, in resource distribution, in status and in the role played in religion has been bound up with gender. Many societies hold reproductive matters as absolutely central and have legal measures for enforcement. Until very recently, legislation and custom regulated access to some events and some activities in terms of gender. Male gender is associated with power, dominance and property rights and the confirmation of status (Low Bobbi 2000).

Gender and Behaviour

Although humans are less restricted by their environment than was previously the case, and notwithstanding the widely held belief that psychological variance is greater within than between males and females, there is clear evidence for psychological differences that accompany the biological differences between the sexes (Blurton-Jones and Konner 1973). Behavioural characteristics differ and are linked to behavioural specialisations in mating, reproducing, territory acquisition and survival, and are known to include differences in physical movement patterns, dominance behaviour and aggression (Freedman 1980). Evidence exists in some species that submissive males have higher stress hormone levels (Clark and Grunstein 2000). In certain situations being less certain of one's right to status or showing behaviour less typical for males can be associated with what biologists call "scramble competition" by other males. Darwinian theories suggest that the male's display of capacity to take risks is presumably used to impress females with the male's gene potential in mate selection (Low Bobbi 2000).

Gender and Parenting

The gender of a child produces differential parental investment patterns, and parents raise sons and daughters differently. There is a complex interaction between genotype and environment, with sensitivity to various forms of environmental experience differing according to genotype of the individual. Phenotype would therefore be a product of environmental influence in which sensitivity to effect is regulated by genotype. This thinking influences current psychological research on shared and non-shared environment in sibs. It is known that parents' behaviour is influenced by a belief in a child's gender. Male children in some cultures are considered of more value than female children.

Parental Perceptions of Maleness

Parental perception of maleness is particularly important in some families and for some individuals. Perhaps men have their own maleness confirmed by the maleness of their sons. A father uncertain about his own maleness may be particularly troubled by a genital anomaly in his son. Similarly, a male child with an absent father, or particularly with a father who is perceived to be unacceptable, might worry about his own maleness and its significance.

The Phallus

The penis or phallus, particularly the erect phallus, has had significance across time as a symbol of power, including resource allocation, fertility and lineage rights. It has been venerated in primitive religions. The modern parent, although possibly not directly aware of the symbolic property of the penis, may be more affected by behavioural anthropological forces than he or she would like to think. The current media exploitation of sexuality and hence sexual organs for commercial gain emphasises the connection between organ superiority and success of every kind and hence creates, for many, a sense of inferiority and dissatisfaction with self. Older children and adolescents are highly susceptible to media pressures.

The psychological experience of organ inferiority and of body dysmorphism by the individual with a normal body is a known powerful source of unhappiness and it is interesting to reflect that the well-managed child with an abnormal body can experience less discontent than the individual with a normal body but an abnormal sense of self-worth.

It is important to seek out covert as well as overt parental and child anxieties, to acknowledge disappointments and to encourage a sense of calm and self-worth. Covert parental attitudes and feeling states have a powerful effect on the child even if not acknowledged or, indeed, actively denied.

The child's anxieties and perceptions differ at different stages, and the child needs the opportunity to disentangle the fears and misperceptions of the stage and to receive developmentally appropriate information and advice. The attempt to assay the child's views at each stage and to take these into account in the psychological management of the child is crucial to success.

Decision Taking, the Rights of the Child, Law on Capacity for Consent

Analysing how the parent or child appraises the situation and offering help in coming to a realistic appraisal is important. Current debate on adult satisfaction with past genital surgery and current sexual function, resulting from decisions taken in childhood, together with discussion on the best timing of surgical intervention, directs the surgeon's attention to the Age of Legal Capacity Act (Scotland) 1991, which states that children under age 16 years can give their own consent in Scotland if the medical practitioner considers the child capable of understanding the nature and possible consequences of a procedure or treatment. The UN Convention on the Rights of the Child similarly directs our attention to the requirements placed on signatory nations to ensure that the child is informed and advised and that the views of the child are sought whilst acting in the child's best interests as the overriding principle. It is technically difficult to inform and advise a child and seek his informed view, but the practice of doing so will support skill increase in this area. Skills for using developmentally appropriate discussion with children about sexual and reproductive function need to be explored. Books are available for children on these topics. These could be used as a basis for discussion. Children in middle childhood have more interest in reproduction than in sex. Adolescents require more specific material. Books which incorporate emphasis on the wider psychological context of relationships and values are important.

Empowerment and Partnership

Informed and empowered partnership between parents, child and medical team is important. Parental feeling states, attitudes and parenting practice have a profound impact on the child and operate to entrench negative impact or consolidate positive impact across childhood into adolescence and young adulthood. The general psychological foundations for each succeeding phase are laid during the preceding phases. A parent who is a calm partner, who seeks information, takes advice, makes thoughtful, informed decisions, develops practical skills, carries out instructions and adapts positively to what cannot be adjusted is the ideal role model for the child. The opportunity for all members of the partnership to express disappointment, anxious concern and sadness is part of the helping process.

Coping Styles

Stress inevitably occurs in association with diagnosis of disorders in childhood, with the attendant exposure to medical intervention, to functional disruption and possible uncertainty of outcome. Coping is defined as the way people deal with stress. Coping varies as a function of situation, i.e. stressful situations perceived as controllable elicit problem-focused coping, whereas stressful situations perceived as outwith one's control evoke emotion-focused coping. It is helpful if the coping style is appropriate to the reality of the situation.

Coping in children varies as a function of age and cognition. Three types of coping have been described in child aged 5–12 years: avoidant or primary coping, or the attempt to alter objective conditions by screaming, hitting etc.; secondary coping, or the attempt to adjust to objective conditions as they are; and relinquished control coping, in which there is no attempt to cope and apathy intervenes. Secondary coping is related to behavioural and emotional adjustment, illness- or disorder-specific adjustment and decreased distress ratings in painful interventions (Thomson and Gustafson 1999).

Children are at risk of developing avoidant coping strategies of an instrumental kind in their attempt to solve the problem by using refusal, oppositional crying, etc. Denial is a common mechanism in adolescents. Depression and conduct disorders are linked to increased use of avoidant coping strategies. Children need help to develop positive practical coping skills in which the problem is approached rather than avoided. Realistic attitudes and behaviour need encouragement. Adults with pre-existing coping disorder require extra help. A sense of control of self, of information and of events helps promote coping in both child and adult.

Pain

Pain management involves using information to regulate the reality of the perception of danger which is commonly associated with the experience of pain. It involves promoting coping strategies, including use of distraction and relaxation techniques and child-focused cognitive and behavioural therapies, including desensitisation and stress inoculation techniques. Parent coaching is an important part of pain management. Children's conceptualisation of pain and illness lies slightly behind general development. A sense of partnership in the management of pain is reassuring to the child. Parent and child need coaching in pain management techniques.

It is the experience of psychologists working in paediatric services that minor pain for minor intrusions requires to be managed carefully in order to minimise the possibility of generalisation of anxiety and the emergence of a phobic reaction that might complicates future interventions. The association at any one point in time of wider unexplored anxiety and minor discomfort during an intrusive procedure can trigger phobic response.

Adherence

Adherence to treatment is more difficult if treatment interferes with normal development or daily activities, or if it produces negative physical or cosmetic side effects. Adherence is best when adherence behaviours bring immediate results such as symptom reduction. It is harder to obtain adherence for future-oriented results or for regimes designed to prevent or forestall complications. Adverse social and emotional events occurring at any time in a person's life may affect temporarily their capacity for self-regulation, producing adherence fluctuation which requires to be understood and managed.

Talking to Children About Elimination Function, About Future Fertility and Sexual Function

The child is introduced to the facts of elimination through the practical activities of toilet training. Numerous books and advisory leaflets on this subject are available for both parents and children. Discussion of genitals in this context needs to be explicit, factual and positive. It is important to avoid the development of a sense of shame or the creation of anxiety.

Talking to the child about reproduction usually is triggered by the child questioning, often in middle childhood, about how babies are made. There are helpful titles available for parents and children. Many parents feel ambivalence about answering their questions in mechanical or sexual detail and generally concentrate on the baby's presence as the focus of pleasant attention. Discussing sexual matters with children causes considerable reserve in many parents and some authors have related this to incest taboo. Parents may instruct female children on menstruation and male and female pubertal children on visible secondary sexual characteristics, often needing to reassure a slow-developing child of his or her normality. Matters to do with sexual arousal, erection and penetration are seldom dealt with in helpful detail by parents, and children often find themselves learning both myths and facts within peer groups in later childhood and adolescence.

Little is known about discussing future fertility with children. Generally the loss of the concept of self as a fertile individual must require considerable adjustment. Discussing matters of future fertility or infertility with the child requires further research.

More is known about the effects of infertility on adult women, where wide-ranging emotional ramifications are reported, including mood change, loss of self-worth and relationship strain (Shaw 1991). Dhillon et al. (2000), despite stating that the psychological response of men perceiving themselves to be infertile can be substantial and include feelings of personal and sexual inadequacy, reports as a general conclusion that men's psychological adjustment to their own infertility is generally healthy.

It is likely that children facing challenge in sexual function or fertility will benefit from early factual information and direction towards prospects of future positive alternatives to the impaired function. It is important for children to know that they will not be totally excluded from all aspects of either of these functions.

Cosmetic Challenge

Great help for children in developing coping strategies for cosmetic challenge is provided by the "Changing Faces" initiative (1 & 2 Junction Mews, London, W2 1PN), which has produced a series of booklets and organised a number of study days for young people. Although the focus is on facial cosmetic challenge, the skills of sharing information, advancing social skills training and offering emotional expression and support are common to all cosmetic challenge. Titles from this series such as "What Happened to You", "Do Looks Count?", "You're in Charge" and "Looking Different, Feeling Good" are designed for children. Bradbury (1993) provides a useful review of literature on psychological approaches for children and adolescents facing embarrassment or stigma.

Solution Focus and Positive Psychology

Solution-focussed approach and positive psychology as described by Seligman (2000) are based on the scientific study of signature strengths, i.e. positive attributes in a person's profile, and the importance for an individual of building on these strengths in order to acquire positive emotional states. Examination of life goals, dreams and aspirations, along with dialogue on specific dilemmas, is helpful to children and adolescents.

Goals for Public Policy and Research

Goals for public policy and research should include promoting adaptation to stress; preventing disruption of normal development, family functioning and parenting; gathering knowledge on how illness-specific and psychological adjustment processes mediate adaptation in individual and family across developmental phase and illness course; promoting support policies to help parents fulfil case manager and nurse roles; identifying high-risk individuals; and supplying efficient and effective interventions.

If helped to be calm, informed, accepting and supportive, parents should be able to help children through the experience of later-treated hypospadias, imperfect technical results and compromised sexual or fertility function. Intersex issues can be more challenging, and this chapter has not attempted to make more than fleeting references to gender insofar as it affects psychological adjustment in genital anomalies.

Parenting the child with hypospadias has got to do with ensuring good self-esteem through acceptance and affection, supporting the child in developing a firm conviction that it is the child himself who is loved and valued, first by parents and then by peers, by helping this child and other children understand that people sometimes have specific illness or morphology deficits which it is important to tackle as effectively as possible, that this can involve inconvenience or discomfort and sometimes disappointment in terms of outcome, but that self-worth and continuity of support, and learning how to realise one's potential as a person, are the key in life. Enjoying aspiration and effort, being socially included and being able to regulate one's inner states to achieve a sense of well-being are successful outcomes.

As medical and surgical treatments advance, as more children with compromising medical conditions are helped, it becomes important to ensure that good psychological health accompanies this process and forms one of the aims of case management.

Quality-of-life measures should be used to commission programmes of care through systematic review of multidimensional issues for the child, including reflecting the impact of treatment from the child's point of view. Audit of well-being, satisfaction and emotional status should accompany other outcome measures.

It is increasingly recognised as a valuable resource for the medical and surgical team to have access to a proactive clinical psychology service with a dedicated skill not only in averting psychological disorder in chronic illness and in treating specific disorders but in supporting sound psychological development and adjustment for the child during the changing stages of childhood. Early intervention and continuity of contact as developmental stages proceed or the course of illness changes across time recognises the nature of development as a dynamic process in which the child learns who he is and how the world relates to him. Clinicians who are aware of the importance of this process have a positive impact throughout the child's life.

> What is vulnerable is less the child than the developmental process itself.
> Anna Freud in foreword of "*The Child in the Family: Vulnerable Children*"

References

Aho MD, Tammela OKT, Tammela TLJ: Sexual and social life of men operated in childhood for hypospadias and phimoses: a comparative study. Eur Urol. 2000; 37:95–100, discussion 101.

Berg G, Berg R: Castration complex: evidence from men operated for hypospadias. Acta Psychiatr Scand. 1983a; 68:143–153.

Berg R, Berg G: Penile malformation, gender identity, and sexual orientation. Acta Psychiatr Scand. 1983b; 68:154–166.

Berg R, Berg G, Svensson J: Penile malformation and mental health: a controlled psychiatric study of men operated for hypospadias in childhood. Acta Psychiatr Scand. 1982; 66:398–416.

Blurton Jones N, Konner MJ: Sex differences in behaviour in Bushmen and London two to five year olds. In: Crook J, Michael R (eds): Comparative ecology and behaviour of primates. Academic, New York; 1973.

Bradbury E: Looking different, feeling good: psychological approaches to children and adolescents with disfigurement. A review of the literature 15(1). ACPP Rev Newslett. 1993; 15:1–6

Changing Faces: Series of booklets for children on coping strategies in cosmetic challenge. Changing Faces, 1 & 2 Junction Mews, London W2 1PN.

Clark WR, Grunstein M: Are we hard wired? The role of human behaviour. Oxford University Press, Oxford; 2000.

Cracco A, Dettin C, Cordaro S, et al: Psychological study of adults surgically treated in childhood for hypospadias. Pediatr Med Chir. 1989; 11:447–450.

Dhillon R, Cumming CE, Cumming DC: Psychological well being and coping patterns in infertile men. Fertil Steril. 2000; 74:702–706.

Freedman DG: Sexual dysmorphism and status hierarchy. In: Omark FF, Strayer S, Freedman DG (eds): Dominance relations. Garland, New York, pp 261–271; 1980.

Kagen J: The second year: the emergence of a self-awareness. Harvard University Press, Harvard; 1981.

Low BS, Mueller U: Why sex matters. A Darwinian look at human behaviour. Princeton Paperbacks. Princeton University Press, Princeton; 2000.

Mureau MA, Slijper FME, Van der Meulen JC, et al: Psychosexual adjustment of men who underwent hypospadias repair: a norm related study. J Urol. 1995; 154:1351–1355.

Mureau MA, Slijper FM, Slob AK, et al: Psychosocial functioning of children, adolescents, and adults following hypospadias surgery: a comparative study. J Pediatr Psychol. 1997; 22:371–387.

Sandberg DE, Meyer-Bahlburg HF, Aranoff GS: Boys with hypospadias: a survey of behavioural difficulties. J Pediatr Psychol. 1989; 14:491–514.

Sandberg DE, Meyer-Bahlburg HF, Hensle TW, et al: Psychosocial adaptation of middle childhood boys with hypospadius after genital surgery. J Pediatr Psychol. 2001; 26:465–475.

Schultz JR Klykylo WM, Wacksman J: Timing of elective hypospadias repair in children. Pediatrics. 1983; 71:342–351.

Seligman M: www.positivepsychology.org (marty@apa.org), 2000.

Shaw P: Infertility counselling. In: Davis A, Fallowfield L (eds): Counselling and communication in health care. Wiley, Chichester; 1991.

Svensson J, Berg R, Berg G: Operated hypospadiacs: late follow-up. Social, sexual, and psychological adaptation. J Pediatr Surg. 1981; 16:134–135.

Thomson RJ, Gustafson KE: Adaptation to chronic childhood illness. American Psychological Association, Washington DC, 1999.

Uncommon Conditions and Complications

34

Amir F. Azmy

Uncommon Conditions

Iatrogenic Hypospadias

Iatrogenic hypospadias is caused by an injury to the ventral male urethra produced by downward pressure of an indwelling urethral catheter (as shown in Fig. 34.1).

Andrews et al. (1998) reported 16 patients with this injury during a 9-year period. They reconstructed the urethra in 6 patients and proposed that patients requiring long-term indwelling catheter should be investigated so that an alternative therapy to catheterisation can be established.

Genitourinary Injuries in the Newborn

Genitourinary trauma in the newborn is rare but often necessitates significant surgical intervention.

Patel et al. (2001) reported seven cases of genitourinary trauma in newborns. Two of these infants suffered degloving injury from a Gomco clamp and required skin grafting. Three had a Mogen clamp, which caused glans injuries: one required haemostasis, one a modified meatal advancement glanuloplasty and the third had a formal hypospadias repair. The sixth patient suffered a ventral slit and division of the ventral urethra before placement of a Gomco clamp, requiring hypospadias repair, and the last suffered a vaginal tear during emergency Caesarean section.

Congenital Urethrocutaneous Fistula Without Hypospadias

Congenital fistula of the penile urethra without hypospadias or chordee (Fig. 34.2) is very rare. It has been postulated to be due to a focal defect in the urethral plate with normal development of the glanu-

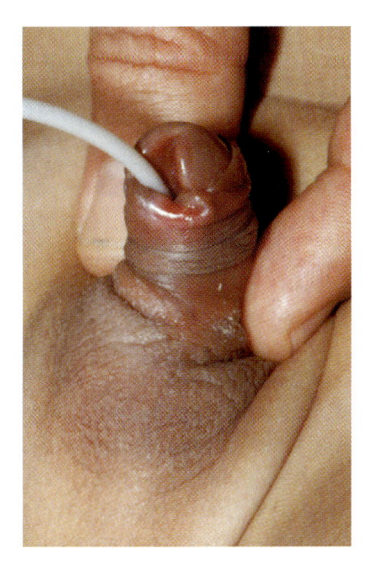

Fig. 34.1. Injury to the ventral urethra due to downward pressure of indwelling catheter

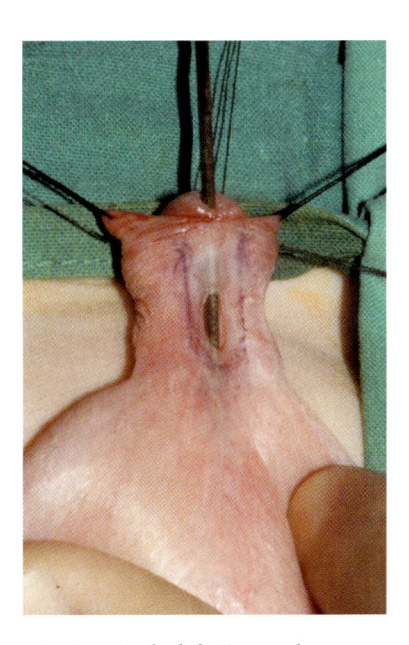

Fig. 34.2. Wide defective urethra

lar urethra, as it develops separately from the surface ectodermal invagination (Ritchey et al. 1994).

The defective urethra should be opened, and urethral reconstruction can be achieved with a vascularised preputial flap (Maarafie and Azmy 1997).

Urethral Duplication With Hypospadias

Urethral duplication is a rare congenital anomaly. Podesta et al. (1998) reported seven boys with incomplete sagittal duplication of the urethra. Duplication involved hypospadias in five patients. They were treated with one-stage urethroplasty, including marsupialisation of the dorsal orthotopic urethra, ventral-to-dorsal urethrourethrotomy and penile island onlay flap repair to cover the open dorsal urethra. One of the five patients developed urethrocutaneous fistula.

Concealed Penis

A concealed penis (synonym: inconspicuous penis) is hidden by an overlying fold of abdominal fat and skin. This uncommon condition is due to poor skin fixation at the base of the penis, cicatricial scarring after penile surgery and excessive obesity. It varies in severity.

Casale et al. (1999) reported 43 patients treated for concealed penis between 1993 and 1998. They identified type 1 congenital concealed penis in 18 cases, type 2 concealed penis due to scarring after previous penile surgery in 18 cases and type 3 complex causes including excessive obesity in 7 cases.

The mean age of type 2 patients at the time of surgery was 19.8 months. All had had previous surgery, including hypospadias repair. All 18 patients underwent complete penile degloving and excision of the cicatricial scar that trapped the penis; penile skin flaps and Z-plasties were used in 12 cases, scrotal skin flaps in 2 cases and skin grafting in 1 case. The penile skin was fixed with sutures to maintain penile length in 10 cases. The results were good in 14 of the 18 type 2 patients. Excessive suprapubic fat could be removed by liposuction or formal excision.

Congenital Buried Penis

Many terms are used to describe an inconspicuous phallus, causing considerable confusion. Maizels and colleagues (1986) proposed a classification system that helps to clarify these entities and their subsequent correction.

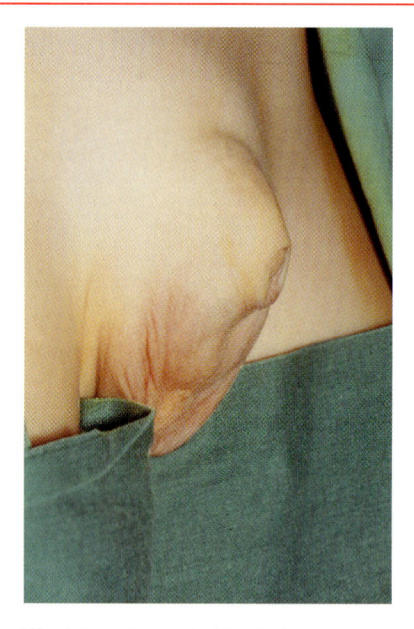

Fig. 34.3. Congenital buried penis

Buried penis refers to a penile shaft buried below the surface of the prepubic skin and also to partial or total obscuring of the penis caused by obesity or by radical circumcision (Fig. 34.3).

The word *micropenis* must not be used interchangeably with buried penis. A micropenis is an otherwise normally formed phallus that is more than two standard deviations below the mean in size. In contrast, a buried penis has normal corporeal length that is palpable under the overlying skin and subcutaneous tissue.

A true buried penis is a rare congenital anomaly that has two components: an abnormally large suprapubic fat pad and dense dysgenetic dartos fascial bands that tether the penis and retract it inward. The fat pad extends from the suprapubic region onto the scrotum, perineum and medial thigh and, combined with a lipoma of each spermatic cord, hides the penis from view. Thick abnormal dysgenetic dartos fascial bands extend from Scarpa's fascia of the abdomen onto the distal penile shaft, tethering the corporeal bodies proximally. The penile skin drapes over the penile shaft, giving the appearance of redundant skin overlying the glans of the penis with concealed corporeal bodies. Circumcision performed by using a Gomco clamp on an unrecognised buried penis can remove normal shaft skin instead of prepuce, thereby worsening the abnormality. The skin and dartos fascia are mobile, causing the corporeal bodies to move proximally without their normal overlying cover. In a normal infant, inadvertent removal of excess shaft skin during circumcision can leave a variable amount of preputial skin. The incision line constricts on healing, burying the penis by pushing it proximally into the pubic fat. A secondary circumcision may frequently be incorrectly performed on patients with different causes of concealment. This may prevent repair, which requires the remaining penile or preputial skin, and may necessitate a skin graft.

A buried penis often exhibits some penoscrotal transposition or penoscrotal webbing, which accentuates the abnormality. Many techniques have been described for the correction of buried penis (Maizels et al. 1986; Donohue and Keating 1986; Boemers and DeJong 1995; Wollin et al. 1990; Shapiro 1987; Kubota et al. 1980).

Correction of Buried Penis With Adequate Skin ▶
Through a lower Pfannenstiel incision, fat is resected inferior to the umbilicus down to the rectus fascia and is tapered cephalad and laterally to prevent a step-off deformity or an unsightly concavity. Care is taken not to make the abdominal flap too thin. Large lipomas are usually removed from the cords. Dense fibrous bands of dartos fascia, which travel from the distal penis to Scarpa's fascia, tether the corporeal bodies. These bands are identified during lipectomy and are easily excised, thereby lengthening the penis. Further lengthening is performed by partially releasing the suspensory ligament of the penis. Several tacking sutures of 2-0 nonabsorbable material are placed from firm subdermal tissue at the pubis to the rectus fascia or pubic periosteum, preventing the suprapubic and penile skin from descending over the corporeal bodies. Other tacking sutures of 3-0 material are placed from the ventral penoscrotal subdermal tissue or dermis bilaterally to the proximal tunica albuginea just lateral to each side of the urethra. Care must be taken with all tacking sutures to prevent dimpling and deformities. Penoscrotal tacking sutures are mandatory to maintain penile shaft skin on the proximal shaft and to prevent retraction of the penis.

Correction of Buried Penis Without Adequate Skin ▶ The increased length of the penile shaft requires coverage with penile skin. If the patient had a previous circumcision with a true buried penis or if he had a radical circumcision without a true buried penis, he may now have inadequate skin available for coverage.

After the circumferential circumcision scar is released, an inner preputial layer is often available for coverage. If enough inner preputial layer remains despite a shortage of shaft skin, the distal circular incision may allow the inner layer to be peeled down to replace the lost external skin. This circular scar is sometimes constricting, thereby preventing proximal advancement of preputial skin. A small Z-plasty may release the constriction and enable the remaining skin to be advanced proximally. This preputial skin is unfolded and wrapped around the shaft, keeping any longitudinal scars on the ventral aspect of the penis whenever possible. If the skin is inadequate, a large Z-plasty or double Z-plasty in the pubis may help to advance skin onto the penile shaft, but this skin is thicker and may not be helpful. A minor deficiency of the ventral skin can be resolved by a Z-plasty at the penoscrotal junction. A full-thickness or thick split-thickness skin graft may be used as a patch to fill a partial deficiency. This should be placed ventrally, if possible, to minimise the cosmetic deformity.

Accessory Scrotum

Accessory scrotum or perineal scrotum is an uncommon anomaly. Balik et al (1990) traced five patients reported in the literature and reported a case of accessory scrotum and glanular hypospadias.

Hair Coil

In occasional cases a hair coil constricts the distal penile shaft, causing pressure necrosis and resulting in hypospadias fistula if the condition is not recognised very early. Immediate release is obtained by dividing the constricting hair; if a fistula occurs, however, it may require formal closure. ◉ Figure 34.4 shows incomplete separation of the glans due to hair coil and its correction. The main principle in treatment is complete excision of any unhealthy scarred tissue and closure with fine sutures; no stenting is carried out. Interestingly, the penis heals nicely and the incidence of recurrent fistula is much lower than with hypospadias fistula.

Female Hypospadias

The natural history of meatal anomalies in girls and the incidence of female hypospadias in the normal population are not known. It is thought that there is an aetiological correlation between the functional voiding disorders and the meatal anomaly. Two types of meatal anomalies have been recognised:
1. Hypospadias in which the urethral meatus is displaced dorsally (female hypospadias)
2. Meatal web or covered hypospadias in which there is a mucosal web on the dorsal side of the urethral meatus that deflects the urinary stream anteriorly.

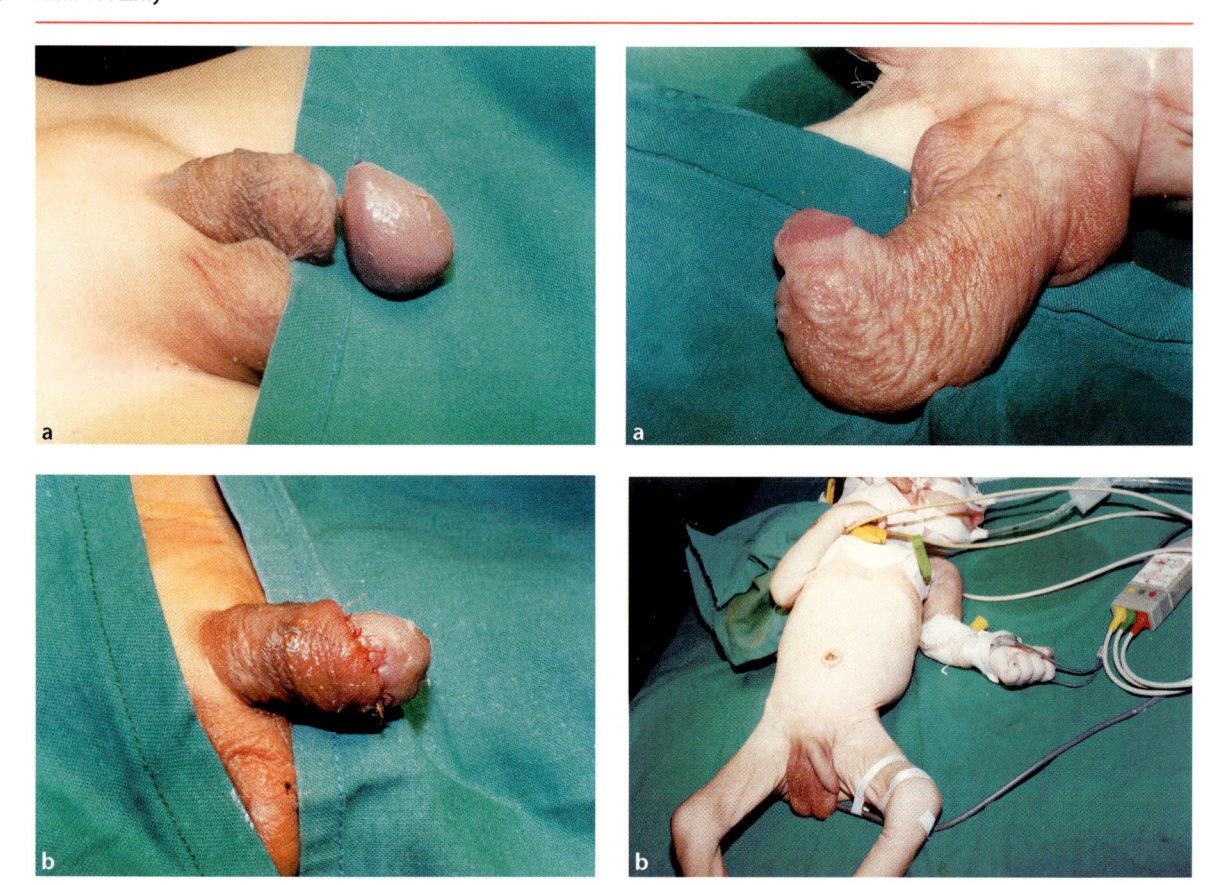

Fig. 34.4a, b. Hair coil (courtesy of Prof. A. Hadidi). **a** Incomplete separation of the glans due to hair coil; **b** postoperative view

Fig. 34.5a, b. Congenital scaphoid megalourethra (courtesy of Prof. A. Hadidi). **a** Preoperative view; **b** postoperative view

Hoebeke et al. (1999) studied the cases of 288 girls who were referred for urodynamic assessment. Eighty-eight had meatal anomalies, female hypospadias was found in 24 and covered hypospadias in 64 girls. Hoebeke and colleagues concluded that girls with meatal anomalies have more severe dysfunction as assessed by video urodynamics and proposed correction of the anomaly.

Hendren (1998) reported the cases of 40 girls in whom he constructed the female urethra using a vaginal wall and a buttock flap. The underlying pathology included bilateral ectopic ureters, cloacal malformation, urogenital sinus anomaly, previous failed surgery of the urethra, severe trauma and female hypospadias. The urethra was reconstructed using tubularised anterior vaginal wall and covered with a buttock flap in patients with urinary incontinence associated with short or absent urethra.

Gonzales and Fernandes (1990) described a single-stage feminisation genitoplasty which combines the Hendren and Crawford pull-through operation and the Kogan clitoroplasty. They used a flap of the preputial skin to construct the vestibule and anterior vaginal wall and advocated universal use of the urogenital sinus to construct the distal urethra and avoid creation of female hypospadias.

Congenital Megalourethra

Congenital megalourethra is defined as congenital diffuse enlargement of the anterior urethra. It was first described by Nesbit in 1955. This disorder is characterised by a nonobstructive urethral dilatation associated with deficiency of corpus spongiosum erectile tissue.

In 1963, Dorairajan classified megalourethra into a scaphoid type and a fusiform variety. In the more common *scaphoid variant*, the corpora cavernosa are intact and a dorsal penile curvature is often noted (Fig. 34.5). Characteristic ballooning of the ventral urethra occurs on micturition. *Fusiform megalourethra* is characterised by absence of both the corpus spongiosum and the corpora cavernosa. The penis is elongated and saclike, and erections are not possible. In 1986, Appel and colleagues reviewed several cases of megalourethra with histological evaluation and observed that atresia of the corpora cavernosa was variable. It was concluded that the classification of megalourethra into scaphoid and fusiform subtypes was arbitrary, and megalourethra is currently recognised as a disorder with a spectrum of presentations (Bloom and Ritchey 1993).

Although the aetiology of megalourethra is controversial, mesodermal dysplasia is a potential cause. This view is supported by the observation that megalourethra is often associated with other congenital anomalies, particularly diffuse mesenchymal disorders. As many as 50% of patients with scaphoid megalourethra have prune-belly syndrome (Caldamone 1994).

The diagnosis of megalourethra is made by physical examination of the external genitalia. Imaging studies such as retrograde urethrography or voiding cystourethrography demonstrate the urethral dilatation and diagnose any associated lower tract anomalies. Upper tract imaging is mandatory. When instrumentation is performed, prophylactic antibiotics are indicated to prevent sepsis.

The initial management of megalourethra includes the initiation of suppressive antibiotics, particularly when upper tract anomalies coexist. When the overall prognosis is good, corrective surgical intervention should be considered. With fusiform megalourethra, the absence of corporeal tissue compromises reconstructive repair, and gender reassignment surgery is generally considered the procedure of choice. The redundant penile skin is excised, gonadal tissue is removed, and labia are developed from the scrotal skin. A promising alternative to gender reassignment may be phallus construction using a forearm free flap. With this technique, a phallus of adequate size and acceptable appearance can be constructed. The patient can void while standing, achieve erections after placement of a prosthesis and experience erogenous sensations (Gilbert et al. 1993).

Patients with scaphoid megalourethra do not always require surgery. When hypospadias is absent, asymptomatic patients can be observed. When minimal postvoid dribbling is the only symptom, the retained urine can be drained by massage of the urethra after urination. Surgical repair of scaphoid megalourethra is usually achieved by mobilisation of the penile shaft skin, ventral vertical incision of the urethra, excision of redundant urethral tissue and suture reapproximation of the urethra over a stent as originally described by Nesbit. Although excision of redundant urethra is the most commonly reported repair (Walker 1992), Heaton and colleagues (1994) described a successful technique using infolding urethral plication rather than excision. The penis is degloved, and fine absorbable inverted Lembert sutures are placed in a vertical row approximately 2–3 mm apart. If necessary, hypospadias repair can be simultaneously performed. Potential advantages of plication include improved preservation of the urethral blood supply and a reduced incidence of urethrocutaneous fistula (Kester et al. 1990; Duckett and Smith 1996).

Uncommon Complications

Partial Dissection of the Epithelium of the Urethral Wall

Wall dissection of the neourethra is a rare complication causing severe infravesical obstruction after hypospadias repair after an initially successful double facial island flap repair. The obstruction is caused by partial dissection of the epithelium of the urethral wall, comparable to intima dissection in an aortic aneurysm (de Gier et al. 1997).

Lymphoedema of the Penis After Hypospadias Surgery

Marked lymphoedema of the penis (Fig. 34.6) may occur after hypospadias repair due to impairment of

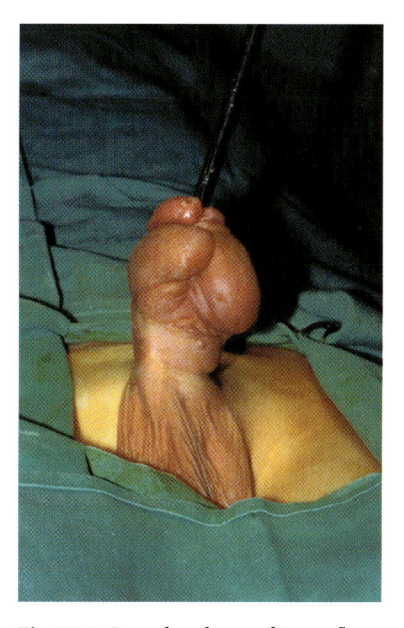

Fig. 34.6. Lymphoedema of Byars flaps

lymph drainage, particularly after construction of Byars flaps. It is rare and has been attributed to postoperative infection. Surgical excision of the lymphoedematous tissue is required to improve the appearance.

Adenoma After Hypospadias Repair

Nephrogenic adenoma is an unusual benign metaplastic lesion of the urothelium.

Weingartner et al. (1997) reported five children and one adult who developed nephrogenic adenoma of the urethra after hypospadias repair using bladder mucosal grafts. Successful treatment consisted of endoscopic resection of the polyps in four patients in whom the tumour is small. However, severe nephrogenic adenoma involving most of the reconstructed urethra may require complete resection of the graft and creation of a new urethra.

Squamous Cell Carcinoma After Hypospadias Repair

Dodd et al. (1996) reported a case of squamous cell carcinoma of the distal urethra in a patient with congenital hypospadias.

Hairy Urethra

Hairy urethra is due to the use of hair-bearing scrotal skin in cases of severe perineal hypospadias. Stones may develop in the hairy segment of the urethra. A new urethroplasty may be required to remove the hairy segment and replace it with non-hair-bearing skin.

References

Andrews HO, Nauth-Misir R, Shah PJ: Iatrogenic hypospadias – a preventable injury? Spinal Cord. 1998; 36: 177–180.

Appel RA, Kaplan GW, Brock WA: Megalourethra. J Urol. 1986; 135:747.

Balik E, Cetinkursum S, Oztop F: Accessory scrotum: report of a case. Z Kinderchir. 1990; 45:253–254.

Bloom DA, Ritchey M: Anomalies of the urethra. In: Hashmat AI, Das S (eds): The penis. Lea and Febiger, Philadelphia, pp 35–59; 1993.

Boemers TML, DeJong TPVM: The surgical correction of buried penis: a new technique. J Urol. 1995; 154:550.

Caldamone AA: Megalourethra. In: Seidmon EJ, Hanno PM (eds): Current urologic therapy. Saunders, Philadelphia, pp 402–403; 1994.

Casale AJ, Beck SD, Caiss MP, et al: Concealed penis in childhood. A spectrum of etiology and treatment. J Urol. 1999; 162:1165–1168.

De Gier RP, Feita WF, de Vries JD: Wall dissection of the neourethra, a rare condition after hypospadias repair. Urology. 1997; 50:462–464.

Dodd M, Lawson P, Hayman J: Squamous cell carcinoma of the distal urethra in a patient with congenital hypospadias. Pathology. 1996; 28:96–97.

Donohue PK, Keating MA: Preputial unfurling to correct the buried penis. J Pediatr Surg. 1986; 21:1055–1057.

Dorairajan T: Defects of spongy tissue and congenital diverticula of the penile urethra. Aust NZ J Surg. 1963; 32:209.

Duckett JW, Smith GHH: Urethral lesions in infants and children. In Gillenwater JY, Grayhack JT, Howards SS, Duckett JW (eds): Adult and pediatric urology. St Louis, Mosby, pp 2411–2413; 1996

Gilbert DA, Jordan GH, Devine CJ Jr, et al: Phallic construction in prepubertal and adolescent boys. J Urol. 1993; 149:1521.

Gonzales R, Fernandes ET: Single stage feminisation genitoplasty. J Urol. 1990; 143:776–778.

Heaton BW, Snow BW, Cartwright PC: Repair of urethral diverticulum by plication. Urology. 1994; 44:749.

Hendren WH: Construction of a female urethra using the vaginal wall and a buttock flap: experence with 40 cases. J Paediatr Surg. 1998; 33:180–187.

Hoebeke P, van Laecke E, Raes A, et al: Anomalies of the external urethral meatus in girls with non-neurogenic bladder sphincter dysfunction. BJU Int. 1999; 83:294–298.

Kester RR, Mooppan UMM, Hyunsook KO, et al: Congenital megalourethra. J Urol. 1990; 143:1213.

Kubota Y, Ishii N, Watanabe H, et al: Buried penis: a surgical repair. Urol Int. 1980; 46:61–63.

Maarafie A, Azmy AF: Congenital fistula of the penile urethra. Br J Urol. 1997; 79:814.

Maizels M, Zaontz M, Donovan J, et al: Surgical correction of the buried penis: description of a classification system and a technique to correct this disorder. J Urol. 1986; 136:268–271.

Nesbit TE: Congenital megalo-urethra. J Urol. 1955; 73:839.

Patel HI, Moriarty KP, Brisson PA: Genito-urinary injuries in the newborn. J Pediatr Surg. 2001; 36:235–239.

Podesta ML, Medel R, Castera R: Urethral duplication in children: surgical treatment and results. J Urol. 1998; 160: 1830–1833.

Ritchey ML, Sinha A, Argueso L: Congenital fistula of the penile urethra. J Urol. 1994; 151:1061–1062.

Shapiro S: Surgical treatment of the "buried" penis. Urology. 1987; 30:554–559.

Walker RD: Megalourethra. In: Resnick MI, Kursh ED (eds): Current therapy in genitourinary surgery. Mosby, St Louis, pp 316–318; 1992.

Weingartner K, Kozakewich HP, Hendren WH: Nephrogenic adenoma after urethral reconstruction using bladder mucosa. Reports of 6 cases and review of the literature. J Urol. 1997; 158:1175–1177.

Wollin M, Duffy PG, Malone PS, et al: Buried penis. A novel approach. Br J Urol. 1990; 65:97–100.

Editorial Overview of the Current Management of Hypospadias

35

Ahmed T. Hadidi, Amir F. Azmy

Hypospadias surgery has developed into a well-defined art and science. Despite major advances in technique, instrumentation and aftercare, the correction of hypospadias remains one of the most technically challenging aspects of paediatric surgery and urology. There is no place for the occasional hypospadias surgeon, even in the so-called "minor" hypospadias. Surgeons should have a detailed understanding of the various basic principles and surgical techniques and maintain a clinical workload that is sufficient to obtain consistently good results. With improving functional outcome, the challenge is now to obtain the optimal cosmetic result to provide patients with a penis of normal function and appearance regardless of the severity of the original abnormality (Wilcox and Mouriquand 2002). For distal hypospadias, a fistula rate of less than 5% is now to be expected (Belman 1994). For proximal hypospadias, the expected incidence of complications is less than 20% (Keating and Rich 1999).

Major changes in the approach to hypospadias surgery over the past 20 years have contributed to the improved functional and cosmetic results of hypospadias surgery. These changes include:
a) Preservation of the urethral plate
b) Technical surgical details
c) Protective intermediate layer
d) New methods for glanuloplasty and meatoplasty
e) Single-stage repair
f) Flaps rather than grafts
g) The role of stenting
h) The role of dressing
i) Preoperative hormonal treatment.

Preservation of the Urethral Plate

In the past decade, the term urethral plate has been commonly applied to the strip of tissue that extends distally from the hypospadiac meatus to near the tip of the glans. Operations that involve use of the plate, such as onlay preputial flap, glans approximation procedure (GAP) and tubularised incised plate (TIP) repair, have gained in popularity, in part because of the perception that such repairs have low complication rate (Snodgrass and Lorenzo 2002a, b; see Chap. 5.2).

Technical Surgical Details

The composition of suture material, suturing technique, and the use of magnification are variables that have had a significant impact on the results. Ulman et al. (1997) documented a statistically significant lower fistula rate (4.9% vs 16.6%) for subcuticular repair than for a full-thickness (through and through) technique. Chromic catgut is favoured for the skin. Polyglycolic acid (Dexon) or polyglactin 910 (Vicryl) are favoured for urethroplasty. Polydioxanone (PDS) may react with urine and has not been advised for hypospadias surgery (Bickerton and Duckett 1984; El-Mahrouky et al. 1987; Duckett and Baskin 1996). Optical magnification is considered essential by most hypospadiologists. The power of magnification varies, according to the surgeon's preference, from 1.5× to operative microscope power. The importance of using fine, delicate instruments cannot be overemphasised (Chap. 8).

Protective Intermediate Layer

One of the most important factors in reducing the incidence of fistula and other complications of hypospadias repair was the introduction of a protective intermediate layer between the neourethra and the skin layer.

Types of protective intermediate layer include Smith's de-epithelialised skin, Snow's tunica vaginalis wrap from the testicular coverings, Retik's dorsal – subcutaneous flap from the foreskin, Motiwala's dartos flap from the scrotum, and the external spermatic fascia flap (Chap. 24).

New Methods for Glanuloplasty and Meatoplasty

The aim of hypospadias surgery today is to achieve a normal-looking glans and meatus following hypospadias surgery. Procedures that help to achieve this aim include the Snodgrass tubularised incised plate repair, Y-V glanuloplasty and MAVIS repair (Chap. 25).

Single-Stage Repair

In the 1950s, the accepted methods for surgical management of hypospadias involved a two-stage approach. The three most popular techniques were the Thiersch–Duplay method, later modified and popularised by Byars, the Nove-Josserand approach, later modified and popularised by Bracka, and the Denis Browne technique. Horton and Devine, Broadbent, DesPrez, Standoli and Duckett were instrumental in popularising the one-stage approach for the correction of hypospadias. By 1988, it has been suggested that all primary hypospadias should be repaired with a single-stage approach (Sadove et al. 1988).

For distal hypospadias, the general concept is to perform a single-stage repair (Borer and Retik 1999). The most popular techniques are the Y-V modified Mathieu method (Chap. 14), MAGPI (Chap. 11) and Snodgrass tubularised incised plate urethroplasty (Chap. 15). However, a few surgeons still recommend two-stage repair in all patients (Bracka 1995a, b; Chap. 23).

Approximately 20% of patients with hypospadias have a proximal defect. The majority can be repaired in a single stage. The most popular techniques are the onlay island flap (Chap. 16.1), the transverse preputial island flap (Chap. 16.2), the Koyanagi method (Chap. 19), the yoke technique (Chap. 20) and the lateral-based flap (Chap. 21).

Patients with scrotal or perineal hypospadias, a small phallus and severe chordee are candidates for two-stage repair. This subset of patients, when treated with a one-stage repair, usually needs a composite graft. Unsatisfactory results have been reported in this group of patients when managed with a one-stage repair (Retik et al. 1994; Kroovand and Perlmutter 1980; Greenfield et al. 1994; Bracka 1995a, b).

Flaps Rather Than Grafts

Flaps are very popular nowadays for hypospadias repair. The most popular flap for distal penile hypospadias is the Y-V modified Mathieu repair. The onlay preputial flap has gained great popularity because of the low complication rate. The controversy of flaps versus grafts is discussed in Chap. 27.1.

The Role of Stenting

Urinary diversion has passed through different stages and methods. Techniques of urinary diversion include perineal urethrotomy, a Foley catheter, Silastic stents, deroofed Silastic stents and catheters. Some investigators report rates of fistula formation and meatal stenosis that are two times greater in stented than in suprapubic diverted hypospadias repair (Demirbilek and Atayurt 1997). Support for unstented repair is not universal. The controversy of stenting is covered in Chap. 27.3.

The Role of Dressing

Dressings are used to provide immobilisation and prevent haematoma and oedema. Tegaderm wrap and the sandwich dressing are popular. However, recent papers have questioned the value of dressings and recommended no dressing in most hypospadias repairs (van Savage et al. 2000; McLorie et al. 2001; Hadidi et al. 2003). The issue of dressing is dealt with in Chap. 27.4.

Preoperative Hormonal Treatment

The results of surgery for severe proximal and perineal hypospadias are still less satisfactory than for other forms of hypospadias. In an attempt to improve the surgical results, androgen stimulation before the repair has been suggested, using testosterone (Guthrie et al. 1973), dihydrotestosterone (Monfort and Lucas 1982) or human chorionic gonadotropin (Koff and Jayanthi 1999). This may help to enlarge the phallus temporarily. Whether preoperative endocrine therapy is really beneficial and whether one should use testosterone propionate cream, parenteral testosterone injection or human chorionic gonadotropin is still controversial. The topic is discussed in Chap. 6.2.

To conclude this chapter, we the editors would like to express our own personal preferences:

Surgery for hypospadias repair is a delicate art. The surgeon should not compromise on the result just because certain techniques are less prone to complications than others. In other words, the surgeon should use the technique that is suitable for the de-

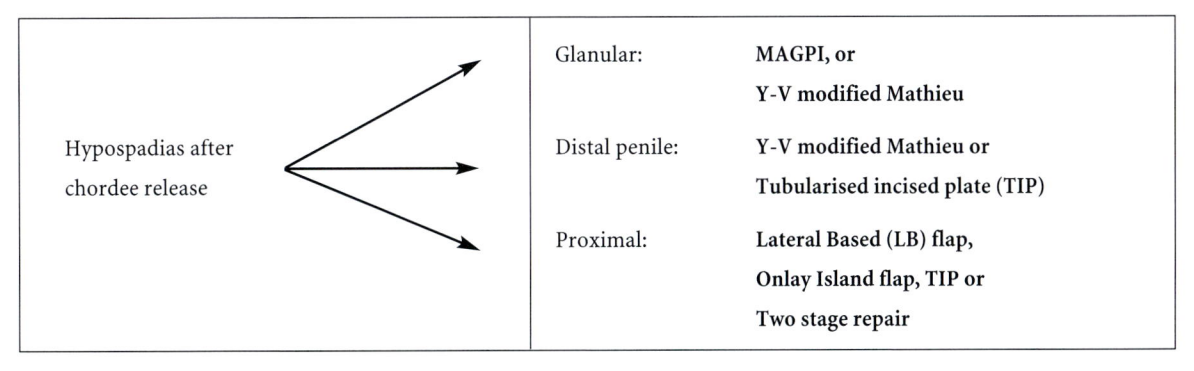

Hypospadias after chordee release	Glanular:	**MAGPI, or**
		Y-V modified Mathieu
	Distal penile:	**Y-V modified Mathieu or**
		Tubularised incised plate (TIP)
	Proximal:	**Lateral Based (LB) flap,**
		Onlay Island flap, TIP or
		Two stage repair

Fig. 35.1. Algorithm for primary hypospadias repair

formity rather than making the hypospadiac deformity suit the repair he prefers. We do not believe that one should use a technique that shortens an already short penis just because it has a lower complication rate. By the same reasoning, one should not shorten the penis dorsally to correct the ventral chordee and, lastly, one should not leave a raw surface if a fully epithelialised neourethra can be achieved.

For glanular hypospadias with mobile meatus or cleft glans, we prefer to use the MAGPI or the GAP technique. For distal hypospadias, we prefer to use the Y-V glanuloplasty modified Mathieu approach. We do not leave a stent inside the urethra. A temporary compression dressing is applied for 6 h, then the wound is left exposed. This has proven very satisfactory to children and parents. We have adopted the lateral-based flap for proximal hypospadias. Two-stage repair is advisable for perineal hypospadias to avoid the use of hair-bearing areas of skin. We believe that not leaving a stent inside the urethra or a dressing on the penis has improved our results dramatically. ◉ Figure 35.1 summarises our recommendations for primary hypospadias repair.

References

Belman AB: The de-epithelialized flap and its influence on hypospadias repair. J Urol. 1994; 152:2332–2334.
Bickerton MW, Duckett JW: Suture material and wound healing. AUA Update Ser. 1984; 3, lesson 15.
Borer JG, Retik AB: Current trends in hypospadias repair. Urol Clin North Am. 1999; 26:15–37.
Bracka A: A versatile two-stage hypospadias repair. Br J Plast Surg. 1995a; 48:345–352.
Bracka A: Hypospadias repair: the two-stage alternative. Br J Urol. 1995b; 76 [Suppl 3]:31–41.
Demirbilek S, Atayurt HF: One-stage hypospadias repair with stent or suprapubic diversion: which is better? J Pediatr Surg. 1997; 32:1711–1712.
Duckett JW, Baskin LS: Hypospadias. In: Gillenwater JY, Grayhack JT, Howards SS, Duckett JW (eds): Adult and pediatric urology, 3rd edn, vol 3, chap 55. Mosby Year Book, St Louis, pp 2549–2589; 1996.
El-Mahrouky A, McElhaney J, Bartone FF, et al: In vitro comparison of the properties of polydioxanone, polyglycolic acid and catgut sutures in sterile and infected urine. J Urol. 1987; 138:913–915.
Greenfield SP, Sadler BT, Wan J: Two-stage repair for severe hypospadias. J Urol. 1994; 152:498.
Guthrie RD, Smith DW, Graham CB: Testosterone treatment for micropenis during early chilhood. J Pediatr. 1973; 87:247.
Hadidi A, Abdaal N, Kaddah S: Hypospadias repair: is dressing important. Kasr El Aini J Surg. 2003; 4 (1):37–44.
Keating MA, Rich MA: Onlay and tubularised preputial island flap. In: Ehrlich RM, Alter GJ (eds): Reconstructive and plastic surgery of the external genitalia, adult and pediatric. Saunders, Philadelphia. p 77; 1999.
Koff SA, Jayanthi VR: Preoperative treatment with human chorionic gonadotrophin in infancy decreases the severity of proximal hypospadias and chordee. J Urol. 1999; 162:1435–1439.
Kroovand RL, Perlmutter AD: Extended urethroplasty in hypospadias. Urol Clin North Am. 1980; 7:431.
McLorie G, Joyner B, Herz D, et al: A prospective randomized clinical trial to evaluate methods of postoperative care of hypospadias. J Urol. 2001; 165:1669–1672.
Monfort G, Lucas C: Dihydrotestosterone penile stimulation in hypospadias surgery. Eur Urol. 1982; 8:201–203.
Retik AB, Bauer SB, Mandell J, et al: Management of severe hypospadias with a 2-stage repair. J Urol. 1994; 152:749–751.
Sadove RC, Horton CE, McRoberts JW: The new era of hypospadias surgery. Clin Plast Surg. 1988; 15:354.
Snodgrass W, Lorenzo A: Tubularized incised plate urethroplasty for hypospadias reoperation. BJU Int. 2002a; 89:98.
Snodgrass W, Lorenzo A: Tubularized incised plate urethroplasty for proximal hypospadias. BJU Int. 2002b; 89:90.
Ulman I, Erikci V, Avanoglu A, et al: The effect of suturing techniques and material on complication rate following hypospadias repair. Eur J Pediatr Surg. 1997; 7:156.
Van Savage JG, Palanca LG, Slaughenhoupt BL: A prospective randomized trial of dressings versus no dressings for hypospadias repair. J Urol. 2000; 164:981–983.
Wilcox DT, Mouriquand PD: Hypospadias. In: Thomas DFM, Rickwood AMK, Duffy PG (eds): Essentials of paediatric urology. Dunitz, London, p 179; 2002.

Potential Techniques and Future Research

Arup Ray, Amir F. Azmy

A wide range of techniques has been described in the management of the hypospadias deformity. Increasing levels of awareness amongst patients and higher expectations are driving forces in the search for results that are not merely satisfactory but meet the criteria of acceptability in terms of form and function.

The advent of techniques such as microsurgical free tissue transfers and tissue expansion has provided a wider range of procedures available to address the reconstructive needs of this group of patients. As the severity of the hypospadias deformity tends to be relatively minor in the vast majority of cases, these complex techniques are applicable in only a small proportion of patients with more severe deformity or those requiring more complex revision surgery. Other body-contouring techniques such as tissue augmentation and liposculpturing have also been usefully employed as adjunctive procedures in the management of the deformity in hypospadias as well as in epispadias.

Hypospadias is often associated with smaller overall penile size. The problem is often compounded by the techniques used to "correct" the deformity by attempting to "advance" the abnormally located urethral meatus to a more terminal position, resulting in further shortening of the shaft. Procedures utilising extensive mobilisation of the urethra or corpus spongiosum in order to achieve an adequate terminal relocation of the meatus may also result in considerable scarring with consequent distortion during erection. Several techniques utilising bulky flaps of tissue or methods attempting to refashion the deficient urethra along the ventral or even the dorsal aspect of the glans penis using the adjacent skin and tissues can also result in grossly abnormal genital appearance as well as function in adulthood. A variety of single- and multiple-stage operations that have been described over the decades have subsequently been discarded as the long-term results became obvious.

These effects were understandably not apparent in the immediate postoperative assessment of the reconstructive techniques employed in childhood. The ever-increasing numbers of patients seeking secondary revision surgery in adulthood, especially in the current day and age, as a result of serious psychological or functional problems is a reflection of the demands and expectations of individuals and society.

Microsurgical Free Tissue Transfers

Microsurgical free tissue transfers have revolutionised the scope of reconstructive surgery, and the refinements in techniques and range of reconstructive options currently available allow a wide selection of procedures which can be tailored to the specific needs of the individual patient. Reconstruction of the penis using the radial forearm flap following traumatic amputation, resection for cancer or gender re-assignment has been extensively reported. Utilising the radial forearm flap (Granato 1974), which is a fasciocutaneous flap based on perforating branches of the radial artery, permits the harvesting of virtually the entire skin and deep fascia of the forearm, which can be fashioned to provide an inner tube to reconstruct the urethra and an outer lining for the penile shaft. Reconstruction with sensate flaps, achieved by identifying the cutaneous sensory nerves in the flap and anastomosing them to the appropriate recipient sensory nerves such as the dorsal nerves of the penis or the pudendal nerves, has also been documented. Alternatively, the sensate skin of a rudimentary penis may be incorporated into the flap to provide appropriate erogenous sensation. Functional rigidity of the reconstruction to permit effective intercourse has been achieved by incorporating a segment of bone, such as a portion of costal cartilage or the shaft of the radial bone, as a vascularised composite osteo-fasciocutaneous free tissue transfer. Other composite free tissue transfers, such as free sensate osteo-cutaneous fibula flaps incorporating a vascularised segment of the fibula wrapped in the overlying skin island with its sensory nerve supply, have also been reported.

Prosthetic stiffeners, such as Silastic filler implants which may be ingeniously inflated or deflated as required, have been employed to simulate erectile function or avoid the need to use bone. Prosthetic implants, however, are very expensive and are associated with a high rate of complications in the long term, such as postoperative infection and extrusion, peri-implant fibrosis or atrophy and eventual implant failure.

A range of other free tissue transfers, such as the lateral arm flap, deltoid flap, dorsalis pedis flap and composite reconstructions with innervated osteo-fascio-cutaneous radial forearm flaps and big toe pulp transfers, have been similarly employed.

Tissue Expansion

The first clinical use of tissue expansion – the reconstruction of an ear using expanded temporal skin – was reported by Neumann in 1957. Tissue expansion may provide a large amount of local skin with pigmentation and properties similar to those of the surrounding skin. Tissue expansion has been successfully used for the reconstruction of the scalp, face, breast and trunk. Various sizes and shapes of expanders made from silicone elastomers have been used. They are inserted in subcutaneous tissue through a small incision at the edge of the defect; the expanders are gradually enlarged by injecting saline at weekly intervals. When expansion is complete, the expander is removed and reconstruction is performed.

Tissue expansion has been used in male-to-female gender reassignment. In the technique of placement of tissue expanders as advocated by Franato, a pocket is created along the entire length of the dorsum of the penis between the dartos fascia and Buck's fascia and a pocket of the port is fashioned beneath Scarpa's fascia of the inguinal area; the expander is then inserted through a small incision into the two cavities created. Injections of saline follow until the volume of expanded skin is sufficient for reconstruction of the vagina (Patil 1994).

The results of vaginoplasty for females with adrenogenital syndrome are disappointing, as the rate of vaginal stenosis is very high, approaching 80%, despite repeated dilatation. Tissue expansion of the labia provides ample skin flaps for vaginoplasty (Patil 1994).

Tissue Expansion for Urethral and Penile Reconstruction

The use of tissue expanders in penile surgery yields adequate amounts of the patient's own penile skin to complete reconstruction in cases of failed hypospadias repair and deficient skin, complex urethral defects and penile malformations. The expander is placed under penile skin and the injection port in the lower abdomen. The abnormal urethra should be excised leaving the meatus in a proximal position on the shaft. Byars flaps are used to cover the ventral defect, and this should be done prior to insertion of the tissue expander. The expander is inserted on the dorsal surface of the penis and expansion is gradual over a period of 4–6 weeks. The excess skin is used for penile reconstruction.

Tissue expansion for the lower abdominal wall in cases of bladder exstrophy will allow satisfactory skin cover in cases of abdominal scars and depression of mons pubis after closure of the bladder exstrophy. The resultant excess skin flaps fill the gap after excision of median scar tissue; excess skin could also be used for epispadias repair.

Penile Enhancement

Penile enhancement can be achieved by division of the suspensory ligaments of the penis and injections of fat cells into the subcutaneous tissues to augment the penile girth. This technique may be applicable in selected cases of hypospadias where the patient is dissatisfied with the resting dimensions of the penis or experiences social embarrassment because of adverse peer remarks or extreme self-consciousness (locker-room envy). However, in such cases it is essential to ensure that the patients are assessed by psychologists and extensively counselled prior to being considered for surgery. Release of the suspensory ligament of the penis, combined if required with a V-Y advancement of the suprapubic skin and underlying soft tissues, increases the apparent visible length of the penile shaft at rest by altering the angulation of the shaft of the penis relative to the pubic symphysis. Interposition of soft tissues to prevent reattachment of the suspensory ligament is recommended.

Liposculpturing Procedures

Liposculpturing of the suprapubic fat by means of liposuction and injection of the harvested fat cells into the penis may be used to increase penile girth if required. Suprapubic lipectomy is generally not recommended in infants unless there are concurrent problems such as hypospadias. Liposculpturing is especially useful in peripubertal patients with excess abdominal fat, who are often acutely conscious of their genital dimensions or experience adverse remarks from their peer group and are very keen to consider any measures that may help to improve their body image. Liposuction and abdominoplasty in adults with a buried penis appearance has also been described to improve the visible projection and shaft length of the penis. The results of this type of procedure that combines a reduction of the abdominal girth with an apparent increase in penile dimensions are often very gratifying for the patient.

Laser Tissue Soldering for Hypospadias Repair

Laser tissue soldering provides effective tissue closure by creating a leak-free anastomosis with minimal scar formation. Experimental and clinical data have supported the concept of laser tissue soldering to improve wound healing. The use of laser soldering in animal models for vascular, skin, intestinal, urethral, corporeal body, dorsal, vesical and vasoepididymal anastomoses have shown technical and wound healing advantages of laser tissue soldering over suturing alone (Poppas et al. 1988)ne. The advantages include minimal tissue handling, maximal alignment, water tight anastomosis, maximal tensile strength during early healing and minimal scar formation (Poppas et al. 1988).

Kirsch et al. (2001) performed a controlled prospective clinical trial. A consecutive group of 138 boys aged 4 months to 8 years (mean age 15 months) were divided into a standard suturing group (84 patients) and a sutureless laser group (54 patients). The method of preparation of the human albumin and indocyanine green dye solder has been described (Kirsch et al. 1995; Oz et al. 1990).

The treatment was performed with diode laser module coupled to a rounded quartz silica fibreoptic with a 600 mm core diameter housed within a plastic hand-piece. The laser system consists of a phased array of gallium–albumin arsenide semiconductor diodes and produces an invisible laser beam. A red pilot beam allows laser spot size to be visualised during activation. A minimal number of sutures is used to align precisely the edges of the neo urethra. This layer of solder is applied along the approximated edges of the neo-urethra and the laser is activated until complete desiccation occurs (Poppas et al. 1993).

Urethral surgery appears to be a good application for laser tissue soldering and provides the rationale for human experimentation. The results in terms of operative time and overall complications are impressive compared to traditional suturing methods and it seems that laser tissue soldering may be performed in a nearly sutureless fashion. Snodgrass tubularised incised plate urethroplasty is more amenable to laser tissue soldering because of the single anterior suture line.

Kirsch et al. (1997) reported on skin flap closure by dermal laser soldering and established an animal wound healing model for sutureless hypospadias repair. They compared the histology and immunohistochemistry of wound healing following laser tissue soldering and suturing in a rat skin flap model. There was no evidence of thermal injury or foreign body reactions in the laser tissue soldering group; solder was incorporated within the dermis in all wounds at 21 days. The authors concluded that sutureless dermal laser tissue soldering of skin flaps provides increased tensile strength for up to 7 days, particularly within the first 3 days, and their laser technique does not appear to alter the normal wound healing process; rather, initial solder–tissue interaction and subsequent extracellular matrix infiltration of solder provide the basis for improved wound strength for hypospadias repair using skin flaps.

Reconstruction of Neourethra from Cultivated Keratinocytes

Keratinocytes cultivated in vitro have been used for skin graft in patients with extensive burns or large skin defects. Use of in vitro-cultivated keratinocytes for urethral reconstruction was reported by Romagnoli et al. (1990): A sample of urethral mucosal biopsy is taken and keratinocytes are enzymatically treated to produce a cell suspension, which is further cultivated by seeding on dishes. Sheets of cultivated epithelium are placed on the prepared bed of the urethra to be reconstructed. In a modification of the Romagnoli technique, a biopsy sample of urethral epithelium is expanded and later placed on the outer side of a tubularised Teflon graft. The tubularised graft, sealed with keratinocytes, is placed through a subcutaneous tunnel. Romagnoli and colleagues (1990) concluded that reconstruction of the neourethra could be achieved with cultivated keratinocytes. However, there is a need for further investigation; greater clinical experience and long-term follow-up are required.

Harvesting Human Urothelial Cells for Urethral Reconstruction

Homologous urothelial substitute is the ideal material for urethral reconstruction and has been successfully harvested, cultivated and extensively expanded in vitro in sufficient quantities for reconstruction (Cilento et al. 1994). Autologous urothelial cells could be collected from human patients, expanded in culture and returned to the human donor in sufficient quantities for reconstruction. Atala et al. (1992) were able to create urothelial tissue grafts using an isolated population of transitional epithelium in concert with a synthetic biodegradable polymer. The polymer is used as a delivery vehicle for the creation of new urothelial structures in vivo from desiccated cells. The biodegradable polymer is a synthetic polymer of hydroxyacetic acid and exists as non-woven meshes of polyglycolic acid. The physical characteristics of the polymer allow for ample surface area for cellular attachment or diffusion of cellular nutrients (the interfibre distance ranges from 0 μm to 200 μm, while the average fibre diameter is 15 μm).

Various experiments in New Zealand white rabbits have shown the possibility of the use of biodegradable polymers for the delivery, survival and expansion of urothelial cells in vivo (Atala et al. 1993a, b). Cilento et al. (1995) used polymers seeded with autologous urothelial cells for urethral replacement in New Zealand white rabbits. They performed partial excision of the urethra and replaced it with a segment of polymer mesh. Retrograde studies showed no stricture, and histology of the reconstructed urethra showed complete re-epithelialisation of the polymer mesh after 2 weeks which persisted at 4 and 6 weeks. The polymer gradually degraded and was completely absorbed by one month. Autologous cells have been proposed for other urological applications, e.g. the use of injectable alginate seeded with chondrocytes as a potential treatment for vesicoureteric reflux (Atala et al. 1993b, 1994).

There is a need for continuing research in animal models to identify suitable autologous tissue culture for clinical application for urological reconstruction, particularly for complex cases of hypospadias where there is insufficient skin suitable for urethral repair.

Inert Collagen Matrix for Hypospadias Repair

In patients with hypospadias where there is insufficient genital skin, an alternative tissue is required for urethral reconstruction. Free skin graft and buccal and bladder mucosal grafts have been used. Atala et al. (1999) used an inert collagen matrix which was trimmed to appropriate size suitable to each patient. The neourethra was created by anastomosing the collagen matrix as an onlay graft to the urethral plate and sutured with 6-0 polyglactin sutures. This procedure was performed in four patients, three of whom had a successful outcome functionally and cosmetically. One patient in whom a 15-cm neourethra was fashioned had a subglanular fistula. Atala and colleagues (1999) concluded that the use of inert collagen matrix appears to be beneficial in patients who have undergone previous repair and lack sufficient genital skin for further reconstruction.

References

Atala A, Vacanti JP, Peters CA, et al: Formation of urothelial structures in vitro from dissociated cells attached to biodegradable polymer scaffolds in vitro. J Urol. 1992; 148:658.

Atala A, Cima LG, Kim W, et al: Injectable alginate seeded with chondrocytes as a potential treatment for vesicoureteric reflux. J Urol. 1993; 150:745–747.

Atala A, Freeman MR, Vacanti JP, et al: Implantation in vivo and retrieval of artificial structures consisting of rabbit and human urothelium and human bladder muscle. J Urol. 1993; 150:608–612.

Atala A, Kim W, Paige KT, et al: Endoscopic treatment of vesicoureteric reflux with a chondrocyte–alginate suspension. J Urol. 1994; 152:641–643.

Atala A, Guzman L, Retik AB: A novel inert collagen matrix for hypospadias repair. J Urol. 1999; 162:1148–1152.

Cilento BG, Freeman MR, Schneck FX, et al: Phenotypic and cytogenic characterisation of human bladder urothelia expanded in vitro. J Urol. 1994; 152:665.

Cilento BG, Retik AB, Atala A: Urothelial reconstruction using a polymer mesh. J Urol. 1995; 153:371A.

Granato R: Surgical approach to male transsexualism. Urology. 1974; 3:792–797.

Kirsch AJ, Miller MI, Chang DT, et al: Laser tissue soldering in urinary tract reconstruction. First human experience. Urology. 1995; 46:261.

Kirsch AJ, Canning DA, Zderic SA: Skin flap closure by dermal laser soldering: a wound healing model for sutureless hypospadias repair. Urology. 1997; 50:263–272.

Kirsch AJ, Cooper CS, Gatti J, et al: Laser tissue soldering for hypospadias repair: results of a controlled prospective clinical trial. J Urol. 2001; 165:574–577.

Neumann C: The expansion of an area of skin by progressive distension of a subcutaneous balloon. Plast Reconstr Surg. 1957; 19:124–130.

Oz MC, Johnson JP, Parangis S, et al: Tissue soldering by use of indocyanine green dye enhanced fibrinogen with the near diode laser. J Vasc Surg. 1990; 11:718.

Patil UB: Role of tissue expanders in genito urinary reconstructive surgery. Urol Annu. 1994; 8:191.

Poppas DP, Schlossberg SM, Richmond IL, et al: Laser welding in urethral surgery: improved results with a protein solder. J Urol. 1988; 139:145.

Poppas DP, Mininberg DT, Hyacinthe L, et al: Patch graft urethroplasty using dye enhanced laser tissue welding with a human protein solder; a pre-clinical canine model. J Urol. 1993; 150:648.

Romagnoli G, Deluca M, Faranda F, et al: Treatment of posterior hypospadias by the autologous graft of cultured urethral epithelium. N Engl J Med. 1990; 32:527.

References

Aaronson IA, Cakmak MA, Key LL: Defects of the testosterone biosynthetic pathway in boys with hypospadias. J Urol. 1997;157:1884–1888.

Aaronson IA, El-Sherbiny M: Testicular enzyme deficiency as a cause of hypospadias. Abstract presented to AAP, Section on Urology, San Francisco; 1998.

Aarskog D: Intersex conditions masquerading as simple hypospadias. Birth Defects Original Article Series. 1971; 7: 122–130.

Aarskog D: Maternal progestins as a possible cause of hypospadias. N Engl J Med. 1979; 300:75–78.

Aarskog D: Clinical and cytogenetic studies in hypospadias. Acta Pediatr Scand (suppl). 1970; 203: 1–61.

Aberg A, Westbom L, Kallen B: Congenital malformations among infants whose mothers had gestational diabetes or pre-existing diabetes. Early Hum Dev. 2001; 61:85–95.

Adachi Y, Nonomura K, Togashi M, et al: Comparison of one stage and two stage urethroplasty for hypospadias. Jpn J Urol. 1987; 78:667–673.

Adams MC, Chalian VS, Rink RC: Congenital dorsal penile curvature: a potential problem of the long phallus. J Urol. 1999;161:1304–1307.

Aeginata P: Seven books of Paulus Aeginata. Sydenham Society, London, 1844.

Ahmed S, Gough DC: Buccal mucosal graft for Secondary hypospadias repair and urethral replacement. Br J Urol. 1997; 80: 328–330.

Aho M, Koivisto AM, Tammela TLJ, et al: Is the incidence of hypospadias increasing? Analysis of Finnish Hospital Discharge Data 1970–1994. Environ Health Perspect. 2000; 108:463–465.

Aho MO, Tammela OKT, Somppi EMJ, et al: Sexual and social life of men operated in childhood for hypospadias and phimosis: a comparative study. Eur Urol. 2000; 37:95–100, discussion 101.

Aho MO, Tammela OKT, Tammela TLJ: Aspects of adult satisfaction with the result of surgery for hypospadias performed in childhood. Eur Urol. 1997; 32:218–222.

Aigen AB, Khawand N, Skoog SJ, et al: Acquired megalourethra: an uncommon complication of the transverse preputial island flap urethroplasty. J Urol. 1987; 137:712–713.

Akporiaye L, Schlossberg S, Jordan G: Fossa navicularis reconstruction in surgical treatment of balanitis xerotica obliterans. J Urol. 1995; 153:372A.

Akre O, Lipworth L, Criattingius S, et al: Risk factor pattern for cryptorchidism and hypospadias. Epidemiology. 1999; 10:364–369.

Aktuğ T, Akgür FM, Olguner M, et al: Outpatient catheterless Mathieu repair: how to cover ventral penile skin defect. Eur J Pediatr Surg. 1992; 2:99–101.

Albers N, Ulrichs C, Gluer S, et al: Etiologic classification of severe hypospadias: implications for prognosis and management. J Pediatr. 1997; 131: 386–392.

Allen TD, Griffin JE: Endocrine studies in patients with advanced hypospadias. J Urol. 1984; 131:310–314.

Allen TD, Roehrborn CG: Pedicled preputial patch in repair of minor penile chordee with hypospadias. Urology. 1993; 42: 63–65.

Allen TD, Spence HM: The surgical treatment of coronal hypospadias and related problems. J Urol. 1968; 100:504–508.

Allera A, Herbst MA, Griffin JE, et al: Mutations of the androgen receptor coding sequence are infrequent in patients with isolated hypospadias. J Clin Endocrinol Metab. 1995; 80: 2697.

Altemus AR, Hutchins GM: Development of the human anterior urethra. J Urol. 1991; 146:1085–1093.

American Academy of Pediatrics: Timing of elective surgery on the genitalia of male children with particular reference to the risks, benefits, and psychological effects of surgery and anaesthesia. Pediatrics. 1996; 97: 590.

American Academy of Pediatrics, Section of Urology: The timing of elective surgery on genitalia of male children with particular reference to undescended testis and hypospadias. Pediatrics. 1975; 56:479.

American Academy of Pediatrics: Varied opinions and treatment as documented in a survey of the American Academy of Pediatrics, Section of Urology. Urology. 1999; 53:608–612.

Anderson CA, Clark RL: External genitalia of the rat: normal development and the histogenesis of 5-alpha-reductase inhibitor-induced abnormalities. Teratology. 1990; 42: 483–496.

Andrews HO, Nauth-Misir R, Shah PJ: Iatrogenic hypospadias – a preventable injury? Spinal Cord. 1998; 36: 177–180.

Andrich DE, Mundy AR: Substitution urethroplasty with buccal mucosal-free grafts. J Urol. 2001; 165:1131–1134.

Andrich DE, Mundy AR: Urethral strictures and their surgical treatment. BJU Int. 2000; 86:571–580.

Anger MT: Hypospadias péno-scrotal, compliqué de coudure de la verge: redressment du pénis et uréthro-plastie par inclusion cutanée: Guérison. Bull Soc Chir Paris. 1875; p 179.

Anger MT: Hypospadias. Bull Soc Chir Paris. 1874; p 32.

Angerpointer TA: Hypospadias – genetics, epidemiology and other possible aetiological influences. Z Kinderchir. 1984; 39:112–118.

Antyl (1st century AD) In: Hauben DJ (ed): The history of hypospadias. Acta Chir Plast. 1984; 26:196–199.

Appel RA, Kaplan GW, Brock WA: Megalourethra. J Urol. 1986; 135:747.

Arap S, Mitre AI, de Goes GM: Modified meatal advancement and glanuloplasty repair of distal hypospadias. J Urol. 1984; 131:1140–1141.

Arey LB: Developmental anatomy, 7th edn. Saunders, Philadelphia; 1965.

Aronoff M: A one stage operative technique for the treatment of subglandular hypospadias in children. Br J Plastic Surgery. 1963; 16: 59–62.

Asopa HS, Elhence EP, Atria SP, et al: One stage correction of penile hypospadias using a foreskin tube. A preliminary report. Int Surg. 1971; 55:435–440.

Asopa R, Asopa HS: One stage repair of hypospadias using double island preputial skin tube. Int J Urol. 1984; 1:41–43.

Atala A, Cima LG, Kim W, et al: Injectable alginate seeded with chondrocytes as a potential treatment for vesico ureteric reflux. J Urol. 1993; 150:745–747.

Atala A, Freeman MR, Vacanti JP, et al: Implantation in vivo and retrieval of artificial structures consisting of rabbit and human urothelium and human bladder muscle. J Urol. 1993; 150:608–612.

Atala A, Guzman L, Retik AB: A novel inert collagen matrix for hypospadias repair. J Urol. 1999; 162:1148–1152.

Atala A, Kim W, Paige KT, et al: Endoscopic treatment of vesico ureteric reflux with a chondrocyte – alginate suspension. J Urol. 1994; 152:641–643.

Atala A, Vacanti JP, Peters CA, et al: Formation of urothelial structures in vitro from dissociated cells attached to biodegradable polymer scaffolds in vitro. J Urol. 1992; 148:658.

Atallah MM, Saied MM, Yahya R, et al: Presurgical analgesia in children subjected to hypospadias repair. Br J Anaesth. 1993; 71:418–421

Attalla ML: Subcoronal hypospadias with complete prepuce: a distinct entity and new procedure for repair. Br J Plast Surg. 1991; 44:122–125.

Avellán L, Knuttson F: Microscopic studies of curvature-causing structures in hypospadias. Scand J Plast Reconstr Surg. 1980; 14:249–258.

Avellán L: Development of puberty, sexual debut and sexual function in hypospadiacs. Scand J Plast Reconstr Surg. 1976; 10:29–34.

Avellán L: The incidence of hypospadias in Sweden. Scand J Plast Reconstr Surg. 1975; 9:129.

Azmy A, Eckstein HB: Surgical correction of torsion of the penis. Br J Urol. 1981; 53:378–379

Backus LH, de Felice CA: Hypospadias – then and now. Plast Reconstr Surg. 1960; 25:146.

Bagshawe HA, Flynn JT, James AN, et al: The use of thio-glycolic acid in hair bearing skin inlay urethroplasty. Br J Urol. 1980; 52:546–548.

Bainbridge DR, Whitaker RH, Shepheard BGF: BXO and urinary obstruction. Br J Urol. 1994; 74:487–491.

Baker LA, Mathews RL, Docimo SG: Radical bulber dissection to correct severe chordee and proximal hypospadias. J Urol. 2000; 164: 1347–1349.

Balik E, Cetinkursum S, Oztop F: Accessory scrotum: report of a case. Z Kinderchir. 1990; 45:253–254.

Barakat AY, Seikaly MG, Kaloustian VM: Urogenital abnormalities in genetic disease. J Urol. 1986; 136: 778.

Baran NK, Çenetoğlu S: Pictorial history of hypospadias repair techniques. Gazi Medical Faculty, Plast Reconstr Surg. 1993; pp 1–50.

Barbagli G, Palminteri E, Lazzeri M, et al: Long-term outcome of urethroplasty after failed urethrotomy versus primary repair. J Urol. 2001; 165:1918–1919.

Barbagli G, Selli C, Tosto A, et al: Dorsal free graft urethroplasty. J Urol. 1996; 155:123–126

Barcat J: Current concepts of treatment of hypospadias. In: Horton CE (ed): Plastic and reconstructive surgery of the genital area. Little Brown, Boston, 1973; pp 249–263.

Barcat J: L'hypospadias. III. Les urethroplasties, les resultats – les complications. Ann Chir Infant. 1969; 10:310.

Barcat J: Symposium sur l'hypospadias. 16th meeting of the French Society of Children's Surgery. Ann Chir Infant. 1969; 10:287

Barnstein NJ, Mossman HW: The origin of the penile urethra and bulbo-urethral glands with particular reference to the red squirrel (*Tamiasciurus hudsonicus*). Anat Rec. 1938; 72:67–85.

Barraza MA, Roth DR, Terry WJ, et al: One-stage reconstruction of moderately severe hypospadias. J Urol. 1987; 137: 714.

Barroso UJ, Jednak R, Spencer Barthold J, et al: Further experience with the double onlay preputial flap for hypospadias repair. J Urol. 2000; 164: 998–1001.

Barthold JS, Tell TL, Rodman JF: Modified Barcat balanic groove technique for hypospadias repair: experience with 295 cases. J Urol. 1996; 155:1735.

Bartone FF, Adickes ED: Chitosan: effects on wound healing in urogenital tissue: preliminary report. J Urol. 1988; 140(pt 2):1134–1137.

Baskin LS: Controversies in hypospadias surgery: penile curvature. Dial Pediatr Urol. 1996; 19:(8).

Baskin LS: Controversies in hypospadias surgery: the urethral plate. Dial Pediatr Urol. 1996; 19:(8).

Baskin LS: Hypospadias and urethral development. J Urol. 2000; 163:951–956.

Baskin LS: Hypospadias: a critical analysis of cosmetic outcomes using photography. BJU Int. 2001; 87:534–539.

Baskin LS, Duckett JW, Ueoka K, et al: Changing concepts of hypospadias curvature lead to more onlay island flap procedures. J Urol. 1994; 151:191–196.

Baskin LS, Duckett JW: Buccal mucosa grafts in hypospadias surgery. Br J Urol. 1995; 76 [Suppl 3]:23–30.

Baskin LS, Duckett JW: Dorsal tunica albuginea plication for hypospadias curvature. J Urol. 1994; 151:1668–1671.

Baskin LS, Duckett JW: Hypospadias. In: Stringer MD, Mouriquand PDE, Oldham KT, et al (eds): Pediatric surgery and urology: long term outcomes. Saunders, Philadelphia, pp 559–567; 1998.

Baskin LS, Duckett JW: Mucosal grafts in hypospadias and stricture management. AUA Update series. 1994; 13: 270–275.

Baskin LS, Erol A, Li Y, et al: Anatomic studies of hypospadias. J Urol. 1998; 160:1108 – 1115.

Baskin LS, Erol A, Li YW, et al: Anatomy of the neurovascular bundle: is safe mobilization possible? J Urol. 2000; 164: 977–980.

Baskin LS, Himes K, Colborn T: Hypospadias and endocrine disruption: is there a connection? Environ Health Perspect. 2001; 109:1175–1183.

Baskin LS, Liu W, Li YW, et al: FGF-10 gene disruption results in hypospadias. In Section on Urology Program for Scientific Sessions (Poster 31). Presented at 2000 Annual Meeting of the American Academy of Pediatrics, October 28, 2000. Chicago, American Academy of Pediatrics, 2000.

Baskin LS, Lue TF: The correction of congenital penile curvature in young men. Br J Urol. 1998; 81: 895–899.

Batch JA, Evans BAJ, Hughes IA, et al: Mutations of the androgen receptor gene identified in perineal hypospadias. J Med Genet. 1993; 30: 198.

Bauer SB, Bull MJ, Retik AB: Hypospadias: a familial study. J Urol. 1979; 121: 474–477.

Bauer SB, Retik AB, Colodny AH: Genetic aspects of hypospadias. Urol Clin North Am. 1981; 8:559–564.

Beasley SW, Hutson JM, Howat AJ, et al: Posterior extopia of penis mimics marsupial anatomy. Case reported in association with a primitive cloacal anomaly. Pediatr Surg Int. 1987; 2:127–130.

Beck C (1897): Cited by Horton CE, Devine CJ, Baran N: Pictorial history of hypospadias repair techniques. In: Horton CE (ed): Plastic and reconstructive surgery of the genital area. Little Brown, Boston, pp 237–248; 1973.

Beck C: A new operation for balanic hypospadias. NY Med J. 1898; 67:147.

Beck C: Hypospadias and its treatment. Surg Gynecol Obstet. 1917; 24:511.

Bellinger MF: Embryology of the male external genitalia. Urol Clin North Am. 1981; 8: 375–382.

Belman AB: Hypospadias Update. Urology. 1997; 49: 166–172.

Belman AB, Kass EJ: Hypospadias repair in children less than 1 year old. J Urol. 1982; 128:1273–1274.

Belman AB: De-epithelialized skin flap coverage in hypospadias repair. J Urol. 1988; 140:1273–1276.

Belman AB: Editorial comment. J Urol. 1994; 152:1237.

Belman AB: Hypospadias and chordee. In: King LR, Belman AB, Kramer SA (eds): Clinical pediatric urology, 4th edn. Dunitz, London, pp 1061–1092; 2001.

Belman AB: Hypospadias and other urethral abnormalities. In: Kelalis PP, King LR, Belman AB (eds): Clinical pediatric urology, vol 1, 3rd edn. Saunders, Philadelphia, pp 619–663; 1992.

Belman AB: Hypospadias. In: Welch KJ, Randolph JG, Ravitch MM, et al (eds): Pediatric surgery, 4th edn, vol 2. Year Book, Chicago, pp 1286–1302; 1986.

Belman AB: The de-epithelialized flap and its influence on hypospadias repair. J Urol. 1994; 152:2332–2334.

Belman AB: The modified Mustarde hypospadias repair. J Urol. 1982; 127:88–90.

Belman AB: Urethroplasty. Soc Pediatr Urol Newslett. 1977; 12: 1–2.

Ben-Ari J, Merlob P, Mimouni F, et al: Characteristics of the male urethra in the newborn penis. J Urol. 1985; 134: 521–522.

Berg G, Berg R: Castration complex: evidence from men operated for hypospadias. Acta Psychiatr Scand. 1983; 68: 143–153.

Berg G, Berg R, Edman G, et al: Androgens and personality in normal men and men operated for hypospadias in childhood. Acta Psychiatr Scand. 1983; 68:167–177.

Berg R, Berg G: Penile malformations, gender identity and sexual orientation. Acta Psychiatr Scand. 1983; 68:154–166.

Berg R, Berg G, Svensson J: Penile malformations and mental health: a controlled psychiatric study of men operated for hypospadias in childhood. Acta Psychiatr Scand. 1982; 66:398–416.

Berg R, Svensson J, Astrom G: Social and sexual adjustment of men operated for hypospadias during childhood: a controlled study. J Urol. 1981; 125: 313–317.

Bettmann OL, Hinch PS: A pictorial history of medicine, 2nd edn. Thomas, Springfield, Illinois, 1956; pp 4–5.

Bevan AD: A new operation for hypospadias. JAMA. 1917; 68:1032–1034.

Bickerton MW, Duckett JW: Suture material and wound healing. AUA Update Ser. 1984; 3, lesson 15.

Bidder A: Eine Operation der Hypospadie mit Lappenbildung aus dem Scrotum. Dtsch Med Wochenschr. 1892; 10:208.

Bitschai J, Brodny ML: A history of urology in Egypt. Riverside, New York; 1956.

Blair VB, Brown JB, Hamm WG: the correction of scrotal hypospadias and of epispadias. Surg Gynecol Obstet. 1933; 57: 646–653.

Blair VP, Byars LT: Hypospadias and epispadias. J Urol. 1938; 40:814.

Bloom DA, Ritchey M: Anomalies of the urethra. In: Hashmat AI, Das S (eds): The penis. Lea and Febiger, Philadelphia, pp 35–59; 1993.

Blurton Jones N, Konner MJ: Sex differences in behaviour in Bushmen and London two to five year olds. In: Crook J, Michael R (eds): Comparative ecology and behaviour of primates. Academic, New York; 1973.

Bocchiotti G, Bruschi S, Bosetti P, et al: Technical considerations using the Horton-Devine technique in distal hypospadias. Ann Plast Surg. 1982; 9:164–166.

Boddy SA, Samuel M: A natural glanular meatus after "Mathieu and V incision sutured" MAVIS. BJU Int. 2000; 86:394–397.

Boddy SA, Samuel M: Mathieu and 'V' incision sutured (MAVIS) results in a natural glanular meatus. J Pediatr Surg. 2000; 35:494–496.

Boehmer AL, Nijman RJ, Lammers BA, et al: Etiological studies of severe or familial hypospadias. J Urol. 2001; 165:1246–1254.

Boemers TML, De Jong TPVM: The surgical correction of buried penis: a new technique. J Urol. 1995; 154:550.

Bologna RA, Noah TA, Nasrallah PF, et al: Chordee: varied opinions and treatments as documented in a survey of the American Academy of Pediatrics, Section of Urology. Urology. 1999; 53:608–612

Bondonnay JM, Barthaburu D, Vergnes P: L'Hypospadias balanique et penien. Les elements de la malformation; implicatins therapeutiques et resultats. A partir de l'etude de cent trent-cinq dossiers. Ann Urol (Paris). 1984; 18: 21.

Borer JG, Bauer SB, Peters CA, et al: Tubularized incised plate urethroplasty: expanded use in primary and repeat surgery for hypospadias. J Urol. 2001; 165:581.

Borer JG, Retik AB: Current trends in hypospadias repair. Urol Clin North Am. 1999; 26:15–37.

Bouisson MF: De l'hypospadias et de son traitment chirurgical. Trib Chir. 1861; 2:484.

Bouisson MF: Remarques sur quelques variétés de l'hypospadias et sur le traitement qui leur convient. Bull Ther. 1860; 59:349–362.

Bracka A: A long-term view of hypospadias. Br J Plast Surg. 1989; 42:251–255.

Bracka A: A versatile two-stage hypospadias repair. Br J Plast Surg. 1995; 48:345–352.

Bracka A: Hypospadias repair: the two-stage alternative. Br J Urol. 1995; 76 [Suppl 3]:31–41.

Bracka A: Sexuality after hypospadias repair. BJU Int. 1999; 83 (suppl. 3): 29–33.

Bradbury E: Looking different, feeling good: psychological approaches to children and adolescents with disfigurement. A review of the literature 15(1). ACPP Rev Newslett. 1993; 15:1–6

Bramwell RG, Manford ML: Premedication of children with trimeprazine tartrate. Br J Anaesth. 1981; 53:821–826

Brazelton B, Als H: Four early stages in the development of mother-infant interaction. Psychoanal Study Child. 1979; 34:349-369.

Bretteville G: Hypospadias: simple, safe and complete correction in two stages. Ann Plast Surg. 1986; 17:526-531.

Brewer C, Holloway S, Zawalnyski P, et al: A chromosomal deletion map of human malformations. Am J Hum Genet. 1998; 63:1153-1159.

Brewer C, Holloway S, Zawalnyski P, et al: A chromosomal duplication map of malformations: Regions of suspected haplo and triplolethality - and tolerance of segmental aneuploidy - in humans. Am J Hum Genet. 1999; 64: 1702-1708.

Broadbent TR, Woolf RM, Toksu E: Hypospadias - one stage repair. Plast Reconstr Surg. 1961; 27:154-159.

Brodsky MA: Reconstruction of the urethra in hypospadias according to Horton-Devine. Ann Chir Gynaecol. 1980; 69:23-31.

Broman I: Normale und abnorme Entwicklung des Menschen: ein Hand- und Lehrbuch der Ontogenie and Teratologie, speziell für praktische ?rzte und Studierende der Medizin. Bergmann, Wiesbaden; 1911.

Bronshtein M, Riechler A, Zimmier GZ: Prenatal sonographic signs of possible fetal genital anomalies. Prenatal diagnosis. 1995; 15: 215-219.

Browne D: A comparison of the Duplay and Denis Browne techniques for hypospadias operation. Surgery. 1953; 34: 787.

Browne D: An operation for hypospadias. Lancet. 1936; i: 141-149.

Browne D: An operation for hypospadias. Proc R Soc Med. 1949; 41:466-468.

Brueziere J: How I perform the Mathieu technique in the treatment of anterior penile hypospadias. Ann Urol. 1987; 21:277-280.

Bucknall RTH: A new operation for penile hypospadias. Lancet. 1907; 2:887

Burbige KA, Connor JP: Postoperative management of hypospadias. In: Ehrlich RM, Alter GJ (eds): Reconstructive and plastic surgery of the external genitalia, adult and pediatric, 1st edn, chap 33. Saunders, Philadelphia, p 163; 1999.

Burbige KA, Hensle TW, Edgerton P: Extra genital split skin graft for urethral reconstruction. J Urol. 1984; 131: 1137-1139.

Burdorf A, Nieuwenhuisen MJ: Endocrine disrupting chemicals and human reproduction: fact or fiction? Ann Occup Hyg. 1999; 43:435-437.

Burger RA, Muller SC, El-Damanhoury H, et al: The buccal mucosa graft for urethral reconstruction: a preliminary report. J Urol. 1992; 147:662-664.

Buson H, Smiley D, Reinberg Y, et al: Distal hypospadias repair without stents: is it better? J Urol. 1994; 151:1059-1060.

Bussemaker UC, Daremberg CV: Oeuvres d'Oribase, texte Gre, en grande partie inedit collationnée sur les manuscrits (6 vols). Imprimerie National, Paris, pp 1851 ;1876.

Büyükünal SNC, Sarı N: Şarafeddin Sabuncuoğlu, the author of the earliest pediatric surgical atlas: Cerrahiye-i Ilhaniye, J Pediatr Surg. 1991; 26:1148-1151.

Byars LT: A technique for consistently satisfactory repair of hypospadias. Surg Gynecol Obstet. 1955; 100:184-190.

Byers LT: Functional restoration of hypospadias deformities: with a report of 60 completed cases. Surg Gynecol Obstet. 1951; 92: 149-154.

Cabot H: The treatment of hypospadias in theory and practice. N Engl J Med. 1936; 214: 871-875.

Caione P, Capozza N, Lais A, et al: Long term results of the distal urethral advancement glanduloplasty for distal hypospadias. J Urol. 1997; 158:1168-1171.

Caldamone AA, Diamond DA: Contemporary hypospadiology. Contemp Urol. 1999; 11: 61-77.

Caldamone AA, Edstrom LE, Koyle MA, et al: Buccal mucosal grafts for uretheral reconstruction. Urology. 1998; 51: 15-19.

Caldamone AA: Megalourethra. In: Seidmon EJ, Hanno PM (eds): Current urologic therapy. Saunders, Philadelphia, pp 402-403; 1994.

Calzolari E, Contiero MR, Roncarati E, et al: Aetiological factors in hypospadias. J Med Genet. 1986; 23:333-337.

Campbell MF: Hypospadias: when to operate. Am J Surg. 1947; 74: 795-796.

Campbell MF: Anomalies of the genital tract. In: Campbell MF, Harrison JH (eds): Campbell's Urology, 2nd edn. Saunders, Philadelphia, p 1749; 1963.

Campbell MF: Anomalies of the genital tract. In: Campbell MF, Harrison JH (eds): Campbell's Urology, 3rd edn. Saunders, Philadelphia, pp 1576-1577; 1970.

Carbajal R: Analgesia using a 50/50 mixture of nitrous oxide/ oxygen in children. Arch Pediatr. 1999; 6:578-585

Casale AJ, Beck SD, Caiss MP, et al: Concealed penis in childhood. A spectrum of etiology and treatment. J Urol. 1999; 162:1165-1168.

Case GD, Glenn JF, Postlethwait RW: Comparison of absorbable suture in urinary bladder. Urology. 1976; 7:165-168.

Cassar P: A medico-legal report of the 16th century from Malta. Med Hist. 1974; 18:354-359.

Castanon M, Munoz E, Carrasco R, et al: Treatment of proximal hypospadias with a tubularized island flap urethroplasty and the onlay technique: a comparative study. J Pediatr Surg. 2000; 35:1453-1455

Cecil AB: Modern treatment of hypospadias. J Urol. 1952; 67: 1006.

Cecil AB: Repair of hypospadias and urethral fistula. J Urol. 1946; 56:237-242.

Cecil AB: Surgery of hypospadias and epispadias in the male. J Urol. 1932; 27: 507-537.

Cendron J, Melin Y: Congenital curvature of the penis without hypospadias. Urol Clin North Am. 1981; 8: 389-395.

Cerasaro TS, Brock WA, Kaplan GW: Upper urinary tract anomalies with congenital hypospadias: is screening necessary? J Urol. 1986; 135:537-538.

Chambers EL, Malone PSJ: The incidence of hypospadias in two English cities: a case-control comparison of possible causal factors. BJU Int. 1999; 84:95-98.

Changing Faces: Series of booklets for children on coping strategies in cosmetic challenge. Changing Faces, 1 & 2 Junction Mews, London W2 1PN.

Chavez GF, Cordero JR, Beccerra JE: Leading major congenital malformations among minority groups in the United States 1981-1986. MMWR. 1988; 37: 17.

Chen S, Wang G, Wang M: Modified longitudinal preputial island flap urethroplasty for repair of hypospadias: results in 60 patients. J Urol. 1993; 149: 814-816.

Chen SC, Yang SS, Hsieh CH, et al: Tubularized incised plate urethroplasty for proximal hypospadias. BJU Int. 2000; 86:1050.

Chhibber AK, Perkins FM, Rabinowitz R, et al: Penile block timing for postoperative analgesia of hypospadias repair in children. J Urol. 1997; 158:1156-1159

Choi J, Cooper KL, Hensle TW, et al: Incidence and surgical repair rates of hypospadias in New York State. Pediatr Urol. 2001; 57:151–153.

Churchill BM, van Savage JG, Khoury AE, et al: The dartos flaps as an adjunct in preventing urethrocutaneous fistulas in repeat hypospadias surgery. J Urol. 1996; 156:2047–2049.

Cilento BG, Freeman MR, Schneck FX et al: Phenotypic and cytogenic characterisation of human bladder urothelia expanded in vitro. J Urol. 1994; 152:665.

Cilento BG, Retik AB, Atala A: Urothelial reconstruction using a polymer mesh. J Urol. 1995; 153:371A.

Cilento BG, Stock JA, Kaplan GW: Pantaloon spica cast: an effective method for postoperative immobilization after free graft hypospadias repair. J Urol. 1997; 157:1882.

Clark WR, Grunstein M: Are we hard wired? The role of human behaviour. Oxford University Press, Oxford; 2000.

Clarnette TD, Sugita Y, Hutson JM: Genital anomalies in human and animal models reveal the mechanisms and hormones governing testicular descent. Br J Urol. 1997; 79:99–112.

Cloutier A: A method for hypospadias repair. Plast Reconstr Surg. 1962; 30:368–373.

Cohen EL, Kirschenbaum A, Glenn JF: Preclinical evaluation of PDS (polydioxanone) synthetic absorbable suture vs chromic surgical gut in urologic surgery. Urology. 1987; 30:369–372.

Colborn T: Environmental estrogens: health implications for humans and wildlife. Environ Health Perspect. 1995; 103 [Suppl 7]:135–136.

Cook WA, Stephens FD: Pathoembryology of the urinary tract. In: King LR (ed): Urological surgery in neonates and young infants. Saunders, Philadelphia, 1988; pp 1–23.

Cooper CS, Noh PH, Snyder HM III: Preservation of urethral plate spongiosum: technique to reduce hypospadias fistulas. Urology. 2001; 57:351–354.

Coplen DE, Manley CB: Timing of Genital surgery. In: Eherlish RM, Alter GJ (eds): Reconstructive and plastic surgery of the external genitalia, adult and pediatric, 1st edn. Philadelphia, Saunders;1999.

Coran AG: A simplified technique for performing perineal urethrostomy. Surg Gynecol Obstet. 1980; 150:735.

Cote GB, Petmezaki S, Bastakis N: A gene for hypospadias in a child with presumed tetrasomy 18p. Am J Med Genet. 1979; 4:141–146.

Cracco A, Dettin C, Cordaro S, et al: Psychological study of adults surgically treated in childhood for hypospadias. Pediatr Med Chir. 1989; 11:447–450.

Creevy CD: The correction of hypospadias: a review. Urol Surv. 1958; 8: 2–47.

Cromie WJ, Bellinger MF: Hypospadias dressings and diversions. Urol Clin North Am. 1981; 8:545.

Cronin TD, Guthrie TH: Method of Cronin and Guthrie of hypospadias repair. In: Horton CE (ed): Plastic and reconstructive surgery of the genital area. Little Brown, Boston, pp 302–314; 1973.

Culp OS: Experiences with 200 hypospadiacs: evolution of a therapeutic plan. Surg Clin North Am. 1959; 39:1007–1013.

Culp OS: Struggles and triumphs with hypospadias and associated anomalies. Review of 400 cases. J Urol. 1966; 96:339–355.

Culp OS, McRoberts JW: Hypospadias. In: Alken CE, Dix VW, Goodwin WE, et al (eds): Encyclopaedia of urology. Springer, Berlin Heidelberg New York, pp 11307–11344; 1968.

Czeizel A: Increasing morbidity in the male reproductive system. Lancet. 1985; 1:462–463.

Daniels L, Visram A: Should parents be present and assist during inhalational induction of their child? A survey of the APA. Paediatr Anaesth. 2002; 12:821

Daskalopoulos BI, Baskin L, Duckett JW, et al: Congenital penile curvature (chordee without hypospadias). Urology. 1993; 42:708.

Davenport H, Werry J: The effect of general anesthesia, surgery, and hospitalization upon the behavior of children. Am J Orthopsychiatry. 1970; 40:806–824.

Davenport M, MacKinnon AE: The value of ultrasound screening for the upper urinary tract in hypospadias. Br J Urol. 1988; 62:595–596.

Davis DM: The pedicle tube graft in the surgical treatment of hypospadias in the male with new method of closing small urethra fistulas. Surg Gynecol Obstet. 1940; 71:790.

Davis DM: The surgical treatment of hypospadias, especially scrotal and perineal. Plast Reconstr Surg. 1950; 5:373.

Davits RJ, Vanden Aker ES, Scholineijer RJ, et al: Effect of parenteral testosterone therapy on penile development in boys with hypospadias. Br J Urol. 1993; 71:593.

Dayanc M, Tan MO, GoKalp A, et al: Tubularized incised plate urethroplasty for distal and mid penile hypospadias. Eur Urol. 2000; 37:102–125.

De Badiola F, Anderson K, Gonzalez R: Hypospadias repair in an outpatient setting without proximal urinary diversion: experience with 113 urethroplasties. J Pediatr Surg. 1991; 26:461–465.

De Gier RP, Feita WF, de Vries JD: Wall dissection of the neourethra, a rare condition after hypospadias repair. Urology. 1997; 50:462–464.

De Grazia E, Cigna RM, Cimador M: Modified Mathieu's technique: a variation of the classical procedure for hypospadias repair. Eur J Pediatr Surg. 1997; 8:98–99.

De Jong T, Boemers TM: Improved Mathieu repair for coronal and distal hypospadias with moderate chordee. Br J Urol. 1993; 72:972–974.

De Negri P, Ivani G, Visconti C, et al: How to prolong postoperative analgesia after caudal anaesthesia with ropivacaine in children: S-ketamine versus clonidine. Paediatr Anaesth. 2001; 11:679–683

De Pasquale I, Park AJ, Bracka A: The treatment of balanitis xerotica obliterans. BJU Int. 2000; 86:459–465.

De Sy WA: aesthetic repair of meatal stricture. J Urol. 1984; 132: 678–679.

De Sy WA, Oosterlinck W: One-stage hypospadias repair by free full-thickness skin graft and island flap techniques. Urol Clin North Am. 1981; 8:491.

De Sy WA, Oosterlink W: Silicone foam elastomer: a significant improvement in postoperative penile dressing. J Urol. 1982; 128:39.

De Vries PA, Friedland GW: The staged sequential development of the anus and rectum in human embryos and fetuses. J Pediatr Surg. 1987; 9:755–769.

Decter RM: Chordee correction by corporal rotation, the split and roll technique. J Urol. 1999; 162:1152–1154

Decter RM: M inverted V glansplasty: a procedure for distal hypospadias. J Urol. 1991; 146:641–643.

Decter RM, Franzoni DF: Distal hypospadias repair by the modified Thiersch–Duplay technique with or without hinging the urethral plate: a near ideal way to correct distal hypospadias. J Urol. 1999 ; 162:1156.

Decter RM, Roth DR, Gonzales JR: Hypospadias repair by bladder mucosal graft: an initial report. J Urol. 1988; 140:1256–1258.

Deibert GA: The separation of the prepuce in the human penis. Anat Rec. 1933; 57:387.

Demirbilek S, Atayurt HF: One-stage hypospadias repair with stent or suprapubic diversion: which is better? J Pediatr Surg. 1997; 32:1711–1712.

Demirbilek S, Kanmaz T, Aydin G, et al: Outcomes of one-stage techniques for proximal hypospadias repair. Urology. 2001; 58:267–270.

Denson CE, Terry WJ: Hypospadias repair. Preoperative preparation, intraoperative techniques, postoperative care. AORN J. 1988; 47:906–915, 918–924

Des Prez JD, Persky L, Kiehn CL: A one stage repair of hypospadias by island flap technique. Plast Reconstr Surg. 1961; 28:405–411.

Desautel MG, Stock J, Hanna MK: Mullerian duct remnants: surgical management and fertility issues. J Urol. 1999; 162:1008–1013.

Dessanti A, Cossu ML, Noya G, et al: Separation and rotation of corpora in the treatment of chordee penis with hypospadias. Eur J Pediatr surg. 1995 ; 5: 92.

Dessanti A, Rigamonti W, Merulla V, et al: Autologous buccal mucosa graft for hypospadias repair: an initial report. J Urol. 1992; 147:1081–1084.

Devesa R, Munoz A, Torrents M, et al: Prenatal diagnosis of isolated hypospadias. Prenat Diagn. 1998 ; 18: 779.

Devine CJ Jr, Gonsalez-Serva L, Stecker JF Jr, et al: Utricle configuration in hypospadias and intersex. J Urol. 1980; 123: 407.

Devine CJ Jr, Horton CE: A one-stage hypospadias repair. J Urol. 1961; 85:166–172.

Devine CJ Jr, Horton CE: Chordee without Hypospadias. J Urol. 1973;110: 264–271.

Devine CJ Jr, Horton CE: Hypospadias repair. J Urol. 1977; 118:188–193.

Devine CJ Jr, Horton CE: Use of dermal graft to correct chordee. J Urol. 1975; 113:56–58.

Devine CJ Jr, Horton CE, Gilbert DA, et al: Hypospadias. In: Mustarde JC, Jackson IT (eds): Plastic surgery in infancy and childhood, 3rd edn, chap 31. Churchill Livingstone, Edinburgh, pp 493–509; 1988.

Devine CJ, Blackly SK, Horton CE, et al: The surgical treatment of chordee without hypospadias in men. J Urol. 1991; 146:325–329.

Dewan PA, Dinneen MD, Duffy PG, et al: Pedicle patch urethroplasty. Br J Urol. 1991; 67: 420–423.

Dewan PA, Dinneen MD, Winkle D, et al: Hypospadias: duckett pedicle tube urethroplasty. Eur Urol. 1991; 20: 39–42.

Dhillon R, Cumming CE, Cumming DC: Psychological well being and coping patterns in infertile men. Fertil Steril. 2000; 74:702–706.

Dieffenbach JF: Die operative Chirurgie. Brockhaus, Leipzig; 1845.

Dieffenbach JF: Guérison des fentes congénitales de la verge, de l'hypospadias. Gaz Hebd Med. 1837; 5:156.

Dieffenbach JF: The simple canalization method. In: Dictionnaire encyclopedie de medecine. Biblioteque Nationale de Paris, France; 1838.

Diez-Garcia R, Banuelos A, Marin C, et al: Penoscrotal transposition. Eur J Pediatr Surg. 1995; 5:222–225.

Dingwall EJ: Male infibulation. Bale and Danielson, London; 1925.

Dionis P: Course of chirurgical operations demonstrated in Royal Garden at Paris, 2nd edn. J Tonson, London, pp 137–155 ; 1733.

Dionis P: In: Haeger K (ed): The illustrated history of surgery. Harold Strake, London, pp 132–134; 1718.

DiSandro M, Palmer JM: stricture incidence related to suture material in hypospadias surgery. J Pediatr Surg. 996; 31: 881–884.

Docimo SG: Subcutaneous frenulum flap (SCFP) for iatrogenic or primary megameatus and re-operative hypospadias repair. Urology. 2001; 58: 261–273.

Dodd M, Lawson P, Hayman J: Squamous cell carcinoma of the distal urethra in a patient with congenital hypospadias. Pathology. 1996; 28:96–97.

Dolatzas T, Chiotopoulos D, Antipas S, et al: Hypospadias repair in children: review of 250 cases. Pediatr Surg Int. 1994; 9:383–386.

Dolk H, Vrijheid M, Armstrong B, et al: Risk of congenital anomalies near hazardous-waste landfill sites in Europe: The EUROHAZCON Study. Lancet. 1998; 352:423–427.

Dolk H: Rise in prevalence of hypospadias. Lancet. 1998; 351:770.

Donnahoo KK, Cain MP, Pope JC, et al: Etiology, management and surgical complications of congenital chordee without hypospadias. J Urol. 1998; 160: 1120–1122.

Donnenfeld AE, Schrager DS, Corson SL: Update on a family with hand – foot- genital syndrome: hypospadias and urinary tract abnormalities in two boys from the fourth generation. Am J Med Genet. 1992; 44: 482.

Donohue PK, Keating MA: Preputial unfurling to correct the buried penis. J Pediatr Surg. 1986; 21:1055–1057.

Dorairajan T: Defects of spongy tissue and congenital diverticula of the penile urethra. Aust NZ J Surg. 1963; 32: 209.

Driscoll SG, Taylor SH: Effects of prenatal maternal estrogen on the male urogenital system. Obstet Gynecol. 1980; 56: 537.

Duckett JW (quoted in Duckett et al): Proceedings of the Annual Meeting of the Society of Paediatric Urological Surgeons. Southampton, UK, 3 June 1986.

Duckett JW: Foreword: Symposium on hypospadias. Urol Clin North Am. 1981; 8: 371–373.

Duckett JW: Hypospadias. Clin Plast Surg. 1980; 7:149.

Duckett JW: Hypospadias. In: Gillenwater JY, Grayhack JT, Howards SS, et al (eds): Adult and pediatric urology, 1st edn, vol II. Year Book Medical Publishers, Chicago, pp 1880–1915; 1987.

Duckett JW: Hypospadias. In: Walsh PC, Gittes RF, Perlmutter AD, et al (eds): Campbell's urology, 5th edn. Saunders, Philadelphia, pp 1969–1999; 1986.

Duckett JW: Hypospadias. In: Webster G, Kirby R, King L, Goldwasser B (eds): Reconstructive urology, vol 2, chap 54. Blackwell Scientific, Boston, 1993; pp 763–780.

Duckett JW: MAGPI (meatal advancement and glanuloplasty): a procedure for subcoronal hypospadias. Urol Clin North Am. 1981; 8:513.

Duckett JW: Repair of hypospadias. In: Hendry WF (ed): Recent advances in urology/andrology, vol 3. Churchill-Livingstone, New York, pp 279–290; 1980.

Duckett JW: Successful hypospadias repair. Contemp Urol. 1992; 4:42–55.

Duckett JW: The current hype in hypospadiology. Br J Urol. 1995; 76 [Suppl 3]:1–7.

Duckett JW: The island flap technique for hypospadias repair. Urol Clin North Am. 1981; 8:503–511.

Duckett JW: Transverse preputial island flap technique for repair of severe hypospadias. Urol Clin North Am. 1980; 7:423–431.

Duckett JW: Use of buccal mucosa urethroplasty in epispadias. Meeting of Society of Pediatric Urology, Southampton, England. 1986.

Duckett JW, Baskin LS: Hypospadias. In: Gillenwater JY, Grayhack JT, Howards SS, et al (eds): Adult and pediatric urology, vol 3, 3rd edn, Chap 55. Mosby, St Louis. pp 2549–2589; 1996.

Duckett JW, Caldamone AA, Snyder HM: Hypospadias fistula repair without diversion (abstract 11). Proceedings of the Annual Meeting of the American Academy of Pediatrics, New York, Oct 1982, pp 23–28.

Duckett JW, Coplen D, Ewalt D, et al: Buccal mucosa urethral replacement. J Urol. 1995; 153:1660–1663.

Duckett JW, Devine CJ Jr, Mitchell ME, et al: Controversies in hypospadias surgery. Dial Pediatr Urol. 1996; 19: 8.

Duckett JW, Kaplan GW, Woodard JR, et al: Complications of hypospadias repair. Urol Clin North Am. 1980; 7:443–454.

Duckett JW, Keating MA: Technical challenge of the megameatus intact prepuce hypospadias variant: the pyramid procedure. J Urol. 1989; 141:1407.

Duckett JW, Smith GHH: Urethral lesions in infants and children. In: Gillenwater JY, Grayhack JT, Howards SS, et al (eds): Adult and pediatric urology, 3rd edn. St Louis, Mosby, pp 2411–2413; 1996.

Duckett JW, Snyder H: The MAGPI hypospadias repair in 1111 patients. Ann Surg. 1991; 213:620–626.

Duckett JW, Snyder HM: Hypospadias "pearls". Soc Pediatr Urol Newslett. 1985; 7:4.

Duckett JW, Snyder HM: Meatal advancement and glanuloplasty hypospadias repair after 1000 cases: avoidance of meatal stenosis and regression. J Urol. 1992; 147:665–669.

Duel BP, Barthold JS, Gonzales R: Management of urethral strictures after hypospadias repair. J Urol. 1998; 160:170–171.

Duffy PG, Ransley PG, Malone PS, et al: Combined free autologous bladder mucosa/skin tube for urethral reconstruction: an update. Br J Urol. 1988; 61:505.

Duplay S: Asselin, Paris; 1874 (also in Arch Gen Med 1:513:1:657, 1874; and in Bull Soc Chir Paris. 49:157).

Duplay S: De l'hypospade périnéo-scrotal et de son traitement chirurgical. Arch Gen Med. 1874; 1:613–657.

Duplay S: De l'hypospadias périnéo-scrotal et de son traitment chirurgical. Asselin, Paris, 1874.

Duplay S: Sur le traitement chirugical de l'hypospadias et de l'épispadias. Arch Gen Med. 1880; 5:257.

Eberle J, Uberreiter S, Radmyr C, et al: Posterior hypospadias: long term follow-up after reconstructive surgery in the male direction. J Urol. 1993; 150:1474–1477.

Edlick RF, Rodeheaver GT, Thacker JG: Considerations in the choice of suture for wound closure of the genitourinary tract. J Urol. 1987; 137:373–379.

Edmunds A: An operation for hypospadias. Lancet. 1913; 1: 447–449.

Edmunds A: Pseudohermaphroditism and hypospadias: their surgical treatment. Lancet. 1926; 1: 323–327.

Ehle JJ, Cooper CS, Peche WJ, et al: Application of the Cecil-Culp repair for treatment of urethrocutaneous fistulas after hypospadias surgery. Urology. 2001; 57:347–350.

Ehrlich RM, Alter G: Split-thickness skin graft urethroplasty and tunica vaginalis flaps for failed hypospadias repairs. J Urol. 1996; 155:131–134.

Ehrlich RM, Reda EF, Koyle MA, et al: Complications of bladder mucosal graft. J Urol. 1989; 142:626–627.

Ehrlich RM, Scardino PT: Surgical correction of scrotal transposition and perineal hypospadias. J Pediatr Surg. 1982; 17:175–177.

Elbakry A: Complications of the preputial island flap tube urethroplasty. BJU Int. 1999; 84:89–94.

Elbakry A: Further experience with the tubularized-incised urethral plate technique for hypospadias repair. BJU Int. 2002; 89:291–294.

Elbakry A: Management of urethrocutaneous fistula after hypospadias repair: 10 years' experience. BJU Int. 2001; 88:590–595.

Elbakry A: Tubularized-incised urethral plate urethroplasty: is regular dilatation necessary for success? BJU Int. 1999; 84:683–688.

Elbakry A, Shamaa M, Al Atrash G: An axially vascularised meatal-based flap for the repair of hypospadias[see comments]. Br J Urol. 1998; 82: 698–703.

Elder JS: Abnormalities of the genitalia in boys and their surgical management. In Walsh PC (ed): Campbell's urology, 8th edn, chap 66. Saunders, Philadelphia, pp 2334–2352; 2002.

Elder JS, Duckett JW: Urethral reconstruction following an unsuccessful one-stage hypospadias repair. World J Urol. 1987; 5:16–19.

Elder JS, Duckett JW, Snyder HM: Onlay island flap in the repair of mid and distal penile hypospadias without chordee. J Urol. 1987; 138:376–379.

Elias ER, Irons MB, Hurley AD, et al: Clinical effects of cholesterol supplementation in six patients with the Smith–Lemli–Opitz syndrome (SLOS). Am J Med Genet. 1997; 68:305–310.

El-Kasaby AW, El-Beialy H, El-Halaby R, et al: Urethroplasty using transverse penile island flap for hypospadias. J Urol. 1986; 136:643–644.

Ellis H: A history of surgery. Greenwich Medical Media, London, pp 4–5; 2001.

El-Mahrouky A, McElhaney J, Bartone FF, et al: In vitro comparison of the properties of polydioxanone, polyglycolic acid and catgut sutures in sterile and infected urine. J Urol. 1987; 138:913–915.

Emir H, Jayanthi VR, Nitahara K, et al: Modification of the Koyanagi technique for the single stage repair of proximal hypospadias. J Urol. 2000; 164:973–976.

England MA: A colour atlas of life before birth. Normal fetal development. Wolfe Medical Publications, Weert, Netherlands; 1983.

Eppley BL, Keating M, Rink R: A buccal mucosal harvesting technique for urethral reconstruction. J Urol. 1997; 157: 1268–1270.

Etker AS, Duffy PG, Ransley PG: Buccal mucosa graft urethroplasty: the first 50 cases. Abstract of the British Association of Urological Surgeons ; 1993.

EUROCAT Working Group: EUROCAT Report 8. Surveillance of congenital anomalies in Europe 1980–1999, University of Ulster, 2002.

EUROCAT Working Group: EUROCAT Special Report, an assessment and analysis of existing surveillance data on hypospadias in UK and Europe, University of Ulster, 2002.

Fabricii ab Aquapendente H: Opera Chirurgica Patavii: Franciscum Bolzettam, 1641.

Fabricii ab Aquapendente H: Opera Chirurgica Venetiis: Apud Robertum Megliettum, 1619.

Fairbanks JL, Sheldon CA, Khoury AE, et al: Free bladder mucosal graft biology: unique engraftment characteristics in rabbits. J Urol. 1992; 148:663–666.
Falkowski WS, Firlit CF: Hypospadias surgery: the X-shaped elastic dressing. J Urol. 1980; 123:904.
Farkas LG: Hypospadias: some causes of recurrence of ventral curvature of the penis following the straightening procedure. Br J Plast Surg. 1967; 20: 199–203.
Fevre M: Technique for anterior hypospadias. J Chir. 1961; 81:562
Fichtner J, Filipas D, Mottrie AM, et al: Analysis of meatal location in 500 men: wide variation questions the need for meatal advancement in all pediatric anterior hypospadias cases. J Urol. 1995; 154:833–834.
Filipas D, Fisch M, Fichtner J, et al: The histology and immunohistochemistry of free buccal mucosa and full-skin grafts after exposure to urine. BJU Int. 1999; 84:108–111.
Filler J: Disease. British Museum Press, London, p 90; 1995.
Firlit CF: The mucosal collar in hypospadias surgery. J Urol. 1987; 127:80–82.
Fisch H, Golden RJ, Libersen GL, et al: Maternal age as a risk factor for hypospadias. J Urol. 2001; 165:934–936.
Flack CE, Walker RD 3rd: Onlay tube onlay urethroplasty technique in primary perineal hypospadias surgery. J Urol. 1995; 154: 837–839.
Flynn JT, Johnston SR, Blandy JP: The late sequelae of hypospadias repair. Br J Urol. 1980; 52:555–559.
Foley SJ, Denny A, Malone PS: Combined buccal mucosal grafting and Snodgrass technique for salvage hypospadias repairs: a promising alternative (abstract). BJU Int. 2000; 85 [Suppl 5]:46.
Forsberg JG: On the development of the cloaca and the perineum and the formation of the urethral plate in female rat embryos. J Anat. 1961; 95:423–435.
Forshall E, Rickham PP: Transposition of penis and scrotum. Br J Urol. 1956; 28:250–252.
Franzoni DF, Decter RM: Distal hypospadias repair by the modified Thiersch – Duplay technique with or without hinging the urethral plate: near ideal way to correct distal hypospadias. J Urol. 1999; 162; 1156.
Fredell L, Iselius L, Collins A, et al: Complex segregation analysis of hypospadias. Hum Genet. 2002; 111:231–234.
Fredell L, Lichtenstien P, Pedersen NL, et al: Hypospadias is related to birth weight in discordant monozygotic twins. J Urol. 1998; 160: 2197–2199.
Freedman AL: Dressings, stents and tubes. In: Ehrlich RM, Alter GJ (eds): Reconstructive and plastic surgery of the external genitalia, adult and pediatric, chap 32, 1st edn. Saunders, Philadelphia, pp 159–162; 1999.
Freedman DG: Sexual dysmorphism and status hierarchy. In: Omark FF, Strayer S, Freedman DG (eds): Dominance relations. Garland, New York, pp 261–271; 1980.
Frey P, Bianchi A: One-stage preputial pedicle flap repair for hypospadias: experience with 100 patients. Prog Pediatr Surg. 1989; 23:181–191.
Friedrich MG, Evans D, Noldus J, et al: The correction of penile curvature with the Essed-Schroder technique: a long-term follow-up assessing functional aspects and quality of life. BJU Int. 2000; 86:1034–1038.
Fritz G, Czeizel AE: Abnormal sperm morphology and function in the fathers of hypospadias. J Reprod Fertil. 1996; 106:63–66.
Frydmen M, Greiber C, Cohen HA: Uncomplicated familial hypospadias: evidence for autosomal recessive inheritance. Am J Med Genet. 1985; 21:51–55.

Galen (c. 130–201 A.D.) In: Opera omnia, vol 10. Kühn, Leipzig, Cnobloch, p 1001
Gallentin ML, Moreu AF, Thompson IM Jr: Hypospadias: a contemporary epidemiologic assessment. Pediatr Urol. 2001; 57:788–790.
Garcia AM, Fletcher T, Benafvides FG, et al: Parental agricultural work and selected congenital malformations. Am J Epidemiol. 1999; 149:64–74.
Garfield JM: Psychologic problems in anesthesia. Am Fam Physician. 1974; 10:60–67.
Garibay JT, Reid C, Gonzalez R: Functional evaluation of the results of hypospadias surgery with uroflowmetry. J Urol. 1995; 154:835–836.
Gaylis FD, Zaontz MR, Dalton D, et al: Silicone foam dressing for penis after reconstructive pediatric surgery. Urology. 1989; 33:296–299.
Gearhart JP, Borland RN: Onlay island flap urethroplasty: variation on a theme. J Urol. 1992; 148:1507–1509.
Gearhart JP, Donohue PA, Brown TR, et al: Endocrine evaluation of adults with mild hypospadias. J Urol. 1990; 144: 274–277.
Gearhart JP, Jeffs RD: The use of parenteral testosterone therapy in genital reconstructive surgery. J Urol. 1987; 138: 1077–1078.
Gearhart JP, Linhard HR, Berkovitz GD, et al: Androgen receptor levels and 5 ? reductase activities in preputial skin and chordee tissue of boys with isolated hypospadias. J Urol. 1988 ; 140: 1243.
Gelbard MK: Correction of penile curvature using tunica albuginea plication, flaps and expansion with fascial grafts. In: Ehrlich RM, Alter GJ (eds): Reconstructive and plastic surgery of the external genitalia, adult and pediatrics, 1st edn. Saunders, Philadelphia, pp 479–488; 1999.
Ghali AMA, El-Malik EMA, Al-Malki T, et al: One-stage hypospadias repair. Eur Urol. 1999; 36:436–442.
Gibbons MD, Gonzales ET: The subcoronal meatus. J Urol. 1983; 130:739–742.
Gibbons MD: Nuances of distal hypospadias. Urol Clin North Am. 1985; 12:169–174.
Gilbert DA, Jordan GH, Devine CJ Jr, et al: Phallic construction in prepubertal and adolescent boys. J Urol. 1993; 149: 1521.
Gill WB, Schumacher GFB, Bibbs M: structural and functional abnormalities in the sex organs of male offspring of mothers treated with diethylestilbestrol (DES). J Reprod Med. 1976; 16: 147.
Gittes RF, McLaughlin AP III: Injection technique to induce penile erection. Urology. 1974; 4:473–474.
Glassberg K, Hansbrough F, Horowitz M: The Koyanagi-Nonomura 1-stage bucket repair of severe hypospadias with and without penoscrotal transposition. J Urol. 1998; 160:1104.
Glassberg KI: Augmented Duckett repair for severe hypospadias. J Urol. 1987; 138: 380–381.
Glassman CN, Machlus BJ, Kelalis PP: Urethroplasty for hypospadias: long term results. Urol Clin North Am. 1980; 7:437.
Glenister TW: A consideration of the processes involved in the development of the prepuce in man. Br J Urol. 1956; 28:243.
Glenister TW: A correlation of the normal and abnormal development of the penile urethra and of the infra-umbilical abdominal wall. Br J Urol. 1958; 30:117–126.
Glenister TW: The origin and fate of the urethral plate in man. J Anat. 1954; 288:413–425.

Glenn JF, Anderson EE: Surgical correction of incomplete penoscrotal transposition. J Urol. 1973; 110:603–605.

Goldman AS, Bongiovanni AM: Induced genital anomalies. Ann N Y Acad Sci. 1967; 141: 755–767.

Goldstein HR, Hensle TW: Simplified closure of hypospadias fistulas. Urology. 1981; 18: 504–505.

Gonsalez ET Jr: Hypospadias repair. In: Glenn JF (ed.): Urologic Surgery. Philadelphia, Lippincott; 1991.

Gonzales E, Veeraraghavan K, Delaune J: The management of distal hypospadias with meatal-based vascularized flaps. J Urol. 1983; 129:119–120.

Gonzales R, Fernandes ET: Single stage feminisation genitoplasty. J Urol. 1990; 143:776–778.

Gonzalez R, Smith C, Denes ED: Double onlay preputial flap for proximal hypospadias repair. J Urol. 1996; 156:832–834; discussion 834–835.

Gough DCS, Dickson A, Tsung T: Mathieu hypospadias repair: postoperative care. In: Thüroff JW, Hohenfellner M (eds): Reconstructive surgery of the lower urinary tract in children. ISIS Medical Media, Oxford, pp 55–58; 1995.

Granato R: Surgical approach to male transsexualism. Urology. 1974; 3:792–797.

Greene RR, Burrill MW, Ivy AC: Experimental intersexuality: the production of feminized male rats by antenatal treatment with estrogens. Science. 1938;88:130–131.

Greenfield SP, Sadler BT, Wan J: Two-stage repair for severe hypospadias. J Urol. 1994; 152:498–501.

Greenwell TJ, Venn SN, Mundy AR: Changing practice in anterior urethroplasty. BJU Int. 1999; 83:631–635.

Griffin JE: Androgen resistance: the clinical and molecular spectrum. N Engl J Med. 1992; 326:611–618.

Griffin JE, Wilson JD: Syndromes of androgen resistance. Hosp Pract Off Ed. 1987; 22: 159–164.

Guthrie RD, Smith DW, Graham CB: Testosterone treatment for micropenis during early chilhood. J Pediatr. 1973; 87: 247.

Gutierrez Segura C: Urine flow in childhood: a study of flow chart parameters based on 1,361 uroflowmetry tests. J Urol. 1997; 157: 1426–1428.

Haberlick A, Schmidt B, Uray E, et al: Hypospadias repair using a modification of Beck's operation: followup. J Urol. 1997; 157:2308–2311.

Hacker V: Zur operativen Behandlung der Hypospadia Glandis. Beitr Z Klin Chir. 1898; 22:271–276.

Hadidi A, Abdaal N, Kaddah S: Hypospadias repair: is dressing important? Kasr El Aini J Surg. 2003; 4(1):37–44.

Hadidi A, Abdaal N, Kaddah S: Hypospadias repair: is stenting important? Kasr El Aini J Surg. 2003:4(2) 3–8.

Hadidi AT: Lateral based flap with dual blood supply: a single stage repair for proximal hypospadias. Egypt. J. Plast. Reconstr. Surg. 2003;27(3).

Hadidi AT: Y-V Glanuloplasty: a new modification in the surgery of hypospadias. Kasr El Aini Med J. 1996; 2:223–233.

Hafez AT, Smith CR, McLorie GA, et al: Tunica vaginalis for correcting penile chordee in a rabbit model: is there a difference in flap versus graft? J Urol. 2001; 166:1429–1432.

Hagner FR: A new method for straightening the penis in hypospadias. JAMA. 1932; 99: 116.

Hakim S, Merguerian PA, Rabinowitz R, et al: Outcome analysis of the modified Mathieu hypospadias repair: comparison of stented and unstented repairs. J Urol. 1996; 156:836–838.

Hamdy H, Awadhi MA, Rasromani KH: Urethral mobilization and meatal advancement: a surgical principle in hypospadias repair. Pediatr Surg Int. 1999; 15:240–242.

Hamilton JM: Island flap repair of hypospadias. South Med J. 1969; 62: 881–882.

Hamilton SA, Clinch PJ, Goodman PJ, et al: The objective assessment of hypospadias repair (abstract). BJU Int. 2000; 85 [Suppl 5]:45–46.

Harris DL: Splitting the prepuce to provide two independently vascularised flaps: A one-stage repair of hypospadias and congenital short urethra. Br J Plast Surg. 1984; 37: 108–116.

Harris DL, Jeffrey RS: One-stage repair of hypospadias using split preputial flaps (Harris). Br J Urol. 1989; 63:401–407.

Harris EL, Beaty TH: Segregation analysis of hypospadias: a reanalysis of published pedigree data. Am J Med Genet. 1993; 45:420–425.

Harrison DH, Grobbelaar AO: Urethral advancement and glanuloplasty (UGPI): a modification of the MAGPI procedure for distal hypospadias. Br J Plast Surg. 1997; 50:206.

Hastie KJ, Deshpande SS, Moisey CU: Long-term follow-up of the MAGPI operation for distal hypospadias. Br J Urol. 1989; 63:320–322.

Hatch DA, Maizels M, Zaontz MR, et al: Hypospadias hidden by a complete prepuce. Surg Gynecol Obstet. 1989; 169: 233–234.

Hatch DJ: New inhalational agents in paediatric anaesthesia. Br J Anaesth. 1999; 83:42–49

Hauben DJ: The history of hypospadias. Acta Chir Plast. 1984; 26: 196–199.

Hayashi Y, Kojima Y, Mizuno K, et al: Tubularized incised-plate urethroplasty for secondary hypospadias surgery. Int J Urol. 2001; 8:444–448.

Hayashi Y, Sasaki S, Kojima Y, et al: Primary and salvage urethroplasty using Mathieu meatal-based flip-flap technique for distal hypospadias. Int J Urol. 2001; 8:10–16.

Hayes MC, Malone PS: The use of a dorsal buccal mucosal graft with urethral plate incision (Snodgrass) for hypospadias salvage. BJU Int. 1999; 83:508–509.

Heaton BW, Snow BW, Cartwright PC: Repair of urethral diverticulum by plication. Urology. 1994; 44:749–752.

Heinen M, Magna C, Corti A: Caudal anesthesia for hypospadias operations in children. Pediatr Med Chir. 1985; 7: 879–880

Heister L: General system of surgery in three parts. Winnys, London, 1743; pp 129–138; 243–250.

Henderson BE, Benton B, Cosgrove M, et al: Urogenital tract abnormalities in sons of women treated with diethylstilbestrol. Pediatrics. 1976; 58:505–507.

Hendren WH: Construction of a female urethra using the vaginal wall and a buttock flap: experence with 40 cases. J Paediatr Surg. 1998; 33:180–187.

Hendren WH: The Belt-Fuqua for repair of hypospadias. Urol Clin North Am. 1981; 8:431.

Hendren WH, Crooks KK: Tubed free skin graft for construction of male urethra. J Urol. 1980; 123:858.

Hendren WH, Horton CE Jr: Experience with one-stage repair of hypospadias and chordee using free graft of prepuce. J Urol 1988; 140:1259.

Hendren WH, Keating MA: Use of dermal graft and free urethral graft in penile reconstruction. J Urol. 1988; 140: 1265–1269

Hendren WH, Reda EF: Bladder mucosa graft for construction of male urethra. J Pediatr Surg. 1986; 21:189.

Hensle TW, Badillo F, Burbige KA: Experience with the MAGPI hypospadias repair. J Paediatr Surg. 1983; 18:692–694.

Hensle TW, Tennenbaum SY, Reiley EA, et al: Hypospadias repair in adults: adventures and misadventures. J Urol. 2001; 165:77–79.

Hermann RE: Early exposure in the management of the postoperative wound. Surg Gynecol Obstet. 1965; 120:503.

Herrlinger R: History of medical illustration: from antiquity to 1600. Medicina Rara, New York; 1970.

Heyns CF: Exstrophy of the testis. J Urol. 1990; 144:724–725.

Hill GA, Wacksman J, Lewis AG: The modified pyramid hypospadias procedure: repair of megameatus and deep glandular groove variants. J Urol. 1993; 150:1208.

Hinderer U: Behandlung der Hypospadie und der inkompletten Hypospadieformen nach eigenen Methoden von 1966 bis 1975. In: Schmied E, Widmaier W, Reichert H (eds): Wiederstellung von Form und Funktion organischer Einheiten der verschiedenen K?rperregionen: Jahrestagung der Deutschen Gesellschaft für Plastische und Wiederherstellungschirurgie. Thieme, Stuttgart, pp 263–290; 1975.

Hinderer U: Hypospadias repair in long-term results. In: Glodwyn RM (ed): Plastic and reconstructive surgery. Little Brown, Boston, pp 378–410; 1978.

Hinderer U: New one-stage repair of hypospadias (technique of penis tunnelization). In: Hueston JT (ed): Transactions of the 5th International Congress of Plastic And Reconstructive Surgery. Butterworth, Stoneham, Mass, pp 283–305; 1971.

Hinman F: The blood supply to preputial island flaps. J Urol. 1991; 145:1232–1235.

Hinmann F Jr: Atlas of pediatric urologic surgery. Saunders, Philadelphia, pp 581–582; 1994.

Hiott O, Klauber G, Cendron M, et al: Molecular characterization of the androgen receptor gene in boys with hypospadias. Eur J Pediatr. 1994 ; 153: 317.

Hodgson NB: Editorial comment. J Urol. 1993; 149: 816.

Hodgson NB: A one stage hypospadias repair. J Urol. 1970; 104:281–287.

Hodgson NB: Commentary: review of hypospadias repair. In: Whitehead ED, Leiter E (eds): The current operative urology, 2nd edn. Harper and Row, New York, pp 1233–1242; 1984.

Hodgson NB: Hypospadias and urethral duplication. In: Harrison JH (ed): Campbell's urology, 4th edn. Saunders, Philadelphia, pp 1566–1595; 1978.

Hodgson NB: Hypospadias repair. In: Glenn JF (ed.): Urologic Surgery. Philadelphia, Lippincott; 1975.

Hodgson NB: In defense of the one-stage hypospadias repair. In: Scott R Jr, Gordon HL, Scott FB et al (eds): Current controversies in urologic management. Saunders, Philadelphia, pp 263–271; 1972.

Hodgson NB: Use of vascularized flaps in hypospadias repair. Urol Clin North Am. 1981; 8:471.

Hoebeke P, van Laecke E, Raes A, et al: Anomalies of the external urethral meatus in girls with non-neurogenic bladder sphincter dysfunction. BJU Int. 1999; 83:294–298.

Holbrook MC: The resistance of polyglycolic acid sutures to attack by infected human urine. Br J Urol. 1982; 53:313–315.

Holland AJA, Smith GHH, Ross FI, et al: HOSE: an objective scoring system for evaluating the results of hypospadias surgery. BJU Int. 2001; 88:255–258.

Holland AJA, Smith GHH: Effect of the depth and width of the urethral plate on tubularized incised urethral plate urethroplasty. J Urol. 2000; 164:489–491.

Hollowell JG, Keating MA, Snyder HM, et al: Preservation of the urethral plate in hypospadias repair: extended applications and further experience with the onlay island flap urethroplasty. J Urol. 1990; 143:98–100; discussion 100–101.

Holmlund DEW: Knot properties of surgical suture materials. Acta Chir Scand. 1974; 140:355–362.

Hook WV: A new operation for hypospadias. Ann Surg. 1896; 3:378.

Horton CE (ed): Plastic and reconstructive surgery of the genital area. Little Brown, Boston; 1973.

Horton CE Jr, Gearhart JP, Jeffs RD: Dermal grafts for correction of severe chordee associated with hypospadias. J Urol. 1993; 150: 452–455.

Horton CE Jr, Horton CE: Complications of hypospadias surgery. Clin Plast Surg. 1988; 15:371–379.

Horton CE, Devine CJ Jr, Baran N: Pictorial history of hypospadias repair techniques. In: Horton CE (ed): Plastic and reconstructive surgery of the genital area. Little Brown, Boston, pp 237–248; 1973.

Horton CE, Devine CJ Jr: A one stage repair for hypospadias cripples. Plast Reconstr Surg. 1970; 45: 425–430.

Horton CE, Devine CJ Jr: Simulated erection of the penis with saline injection: A diagnostic maneuver. Plast Reconstr Surg. 1977; 59: 138–139.

Horton CE, Devine CJ Jr: One stage repair. In: Horton E (ed): Plastic and reconstructive surgery for the genital area. Little Brown, Boston, p 278; 1973.

Horton CE, Devine CJ, Graham JK: Fistulas of the penile urethra. Plast Reconstr Surg. 1980; 66:407.

Horton CE, Devine CJ: Film: a one-stage hypospadias repair. Eaton Laboratories, 1959.

Horton CE, Devine CJ: Urethral fistula. In: Horton CE (ed): Plastic and reconstructive surgery of the genital area. Little Brown, Boston, pp 397–403; 1973.

Howells CH, Young HB: A study of completely undressed surgical wounds. Br J Surg. 1966; 53:436.

Humby G: A one-stage operation for hypospadias. Br J Surg. 1941; 29:84–92.

Hunter RH: Notes on the development of the prepuce. J Anat. 1936; 70:68.

Hurwitz RS: Chordee without hypospadias. Dial Pediatr Urol. 1986:1–8.

Husmann DA: Microphallic hypospadias: the use of human chorionic gonadotropin and testosterone before surgical repair (editorial; comment). J Urol. 1999; 162:1440–1441.

Ikoma F, Shima H, Yabumoto H, et al: Surgical management for enlarged prostatic utricle vagina masculina in patients with hypospadias. Br J Urol. 1986; 58:423.

Ikoma F, Shima H, Yabumoto H: Classification of enlarged prostatic utricle in patients with hypospadias. Br J Urol. 1985; 57: 334.

Irgens A, Kruger K, Skorve AH, et al: Birth defects and paternal occupational exposure. Hypotheses tested in a record linkage based dataset. Acta Obstet Gynecol Scand. 2000; 79:465–470.

Issa MM, Gearhart JP: The failed MAGPI: management and prevention. Br J Urol. 1989; 64:169–171.

Jackson K: Psychological preparation as a method of reducing the emotional trauma of anesthesia in children. Anesthesiology. 1951; 12:293–300.

Jayanthi VR, McLorie GA, Khoury AE, et al: Functional characteristics of the reconstructed neourethra after island flap urethroplasty [see comments]. J Urol. 1995; 153: 1657–1659.

Jayanthi VR, McLorie GA, Khoury AE, et al: Can previously relocated penile skin be successfully used for salvage hypospadias repair? J Urol. 1994; 152:740–743.

Jensen BH: Caudal block for postoperative pain relief after genital operations. A comparison between morphine and bupivacaine. Acta Anesthesiol Scand. 1981; 25:373–375.

Joffe M: Are problems with male reproductive health caused by endocrine disruption? Occup Environ Med. 2001; 58: 281–288.

Johanson B, Avellan L: Hypospadias: a review of 299 cases operated 1957–1969. Scand J Plast Reconstr Surg. 1980; 14:259–267.

Johanssen B: Reconstruction of the male urethra in strictures: application of the buried intact epithelium tube. Acta Chir Scand Suppl. 1953 ; 176:1.

Johnson D, Coleman DJ: The selective use of a single-stage and a two-stage technique for hypospadias correction in 157 consecutive cases with the aim of normal appearance and function. Br J Plast Surg. 1998; 51:195–201.

Johnson T: The works of that famous chirurgion Ambrose Paré, translated out of Latine and compared with the French by T Johnson. Cotes TH, Young R, London, 1634. Reprinted by Milord, Boston, 1968.

Jones KL: Smith's Recognizable patterns of human Malformation, 5th edn, vol 1. Philadelphia. WB Sounders; 1997.

Jordan GH: Penile reconstruction, Phallic construction, and urethral reconstruction. Urol Clin North Am. 1999; 26: 1–13.

Jordan GH: Techniques of tissue handling and transfer. J Urol. 1999; 162: 1213–1217.

Jordan GH: Reconstruction of the fossa navicularis. J Urol. 1987; 138:102–104.

Joseph DB, Perez LM: Tunica vaginalis onlay urethroplasty as a salvage repair. J Urol. 1999; 162: 1146–1147.

Joseph JV, Andrich DE, Leach CJ, et al: Urethroplasty for refractory anterior urethral stricture. J Urol. 2002; 167: 127–129.

Joseph VT: Concepts in surgical technique of one-stage hypospadias correction. Br J Urol. 1995; 76:504–509.

Juskiewenski S, Vaysse P, Guitard J, et al: Traitement des hypospadias anterieurs. Chir Pediatr. 1983; 24:75.

Juskiewenski S, Vaysse P, Moscovici J: A study of the arterial blood supply to the penis. Anat Clin. 1982; 4:101.

Kaefer M, Diamond D, Hendren WH, et al: The incidence of inter-sexuality in children with cryporchidism and hypospadias. Stratification based on gonadal palpability and meatal position. J Urol. 1999; 162:1003–1006.

Kagen J: The second year: the emergence of a self-awareness. Harvard University Press, Harvard; 1981.

Kallen B, Bertollin R, Castilla E, et al: A joint international study on the epidemiology of hypospadias. Acta Paediatr Scand. 1986; 324 [Suppl]:5–52.

Kallen B, Castilla EE, Kringelbach M, et al: Parental fertility and infant hypospadias: an international case-control study. Teratology. 1991; 44:629–634.

Kallen B, Mastoiavcovo P, Lancaster PAL, et al: Oral contraceptives in the etiology of isolated hypospadias. Contraception. 1991; 44: 173.

Kallen B, Winberg J: An Epidemiological study of hypospadias in Sweden. Acta Paediatr Scand. 1982; 293 [Suppl]:1–21.

Kanagasuntheram R, Anandaraja S: Development of the terminal urethra and prepuce in the dog. J Anat. 1960; 94:121–129.

Kang S, Graham JM, Olney AH, et al: GLI3 frame shift mutations cause autosomal dominant Pallister-Hall syndrome. Nat Genet. 1997; 15:266–268.

Kaplan GW: Repair of proximal hypospadias using a preputial free graft for neourethral construction and preputial pedicle flap for ventral skin coverage. J Urol. 1988; 140: 1270.

Kaplan W, Lamm DL: Embryogenesis of chordee. J Urol. 1975; 114:769.

Kass E, Kogan SJ, Manley C: Timing of elective surgery on the genitalia of male children with particular reference to the risks, benefits, and psychological effects of surgery and anaesthesia. Pediatrics. 1996: 97: 590–594.

Kass EJ: Dorsal corporeal rotation: An alternative technique for the management of severe chordee. J Urol. 1993; 150: 635–636.

Kass EJ, Bolong D: Single stage hypospadias reconstruction without fistula. J Urol. 1990; 144:520–522.

Kass EJ, Chung AK: Glanuloplasty and in situ tubularisation of the urethral plate: long term follow-up. J Urol. 2000; 164:991–993.

Katz AR, Turner RJ: Evaluation of tensile and absorption properties of polyglycolic acid suture. Surg Gynecol Obstet. 1970; 131:701–716.

Katz J: Pre-emptive analgesia: evidence, current status and future directions. Eur J Anaesthesiol Suppl. 1995; 10:8–13

Keating MA, Cartwright PC, Duckett JW: Bladder mucosa in urethral reconstructions. J Urol. 1990; 144:827–834.

Keating MA, Duckett JW: Failed hypospadias repair. In Cohen MS, Resnick MI (eds.): Reoperative Urology. Boston, Little Brown, pp 187–204; 1995.

Keating MA, Rich MA: Onlay and tubularised preputial island flaps. In: Ehrlich RM, Alter GJ (eds): Reconstructive and plastic surgery of the external genitalia: adult and pediatric, 1st edn. Saunders, Philadelphia, p 77; 1999.

Kelalis P, Bunge R, Barkin M, et al: The timing of elective surgery on the genitalia of male children with particular reference to undescended testes and hypospadias. Pediatrics. 1975; 56:479–483.

Kelalis PP, Benson RC Jr, Culp OS: Complications of single and multistage operations for hypospadias: a comparative review. J Urol. 1977; 118:657–658.

Kelalis PP, Benson RC Jr, Culp OS: Complications of single and multistage operations for hypospadias: a comparative review. Trans Am Assoc Genitourin Surg. 1977; 68:88–90.

Kelly D, Harte FB, Rose P: Urinary tract anomalies in patients with hypospadias. Br J Urol. 1984; 56:316–318.

Kenawi MM: Sexual function in hypospadiacs. Br J Urol. 1976; 47:883–890.

Keramidas DC, Soutis ME: Urethral advancement, glanduloplasty and preputioplasty in distal hypospadias. Eur J Pediatr Surg. 1995; 5:348–351.

Kester RR, Mooppan UMM, Hyunsook KO, et al: Congenital megalourethra. J Urol. 1990; 143:1213.

Khoury AE, Olson ME, McLorie GA, et al: Urethral replacement with tunica vaginalis: a pilot study. J Urol. 1989; 142:628–630; discussion 631.

Khuri FJ, Hardy BE, Churchill BM: Urologic anomalies associated with hypospadias. Urol Clin North AM. 1981; 8: 565–571.

Kim KS, King LR: Method for correcting meatal stenosis after hypospadias repair. Urology. 1992; 39:545–546.

Kim SH, Hendren WH: Repair of mild hypospadias. J Pediatr Surg. 1981; 16:806–811.

Kinahan TJ, Johnson HW: Tisseel in hypospadias repair. Can J Surg. 1992; 35:75.

King LR: Bladder mucosal grafts for severe hypospadias: a successful technique. J Urol. 1994; 152:2338–2340.

King LR: Cutaneous chordee and its implications in hypospadias repair. Urol Clin North Am. 1981; 8:397–402.

King LR: Hypospadias – a one stage repair without skin graft based on a new principle: chordee is sometimes produced by the skin alone. J Urol. 1970; 103:660–662

King LR: Hypospadias. In: King LR (ed): Urologic surgery in infants and children. Saunders, Philadelphia, pp 194–208; 1998.

King LR: Overview: Hypospadias repair. In: Whitehead ED, Leiter E (eds): The current operative urology, 2nd edn. Harper and Row, New York, pp 1265–1271; 1984.

Kinkead TM, Borzi PA, Duffy PG, et al: Long-term followup of bladder mucosa graft for male urethral reconstruction. J Urol. 1994; 151:1056–1058.

Kirkali Z: Tunica vaginalis: An aid in Hypospadias surgery. Br J Urol. 1990; 65; 530 – 532.

Kirsch AJ, Canning DA, Zderic SA: Skin flap closure by dermal laser soldering: a wound healing model for sutureless hypospadias repair. Urology. 1997; 50:263–272.

Kirsch AJ, Cooper CS, Gatti J et al: Laser tissue soldering for hypospadias repair: results of a controlled prospective clinical trial. J Urol. 2001; 165:574–577.

Kirsch AJ, DE Vries GM, Chang DT, et al: Hypospadias repair by tissue soldering: intraoperative results and follow up in 30 children. Urology. 1996; 48: 616–623.

Kirsch AJ, Miller MI, Chang DT, et al: Laser tissue soldering in urinary tract reconstruction. First human experience. Urology. 1995; 46:261.

Klevmark B, Andersen M, Schultz A, et al: Congenital and acquired curvature of the penis treated surgically by plication of the tunica albuginea. Br J Urol. 1994; 74: 501–506.

Klijn AJ, Dik P, de Jong TPVM: Results of preputial reconstruction in 77 boys for distal hypospadias. J Urol. 2000; 165:1255–1257.

Klip H, Verloop J, Van Gool J, et al: Increased risk of hypospadias in male offspring of women exposed to diethylstilbestrol in utero. Paediatr Perinatal Epidemiol. 2001; 15:A1–A38.

Kluth D, Lambrecht W, Reich P: Pathogenesis of hypospadias – more questions than answers. J Pediatr Surg. 1988; 23: 1095–1101.

Kocvara R, Dvoracek J: Inlay- onlay flap urethroplasty for hypospadias and stricture repair. J Urol. 1997; 158: 2142–2145.

Koff S, Brinkman J, Ulrich J, et al: Extensive mobilization of the urethral plate and urethra for repair of hypospadias. The modified Barcat technique. J Urol. 1994; 151:466–469.

Koff S, Eakins M: The treatment of penile chordee using corporal rotation. J Urol. 1984; 131:931.

Koff S, Jayanthi VR: Preoperative treatment with human chorionic gonadotrophin in infancy decreases the severity of proximal hypospadias and chordee. J Urol. 1999; 162: 1435–1439

Koff S: Mobilization of the urethra in the surgical treatment of hypospadias. J Urol. 1981; 125:394–397.

Kogan BA: Intraoperative pharmacological erection as an aid to pediatric hypospadias repair. J Urol. 2000; 164: 2058–2061.

Koyanagi T, Imanaka K, Nonomura K, et al: Further experience with one-stage repair of severe hypospadias and scrotal transposition. Modifications in the technique and its result in eight cases. Int Urol Nephrol 1988; 20:167–177.

Koyanagi T, Matsuno T, Nonomura K, et al: Complete repair of severe penoscrotal hypospadias in 1 stage: experience with urethral mobilization, wing flap-flipping urethroplasty and »glanulomeatoplasty«. J Urol. 1983; 130D: 1150–1154.

Koyanagi T, Nonomura H, Kakizaki H, et al: Hypospadias repair. In: Thüroff JW, Hohenfellner M (eds): Reconstructive surgery of the lower urinary tract in children. Isis Medical Media, Oxford, pp 1–21; 1995.

Koyanagi T, Nonomura K, et al: One-stage urethroplasty with parameatal foreskin-flap (OUPF) for severe proximal hypospadias associated with bifid scrotum (abstract). J Urol. 1987; 137:152A.

Koyanagi T, Nonomura K, Gotoh T, et al: One stage repair of perineal hypospadias and scrotal transposition. Eur Urol. 1984; 10:364–367.

Koyanagi T, Nonomura K, Kakizaki H, et al: Experience with stage repair of severe proximal hypospadias: operative technique results. Eur Urol. 1993; 24:106–110.

Koyanagi T, Nonomura K, Yamashita T, et al: One-stage repair of hypospadias: is there no simple method universally applicable to all types of hypospadias? J Urol. 1994; 152:1232–1237.

Koyanagi T, Nonomura K: Hypospadias repair: one-stage urethroplasty with parameatal foreskin flap for all types of hypospadias. In: Ehrlich RM, Alter GJ (eds): Reconstructive and plastic surgery of the external genitalia: adult and pediatric, 1st edn, chap 19. Saunders, Philadelphia, pp 92–100; 1999.

Koyle MA, Ehrlich RM: The bladder mucosal graft for urethral reconstruction. J Urol. 1987; 138:1093–1095.

Kramer SA, Aydin G, Kelalis PP: Chordee without hypospadias in children. J Urol. 1982; 128:539.

Kristensen P, Irgens LM, Andersen A, et al: Birth defects among offspring of norwegian farmers, 1967–1991. Epidemiology. 1997; 8:537–544.

Kroovand RL, Perlmutter AD: Extended urethroplasty in hypospadias. Urol Clin North Am. 1980; 7:431.

Kubota Y, Ishii N, Watanabe H, et al: Buried penis: a surgical repair. Urol Int. 1980; 46:61–63.

Kumar MV, Harris DL: A long term review of hypospadias repaired by split preputial flap technique (Harris). Br J Plast Surg. 1994; 47:236–240.

Kumar MV, Harris DL: Balanitis xerotica obliterans complicating hypospadias repair. Br J Plast Surg. 1999; 52: 69–71.

Kurzrock EA, Baskin LS, Cunha GR: Ontogeny of the male urethra: Theory of endodermal differentiation. Differentiation. 1999; 64:115–122.

Landerer: Dtsch Z Chir. 1891; p 32.

Lane RW: The effect of pre-operative stress on dreams. Doctoral dissertation, University of Oregon, Eugene, OR; 1966.

Lascaratos J, Kostakopoulos A, Louras G: Penile surgical techniques described by Oribasius (4th century CE). BJU Int. 1999; 84:16–19.

Lauenstein C: Zur Plastik der Hypospadie. Arch Klin Chir. 1892; 43:203.

Law NW, Ellis H: Exposure of the wound – a safe economy in the NHS. Postgrad Med J. 1987; 63:27.

Lenzi R, Barbagli G, Stomaci N: One stage skin-graft urethroplasty in anterior middle urethra: a new procedure. J Urol. 1984; 131:660–663.

Lepore AG, Kesler RW: Behavior of children undergoing hypospadias repair. J Urol. 1979; 122:68–70

Levy D: Psychic trauma of operations in children. Am J Dis Child. 1945; 69:7–25.

Lindgren BW, Reda EF, Levitt SB, et al: Single and multiple dorsal grafts for the management of severe penile curvature. J Urol. 1998; 160:1128–1130.

Livne P, Gibbons D, Gonzales E Jr: Meatal advancement and glanduloplasty: an operation for distal hypospadias. J Urol. 1984; 131:95–98.

Long-Cheng L, Xy Z, Si-Wei Z, et al: Experience of hypospadias using bladder mucosa in adolescents and adults. J Urol. 1995; 153:1117–1119.

Lorenzo AJ, Snodgrass WT: Regular dilatation is unnecessary after tubularized incised-plate hypospadias repair. BJU Int. 2002; 89:94–97.

Low BS, Mueller U: Why sex matters. A Darwinian look at human behaviour. Princeton Paperbacks. Princeton University Press, Princeton; 2000.

Lowsley OS, Begg CL: A three stage operation for the repair of hypospadias. Report of cases. JAMA. 1938; 110:487.

Maarafie A, Azmy AF: Congenital fistula of the penile urethra. Br J Urol. 1997; 79:814.

Macrab AJ, Zouves C: Hypospadias after assisted reproduction incorporating in vitro fertilization and gamete intrafallopian transfer. Fertil Steril. 1991:56:918–922.

Maizels M, Zaontz M, Donovan J, et al: Surgical correction of the buried penis: description of a classification system and a technique to correct this disorder. J Urol. 1986; 136:268–271.

Malyon AD, Boorman JG, Bowley N: Urinary flow rates in hypospadias. Br J Plast Surg. 1997; 50:530–535.

Mammelaar J: Use of bladder mucosa in a one stage repair of hypospadias. J Urol. 1947; 58:68.

Man DWK, Hamdy MH, Bisset WH: Experience with meatal advancement and glanduloplasty (MAGPI) hypospadias repair. Br J Urol. 1984; 56:70–72.

Man DWK, Vorderwark JS, Ransley PG: Experience with single stage hypospadias reconstruction. J Pediatr Surg. 1986; 21:338.

Mandell J, Bromley B, Peters CA, et al: Prenatal sonographic detection of genital malformations. J Urol. 1995; 153: 1994–1996.

Manley CB, Epstein ES: Early hypospadias repair. J Urol. 1981; 125:698–700.

Manzoni GM, Ransley PG: Buccal mucosa graft for hypospadias. In: Ehrlich RM, Alter GJ (ed): Reconstructive and plastic surgery of the external genitalia: adult and pediatrics. Saunders, Philadelphia, pp 121–125; 1999

Marberger H, Pauer W: Experience in hypospadias repair. Urol Clin North Am. 1981; 8:403.

Marshall M Jr, Beh WP, Johnson SH, et al: Etiologic considerations in penoscrotal hypospadias repair. J Urol. 1978; 120:229–231.

Marshall M Jr, Johnson SH III, Price SE Jr, et al: Cecil urethroplasty with concurrent scrotoplasty for repair of hypospadias. J Urol. 1979; 121:335.

Marshall VF, Spellman RM: Construction of urethra in hypospadias using vesical musocal grafts. J Urol. 1955; 73: 335–342.

Marte A, Di Iorio G, De Pasquale M, et al: Functional evaluation of tubularised incised plate repair of mid shaft – proximal hypospadias using uroflowmetry. BJU Int. 2001; 87:540–543.

Marte A, Di Iorio G, De Pasquale M: MAGPI procedure in meatal regression after hypospadias repair. Eur J Paediatr Surg. 2001; 11:259–262.

Mathieu P: Traitement en un temps de l'hypospade balanique et juxta-balanique. J Chir (Paris). 1932; 39:481–484.

Matlay P, Beral V: Trends in congenital malformations of external genitalia. Lancet. 1985; 1:108.

Mau G: Progestins during pregnancy and hypospadias. Teratology. 1981;2:285–287.

Mayhew JF, Guiness WS: Cardiac arrest due to anesthesia in children (letter). JAMA. 1986; 256:216.

Mayo CH: JAMA. 1901; 36:1157.

Mays HB: Hypospadias: a concept of treatment. J Urol. 1951; 65:279.

McAleer IM, Kaplan GW: Is routine karyotyping necessary in the evaluation of hypospadias and cryptorchidism? J Urol. 2001; 165:2029–2031.

McArdle F, Labowitz R: Uncomplicated hypospadias and anomalies of upper urinary tract: need for screening? Urology. 1975; 5: 712–716.

McCarthy JG: Introduction to plastic surgery. In: McCarthy JG (ed): Plastic surgery, vol 1: general principles. Saunders, Philadelphia, pp 48–66; 1990.

McCormeck M, Homsy Y, Laberge Y: "no stent, no diversion"; mathieu hypospadias repair. Can J Surg. 1993; 36: 152–154.

McGowan AJ Jr, Waterhouse RK: Mobilization of the anterior urethra. Bull NY Acad Med. 1964; 40:776–782.

McGregor IA, McGregor AD (eds): Fundamental techniques of plastic surgery and their surgical applications. Churchill Livingstone, Edinburgh, pp 21–121; 1995.

McIlvoy DB, Harris HS: Transposition of the penis and scrotum: case report. J Urol. 1955; 73:540–543.

McIndoe AH: The treatment of hypospadias. Am J Surg. 1937; 38:176–185.

McIndoe AH: An operation for cure of adult hypospadias. Br Med J. 1937; 1:385.

McKusick VA, Bauer RL, Koop CE, et al: Hydrometrocolpos as a simply inherited malformation. JAMA. 1964; 189: 816.

McLorie G, Joyner B, Herz D, et al: A prospective randomized clinical trial to evaluate methods of postoperative care of hypospadias. J Urol. 2001; 165:1669–1672.

McQuay HJ: Pre-emptive analgesia: a systematic review of clinical studies. Ann Med. 1995; 27:249–256

Memmelaar J: Use of bladder mucosa in a one stage repair of hypospadias. J Urol. 1947; 58:68–73.

Metro MJ, Hsi-Yang W, Snyder HM, et al: Buccal mucosal grafts: lessons learned from an 8-year experience. J Urol. 2001; 166:1459–1461.

Mettauer JP: Practical observations on those malformations of the male urethra and penis, termed hypospadias and epispadias, with an anomalous case. Am J Med Sci. 1842; 4:43.

Michell ME, Kulb TB: Hypospadias repair without a bladder drainage catheter. J Urol. 1986; 135:321.

Miller MAW, Grant DB: Severe hypospadias with genital ambiguity: adult outcome after staged hypospadias repair. Br J Urol. 1997; 80:485–488.

Mills C, McGovern J, Mininberg D, et al: An analysis of different techniques for distal hypospadias repair: the price of perfection. J Urol. 1981; 125: 701.

Minevich E, Pecha BR, Wacksman J, et al: Mathieu hypospadias repair: An experience in 202 patients. J Urol. 1999; 162:2141–2143.

Mirabet Ippolito V: Modification de la técnica de McIndoe para el tratamiento de los hipospadias. Doctoral thesis, Valencia, 1964.

Mitchell M: Experience with the MAGPI hypospadias repair. J Pediatr Surg. 1993; 18:692–694.

Mitchell ME, Kulb TB: Hypospadias repair without a bladder drainage catheter. J Urol. 1986; 135:321.

Moir GC, Stevenson JH: A modified Bretteville technique for hypospadias. Br J Plast Surg. 1996; 49:223–227.

Mollard P, Castagnola C: Hypospadias: the release of chordee without dividing the urethral plate and onlay island flap (92 cases). J Urol. 1994; 152:1238–1240.

Mollard P, Mouriquand P, Bringeon G, et al: Repair of hypospadias using a bladder mucosa graft in 76 cases. J Urol. 1989; 142:1548–1550.

Mollard P, Mouriquand P, Felfela T: Application of the onlay island flap urethroplasty to penile hypospadias with severe chordee. Br J Urol. 1991; 68:317–319.

Mollard P, Mouriquand PDE, Basset T: Le traitement de l'hypospade. Chir Pediatr. 1987; 28:197–203.

Moller H, Weidner IS: Epidemiology of cryptorchidism and hypospadias. Epidemiology. 1999; 10:352–354.

Money J, Ehrhardt A: Man and woman, boy and girl. Johns Hopkins University Press, Baltimore, MD; 1972.

Money J, Norman BF: Gender identity and gender transposition: longitudinal outcome study of 24 male hermaphrodites assigned as boys. J Sex Marital Ther. 1987; 13:75–92.

Monfort G, Jean P, Lacoste M: Correction des hypospadias posterieurs en un temps par lambeau pedicule transversal (intervention de Duckett). A propos de 50 observations. Chir Pediatr. 1983; 24:71.

Monfort G, Lucas C: Dihydrotestosterone penile stimulation in hypospadias surgery. Eur Urol. 1982; 8:201–203.

Montagnani CA: Pediatric surgery in Islamic medicine from the middle ages to renaissance. In: Rickam PP (ed): Historical aspects of pediatric surgery. Prog Pediatr Surg, vol 20. Springer, Berlin Heidelberg New York, pp 39–51; 1986.

Montagnino BA, Gonzales ET Jr, Roth DR: Open catheter drainage after urethral surgery. J Urol. 1988; 140:1250.

Moore CC: The role of routine radiographic screening of boys with hypospadias: a prospective study. J Paediatr Surg. 1990; 25:339–341.

Moore KL, Persaud TVN: The developing human, 5th edn. Saunders, Philadelphia; 1993.

Mor Y, Ramon J, Jonas P: Is only meatoplasty a legitimate surgical solution for extreme distal hypospadias? A long term follow up. BJU Int. 2000; 85:501–503.

Morey AF, McAninch JW: Technique of harvesting buccal mucosa for urethral reconstruction. J Urol. 1996; 155: 1696–1697.

Mori Y, Ikoma F: Surgical correction of incomplete penoscrotal transposition associated with hypospadias. J Pediatr Surg. 1986; 21:46–48.

Morton NS: Prevention and control of pain in children. Br J Anaesth. 1999; 83:118–129

Motiwala HG: Dartos flap: an aid to urethral reconstruction. Br J Urol. 1993; 72:260.

Mouriquand PDE, Mure PY: Hypospadias. In: Gearhart JP, Rink RC, Mouriquand PDE (eds): Pediatric urology. Saunders, Philadelphia, pp 713–728; 2001.

Mouriquand PDE, Persad R, Sharma S: Hypospadias repair: current principles and procedures. Br J Urol. 1995; 76 [Suppl 3]: 9–22.

Mouriquand PDE: Hypospadias. In: Atwell JD (ed): Paediatric surgery. Arnold, London, pp 603–616; 1998.

Moutet: De l'uréthroplastie dans hypospadias scrotal. Montpellier Méd, May, 1870.

Mulvihill SJ, Pellegrini CA: Postoperative care. In: Way LW (ed): Current surgical diagnosis and treatment, 10th edn, chap 3. Lange, Connecticut, p 16; 1994.

Mundy AR, Stephenson TP: Pedicled preputial patch urethroplasty. Br J Urol. 1988; 61:48–52.

Mundy AR: The long-term results of skin inlay urethroplasty. BJU Int. 1995; 75:59–61.

Murat I, Constant I: Excitation phenomena during induction and recovery using sevoflurane in paediatric patients. Acta Anaesthesiol Belg. 2000; 51:229–232

Mureau MA, Slijper FM, Slob AK, et al: Psychosexual adjustment of men who underwent hypospadias repair: a norm related study. J Urol. 1995; 154:1351–1355.

Mureau MA, Slijper FM, Slob AK, et al: Psychosocial functioning of children, adolescents, and adults following hypospadias surgery: a comparative study. J Pediatr Psychol. 1997; 22:371–387.

Mureau MA, Slijper FM, Van der Meulen JC, et al: Psychological adjustment of men who underwent hypospadias repair: a norm –related study. J Urol. 1995; 154: 1351–1355.

Mureau MA, Slijper FME, Nijman RJM, et al: Psychosexual adjustment of children and adolescents after different types of hypospadias repair: a norm related study. J Urol. 1995; 154:1902–1907.

Mureau MA, Slijper FME, Slob AK, et al: Satisfaction with penile appearance after hypospadias surgery: the patient and surgeon view. J Urol. 1996; 155:703–706.

Murphy JP: Hypospadias. In: Ashcraft KW, Murphy JP, Sharp RJ, et al (eds): Pediatric surgery, 3rd edn. Saunders, Philadelphia, pp 763–782; 2000.

Murphy LJT: The urethra. In Murphy LJT (ed.): The history of urology. Springfield, Charles C Thomas. pp 453–481; 1972.

Mustarde JC: One stage correction of distal hypospadias and other people's fistulae. Br J Plast Surg. 1965; 18: 413–422.

Myers JP: Endocrine disruption: emerging science vitally important for pediatric urologists. Dial Pediatr Urol. 2000; 23: 8. [special issue].

Nahas BW, Nahas WB: The use of buccal mucosa patch graft in the management of a large urethro-cutaneous fistula. Br J Urol. 1994; 74:679–681.

Nasrallah PF, Minnot HB: Distal hypospadias repair. J Urol. 1984; 131:87–91

Nesbit RM: Congenital curvature of the phallus: report of three cases with description of correction operation. J Urol. 1965; 93:230–232.

Nesbit RM: Operation for correction of distal penile ventral curvature with and without hypospadias. Trans Am Assoc Genitourin Surg. 1966; 58:12–14.

Nesbit RM: Operation for correction of distal penile ventral curvature with or without hypospadias. J Urol. 1967; 97: 720–722.

Nesbit RM: Plastic procedure for correction of hypospadias. J Urol. 1941; 45: 699–702.

Nesbit TE: Congenital megalo-urethra. J Urol. 1955; 73:839.

Neumann C: The expansion of an area of skin by progressive distension of a subcutaneous balloon. Plast Reconstr Surg. 1957; 19:124–130.

Nicolle F: Improved repairs in 100 cases of penile hypospadias. Br J Plast Surg. 1976; 29:150–157.

Nievelstein RAJ, van der Werff JFA, Verbeek FJ, et al: Normal and abnormal embryonic development of the anorectum in human embryos. Teratology. 1998; 57:70–78.

Nonomura K, Fuijeda K, Sakakibara N, et al: Pituitary and gonadal function in prepubertal boys with hypospadias. J Urol. 1984; 132: 595.

Nonomura K, Kakikazia H, Shomoda N, et al: Surgical repair of anterior hypospadias with fish-mouth meatus and intact prepuce based on an anatomical characteristics. Eur Urol. 1998; 34: 368–371.

Nonomura K, Koyanagi T, Imamaka K, et al: Measurement of blood flow in the parameatal foreskin flap for urethroplasty in hypospadias repair. Eur Urol. 1992; 21:155–159.

North K, Golding J, The ALSPAC Study Team: a maternal vegetarian diet in pregnancy is associated with hypospadias. BJU Int. 2000; 85:107–113.

Nove-Josserand G: Hypospadias perineo scrotal total gueri par le procede de la greffe autoplastique. Lyon Med. 1906; 93:322.

Nové-Josserand G: Résultates éloignés de l'uréthroplastie par la tunnelisation et la greffe dermo-épidermique dans les formes graves de l'hypospadias et de l'épispadias. J Urol Med Chir. 1914; 5:393.

Nové-Josserand G: Traitement de l'hypospadias: nouvelle method. Lyon Med. 1897; 85:198.

Numanoğlu I: Cerrahiye-i Ilhaniye: the earliest known book containing pediatric surgical procedures. J Pediatr Surg. 1973; 8:547–548.

Nunn JF: Ancient Egyptian medicine. Chapter 8: Surgery, trauma and dangerous animals. British Museum Press, London, 1996; pp 163–190.

O'Hara K, O'Hara J: The effect of male circumcision on the sexual enjoyment of the female partner. BJU Int. 1999; 83 [Suppl 1]:79–84.

Olshan AF, Teschke K, Baird PA: Paternal occupation and congenital anomalies in offspring. Am J Ind Med. 1991; 20:447–475.

Ombrédanne L: Hypospadias pénien chez l'enfant. Bull Mem Soc Chir Paris. 1911; 37:1076.

Ombrédanne L: Precis clinique et operation de chirurgie infantile. Masson, Paris, p 851; 1932.

Ombrédanne L: Précis clinique et opératoire de chirurgie infantile. Collection de Précis Médicaux Masson et ?diteurs, Paris, pp 654–689 ; 1925.

Online Mendelian Inheritance in Man (OMIM) http://www.ncbi.nlm.nih.gov/Omim

Orandi A: One stage urethroplasty: four year follow up. J Urol. 1972; 107:977–980.

Oswald J, K?rner I, Riccabona M: Comparison of the perimeatal-based flap (Mathieu) and the tubularized incised-plate urethroplasty (Snodgrass) in primary distal hypospadias. BJU Int. 2000; 85:725–727.

Oz MC, Johnson JP, Parangis S, et al: Tissue soldering by use of indocyanine green dye enhanced fibrinogen with the near diode laser. J Vasc Surg. 1990; 11:718.

Ozen HA, Whitaker RH: Scope and limitations of the MAGPI hypospadias repair. Br J Urol. 1987; 59:81–83.

Paidas CN, Morreale RF, Holoski KM, et al: Septation and differentiation of the embryonic human cloaca. J Pediatr Surg. 1999; 34:877–884.

Pancoast J: Hypospadias. In: Pancoast J(ed): Treatise on operative surgery. Carrey and Hart, Philadelphia, pp 317–318; 1844.

Pancoast J: In: Murphy LJT (ed): The history of urology. Thomas, Springfield, Ilinois, p 456;1972.

Paparel P, Mure PY, Garignon C, et al: Translation uréthrale de Koff: a propos de 26 hypospades présentant une division distale du corps spongieux. Prog Urol. 2001; 11:1327–1330.

Paparel P, Mure PY, Margarian M, et al: Approche actuelle de l'hypospade chez l'enfant. Prog Urol. 2001; 11:741–751.

Paré A: Les oeuvres de M. Ambroise Paré. Chez Gabriel Buon, Paris; 1575.

Paré A: The works of that famous chirurgion Ambroise Parey, translated out of Latin and compared with the French by Th Johnson. Cotes and Young, London, p 419; 1634 (2nd edn, p 655; 1649). Academy-HMB-L (Vault) WZ 250.

Park JM, Faerber GJ, Bloom DA: Long-term outcome evaluation of patients undergoing the meatal advancement and glanuloplasty procedure. J Urol. 1995; 153:1655–1656.

Parsons KF, Abercrombie GF: Transverse preputial island flap neo-urethroplasty. Br J Urol. 1982; 54:745–747.

Patel HI, Moriarty KP, Brisson PA: Genito-urinary injuries in the newborn. J Pediatr Surg. 2001; 36:235–239.

Patel RI, Hanallah RS: Anesthetic complications following pediatric ambulatory surgery: a 3-year study. Anesthesiology. 1988; 69:1009–1012.

Patil UB, Alvarez J: Simple effective hypospadias repair dressing. Urology. 1989; 34:49.

Patil UB: Role of tissue expanders in genito urinary reconstructive surgery. Urol Annu. 1994; 8:191.

Paul M, Kanagasuntheram R: The congenital anomalies of the lower urinary tract. Br J Urol. 1956; 28: 118.

Paulozzi LJ: Is hypospadias an "environmental" birth defect. Dial Pediatr Urol. 2000; 23: 8. [special issue].

Paulozzi LJ, Erickson JD, Jackson RJ: Hypospadias trends in two US surveillance systems. Pediatrics. 1997; 100:831–834.

Paulozzi LJ: International trends in rates of hypospadias and cryptorchidism. Environ Health Perspect. 1999; 107:297–302.

Paulus C, Dessouki T, Chelade M, et al: 220 cases of distal hypospadias. Results of MAGPI and Duplay procedures. Retrospective place of glanduloplasty and urethroplasty. Eur J Pediatr Surg. 1993; 3:87–91.

Penington EC, Hutson JM: The cloacal plate – the missing link in anorectal and urogenital development. BJU Int. 2002; 89: 726–732.

Penington EC, Hutson JM: The urethral plate – does it grow into the genital tubercle or within it? BJU Int. 2002; 89: 733–739.

Penington EC: MD Thesis, University of Melbourne, 2002.

Permutter AD, Montgomery BT, Steinhardt GF: Tunica vaginalis free graft for the correction of chordee. J Urol. 1985; 134: 311–313.

Perovic S, Djordjevic ML, Djakovic N: Natural erection induced by prostaglandin-E1 in the diagnosis and treatment of congenital penile anomalies. Br J Urol. 1997; 79: 43–46.

Perovic S, Vukadinovic V: Onlay island flap urethroplasty for severe hypospadias: a variant of the technique. J Urol. 1994; 151: 711–714.

Perovic SV, Vukadinovic V, Djordjevic MLJ, et al: The penile disassembly technique in hypospadias repair. Br J Urol. 1998; 81:479–487.

Perovic SW, Djordjevic ML, Djakovic NG: A new approach to the treatment of penile curvature. J Urol. 1998; 160:1123–1127.

Physick: Cited by Pancoast JA: Treatise on operative surgery. Carrey and Hart, Philadelphia, pp 317–318; 1844.

Pierik FH, Burdorf A, Nijman JMR, et al: A high hypospadias rate in the Netherlands. Hum Reprod. 2002; 17:1112–1115.

Pike LA, Rathbun SR, Husmann DA, et al: Penoscrotal transposition: review of 53 patients. J Urol. 2001; 166:1865–1868.

Podesta ML, Medel R, Castera R: Urethral duplication in children: surgical treatment and results. J Urol. 1998; 160:1830–1833.

Pohlman AG: The development of the cloaca in human embryos. Am J Anat. 1911; 12:1–26.

Pope JC 4th, Kropp BP, McLaughlin KP, et al: Penile orthoplasty using dermal grafts in the outpatient setting. Urology. 1996; 48:124–127

Poppas DP, Mininberg DT, Hyacinthe L, et al: Patch graft urethroplasty using dye enhanced laser tissue welding with a human protein solder; a pre-clinical canine model. J Urol. 1993; 150:648.

Poppas DP, Schlossberg SM, Richmond IL, et al: Laser welding in urethral surgery: improved results with a protein solder. J Urol. 1988; 139:145.

Portman I: A guide to the Temple of Kom Ombo. Palm Press, Cairo, 2001; p 19.

Powell CR, McAleer I, Alagiri M, et al: Comparison of flaps versus grafts in proximal hypospadias surgery. J Urol. 2000; 163:1286–1288; discussion 1288–1289.

Qi BQ, Williams A, Beasley S, et al: Clarification of the process of separation of the cloaca into rectum and urogenital sinus in the rat embryo. J Pediatr Surg. 2000; 35:1810–1816.

Quartey JKM: Microcirculation of penile and scrotal skin. Atlas Urol Clin North Am. 1997; 5:1

Rabinovitch HH: Experience with a modification of the Cloutier technique for hypospadias repair. J Urol. 1988; 139:1017–1019.

Rabinowitz R, Hulbert WC: Meatal-based flap Mathieu procedure. In: Ehrlich RM, Alter GJ (eds): Reconstructive and plastic surgery of the external genitalia: adult and pediatric, 1st edn. Saunders, Philadelphia, pp 39–43; 1999.

Rabinowitz R: Outpatient catheterless modified Mathieu hypospadias repair. J Urol. 1987; 138:1074–1076.

Rajfer J, Walsh PC: The incidence of intersexuality in patients with hypospadias and cryptorchidism. J Urol. 1976 ; 116: 769–770.

Raman-Wilms L, Lin-in Tseng A, Wignardt S, et al: Fetal genital effects of first-trimester sex hormone exposure: a meta-analysis. Obstet Gynecol. 1995; 85:141–149.

Ransley PG, Duffy PG, Oesch IL, et al: Autologous bladder mucosa graft for urethral substitution. Br J Urol. 1987; 59:331.

Ransley PG, Duffy PG, Oesch IL, et al: The use of bladder mucosa and combined bladder mucosa/preputial skin grafts for urethral reconstruction. J Urol. 1987; 138:1096–1099.

Ratan SK, Sen A, Ratan J, et al: Mercurochrome as a adjunct to local preoperative preparation in children undergoing hypospadias repair. BJU Int. 2001; 88:259–262.

Ravasse P, Petit T, Delmas P: Anterior hypospadias: Duplay or Mathieu? Prog Urol. 2000; 10:653–656.

Ravasse P, Petit T: Mathieu's urethroplasty in surgery for hypospadias: postoperative complications. Ann Urol. 2000; 34:271–273.

Reddy LN: One stage repair of hypospadias. Urology. 1975; 5:475.

Redman JF: A dressing technique that facilitates outpatient hypospadias surgery. Urology. 1991; 37:248–250.

Redman JF: Dorsal curvature of penis. Urology. 1983; 21: 479–481.

Redman JF: Experience with 60 consecutive hypospadias repairs using the Horton-Devine techniques. J Urol. 1983; 129:115–118.

Redman JF: The Barcat balanic groove technique for the repair of distal hypospadias. J Urol. 1987; 137:83.

Redman JF: Tourniquet as hemostatic aid in repair of hypospadias. Urology. 1986; 28:241–245.

Redman JF, Smith JP: Surgical dressing for hypospadias repair. Urology. 1974; 4:739–740

Rees MJW, Sinclair SW, Hiles RW, et al: A 10-years prospective study of hypospadias repair at Frenchay Hospital. Br J Urol. 1981; 53:637.

Reeves C: Egyptian medicine. Shire Publications, Buckinghamshire, UK. pp 26–27, 29–31;2001.

Retick AB: Proximal Hypospadias. In Marshall FF (ed.): Textbook of operative Urology, Philadelphia, WB Saunders, pp. 977–984; 1996.

Retik AB, Bauer SB, Mandell J, et al: Management of severe hypospadias with a 2-stage repair. J Urol. 1994; 152:749–751.

Retik AB, Borer JG: Primary and reoperative hypospadias repair with the sondgrass technique. J Urol. 1998; 16: 186–191.

Retik AB, Keating M, Mandell J: Complications of hypospadias repair. Urol Clin North Am. 1988; 15:223–236.

Retik AB, Mandell J, Bauer SB, et al: Meatal based hypospadias repair with the use of dorsal subcutaneous flap to prevent urethrocutaneous fistula. J Urol. 1994; 152:1229– 1231.

Rich MA, Keating MA, Snyder HM, et al: »Hinging« the urethral plate in hypospadias meatoplasty. J Urol. 1989; 142:1551.

Rich MA, Keating MA: Hinging the urethral plate. In: Ehrlich RM, Alter GJ (eds): Reconstructive and plastic surgery of the external genitalia, adult and pediatric. Saunders, Philadelphia, pp 63–65; 1999.

Ricketson G: A method of repair of hypospadias. Am J Surg. 1958; 95:279.

Rickwood AMK: Hypospadias repairs. BJU Int. 1997; 79:662.

Rickwood AMK, Anderson PA: One stage hypospadias repair: experience of 367 cases. Br J Urol. 1991; 67:424.

Rickwood AMK, Fearne C: Pedicled penile skin for hypospadias 'rescue'. Br J Urol. 1997; 80:145–146.

Riley MM, Halliday JL, Lumley JM: Congenital malformations in Victoria, Australia 1983–1995: an overview of infant characteristics. J Paediatr Child Health. 1998; 34:233– 240.

Ritchey ML, Sinha A, Argueso L: Congenital fistula of the penile urethra. J Urol. 1994; 151:1061–1062.

Rober PE, Perlmutter AD, Reitelman C: Experience with 81, 1-stage hypospadias/chordee repairs with free graft urethroplasties. J Urol. 1990; 144:526–529; discussion 530.

Roberts CJ, lloyd S: Observations on epidemiolgy of simple hypospadias. BMJ. 1973; 1: 768–770.

Robertson M, Walker D: Psychological factors in hypospadias repair. J Urol. 1975; 113:698–700

Rochet V: Nouveau procédé pour réfaire le canal pénien dans l'hypospadias. Gaz Hebd Med Chir. 1899; 4:673.

Rogers BO: History of external genital surgery. In: Horton CE (ed): Plastic and reconstructive surgery of the genital area. Little Brown, Boston, pp 3–47; 1973.

Rogers HS, McNicholas TA, Blandy JP: Long-term results of one-stage scrotal patch urethroplasty. Br J Urol. 1992; 69:621–628.

Romagnoli G, Deluca M, Faranda F, et al: Treatment of posterior hypospadias by the autologous graft of cultured urethral epithelium. N Engl J Med. 1990; 32:527.

Rosenberger: Dtsch Med Wochenschr. 1891; 9:1250.

Ross JH, Kay R: Use of de-epithelialized local skin flap in hypspadias repairs accomplished by tubularization of the incised urethral plate. Urology. 1997; 50:110.

Roth DR: Hypospadias. In: Gonzales ET, Bauer SB (eds): Pediatric urology practice. Lippincott Williams and Wilkins, Philadelphia, pp 487–497; 1999.

Rowsell AR, Morgan BDE: Hypospadias and the embryogenesis of the penile urethra. Br J Plastic Surg. 1987; 40:201–206.

Rushton HG, Belman AB: The split prepuce in situ onlay hypospadias repair. J Urol. 1998; 160:1134–1136; discussion 1137.

Russell RH: Operation for severe hypospadias. Br Med J. 1900; ii:1432–1435.

Saalfeld J, Eherlich RM, Gross JM, et al: Congenital curvature of the penis: successful results with variations in corporoplasty. J Urol. 1973; 109: 64–65.

Sabuncuoğlu I: Cerrahiye-i Ilhaniye, Istanbul Fatih National library, 1465; no 79 (1st manuscript).

Sadler TW: Langman's medical embryology, 6th edn. Williams and Wilkins, Baltimore, 1990; pp 237–259.

Sadove RC, Horton CE, McRoberts JW: The new era of hypospadias surgery. Clin Plast Surg. 1988; 15:354.

Sakakibara N, Nonomura K, Koyanagi T, et al: Use of testosterone ointment before hypospadias repair. Urol Int. 1991; 47:40–43

Sandberg DE, Meyer-Bahlburg HF, Aranoff GS: Boys with hypospadias: a survey of behavioural difficulties. J Pediatr Psychol. 1989; 14:491–514.

Sandberg DE, Meyer-Bahlburg HF, Hensle TW, et al: Psychosocial adaptation of middle childhood boys with hypospadias after genital surgery. J Pediatr Psychol. 2001; 26:465–475.

Sandberg DE, Meyer-Bahlburg HF, Yager TJ, et al: Gender development in boys born with hypospadias. Pschoneuroendocrinology. 1995; 20: 693–709.

Sanders AR, Schein CJ, Orkin LA: Total mucosal denudation of the canine bladder: experimental observations and clinical implications. Final report. J Urol. 1958; 79:63–68.

Sauvage P, Becmeur F, Geiss S, et al: Transverse mucosal preputial flap for repair of severe hypospadias and isolated chordee without hypospadias: a 350-case experience. J Pediatr Surg. 1993; 28:435–438.

Sauvage P, Rougeron G, Bientz J, et al: L'utilisation du lambeau preputial transverse pedicule dans la chirurgie de l'hypospadias. A propos de 100 cas. Chir Pediatr. 1987; 28:220.

Schaeffer DD, Erbes J: Hypospadias. Am J Surg 1950; 80:183.

Scherr DS, Poppas DP: Laser tissue welding. Urol Clin North Am. 1998; 25: 123–135.

Scherz H: Preputial graft in hypospadias. In: Ehrlich RM, Alter GJ (ed): Reconstructive and plastic surgery of the external genitalia: adult and pediatric, 1st edn. Saunders, Philadelphia, pp 83–86; 1999.

Scherz HC, Kaplan GW, Packer MG, et al: Post-hypospadias repair urethral strictures: a review of 30 cases. J Urol. 1988; 140:1253–1255.

Schinzel A: Human Cytogenetics Database. Oxford University Press, Oxford; 1994.

Schneider CS: An analysis of presurgical anxiety in boys and girls. University of Michigan, Ann Arbor MI, 1960. Doctoral dissertation.

Schonfeld WA: Primary and secondary sexual characteristics. Am J Dis Child. 1943; 65:535–549.

Schonfeld WA, Beebe CW: Normal growth and variation in the male genitalia from birth to maturity. J Urol. 1942; 48:759

Schreiter F, Noll F: Mesh graft urethroplasty. World J Urol. 1987; 5:41–46.

Schrieter F, Noll F: Mesh Graft urethroplasty using split thickness skin graft or foreskin. J Urol. 1989; 142: 1223–1226.

Schultz JR, Klykylo WM, Wacksman J: Timing of elective hypospadias repair in children. Pediatrics. 1983; 71:342–351.

Schwartz DA, Newsum LA, Markowitz Heifetz R: Parental occupation and birth outcome in an agricultural community. Scand J Work Environ Health. 1986; 12:51–54.

Schwartz GS: Infibulation, population control and the medical profession. Bull NY Acad Med. 1970; 46:964.

Sebeseri O, Keller U, Spreng P, et al: The physical properties of polyglycolic acid suture (dexon) in sterile and infected urine. Invest Urol. 1975; 12:490–493.

Secrest CL, Jordan GH, Winslow BH, et al: Repair of complications of hypospadias surgery. J Urol. 1993; 150:1415–1418.

Seligman M: www.positivepsychology.org (marty@apa.org), 2000.

Sensöz Ö, Celebioglu S, Baran CN, et al: A new technique for distal hypospadias repair: advancement of a distally de-epithelialized urethrocutaneous flap. Plast Reconstr Surg. 1997; 99: 93–99.

Setchell BP: Reproduction in male marsupials. In: Stonehouse B, Gilmore G (eds): The biology of marsupials. Macmillan, London, 1977; pp 411–455.

Shanberg AM, Rosenberg MT: Partial transposition of the penis and scrotum with anterior urethral diverticulum in a child born with the caudal regression syndrome. J Urol. 1989; 142:1060–1062.

Shanberg AM, Sanderson K, Duel BP: Re-operative hypospadias repair using the Snodgrass incised urethral plate. BJU Int. 2001; 87:544–547.

Shankar KR, Losty PD, Hopper M, et al: Outcome of hypospadias fistula repair. BJU Int. 2002; 89:103–105.

Shapiro S: Surgical treatment of the "buried" penis. Urology. 1987; 30:554–559.

Shapiro SR: Complications of hypospadias repair. J Urol. 1984; 131:518.

Shapiro SR: hypospadias repair: optical magnification versus Ziess reconstruction microscope. Urology. 1989; 33: 43–46.

Sharpe RM, Skakkebaek NE: Are oestrogens involved in falling sperm counts and disorders of the male reproductive tract? Lancet. 1993; 341:1392–1395.

Shaw P: Infertility counselling. In: Davis A, Fallowfield L (eds): Counselling and communication in health care. Wiley, Chichester; 1991.

Sheldon CA, Duckett JW: Hypospadias. Pediatr Clin North Am. 1987; 34:1259.

Shelton TB, Noe HN: The role of excretory urography in patients with hypospadias. J Urol. 1985; 134: 97.

Shima H, Ikoma F, Terakawa T, et al: Developmental anomalies associated with hypospadias. J Urol. 1979; 122: 619.

Shima H, Ikoma F, Yabumoto H, et al: Gonadotropin and testosterone response in prepubertal boys with Hypospadias. J Urol. 1986; 135: 539–542.

Shima H, Yabumoto H, Okamoto E, et al: Testicular function in patients with hypospadias associated with enlarged prostatic utricle. Br J Urol. 1992; 69: 192.

Shokeir AA, Hussein MI: The urology of Pharaonic Egypt. BJU Int. 1999; 84:755–761.

Siever R: Anomalien auf Penis: ihre Beziehung zur Hypospadie und ihre Deutung. Z Chir. 1926; 199:286.

Silver RI, Rodriguez R, Chang TS, et al: In Vitro fertilization is associated with an increased risk of hypospadias. J Urol. 1999; 161:1954–1957.

Silver RI, Russell DW: 5 ? reductase type 2 mutations are present in some boys with isolated hypospadias. J Urol. J Urol. 1999; 162: 1142.

Simmons GR, Cain MP, Casale AJ, et al: Repair of hypospadias complications using the previously utilized urethral plate. Urology. 1999; 54:724–726.

Slate RK: Principles of plastic surgery. In: Ehrlich RM, Alter GJ (eds): Reconstructive and plastic surgery of the external genitalia, adult and pediatric. Saunders, Philadelphia, pp 1–5; 1999.

Smith CK: Surgical procedures for correction of hypospadias. J Urol. 1938; 40:239.

Smith DP: A comprehensive analysis of a tubularized incised plate hypospadias repair. Urology. 2001; 57:778.

Smith DR: Hypospadias: Its anatomic and therapeutic considerations. J Int Coll Surg. 1955; 24:64.

Smith DR: Repair of hypospadias in pre-school child. A report of 150 cases. J Urol. 1967; 97:723–730.

Smith DR, Blackfield HM: A critique on the repair of hypospadias. Surgery. 1952; 31: 885.

Smith DW, Lemli L, Opitz JM: A newly recognized syndrome of multiple congenital anomalies. J Pediatr. 1964; 64:210–217.

Smith ED: A de-epithelialised overlap flap technique in the repair of hypospadias. Br J Plast Surg. 1973; 26:106–114.

Smith ED: Durham Smith repair of hypospadias. Urol Clin North Am. 1981; 8:451–455.

Smith ED: Hypospadias. In: Ashcraft KW (ed): Pediatric urology. Saunders, Philadelphia, pp 353–395; 1990.

Smith ED: The history of hypospadias. Pediatr Surg Int. 1997; 12:81–85.

Smith EP, Wacksman J: Evaluation of severe hypospadias (editorial comment). J Pediatr. 1997; 131: 344–346.

Smith EP, Wacksman J: Evaluation of severe hypospadias. J Pediatr. 1997; 131: 334.

Smith RM: Anesthesia for infants and children, 4th edn. Mosby, St Louis, 1980; pp 653–661.

Smulian JC, Scorza WE, Guzman ER, et al: Prenatal sonographic diagnosis of midshaft hypospadias. Prenat Diagn. 1996; 16: 276.

Snodgrass W: Does tubularized incised urethral plate hypospadias repair create neourethral strictures? J Urol. 1999; 162:1159–1161.

Snodgrass W: Reoperative hypospadias: a spectrum of challenges. Dial Pediatr Urol. 2002; 25:1–8.

Snodgrass W: Suture tracts after hypospadias surgery. BJU Int. 1999; 84:843

Snodgrass W: Tubularized incised plate hypospadias repair: indications, technique, and complications. Urology. 1999; 54:6–11.

Snodgrass W: Tubularized incised plate urethroplasty for distal hypospadias. J Urol. 1994; 151:464–465.

Snodgrass W, Baskin LS, Mitchell ME: Hypospadias. In: Gillenwater JY, Grayhack JT, Howards SS, et al (eds): Adult and pediatric urology, vol III, 4th edn. Lippincott, Williams and Wilkins, Philadelphia, pp 2509–2532; 2002.

Snodgrass W, Decter RM, Roth DR, et al: Management of the penile shaft skin in hypospadias repair: alternatives to Byers Flap. J Pediatr Surg. 1988; 23: 181.

Snodgrass W, Koyle M, Manzoni G, et al: Tubularized incised plate hypospadias repair: results of a multicenter experience. J Urol. 1996; 156:839.

Snodgrass W, Koyle M, Manzoni G, et al: Tubularized incised plate hypospadias repair for proximal hypospadias (see comments). J Urol. 1998; 159:2129–2131.

Snodgrass W, Lorenzo A: Tubularized incised-plate urethroplasty for proximal hypospadias. BJU Int. 2002; 89:90–93.

Snodgrass W, Lorenzo A: Tubularized incised-plate urethroplasty for hypospadias reoperation. BJU Int. 2002; 89: 98–100.

Snodgrass W, Patterson K, Plaire JG, et al: Histology of the urethral plate: implications for hypospadias repair. J Urol. 2000; 164:988.

Snow BW: Transverse corporeal plication for persistent chordee. Urology. 1998; 34: 360–361.

Snow BW: Use of tunica vaginalis to prevent fistula in hypospadias surgery. J Urol. 1994; 151:464–465.

Snow BW: Use of tunica vaginalis to prevent fistulas in hypospadias surgery. J Urol. 1986; 136:861–863.

Snow BW, Cartwright PC, Unger K: Tunica vaginalis blanket wrap to prevent urethrocutaneous fistulas: an eight-year experience. J Urol. 1995; 153:472–473.

Snow BW, Cartwright PC: The yoke hypospadias repair. J Pediatr Surg. 1994; 29:557–560.

Snow BW, Cartwright PC: Tunica vaginalis urethroplasty. Urology. 1992; 40: 442–445.

Snow BW, Cartwright PC: Tunica vaginalis wrap. In: Ehrlich RM, Alter GJ (eds): Reconstructive and plastic surgery of the external genitalia: adult and pediatric, 1st edn. Saunders, Philadelphia, pp 109–112; 1999.

Sommerlad BC: A long-term follow-up of hypospadias patients. Br J Plast Surg. 1975; 28:324–330.

Sorber M, Feitz WF, De Vries JD: Short and mid term outcome of different types of one stage hypospadias corrections. Eur Urol. 1997; 32: 475–479.

Sorensen HR: Hypospadias with special reference to aetiology. Munksgaard, Copenhagen; 1953.

Speakman MH, Azmy AF: Skin chordee without hypospadias – an under-recognised entity. Br J Urol. 1992; 69:428–429.

Spinks MS, Lewis GL: Albucasis: on surgery and instruments. A definitive edition of the Arabic text with English translation and commentary. The Wellcome Institute of the History of Medicine, London; pp 170, 827; 1973.

Spiro SA, Seitzinger JW, Hanna MK: Hypospadias with dorsal chordee. Urology. 1992; 39:389–392.

Standoli L: Vascularised urethroplasty flaps: The use of vascularised flaps of preputial and penopreputial skin for urethral reconstruction in hypospadias. Clin Plast Surg. 1988; 15: 355–370.

Standoli L: Correzione dell'ipospadia in tempo unico: tecnica dell'uretroplastica con lembo ad isola prepuziale. Rass IT Chir Ped. 1979; 21:82–91.

Standoli L: One-stage repair of hypospadias: preputial island flap technique. Ann Plast Surg. 1982; 9:81–88.

Stecker JF, Horton CE, Devine CJ, et al: Hypospadias cripples. Urol Clin North Am. 1981; 8:539–544.

Steckler RE, Zaontz MR: Stent-free Thiersch-Duplay hypospadias repair with the Snodgrass modification. J Urol. 1997; 158:1178.

Stephens FD, Smith ED, Hutson JM: Congenital anomalies of the kidney, urinary and genital tracts, 2nd edn. Dunitz, London; 2002.

Stern DN: The interpersonal world of the infant. Basic Books, New York; 1985.

Stewart DW, Buffington PJ, Wacksman J: Suture material in bladder surgery: a comparison of polydioxanone, polyglactin, and chromic catgut. J Urol. 1990; 143:1261–1263.

Stewart TS, Bartkowski DP, Perlmutter AD: Tunica vaginalis patch graft for treatment of severe chordee. J Urol. 1995; 153(suppl.)340.

Stock JA, Hanna MK: Distal urethroplasty and glanuloplasty procedures: results of 512 repairs. Urology. 1997; 49:449.

Stock JA, Kaplan GW: Ketoconazole for prevention of postoperative penile erection. Urology. 1995; 45: 308–309.

Stock JA, Scherz HC, Kaplan GW: Distal hypospadias. Urol Clin North Am. 195; 22: 131–138.

Stoll C, Alembik Y, Roth MP, et al: Genetic and environmental factors in hypospadias. J Med Genet. 1990; 27:559–563.

Stone DL, Slavotinek A, Bouffard GG, et al: Mutation of a gene encoding a putative chaperonin causes McKusick-Kaufman syndrome. Nat Genet. 2000; 25:79–82.

Sugar EC, Firlit CF: Urinary prophylaxis and postoperative care of children at home with an indwelling catheter after hypospadias repair. Urology. 1989; 32:418.

Sugita Y, Tanikaze S, Yoshino K, et al: Severe hypospadias repair with meatal based paracoronal skin flap: the modified Koyanagi repair. J Urol. 2001; 166:1051–1053.

Sussman M: Diseases in the bible and the Talmud. In: Brothwell D, Sandison AT (eds): Diseases in antiquity: a survey of the diseases. Injuries and surgery of early population. Thomas, Springfield, Illinois. p 209; 1967.

Sutherland RS, Kogan BA, Baskin LS, et al: The effects of prepubertal androgen exposure on adult penile length. J Urol. 1996; 156: 783–787.

Svensson J, Berg R, Berg G: Operated hypospadiacs: late follow-up. Social, sexual, and psychological adaptation. J Pediatr Surg. 1981; 16:134–135.

Svensson J, Berg R: Micturition studies and sexual function in operated hypospadias. Br J Urol. 1983; 55:422–426.

Sweet RA, Schrott HG, Kurland R, et al: Study of the incidence of hypospadias in Rochester, Minnesota, 1940–1970, and a case-control comparison of possible aetiological factors. Mayo Clin Proc. 1974; 49:52–58.

Tan KK, Reid CD: A simple penile dressing following hypospadias surgery. Br J Plast Surg. 1990; 43:628–629

Tekand G, Beçik C, Emir H, et al: Is it possible to create slit-like meatus without incising urethrael plate? IIIrd congress of Mediterranean Association of Pediatric Surgeons, Corfu, Greece, 12–15 Oct, abstracts, 2000, p 67.

Telfer JRC, Quaba AA, Kwai Ben I, et al: An investigation into the role of waterproofing in a two-stage hypospadias repair. Br J Plast Surg. 1998; 51:542–546.

Thacker JG, Rodeheaver G, Moore JW, et al: Mechanical performance of surgical sutures. Am J Surg. 1975; 130:374–380.

Thiersch C: On the origin and operative treatment of epispadias. Arch Heilkd. 1869; 10:20.

Thiersch C: Über die Entstehungsweise und operative Behandlung des Epispadie. Arch Heilkd. 1869; 10:20–25.

Thomson RJ, Gustafson KE: Adaptation to chronic childhood illness. American Psychological Association, Washington DC; 1999.

Tint GS, Irons M, Elias ER, et al: Defective cholesterol biosynthesis associated with the Smith-Lemli-Opitz syndrome. N Engl J Med. 1994; 330:107–113.

Tiret L, Nivoche TY, Hatton R, et al: Complications related to anesthesia in infants and children: prospective survey of 40240 anaesthetics. Br J Anaesth. 1988; 61:263–269.

Toksu E: Hypospadias: one-stage repair. Plast Reconstr Surg. 1970; 45:365.

Toppari J, Kaleva M, Virtanen HE: Trends in the incidence of cryptorchidism and hypospadias, and methodological limitations of registry based data. Hum Reprod Update. 2001; 7:282–286.

Toppari J, Larsen JC, Chrostiansen P, et al: Male reproductive health and environmental xenoestrogens. Environ Health Perspect. 1996; 104 [Suppl 4]:741–803.

Tourneux F: Sur les premiers développements du cloaque du tubercule génital et de l'anus chez l'embryon de mouton. Anat Physiol. 1888; 24:503–517.

Tsur M, Linder N, Cappis S: Hypospadias in a consanguineous family (letter). Am J Med Genet. 1987; 27:487–489.

Turnbull RB Jr, Fazio V: Advances in the surgical technique and ulcerative colitis surgery. In: Nybus L (ed): Surgery annual. Appleton Century-Crofts, California, USA, p 315; 1975.

Turner-Warwick R, Parkhouse H, Chapple CR: Bulbar elongation anastomotic meatoplasty (BEAM) for subterminal and hypospadiac urethroplasty. J Urol. 1997; 158: 1160–1167.

Turner-Warwick R: Observations upon techniques for reconstruction of the urethral meatus, the hypospadiac glans deformity and the penile urethra. Urol Clin North Am. 1979; 6:643–655.

Udall DA: Correction of 3 types of congenital curvature of the penis, including the first reported case of dorsal curvature. J Urol. 1980; 124: 50–52.

Uemura S, Hutson JM, Woodward AA, et al: Balanitis xerotica obliterans with urethral stricture after hypospadias repair. Pediatr Surg Int. 2000; 16:144–145.

Ulman I, Erikci V, Avanoglu A, et al: The effect of suturing techniques and material on complication rate following hypospadias repair. Eur J Pediatr Surg. 1997; 7:156.

Ünver AS: Şerafeddin Sabuncuoğlu: Kitabül Cerrahiye-i İlhaniye (Cerrahname), Istanbul, İ.Ü Tıp Tarihi Enstitüsü, Adet. 1939; 12:870–1465.

Uzel I: Şerafeddin Sabuncuoğlu: Cerrâhiyyetü'l-hâniyye, vol-I, Atatürk Kültür Dil ve Tarih Yüksek Kurumu Yayınları, III. Dizi. 1992; pp 280–281.

Van der Putte SCJ, Neeteson FA: The normal development of the anorectum in the pig. Acta Morphol Neerl Scand. 1983; 21:107–132.

Van der Werff JF, Boeve E, Brusse CA, et al: Urodynamic evaluation of hypospadias repair. J Urol. 1997; 157:1344–1346.

Van der Werff JFA, Nievelstein RAJ, Brands E, et al: Normal development of the male anterior urethra. Teratology 2000; 61:172–183.

Van Hook W: A new operation for hypospadias. Ann Surg. 1896; 23:378.

Van Horn AC, Kass FJ: Glanuloplasty and in situ tubularization of the urethral plate: simple reliable technique for the majority of boys with hypospadias. J Urol. 1995; 154:1505.

Van Savage JG, Palanca LG, Slaughenhoupt BL: A prospective randomized trial of dressings versus no dressings for hypospadias repair. J Urol. 2000; 164:981–983.

Van Winkle W, Hastings JC: Considerations in the choice of suture material for various tissues. Surg Gynecol Obstet. 1972; 135:113–126.

Vandersteen DR, Husmann DA: Late onset recurrent penile chordee after successful correction of hypospadias repair. J Urol. 1998; 160:1131–1133.

Vasconez LO, Vasconez HC: Plastic and reconstructive surgery. In: Way LW, Doherty GM (eds): Current surgical diagnosis and treatment, 11th edn. McGraw-Hill, USA, pp 1230–1242; 2003.

Velasquez-Uzola A, Leger Jr, Aigrain Y, et al: Hypoplasia of the penis: etiologic diagnosis and results of treatment with delayed-action testosterone. Arch Pediatr. 1998; 5:844– 850.

Venn SN, Mundy AR: Early experience with the use of buccal mucosa for substitution urethroplasty. Br J Urol. 1998; 81:738–740.

Venn SN, Mundy AR: Urethroplasty for balanitis xerotica obliterans. Br J Urol. 1998;81:735–737.

Vermeij-Keers C, Hartwig NG, vander Werff JFA: Embryonic development of the ventral body wall and its congenital malformations. Semin Pediatr Surg. 1996; 5:82–89.

Vernon D, Foley JM, Schulman JL: Effect of mother-child separation and birth order on young children's responses to two potentially stressful experiences. J Pers Soc Psychol. 1967; 5:162–174.

Vernon DTA, Foley JM, Sipowics RR, et al: The psychological responses of children to hospitalization and illness. Thomas, Springfield, Illinois; 1965.

Vordermark JS Jr: Adhesive membrane; a new dressing for hypospadias. Urology. 1982; 20:86.

Vrijheid M, Dolk H, Armstrong B, et al: Hazard potential ranking of landfill sites and risk of congenital anomalies. Occup Environ Epidemiol. 2002; 59:768–776.

Vyas PR, Roth DR, Perlmutter AD: Experience with free grafts in urethral reconstruction. J Urol. 1987; 137:471.

Wacksman J: Modification of one-stage flip-flap procedure to repair distal penile hypospadias. Urol Clin North Am. 1981; 8:527–530.

Wacksman J: Repair of hypospadias using new mouth-controlled microscope. Urology. 1987; 29: 276–278.

Wacksman J: Results of early hypospadias surgery using optical magnification. J Urol. 1984; 131:516.

Wacksman J: Use of the Hodgson XX (modified Asopa) procedure to correct hypospadias with chordee: surgical technique and results. J Urol. 1986; 136:1264–1265.

Walker RD: Megalourethra. In: Resnick MI, Kursh ED (eds): Current therapy in genitourinary surgery. Mosby, St Louis, pp 316–318; 1992.

Warwick RT, Parkhouse H, Chapple CR: Bulbar elongation anastomotic meatoplasty (BEAM) for subterminal and hypospadiac urethroplasty. J Urol. 1997; 158:1160–1167.

Waterhouse K, Glassberg KI: Mobilization of the anterior urethra as an aid in the one-stage repair of hypospadias. Urol Clin North Am. 1981; 8:521.

Watson A, Srinivas J, Daniels L, et al: An interim analysis of a cohort study on the preoperative anxiety and postoperative behavioural changes in children having repeat anaesthetics. Paediatr Anaesth. 2002; 12:824

Webster GD, Brown MW, Koefoot RJ, et al: Suboptimal results in full thickness skin graft urethroplasty using an extrapenile skin donor site. J Urol. 1984; 131:1082–1083.

Wehrbein HI: Hypospadias. J Urol. 1943; 50: 335–340.

Weidner IS, Moller H, Jensen TK, et al: Cryptorchidism and hypospadias in sons of gardeners and farmers. Environ Health Perspect. 1998; 106:793–796

Weinder IS, Moller H, Jensen TK, et al: Risk factors for cryptorchidism and hypospadias. J Urol. 1999; 161: 1606.

Weingartner K, Kozakewich HP, Hendren WH: Nephrogenic adenoma after urethral reconstruction using bladder mucosa. Reports of 6 cases and review of the literature. J Urol. 1997; 158:1175–1177.

Welch KJ: Hypospadias. In: Ravitch MM, Welch KJ, Benson CD, et al (eds): Pediatric surgery, 3rd edn. Year Book Medical Publishers, Chicago, pp 1353–1376; 1979.

Wennerholm U, Bergh C, Hamberger L, et al: Incidence of congenital malformations in children born after ICSI. Hum Reprod. 2000; 15:944–948.

Wessells H, McAninch JW: Current controversies in anterior urethral stricture repair: free-graft versus pedicled skin-flap reconstruction. World J Urol. 1998; 16: 175–180.

Wheeler R, Malone P: The role of the Mathieu repair as a salvage procedure. Br J Urol. 1993; 72:52–53.

Wheeler RA, Malone PS, Griffiths DM, et al.: The Mathieu operation. Is urethral stent mandatory? Br J Urol. 1993; 71: 492–495.

Wiener JS, Sutherland RW, Roth DR, et al: Comparison of onlay and tubularised island flaps of inner preputial skin for the repair of proximal hypospadias. J Urol. 1997; 158: 1172–1174.

Wilcox DT, Mouriquand PD: Hypospadias. In: Thomas DFM, Rickwood AMK, Duffy PG (eds): Essentials of paediatric urology. Dunitz, London, p 179; 2002.

Williams DI: The development and abnormalities of the penile urethra. Acta Anatomie. 1952; 15: 176.

Wilson GN, Oliver WJ: Further delineation of the G syndrome; a manageable genetic cause of infantile dysphagia. J Med Genet. 1988; 25:157–163.

Winslow BH, Devine CJ Jr: Principles in repair of hypospadias. Semin Pediatr Surg. 1996; 5: 41–48.

Winter R, Baraitser M: London Dysmorphology Database. Oxford University Press, Oxford.

Wollin M, Duffy PG, Malone PS, et al: Buried penis. A novel approach. Br J Urol. 1990; 65:97–100.

Wood J (1875): Cited by Mayo CH: JAMA. 1901; 36:1157.

Woodard JR, Cleveland R: Application of Horton-Devine principles to the repair of hypospadias. J Urol. 1982; 127: 1155–1158.

Woodard JR, Parrott TS: Management of severe perineal hypospadias with bifid scrotum (abstract). J Urol. 1991; 145: 245A.

Woodhouse CR: Sexual function in boys born with exstrophy, myelomeningocoele and micropenis. Urology. 1998; 52: 3–11.

Woodhouse CR: The sexual and reproductive consequences of congenital genitourinary anomalies. J Urol. 1994; 152: 645–651.

Wood-Jones F: The nature of the malformations of the rectum and urogenital passages. BMJ. 1904; 2:1630–1634.

Yamaguchi T, Kitoda S, Osada Y: Chromosomal anomalies in cryptorchidism and hypospadias. Urol Int. 1991; 47: 60–63.

Yamataka A, Ando K, Lane G, et al: Pedicled external spermatic fascia for urethroplasty in hypospadias and closure of urethrocutaneous fistula. J Pediatric Surg. 1998; 33: 1788–1789.

Yang CC, Bradley WE: Innervation of the human glans penis. J Urol. 1999; 161: 97.

Yang S, Chen SC, Hsieh CH, et al: Reoperative Snodgrass procedure. J Urol. 2001; 166:2342.

Yavuzer R, Baran C, Latifoglu O, et al: Vascularised double-sided preputial island flap with W flap glanuloplasty for hypospadias repair. Plast Reconstr Surg. 1998; 101: 751– 755.

Yerkes E, Adams M, Miller DA, et al: Y to I wrap: use of distal spongiosum for hypospadias repair. J Urol. 2000; 163: 1536.

Yerkes EB, Cain MP, Casle AJ, et al: Experience with split-prepuce in situ island onlay for anterior hypospadias. J Urol. 2000; 163 (suppl.): 138.

Young F, Benjamin JA: Repair of hypospadias with free inlay skin graft. Surg Gynecol Obstet. 1948; 86:439.

Young F, Benjamin W: Preschool-age repair of hypospadias with free inlay skin grafts. Surgery. 1949; 26:384.

Zaidi SZ, Hodapp J, Cuckow P, et al: Spongioplasty in hypospadias repair. Abstract of the British Association of Urological Surgeons, 1997.

Zaontz MR, Kaplan WE, Maizels M: Surgical correction of anterior urethral diverticula after hypospadias repair in children. Urology. 1989; 33:40–42.

Zaontz MR, Packer MG: Abnormalities of the external genitalia. Pediatr Clin North Am. 1997; 44:1267–1297.

Zaontz MR: The GAP (glans approximation procedure) for glanular/coronal hypospadias. J Urol. 1989; 141:359.

Zeis E: Die Literatur und Geschichte der plastischen Chirurgie. Englemann, Leipzig, 1963; pp 145–173.

Zhong-Chu L, Yu-Hen Z, Ya-Xiong S, et al: One-stage urethroplasty for hypospadias using a tube constructed with bladder mucosa – a new procedure. Urol Clin North Am. 1981; 8:457–462.

Zubowska J, Jankowska J, Kula K, et al: Clinical, hormonal and semiological data in adult men operated in childhood for hypospadias. Endokrynol Polska. 1979; 30:565–573.

Subject Index

A
Abdominoplasty 345
Accessory scrotum 335
Acquired
- detrusor instability 297
- hypospadias 4, 333
Adenoma 338
Adolescent sexual function 317
Adrenogenital syndrome 344
Advancement flap 97
Allantoic diverticulum 63
Ambiguous genitalia 90
Amputation 3, 4
Anaesthesia 109
- anxiety reaction 84, 107
- combined consultation 107
- hysterical reaction 84
- phobias 84
- psychological effect 84
Analgesia
- caudal 110
- epidural 110
- pre-emptive 109
Androgen
- insensitivity syndrome 61, 318
- receptor 89
- sensitivity syndrome 91
Anterior urethral valve 166
Apoptosis 68
Artifical erection test 14, 19, 115, 157
- test 14, 115
Asopa-Duckett tube 308
Asymptomatic strictures 297
Axial flap 98

B
Balanic
- groove technique 20
- hypospadias 23
Balanitis Xerotica Obliterans (BXO) 234, 296, 297, 299, 306, 316, 318
Barcat technique 128
Baskin's dorsal plication 142
Behavioural regulation 325
Bifid 191
- scrotum 254
Biodegradable polymer 346
Bioocclusive membrane dressing 104
Bipedicled suprapubic abdominal skin flap 7

Bipediculated preputial flap 10
Bladder
- mucosa 13
- - graft 296
- - - urethroplasty 308
- scanning 297
- spasm 276, 290
Bovalved scrotum 191
Buccal mucosa 13, 219, 296
- graft 219
- - urthroplasty 309
Buck's fascia 68, 75
Bucket-handle meatus 146
Buried
- penis 183, 334
- strip of skin method 10
Buttonhole technique 10, 203
BXO 234, 296, 297, 299, 306, 316, 318
Byars flap 115, 262

C
Cadaveric pericardial graft 177
Calibration 91
Canalisation 47
Catheter blockage 276
Cecil-culp urethroplasty 283
- three-stage modification 283
Centile growth chart 313
Chemical exposure 55
Chordee 4, 5, 71
- deep 19, 23, 187
- with hypospadias 115
- without hypospadias 115
- recurrent 316
- - penile 118
- release 9, 10
- residual 316
- skin 19
- superficial 19, 21, 187
Chromosome abnormality 59, 90
Circumcision 3, 314
- erroneous 4
Circumcoronal incision 121
Classification 79
Cleft 79,80
- glans 79, 80, 243, 244
- incomplete 79, 80, 243, 244
Cloaca 63, 65
Cloacal
- membrane 63

- plate 64
Colles fascia 73
Combination flap 173
Complex
- genetic syndrome 59
- hypospadias repair 43, 221, 305
Compound tube 221
Concealed penis 334
Congenital
- adrenal hyperplasia 91
- buried penis 334
- fistula 333
- megalourethra 336
Consent 89
Cornu 279
Coronary sulcus 4
Corpora cavernosa 118
Corporal
- disproportion 14
- rotation 19
Corpus spongiosum 177
Crippled hypospadias, 221, 305, 316
Cryptorchidism 90
Cultivated keratinocytes 345
Cultured epithelial and dermal graft 94, 345, 346
Cyproterone acetate 233
Cystoscopy 90

D
Dartos
- fascia 115
- flap 43, 240
- mobilization 191, 194
Deep chordee 23
De-epithelialisation 20, 43, 172, 212, 130, 135, 237
- flap 20, 43, 172, 212, 130, 135, 237
- skin 20, 43, 172, 212, 130, 135, 237
Degloving 115, 157
Dehiscene 90, 306
Deltoid flap 344
Dermal
- graft 117, 317
- laser soldering 345
Desipramine 233
Development theory 20
Distal
- hypospadias 19
- urethroplasty 25

Dog-ear 68, 150
- of prepuce 70
Dorsal
- penile skin 37
- plication 14, 19, 116
- preputial flap 10
- subcutaneous flap 43, 240
Dorsalis pedis flap 344
Double-faced preputial flap 13, 175
Dressing 104, 189, 271, 340
Dripping stent 103
Dundee modification 235
Dysuria 275, 297, 301

E
Eber papyrus 3
Ectopic orifice 68
Ejaculation 4, 318
Emotional
- satisfaction 318
- trauma 84
Emotional regulation 325
Endocrine-disrupting chemicals 54, 55
Environmental exposure 55
Epispadias 5
Epithelium of the urethral wall 337
- partial dissection 337
Erection 14, 19, 109, 115, 157, 275
- test 14, 19, 109, 115, 139, 157
EUROCAT congenital anomaly register 51
External spermatic fascia flap 43, 240

F
Fascia
- Buck's 68, 75
- Colles 73
- Scarpa 73
Fasciocutaneous flap 98
Ferlit skirt flap 167
Fibrin sealant 241
Fistula 29, 128, 160, 206, 234, 261, 199
- formation 267
- rate 189
Flap 5, 96, 257
- advancement 97
- axial 98
- bipedicled suprapubic abdominal skin 7
- bipediculated preputial 10, 37, 191, 203
- Byars 115, 197, 262
- dartos 43, 240
- de-epithelialized skin 20, 43, 172, 212, 130, 135, 237
- deltoid 344
- dorsal
- - preputial 10
- - subcutaneous 43, 240
- dorsalis pedis 344
- double-face prepuce 13
- double-faced preputial 175
- external spermatic fascia 43, 240

- fasciocutaneous 98
- glanular 10
- - triangular 13
- horizontal preputial 13
- interpolation 97
- large round 10
- lateral arm 344
- lateral oblique 37
- lateral-based (LB) 20, 37, 209
- longitudinal 5
- meatal-based 7, 10, 14, 29, 149, 139
- parameatal-based foreskin 20, 135
- pedicled scrotal 139
- perimeatal 29
- radial forearm 343
- random 97
- rectangular 11
- rotation 97
- scrotal 5
- sensate osteo-cutaneous fibula 343
- transposition 97
- triangular 11
- tunica vaginalis 177
- vascularised
- - dorsal preputial 9
- - preputial island 163
- vertical preputial vascularised 13
- Ferlit skirt 167
Flat
- glans 79, 80, 243, 244
Flip-flap technique 10, 139, 149
Foreskin 14, 73
Free-graft preputial urethroplasty 217, 311
Frenulum 68, 75
Full-thickness skin 321
- graft 43, 93
Fusiform megalourethra 336

G
G syndrome 60
Gender assignment 91
Genital
- perception score 314
- tubercle 63, 65, 67
Genitography 90
Genitourinary sinus 65
Gland clefting 226
Glans
- approximation procedure 25
- channel 43
- cleft 79, 80, 243, 244
- flat 79, 80, 243, 244
- groove 121
- incomplete 79, 80, 243, 244
- lamellae 68
- normal 243
- penis 181
- split 43, 245
- tilt 119
- tunnelling 47

Glanular
- dehiscence 199
- flap 10
- tilt 116
- triangular flap 13
- wings 139
Glanulomeatoplasty 212
Glanuloplasty 19, 25, 43, 121, 158, 163, 177, 245, 306
Gonadal dysgenesis 91
Gonadotrophin 88
Graft 9, 44, 257
- buccal mucosa 219
- cultured epithelial 94
- dermal 94
- free inlay 217
- free preputial 217
- full-thickness skin 43, 93
- inner preputial free skin 13
- meshed 94
- skin 93
- split skin 93
- split-thickness
- - free skin 9
- - skin 43
vascularised preputial skin onlay

H
Haematuria 301
Haemorrhage 275
Haemostasis 101
Hair coil 335
Hairy urethra 37, 321, 338
Half-moon meatus 146, 159
Harvested fat cells 345
Heineke-Mikulicz
- meatoplasty 128
- technique 19
Hermaphrodite 3, 90
Hinging 43
Homologous urothelial substitute 346
Horizontal preputial flap 13
Hormonal stimulation, preoperative 88, 307
HOSE system 92, 314
Human chorionic gonadotrophin 88
Hypo 3
Hypoplasia of the penis 88
Hypospadias
- acquired 4, 333
- anatomical classification 14
- classification 79
- cosmetic results 92, 313
- cripple 221, 305, 316
- double-diaper technique 182
- female 335
- iatrogenic 333
- incidence 319
- objective scoring
- - evaluation (HOSE) 314
- - system 92
- onlay-tube-onlay repair 181
- perineal 88, 169, 173, 187, 191, 203, 209

- screening   79, 87,
- severe   203, 209
- surgery
  - – behavioural regulation   325
  - – dressing   104, 189, 271
  - – emotional regulation   325
  - – instruments   100
  - – magnification   99
  - – one-stage approach   261, 174
  - – positioning   99
  - – psychological adaptation   325
  - – self-esteem   325
  - – tension   99
  - – tissue handling   100
  - – two-stage approach   174, 261
- timing of elective repair   83
- ventral lengthening procedure   183

I

Immunohistochemistry   226
Incomplete
- cleft glans   243
- masculinisation   91
Inert collagen matrix   346
Infection   275
Infibulation   3
Infraumbilical mesenchyme   68
Inheritance   59
Inner preputial free skin graft   13
Insoculation   95
Instruments   100
Intermediate layer   237
Interpolation flap   97
Intercourse   318
Intersexuality   90
Intracytoplasmic sperm injection   319
Ischaemia time   102

K

Kendal catheter   167
Keratinocytes   345
Koff urethral mobilisation   308

L

Labioscrotal fold   251
Laser
- Doppler   200
- tissue soldering   345
Lateral
- arm flap   344
- oblique flap   37
Lateral-based (LB) flap   20, 37, 209
Liposculpturing   345
Liposuction   345
Littre's glands   68
Local anaesthetic   109
London Dysmorphology Database   60
Lymphoedema   337

M

M configuration   25
Magnification   99
Male-to-female gender reassignment   344

Male-to-male transmission   59
Mathieu procedure   29, 139, 149, 307
MAVIS technique   144
McKusick-Kaufman syndrome   60
Meatal
- advancement   43
- – and glanuloplasty incorporated (MAGPI)   25
- regression   119
- retraction   122
- stenosis   160, 275, 295
- stricture   199
Meatal-based flap   7, 10, 14, 139, 149
Meatoplasty   19, 43, 245, 306
Meatus   19, 79, 243
Median raphe   68
Megalourethra   301
- acquired   301, 302
- primary   302, 336
Megameatus intact prepuce   25, 135
Mercurochrome   88
Mesenchyme duct   63
Meshed graft   94
Metanephric blastema   63
Mibza   4
Micropenis   88, 334
Microsurgical
- free tissue transfer   343
- technique   98
Micturating cystourethrography   87, 297
Monogenic factor   59
Mori-Ikoma technique   252
Mother-father-child relationship   83
Mucosal protrusion   223
Müllerian duct remnant   87, 88
Mustardé's technique   139

N

Neo-meatus   4
Nephrogenic adenoma   338
Nesbit's
- dorsal plication   19, 116, 142
- modified procedure   187
Nitrofurantoin   275
Non-stenting   102, 269, 340
Normal glans   243

O

Occupational exposures   55
Oedema   275
Onlay
- island flap urethroplasty   33, 308
- patch   33, 221
Opitz
- BBB syndrome   60
- G syndrome   60
Optic magnification   14, 99
Oral contraceptive use   55
Orthoplasty   19, 115

P

Pallister-Hall syndrome   60
Pants over vest   302

Parameatal-based foreskin flap   20, 135
Parental perceptions of maleness   328
Parenting   328
Partial glans dehiscence   161
Pedicled scrotal flap   139
Penile
- block   110
- disassembly technique   14, 117
- dressing   307
- enhancement   344
- skin   73
- – blood supply   73
- torsion   189, 255
Penoscrotal
- angle   212
- transposition   90, 251
Perimeatal flap   29, 139, 149, 209
Perineal
- raphe   67
- urethrostomy   102
Peyronie's disease   317
Phallus   68
Plasma imbibition   95
Plaster of Paris   169
Plication   14, 19, 116, 304
Point mutation   91
Positioning   99
Pre-emptive analgesia   109
Premedication   108
Preoperative
- androgen therapy   88
- hormonal stimulation   88
Prepuce   73
- arterial supply   76
- preservation   125
- reconstruction   19, 123
Preputial skin   14, 33
Preputioplasty   123
Prevalence   51, 54
Progestagen   55
Prostate   65
Prosthetic
- implant   344
- stiffener   344
Protective intermediate layer   43, 45, 212, 237, 339
Proximal hypospadia   37
Psychological adaptation   325
Psychological problems
- adherence   329
- anxiety   327
- behaviour   327
- changing faces initiative   330
- coping   329
- empowerment   329
- gender   327
- phallus   328
- selfhood   326
- society   327
- solution-focussed approach   330
Purse-string suture   31
Pyramid repair   25, 135

R

Radial forearm flap 343
Random flap 97
Rectangular flap 11
Recurrence
- risk 59
- fistula 292
Re-do surgery 90, 226, 306
Regressed meatus 119
Reoperation 155, 159
Retrusive meatus 276
Rotation flap 97

S

Sandwich dressing 167
Scaphoid 336
Scarpa fascia 73
Schaefer classification 79
Screening 79, 87
Scrotal
- flap 5
- hair 37, 292, 321, 338
Scrotum 37, 283, 289
Self-esteem 325
Sensate osteo-cutaneous fibula flap 343
Sexual
- outcome 313
- satisfaction 317
Shanberg-Rosenberg technique 252
Silastic tubing 14, 103, 269
Silicone foam
- dressing 14
- elastomer 104, 271
Silver cannula 4
Single stage repair 261, 340
Skin 93
- colonization 190
- extragenital 43, 217
- graft 43, 93, 217
- - failure 95
- - survival 95
- loss of flap 275
Slit-like vertical meatus 43, 243
SLO 60
Smith's classification 79
Smith-Lemli-Opitz syndrome (SLO) 60
Snodgrass urethroplasty 308
Spadon 3
Split and roll technique 19, 23, 116
Split skin graft 93
Split-thickness
- free skin graft 9
- graft method 13
- skin graft 43
- - urethroplasty 311
Spongioplasty 307
Spongiosum 115, 166, 169
Spraying stream 315
Squamous cell carcinoma 338
Stay suture 99
Stenosis 29
Stenting 102, 269, 340
Stricture 234, 315
Subcutaneous incision 9
Superficial chordee 19, 21
Supplementary pain management 111
Suprapubic
- diversion 103, 269
- lipectomy 345
Surgery
- anxiety reactions 84
- hysterical reactions 84
- phobias 84
- psychological effects 84
Suture
- material 100
- track 281, 282
Suturing technique 101
Syndrome
- androgen insensitivity 61
- androgen sensitivity 91
- chromosomal anomalies 59
- G (see also Opitz G, Opitz BBB) 60
- McKusick-Kaufman 60
- Opitz BBB 60
- Opitz G 60
- Pallister-Hall 60
- Smith-Lemli-Opitz (SLO) 60
System of Browne 79

T

Techniques
- balanic groove 20
- buttonhole 10
- Cecil –Culp 283
- Denis Browne 266
- dorsal plication 14
- Durham Smith 262
- flip-flap 10
- Heineke-Mikulicz 19
- lateral based flap 209
- MAGPI 119
- microsurgical 98
- Mori-Ikoma 252
- Mustardé's 139
- penile disassembly 14, 117
- Shanberg-Rosenberg 252
- split and roll 19, 23, 116
- tubularised incised plate 155
- Y-V glanuloplasty modified Mathieu 149
Tegaderm 121
Tenotomy scissor 158
Tension 99
Testosterone 88, 89, 155
- biosynthesis 61
- injection 142
- stimulation 20
Thiersch-Duplay urethroplasty 308
Timing of elective surgery 83
Tissue expansion 344
Tissue handling 100
Torsion 187
Tourniquet 101
Traction suture 99
Transposition flap 97
Triangular flap 11
Trimethoprim-sulfa 275
Tube urethroplasty 221
Tubularised incised plate 25, 155, 245
- technique 14
- urethroplasty 20
Tunica
- albuginea 115
- vaginalis 43
- - blanket 144
- - flap 177
- - wrap 20
Turnbull modification 206
Twins 90
Two stage repair 174, 261

U

Underascertainment 51
Urethra
- paper-thin 116
- imperforate 4
Urethral
- advancement 25, 123
- ballooning 301
- calculus 301
- catheterisation 103
- development 67
- diverticulum 223, 301
- duplication 334
- groove 7
- meatus 267
- - retrogression 267
- mobilisation 23
- mucosa 67
- plate 20, 67, 128, 142, 157, 173, 174, 306
- - hinging 20, 45, 142
- - incising 142
- plication 304
- prolapse 309
- splint 269
- stricture 295
Urethrocutaneous fistula 145, 289
Urethroplasty 5, 19, 179
- buccal mucosa graft 309
- free-graft preputial 311
- onlay island flap 308
- onlay-tube-onlay 183
- Snodgrass 308
- split-thickness skin graft 311
- Thiersch-Duplay 308
Urinary
- diversion 102, 269
- infection 297
Uroflowmetry 91, 295–297, 299
Urorectal septum 64
Utricle 88
Utriculus masculinus 88

V

V incision 29
Vaginoplasty 344
Vascularised
- dorsal preputial flap 9

– preputial island flap 163
Vegetarian diet 55
Vertical preputial vascularised flap 13
Vesicoureteric reflux 87
Vinegar 4
Voiding cystourethrography 301
V-shaped flap meatoplasty 298

W
White line test 175
Wing rotation 43, 47, 244
Wings 121

X
Xenograft 93
Xeno-oestrogen 54

Y
Y to I closure 159
Yoke 37, 203
Y-shaped incision 149, 169, 209, 245
Y-V glanuloplasty 20, 32, 37, 149, 245

Z
Z-plasty 97, 212